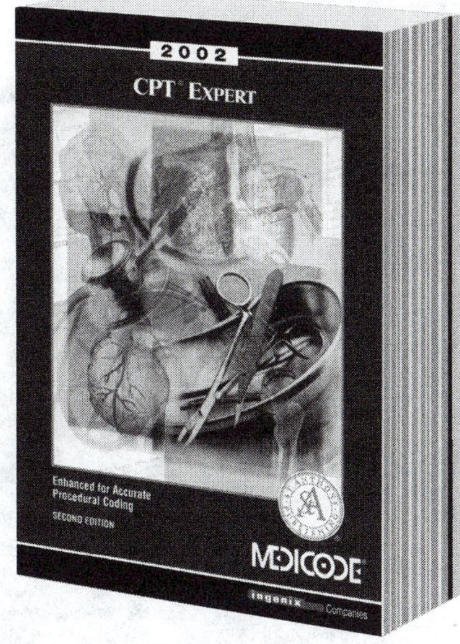

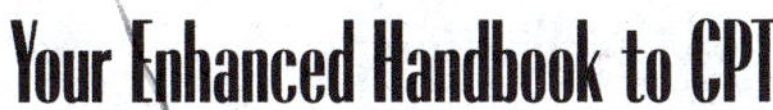

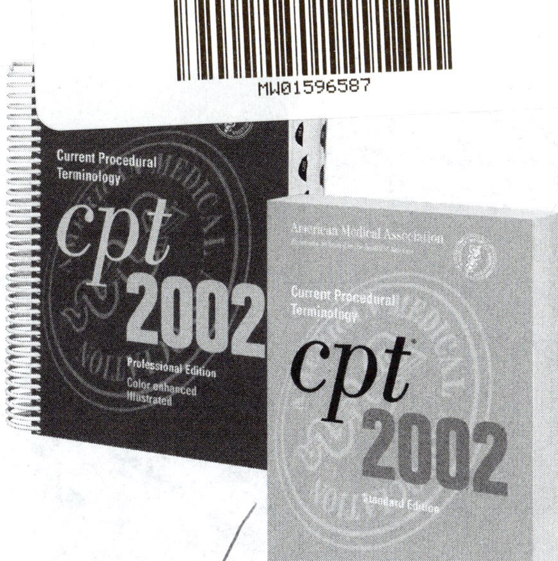

Your Enhanced Handbook to CPT

2002 CPT Expert

A fantastic tool that helps experienced coders take procedural coding to a new level. *CPT Expert* is designed to help maximize reimbursement and save your office time and money. You get each CPT code with comprehensive coding tips, illustrations and definitions.

- **NEW — Special Reports Via E-mail.** Keep up-to-date with quarterly CPT changes.

- **NEW — Complete Description.** Includes all CPT codes and full official descriptions.

- **NEW — Deleted Codes.** 2002 deleted codes with strikeouts that help you finish claims from last year.

- **NEW — Appendix of Codes Most Frequently Miscoded.** Know which codes to watch out for and learn why they can be miscoded.

8 1/2 x 11 Spiral bound
ISBN: 1-56329-830-9   Item No. 4509 **$79.95**

6 x 9 Perfect bound
ISBN: 1-56329-831-7   Item No. 4507 **$69.95**

Available: December 2001

Official industry CPT™ Code books

American Medical Association's (AMA) CPTs™

Many of the changes you've anticipated from CPT-5 project will be seen in CPT 2002, including revamped Category I procedural and service codes and terms, new Category II "Performance Measure" codes, and new Category III "Emerging Technology" codes. New icons refer to the AMA's CPT Changes 2000, 2001, and 2002 books. Don't code without this book which unveils the work of the CPT-5 project! All St. Anthony Publishing/Medicode CPT 2002 buyers who provide an e-mail address will receive e-mail special reports that provide code updates and changes.

CPT 2002 Standard

The AMA's economical, perfect bound classic. Features self-stick tabs and an extensive index.

ISBN: 1-57947-220-6   Item No. 4368 **$49.95**

Available: December 2001

CPT 2002 Professional

Color coded and spiral bound for ease of use, this product includes illustrations, preinstalled thumbtabs, and references to CPT Assistant along with the features of the CPT 2002 Standard.

ISBN: 1-57947-221-4   Item No. 4372 Price **$74.95**

Available: December 2001

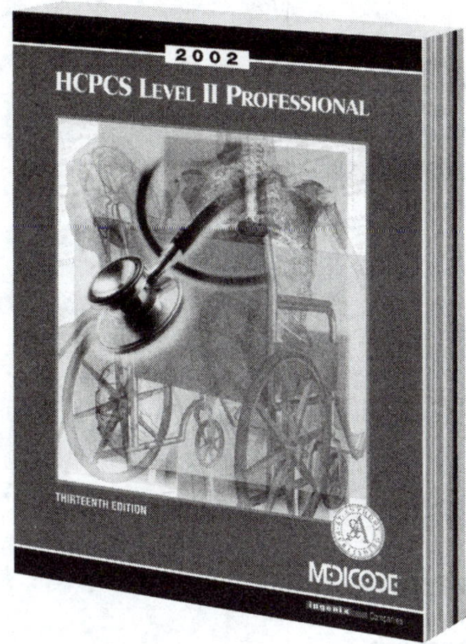
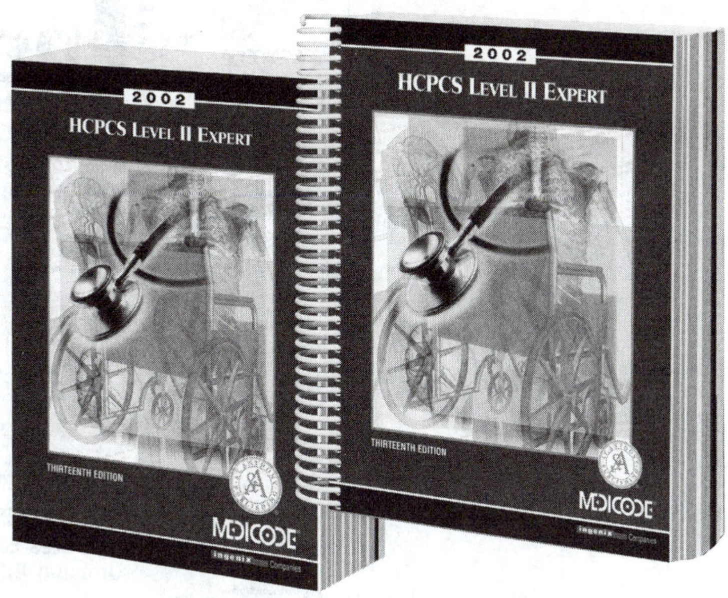

The Best HCPCS Code Books in the Marketplace

Need guidance on how to guarantee your facility receives timely and appropriate reimbursement on DME, drugs, and other medical supplies? Our new *HCPCS Level II Professional* and *Expert* code books can assist you.

Both *Professional* and *Expert* editions include:

- All HCPCS codes and modifiers, including deleted codes for 2002.

- Easy-to-use color-key bars, icons, and tabs help you know which codes are governed by which Medicare coding rule.

- Organized, detailed, and cross-referenced indexes that make it easy to find what you need.

- Modifiers explained to enhance coding accuracy.

- Tables that include codes and other helpful information.

- *Medicare Carriers Manual* and *Coverage Issues Manual* excerpts that indicate drugs and services that are not reimbursed.

- Deleted HCPCS codes before 2002 to help manage old claims and audits.

The *HCPCS Expert* includes all the exclusive features of the *Professional*, plus:

- Medicare fees for HCPCS codes.

- Appendix of payers who accept HCPCS Level II codes.

- E-mail service.

HCPCS Level II Professional
ISBN: 1-56329-827-9   Item No. 4505 **$59.95**
Available: December 2001

HCPCS Level II Expert
Compact
ISBN: 1-56329-828-7   Item No. 4503 **$69.95**

Spiral
ISBN: 1-56329-829-5   Item No. 4501 **$79.95**
Available: December 2001

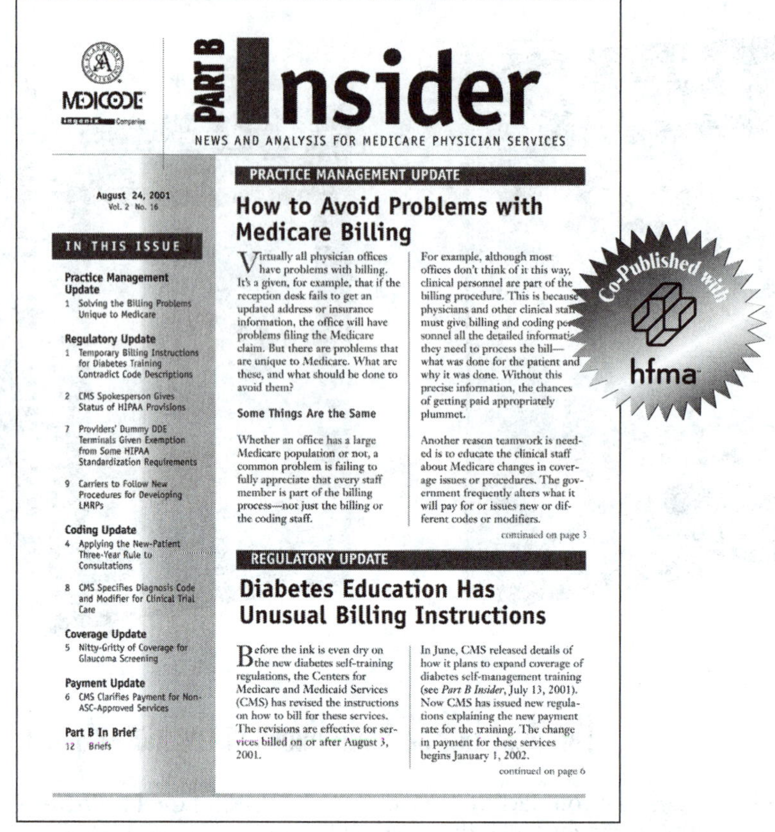

Bi-weekly Guidance You Need to Survive Part B Changes

Part B Insider

Introducing…*PART B INSIDER*, an in-depth and straight-forward biweekly regulatory newsletter. The first newsletterdeveloped exclusively to meet the needs of health care executives, this critical resource will keep you informed andready to act with comprehensive coverage of ongoing changes to Medicare physician services.

St. Anthony Publishing/Medicode, the leading publisher of Medicare Part B resources, has created this unique new service for health care managers and directors. It provides clear and current coverage of the changing legal and regulatory environment with the most authoritative and accurate coding, billing, and compliance strategies in the industry.

Part B Insider is your guide to:

- **NEWS.** Explains new and proposed regulations, coding and billing guidelines, judicial decisions, compliance developments, and more.

- **IMPACT.** Learn from our top-notch editorial advisory board of healthcare executives how these developments will affect your organization and your bottom line.

- **ACTION.** Discover ways to implement the new policies and procedures you need to survive-with nuts-and-bolts, "how-to" guidance to help you direct your staff.

Your subscription also includes:

- **E-mail Alert Service.** When breaking news happens — you'll hear about it immediately!

Item No. 4272 **$349.95**

Available: Now   Up to 10 CEUs from AAPC

Unparalleled Clinical Coding Expertise

Our in-house technical staff includes nurses, medical records experts, billing service managers, consultants, and auditors who are credentialed, field-tested experts. (CPC, CPC-H, CCS, CCS-P, RHIT, RHIA, RN, LPN)

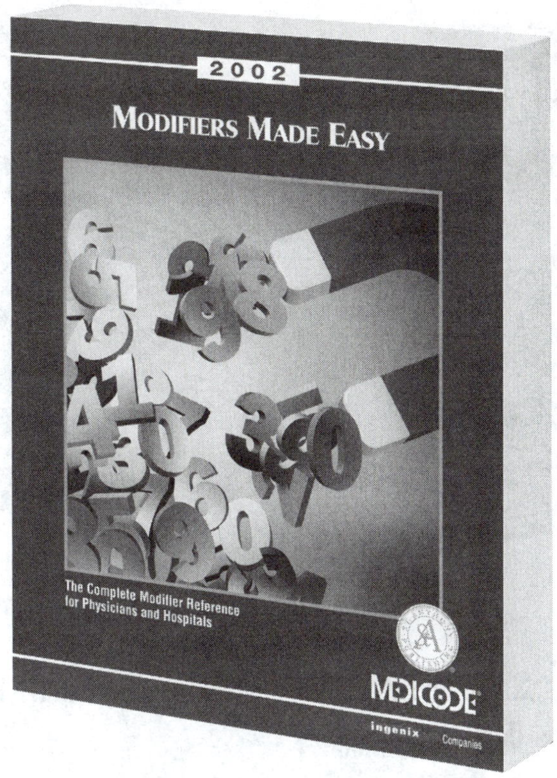

Apply Modifiers Right the First Time!

Modifiers Made Easy

Easy-to use for billing both commercial payers and Medicare, *Modifiers Made Easy* is a "must have" reference to add to your training library. It can be used as a stand-alone training guide or as a supplement to our popular *Code It Right.*

- **Fully Updated 2002 CPT and HCPCS Level II Codes.** Apply the right modifier when more than one could apply.

- **Decision Tree Flow Charts.** Helps you choose the correct modifier when more than one could apply.

- **Real-Life Clinical Examples with Correctly Completed HCFA-1500 Claim Forms.** Helps reduce claim denials by giving scenarios showing modifiers being used correctly.

- **Special Guidance on Modifiers for Nonphysician Practitioners.** Learn to accurately use modifiers for NPs, Pas, and CNSs.

- **CPT Modifiers Arranged by Type of Service:** E/M, Anesthesia, Surgery, etc. Quickly find the applicable modifier. Now includes cross-references between sections.

- **HCPCS Level II Modifiers Arranged Alphabetically, "A-V".** Identify the right modifier at a glance.

- **Special Hospital Section Lists that Outpatient-Applicable Modifiers.** Zero in on just the modifiers you need for outpatient services.

- **Listing of Specific Web Sites That Show How to Apply Modifiers Correctly.** Quickly access information at the AMA, CMS (formerly HCFA), and other sources.

- **Discussion Questions at the End of Each Chapter.** Sharpen yours or any other coder's modifier coding skills.

ISBN: 1-56337-395-5   Item No. 3986 **$79.95**

Available: December 2001   4 CEUs from AAPC 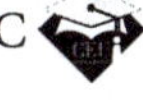

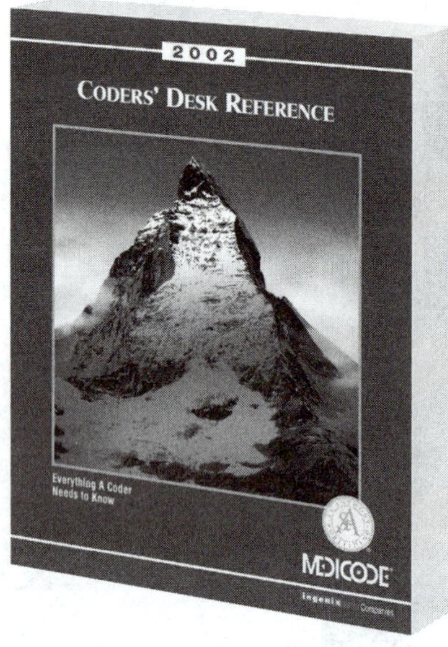

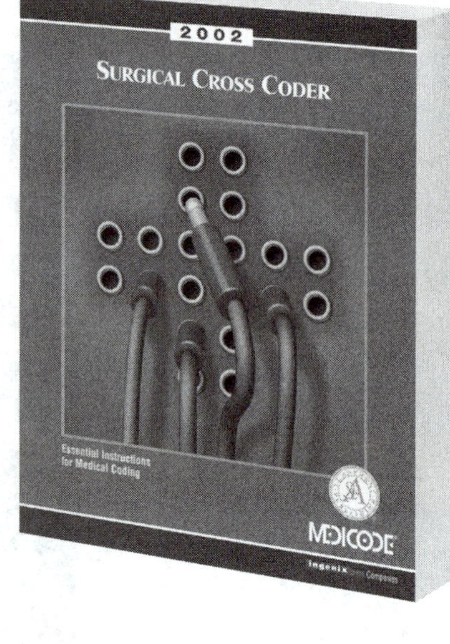

8 Out of 10 Surveyed Coders Prefer the St. Anthony/Medicode Coders' Desk Reference

Coders' Desk Reference

- **NEW! Laboratory and Pathology Codes.** Now you will find lay descriptions for these complicated chapters.

- **Updated CPT Codes.** Includes accurate descriptions for more than 7,000 CPT procedures, plus an anesthesia crosswalk and an E/M chapter.

- **Updated Glossary of Syndromes with Cross-References to the Applicable ICD-9-CM Code.** Understand and identify more than 1,000 medical syndromes found in ICD-9-CM.

- **CPT-5, ICD-10-CM and ICD-10-PCS Preparation.** Learn how each will affect you and discover ways to make the transitions as smooth as possible.

ISBN: 1-56337-390-4   Item No. 5761 **$99.95**

Available: December 2001   5 CEUs from AAPC

Simplify Your Coding Process with This Surgical Code Link Tool

Surgical Cross Coder

You face a myriad of codes and coding systems. How do you connect? This comprehensive illustrated coding guide links more than 4,000 CPT surgical codes to their corresponding diagnostic, procedural and supply codes. Based on sound clinical assumptions and with the input of extensive data and clinical expertise, *Surgical Cross Coder* is a one-source cross-coding book that simplifies the coding of surgical procedures.

- **Organized by CPT Surgical Codes.** Provides a one-step source for coders who need information on a variety of code sets based on surgical procedures.

- **Complete Code Descriptions.** Prevent miscoding and time-consuming corrective action.

- **Comprehensive Appendices.** Includes notes on exempt and excluded codes, modifiers, as well as recommendations for inpatient and outpatient diagnostic coding.

- **Notations.** Serve as a reminder to coders to seek out the causes of the infection, their manifestations and underlying diseases.

ISBN 1-56337-400-5   Item No. 3237 **$149.95**

Available: December 2001   5 CEUs from AAPC

Order Toll-Free 1-800-765-6588
Also Available from your Medical Bookstore or Distributor

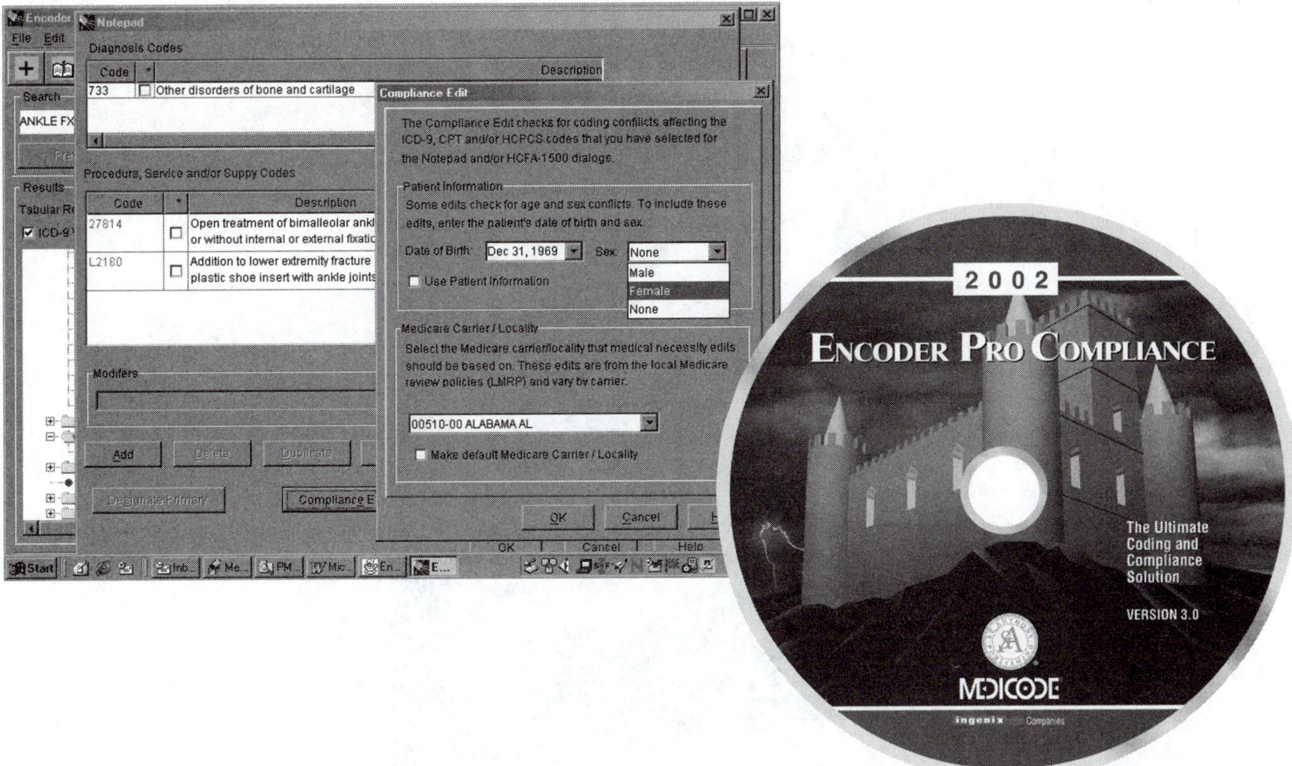

The Ultimate Coding Software Solution

Encoder Pro Compliance

EncoderPro Compliance is the ultimate electronic solution for complete coding. Developed to support all types of network and Intranet installations, EncoderPro Compliance gives the coder or consultant the power of CodeLogic™ search technology, a complete reference library, and a robust compliance tool at their fingertips.

- **CodeLogic™ Technology.** New search capabilities help code simultaneously across all ICD-9-CM, CPT and HCPCS code sets with built in spell-check, abbreviation, and narrow functions for finding the right codes fast.

- **Compliance Editor.** Automated edit of selected claims helps ensure compliance with CCI unbundle policies, Local Medicare Review Policies (LMRPs), age/sex conflicts, and more.

- **Medicare Fees by Locality**. Helps you stay on top of Medicare reimbursement rates. Find the adjusted are fee for any CPT code in the Medicare Physician Fee Schedule.

- **Medicare Color Coding Symbols and Coverage Summaries.** Helps you quickly spot CPT codes effected by Medicare policies for consistent compliance.

- **E/M Calculator.** Helps you review the appropriate CPT Evaluation and Management decision making based on HCFA guidelines or CPT guidelines.

- **Procedural Cross Codes.** View which ICD-9 diagnosis and procedure, HCPCS, ADA, Anesthesia, and PATH/LAB codes are related to your CPT selection.

- **Primary Procedures for Add-on Codes.** Find applicable primary codes for CPT add-on codes CPT and HCPCS Modifiers. Easily find all of the modifier information you need for each code lookup.

- **Notepad Functionality.** Helps you make the most out of your searches. Notepad allows you to export your results to the Windows Clipboard or HCFA 1500 form.

- **Bookmarks and Sticky Notes.** Add reminders and coverage notes to specific codes just like you would in your codebook.

$899.95 (Single User Pricing)

◆*Call for multi-user pricing*

Local Deployment (CD)

Item No. 3460

ASP Deployment (Online)
Available: October 2001

Item No. 7600

LOCAL DEPLOYMENT Recommended Hardware	ASP DEPLOYMENT Recommended Hardware
• 256 MB of RAM	• 128 MB of RAM
• PlII 800 MHZ	• PlI 233 MHZ
• 800X600 SVGA	• 800X600SVGA
• 380 MB Disk Space	• 60 MB Disk Space

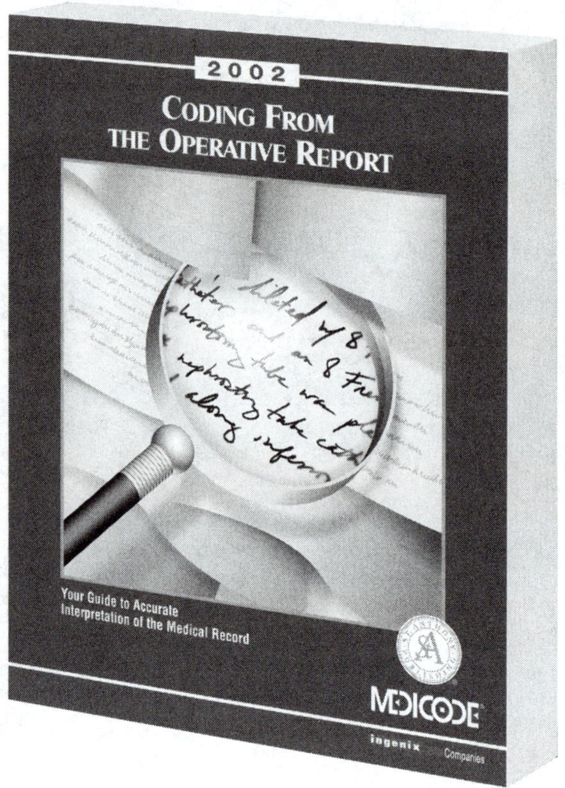

Accurate Coding Using Actual Operative Reports and Notes!

Coding From The Operative Report

This manual provides instruction on gathering the proper information from physician's documentation. Beginning with a discussion of operative reports and their importance to the coding process, this book gives you information you need to successfully and accurately code, from different situations based on specialty, and the CPT chapter in which the service falls.

- **Real Operative Reports and Operative Notes.** This manual reveals the complexities of accurate procedural coding and provides the solutions.

- **Organized by CPT Chapter.** Gives you an overview of each CPT category and its specialty.

- **Definitions, Key Points, Tips and Glossaries.** Helps you interpret cryptic shortcuts, abbreviations and nomenclature used by physicians.

- **Checklists, Guidelines, and Special Situations.** Foolproof guidance through the entire operative report interpretation, abstracting and coding process. Includes scenarios for CPT, ICD-9-CM, HCPCS, DRG and more.

ISBN: 1-56337-396-X   Item No. 4268 **$99.95**

Available: October 2001

Educators: Call for multi-copy discounts

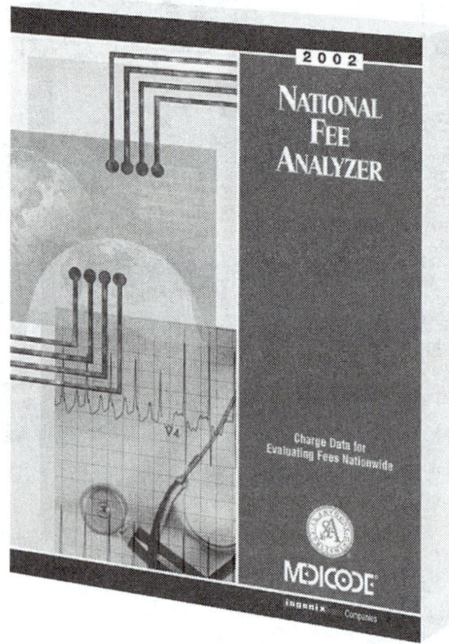

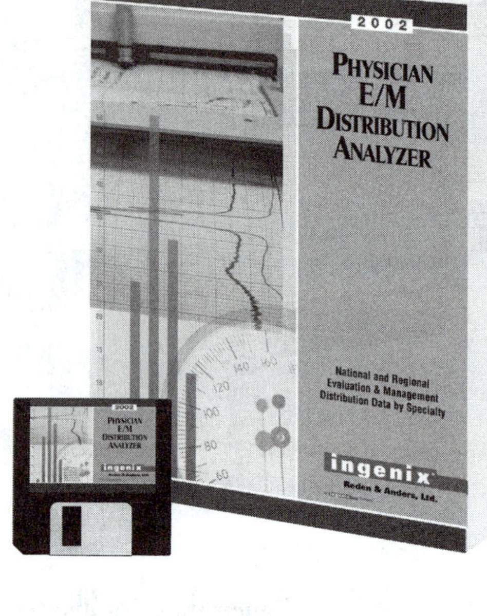

Compare Your Fees Against National Benchmarks

National Fee Analyzer

This important benchmarking resource provides you with national averages of charges based on over 400 million charge transactions. And it is easy to convert the national averages to local estimates with the easy-to-use conversion table featured in the introduction.

- Rely on data from actual claims when analyzing or developing a defensible fee schedule.

- Analyze data broken down into 50th and 75th percentiles for easier benchmarking and decision making.

- Determine relative value based fees with your choice of Ingenix or Medicare relative value units.

- Reference the comprehensive introduction for answers to your reimbursement questions.

ISBN: 1-56337-403-X   Item No. 2493 **$149.95**

Available: February 2002   3 CEUs from AAPC

Regional and National E/M Coding Patterns

Physician E/M Distribution Analyzer

Not knowing how your E/M services stack up against those of your peers can have serious consequences. Now there is a quick way to benchmark your E/M coding history and pinpoint revenue projections in preparation for contract negotiation…*Physician E/M Distribution Analyzer*.

- Depend on data compiled by **Reden & Anders**.

- Compare your E/M distribution against established benchmarks.

- Understand your billing patterns and correct those patterns that vary significantly from established industry benchmarks.

- Evaluate data that is specialty specific as E/M coding patterns can vary significantly by specialty.

ISBN: 1-56337-421-8   Item No. 3346 **$399.95**

ASCII Data File (Includes Book): Item No. 3347 **$599.95**

Available: February 2002   ◆*Call for multi-user pricing*

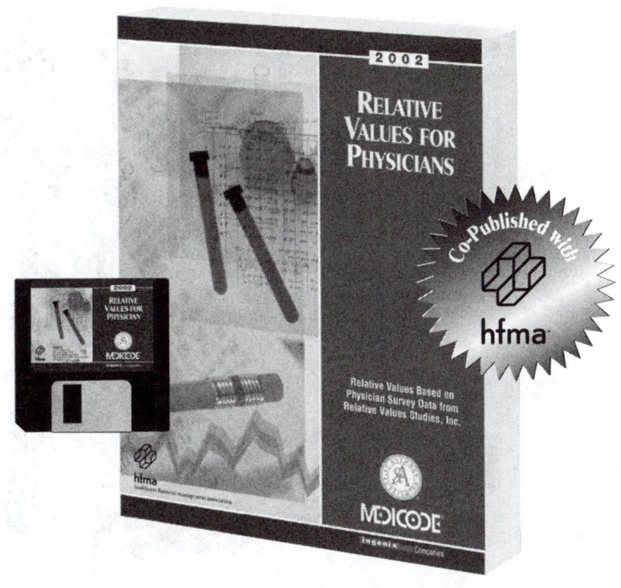
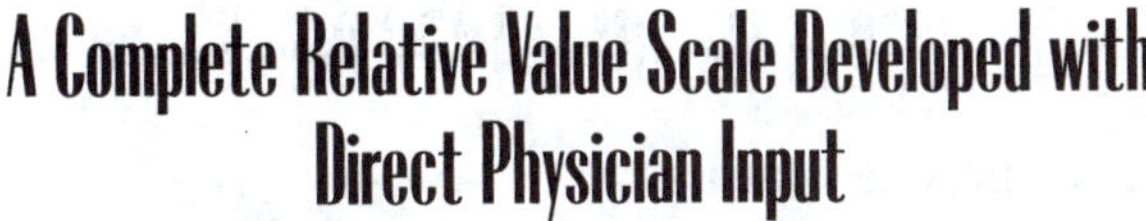
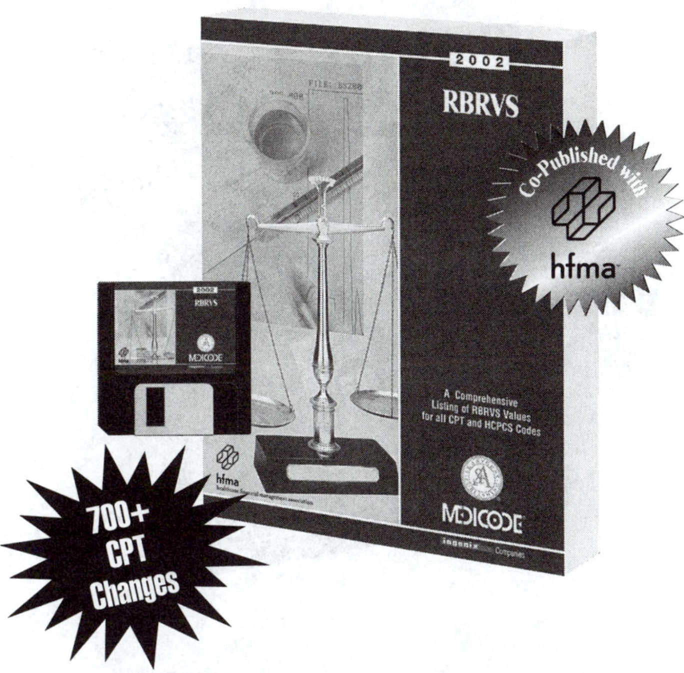

A Complete Relative Value Scale Developed with Direct Physician Input

Relative Values for Physicians

Establish, defend, and negotiate fees using a resource that physician offices like yours have relied on for over 15 years.

- Reference relative values for CPT and HCPCS Level II codes.

- Incorporate relative value units developed through physician surveys.

- Establish relative values based on the clinical skill and knowledge needed to perform a procedure. Subjective charge data is eliminated.

- Value codes relative to one another. Surgery codes are valued relative to surgery codes, E/M codes are valued relative to E/M codes, etc.

ISBN: 1-56337-401-3   Item No. 4322 **$269.95**

ASCII Data File (Includes Book):   Item No. 4320 **$599.95**

Available: December 2001   5 CEUs from AAPC

The Most Comprehensive RBRVS Available

RBRVS

RBRVS is now the most widely used relative value scale in existence and is the system CMS (formerly HCFA) uses to calculate Medicare fees. This is the data you need to reference when negotiating contracts with your payers, conducting fee schedule reviews, or auditing current reimbursements.

RBRVS contains relative value units for all procedures valued by CMS in the *Medicare Physician Fee Schedule*, as well as the relative values for those codes not valued by CMS ("gap" codes). These "gap" codes have been developed using the same methodology used to develop the values for Medicare covered services.

- Reference the same relative value units used by over 60% of the major U.S. HMOs.

- Access CPT and HCPCS Level II codes.

- Analyze the cost and effort associated with a service with work, practice, and malpractice expense components.

- Reference the easy-to-understand tutorial of RBRVS.

ISBN: 1-56337-402-1   Item No. 4206 **$199.95**

ASCII Data File (Includes Book):   Item No. 4323 **$599.95**

Available: December 2001   5 CEUs from AAPC

Order Toll-Free 1-800-765-6588

Also Available from your Medical Bookstore or Distributor

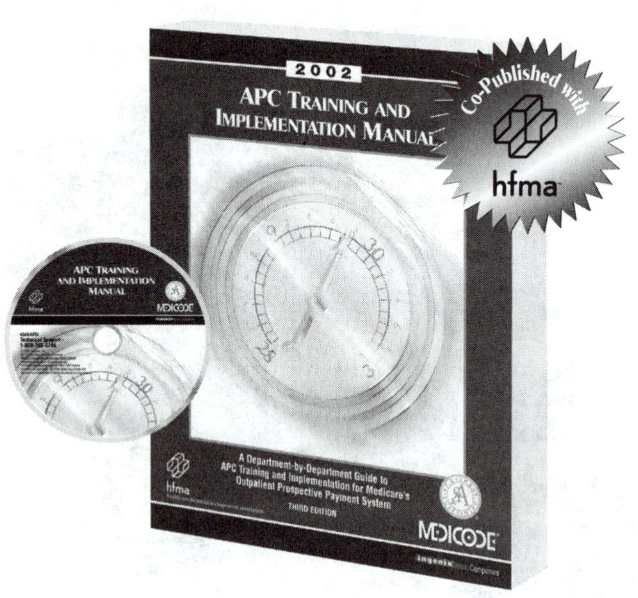

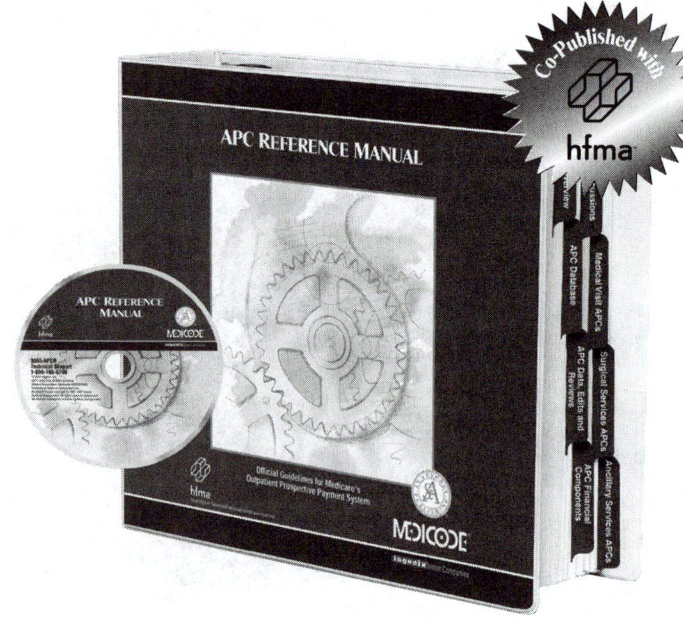

The NEW 2002 edition includes APC Assessment & Ongoing Monitoring for Compliance.

APC Training and Implementation Manual

This manual provides advice, easy-to-follow instructions, and strategies for performing the initial and ongoing assessment, and includes department-by-department training tools to help you develop action plans.

- **Easy-to-Use CD.** Get reproducible forms, exhibits, handouts and other time-saving tools to simplify training.

- **Detailed Plans for Conducting an Operational Assessment.** Get expert advice from our field experts on assessing your facility's performance under APCs.

- **Departmental Strategies for Maintaining Outpatient Revenue.** Includes ED, medical visits/observations, ASU, Radiology, Cardiology.

- **Understand the Impact of Medical Necessity/Orders.** Covering ABN process review & compliance issues, dx coding guidelines & payment implications.

ISBN: 1-56329-815-5   Item No. 4339 **$199.95**

Available: November 2001   6 CEUs from AAPC

Track All of the Official APC Documents

APC Reference Manual

Medicare's rules and instructions for hospitals on APCs are spread over a wide range of documents and make it difficult to find crucial information. This time-saving reference tool arranges key APC information alphabetically, by topic and provides full text of official documents.

- **APC Topics Arranged Alphabetically.** Easily find key topics that explain how the new payment system works.

- **Authoritative Comprehensive Reference.** Includes official guidelines on APCs from Medicare source documents in a handy binder.

- **Full text of Manual on CD-ROM.** Allows for quick searches. Includes hypertext links and resource documents from the manual.

- **Updates For One Full Year.** Keeps you current with APC changes.

Item No. 3055 **$149.95**

Available: Now   5 CEUs from AAPC

St. Anthony Consulting

An **ingenix** Company

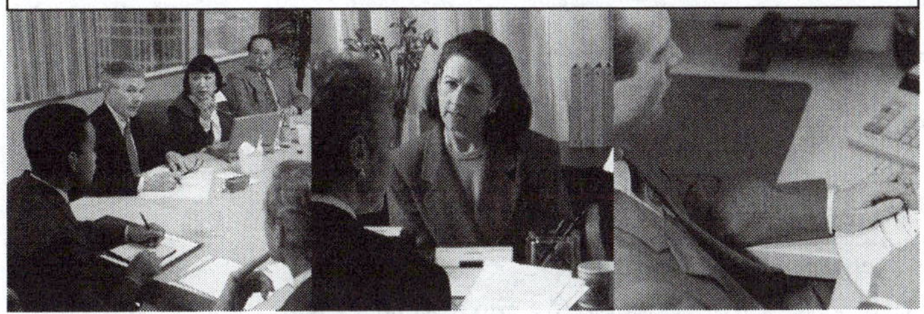

Where There's a Need, St. Anthony Consulting Has a Solution.

St. Anthony Consulting

St. Anthony Consulting, an Ingenix company, offers a full spectrum of healthcare issues from billing, compliance, auditing to coding. Our mission is simple: to help our clients ensure efficient work practices, effective regulatory compliance, and correct reimbursement. Our consulting staff is comprised of former Medicare managers, CEOs, nurses, practice administrators, and more, with a combined experience of over 100 years. Trust the experts who write the books the other consultants are using.

Just a sample of the hospital services we provide:

Hospital Inpatient Revenue Services

- Chargemaster Review and Maintenance
- DRG assignment
- Compliance education
- Billing Procedures
- Record Auditing
- Documentation of Services
- And more.

Hospital Outpatient Revenue Services

- APC Appropriateness
- CPT-4 Educational Programs
- ICD-9 Educational Programs
- Billing Procedures
- Emergency Room Services
- Rehabilitation Services
- Home Health Compliance
- Physician Documentation
- And more.

Call today for more information and put our expertise to work for you.

800-348-2633

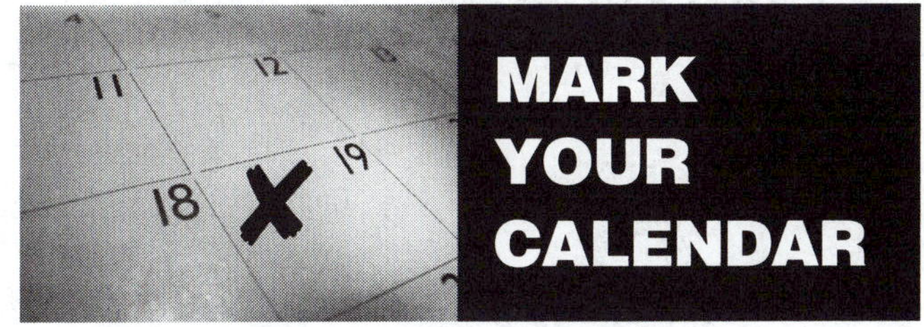

2 Great Ways to Train

1. Live Audioseminars via High Tech Conference Calls
2. Seminars on Tape

We Invite top-notch professionals from all over the nation to present the latest tips, techniques and best practices in coding, billing, and compliance. Train 1, 10, 50 or more, all for the same low rate. You will save hundreds if not thousands of dollars in registration, travel, and lodging expenses.

Our 90-minute audioseminars are the perfect way to learn what you need to know, without losing excessive time away from work. You can rely on St. Anthony Publishing/Medicode for accurate information and a quality experience. Select events are co-sponsored by American Academy of Professional Coders (AAPC) or American Health Information Management Association (AHIMA).

Audioseminar topics include:

- Specialty Coding for Radiology and Laboratory/Pathology
- ICD-9-CM Coding Update for Hospitals and Physicians
- DRG Compliance and Payment
- CPT Coding Update for Hospitals and Physicians
- Part A Billing and Compliance
- Hospital Coding Essentials: Surgical, Medical, Anesthesia
- Hospital Billing Essentials
- Nonphysician Practitioners
- Medical Record Documentation

Visit www.IngenixOnline.com to find a complete list of the latest audioseminars and audiocassettes for your in-house training needs. To find out if you qualify for subscriber or member discounts call (800) 765-6588 today!

4 Easy Ways to Order

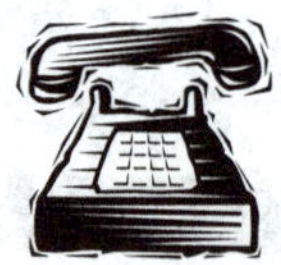

CALL toll-free
800.765.6588 and mention the source code from your mailing label

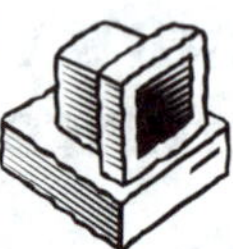

SHOP on line at
www.IngenixOnLine.com

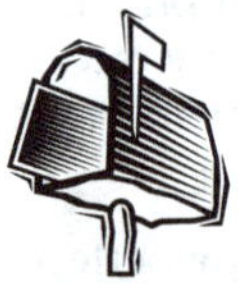

MAIL this form with
payment and/or purchase order to:
PO Box 27116
Salt Lake City, UT 84127-0116

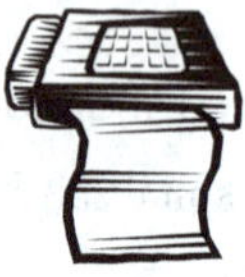

FAX this order form
with credit card information and/or purchase order to
801.982.4033

| Shipping and Handling ||
No. of Items	Fee
1	9.95
2-4	11.95
5-7	14.95
8-10	19.95
11+	Call

Customer No._____________   Purchase Order No.____________
(Attach copy of Purchase Order)

Contact Name _____________________________________

Company___________________________ Title________________

Address ____
(no P.O. Boxes, please)

City_________________________________ State_____ Zip___________

Phone (______)_____________   Fax (______)________________
(in case we have questions about your order)

IMPORTANT: EMAIL REQUIRED FOR ORDER CONFIRMATION AND SELECT PRODUCT DELIVERY.
Email ____
❑ YES, I WANT TO RECEIVE PRODUCT UPDATES AND INFORMATION
❑ YES, I WANT TO RECEIVE INGENIX NEW PRODUCT ANNOUNCEMENTS AND SPECIAL OFFERS

Item #	Qty	Item Description	Price	Total
4025	1	(SAMPLE) DRG Guidebook	$89.95	$89.95
			Sub Total	
		OH and VA residents please add applicable sales tax		
		Shipping & handling (see chart) *(11 plus units, foreign and Canadian orders, please call for shipping costs)*		
		Total enclosed		

Payment Options:

○ Bill Me. *(St. Anthony, Medicode, CHIPS & St. Anthony Consulting are doing business as Ingenix).*

○ Check enclosed. *(Make payable to Ingenix, Inc.)* Check #___________

○ Charge my: ○ MasterCard   ○ VISA   ○ AMEX   ○ Discover

Card # | | | | | | | | | | | | | | | | | | | Exp. Date: | | | |
MM   YR

Signature ____

100% Money Back Guarantee

If our merchandise ever fails to meet your expectations, please contact our Customer Service Department at (800) 765-6588 for an immediate response. We will resolve any concern without hesitation.

2 0 0 2
CPT® EXPERT

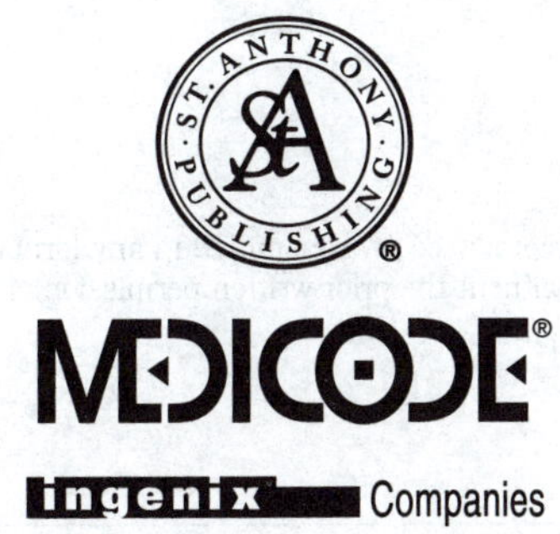

MEDICODE®

ingenix Companies

ACKNOWLEDGEMENTS

Elizabeth Boudrie	*Vice-President, Regulatory Services*
Lynn Speirs	*Senior Director of Publishing Services Group*
Sheri Poe Bernard, CPC	*Director of Essential Regulatory Products*
Brad Ericson, MPC	*Product Manager*
Christine B. Fraizer, MA, CPC	*Project Editor*
Cathy Hopkins, CPC	*Clinical Editor*
Marianne Randall, CPC	*Clinical Editor*
Stacy Perry	*Desktop Publishing Manager*
Kerrie Hornsby	*Desktop Publishing Manager*
Kathy Goebel	*Desktop Publishing Specialist*
Lisa Singley	*Editorial Assistance*
Jennifer Spetsas	*Editorial Assistance*

AAPC CONTINUING EDUCATION UNITS

This publication has prior approval by the American Academy of Professional Coders for one continuing education unit per scenario with a maximum of five units. Granting of prior approval in no way constitutes endorsement by AAPC of the publication content nor the publisher. Please contact the AAPC for the appropriate form to apply for these CEUs. (800) 626-2633 or Fax (801) 236-2258.

CONTENTS

INTRODUCTION

Welcome to Ingenix Publishing's *CPT Expert*, the definitive procedural coding source that combines the work of the American Medical Association (AMA) with the technical components you need for proper reimbursement and coding accuracy. *CPT Expert* not only provides you with the most recent version of the AMA's *Current Procedural Terminology* (CPT), but also detailed coding instructions, clinical guidelines, lay definitions of complex procedures and medical terms, and summaries of the coverage policies used by Federal and commercial payers.

Medical coding and reimbursement professionals developed *CPT Expert* according to their "wish list" for a single, comprehensive coding resource. Like you, they wanted an easy to use coding manual that supplied the most current procedural codes in addition to the regulations governing reimbursement. *CPT Expert* does that in addition to other features found to complement the coding process. Experienced and novice coders will benefit from the extensive glossary of terms scoured from Medicare and commercial payer publications. Illustrations throughout help you visualize the information reported by the physician for documentation in the medical record. Anyone using the index developed specially for *CPT Expert* will be amazed at how simple it is to match a procedure to proper code selection. In addition, you will find that the index in *CPT Expert* has been moved to the front of the book. This was done based on repeated requests from our subscribers to accommodate the coder's approach to coding. It allows the user to locate the code in the index, then confirm in the code section of the manual more easily.

CPT Expert is not intended to replace the AMA's CPT manual. It does not include the AMA's official rules and guidelines, and Ingenix recommends you use this in conjunction with the AMA's 2002 CPT.

CPT Expert is more than just a list of CPT codes and their descriptions. It is an amalgam of coding-valuable material from a number of sources. Developed by the same team that brought you the popular *Coders' Desk Reference*, *CPT Expert* combines material from the American Medical Association (AMA) CPT 2002, Medicare carrier and coverage manuals, the Correct Coding Initiative, Centers for Medicare and Medicaid Services (CMS) fee schedules and rules, and Ingenix's own coding expertise. Designed to be easy-to-use and full of information, this product is an excellent companion to your CPT book, Medicare, Ingenix, or other resources.

FEATURES

Understanding *CPT Expert* begins with an explanation of how the book is organized and the features that will assist you through the steps of code selection and claims submission. However, the *CPT Expert* listing of a service or procedure does not restrict its use to a specific specialty group and any service or procedure code may be used to designate the services rendered by any qualified physician. In terms of coverage, the mere existence of a procedural code does not imply coverage under any given insurance plan. In other words, just because a procedure is identified by code doesn't mean a payer is obligated to reimburse the physician. Commercial payers generally follow the lead of Medicare coverage policies described later in this introduction.

New to CPT 2002 is the addition of Category III codes, which the AMA considers temporary codes for emerging technology, services, and procedures. The codes in this section, which follows the Medicine section, use alphanumeric combinations (0001T-0026T) and must reported in lieu of an unlisted code when appropriate. Category III codes are part of the AMA plans to modify CPT for future use. These codes may eventually be moved to Category I status (e.g., the accustomed five-digit numerical code) once approved by the Food and Drug Administration, as an appropriate, proven technology, service, or procedure performed by health care providers in clinical practice.

ORGANIZATION

CPT Expert follows the same organization as CPT, which is arranged in six major sections as follows:

- Evaluation and Management (99201-99499)

- Anesthesiology (00100-01999)
- Surgery (10021-69990)
- Radiology (including nuclear medicine, radiation oncology, diagnostic ultrasound) (70010-79999)
- Pathology and Laboratory (80048-89399)
- Medicine (90281-99569)

The six major sections of *CPT Expert* are further arranged in subsections. Subsections pertaining to a section are listed within the section guidelines. For example, the surgery subsections are:

- General
- Integumentary System
- Musculoskeletal System
- Respiratory System
- Cardiovascular System
- Hemic and Lymphatic Systems
- Mediastinum and Diaphragm
- Digestive System
- Urinary System
- Male Genital System
- Intersex Surgery
- Female Genital System
- Maternity Care and Delivery
- Endocrine System
- Nervous System
- Eye and Ocular Adnexa
- Auditory System
- Operating Microscope

Appendices in *CPT Expert* that follow the six major sections are:

- Appendix A -HCPCS Level I (CPT) and Level II (National) Modifiers
- Appendix B - Summary of Additions, Deletions, and Revisions
- Appendix C - Glossary
- Appendix D - Commonly Miscoded Procedures

FORMAT

CPT Expert follows the same format for codes found in the CPT book, as shown in the following example. Codes 67005 and 67010 share the common description of *Removal of vitreous, anterior approach (open sky technique or limbal incision);* The difference between the codes is that 67005 is a partial removal of the vitreous using the anterior approach, while 67010 describes a subtotal removal of the vitreous using the anterior approach and a mechanical vitrectomy. The key to interpreting these codes correctly is the semicolon (;) in 67005. The semicolon separates the common portion of the description from the portion unique to that code. Whenever a code is indented, the text that appears before the semicolon in the preceding unindented code is the common portion of the description. The indented 67010 code does not repeat the common portion (that part immediately before the semicolon), but instead supplies its own unique information.

67005   *Removal of vitreous, anterior approach (open sky technique or limbal incision); partial removal*

67010   *subtotal removal with mechanical vitrectomy*

The entire description for 67010 is *Removal of vitreous, anterior approach (open sky technique or limbal incision); subtotal removal with mechanical vitrectomy*

CLINICAL INFORMATION

CODING INFORMATION

Ingenix generated coding information appears in blue at the beginning of the six major sections of *CPT Expert*. However, the information found in *CPT Expert* goes beyond the familiar definitions, explanations of terms, and factors relevant to the section. Each section in *CPT Expert* provides coding tips and other information that enriches your understanding of procedural coding. For example, the introductory paragraphs in the anesthesia section compare the two organizations responsible for developing anesthesia codes and guidelines—the AMA and the American Society of Anesthesiologists (ASA) - and the similarities when using either set of guidelines and codes. The Evaluation and Management (E/M) section gives the background to the documentation guidelines that have been a source of debate since introduced in 1995. The radiology section in *CPT Expert* describes the technical component and professional component appended to codes for differentiating the supplier of services. According to these guidelines, the technical component includes the provision of the equipment, supplies, technical personnel, and costs attendant to the performance of the procedure other than the professional services. The professional component encompasses the physician's work in providing the service, including supervision, interpretation, and report of the procedure. Education, malpractice insurance, and other expenses incident to maintaining a practice are also part of the professional component. The eponyms in blue listed under some of the codes are so noted because of their common association with the procedure.

CODE SPECIFIC COMMENTS

Comments that provide information unique to a particular code appear with that code. For example, the following guidelines are included within the overall description of the vitreous codes 67005 and 67010:

If paracentesis is performed on the anterior chamber of the eye, with removal of the vitreous, consult CPT code 65810. If corneovitreal adhesions are removed, consult CPT code 65880.

SUMMARIES OF COVERAGE POLICIES

MEDICARE MANUALS

The *Coverage Issues Manual* (CIM) and the *Medicare Carriers Manual* (MCM) tell you what's reimbursed, at what amount, under what circumstances, and why, with the criteria of "reasonable and necessary" as the decisive factors. According to Medicare regulations, Medicare Part B helps pay for the provider's services, outpatient hospital care, blood, medical equipment and some home health services. It also pays for other medical services such as lab tests and physical and occupational therapy. Some preventive services such as mammograms and flu shots are also covered. Medicare Part B does NOT cover routine physical exams; eye glasses; custodial care; dental care; dentures; routine foot care; hearing aids; orthopedic shoes; or cosmetic surgery. It also does not cover most prescription drugs or healthcare you receive while traveling outside the United States (except under limited circumstances).

CPT Expert also summarizes the coverage policies that can take hours to find when wading through the program manuals. The CIM and MCM policies appear in blue along with the overall description of the code. For example, the coverage policies applying to codes 67005 and 67010 are as follows:

CIM 35-16 VITRECTOMY

Vitrectomy may be considered reasonable and necessary* for the following conditions:

- Vitreous loss incident to cataract surgery
- Vitreous opacities due to vitreous hemorrhage or other causes
- Retinal detachments secondary to vitreous strands
- Proliferative retinopathy

reasonable and necessary are the criteria government and commercial payers use for determining coverage

BALANCED BUDGET ACT (BBA) OF 1999

The BBA of 1999 continues to impact Medicare coverage of services and supplies, as noted in *CPT Expert*, in areas such as diabetes self-management benefits, physical and occupational therapy, prostate cancer screening tests, and vaccinations. These BBA requirements are summarized in the following sections.

DIABETES SELF-MANAGEMENT BENEFITS

The BBA provides coverage for diabetes outpatient self-management training to include services furnished in non-hospital-based programs (already covered in hospital-based programs). A physician managing the patient's condition must certify that the services are needed under a comprehensive plan of care. In addition, the BBA provides coverage for blood glucose monitors and testing strips for all diabetics (already covered for insulin-dependent diabetics). Payment for testing strips used with blood glucose monitors are reduced by 10 percent.

PHYSICAL AND OCCUPATIONAL THERAPY

Prior to BBA, there were two annual per beneficiary limits of $900 each for physical therapy and occupational therapy furnished by independent practitioners of therapy. The BBA broadened the scope of these limits by establishing two annual payment limits for all outpatient Part B therapy services, except for therapy services furnished in hospital outpatient departments. The limits were established as follows: a $1,500 per beneficiary annual cap for all outpatient physical therapy and speech language pathology services and a $1,500 per beneficiary annual cap for all outpatient occupational therapy services.

PROSTATE CANCER SCREENING TESTS

The BBA covers an annual prostate cancer screening for men over age 50. Covered procedures include: (1) digital rectal exam, (2) prostate-specific antigen (PSA) blood test, and (3) after 2002, other procedures the Secretary of the Department of Health and Human Services (HHS) finds appropriate. Payment for PSA blood test is made under the clinical laboratory fee schedule, and other services are paid under the physician fee schedule.

VACCINATIONS

The BBA extends the Influenza and Pneumococcal Vaccination Campaign through September 30, 2002. The campaign authorizes $8 million for each fiscal year from 1998 through 2002 (60 percent payable from the Part A Trust Fund and 40 percent from the Part B Trust Fund).

GRAPHIC SYMBOLS

Icons throughout *CPT Expert* relay code specific facts regarding CPT conventions such as 2002 code changes, Medicare coverage policies, and codes identified by the Correct Coding Initiative (CCI). The list of icons by category and their related descriptions follow:

Code Changes

The symbol ● placed before the code number designates new procedure codes added to CPT 2002. The symbol ▲ designates an existing code number that has had a revision made to its code narrative for CPT 2002.

Modifier Rules

TC   **Technical Component Only**

Codes with this icon represent only the technical component (staff and equipment costs) of a procedure or service. Do not use either modifier -26 or -TC with these codes.

26   **Professional Component Only**

Codes with this icon represent the physician's work or professional component of a procedure or service. Do not use either modifier -26 or -TC with these codes.

INTRODUCTION

50 **Bilateral Procedure**

This icon identifies codes that can be reported bilaterally when the same surgeon provides the service for the same patient on the same date. Medicare allows payment for both procedures at 150 percent of the usual amount for one procedure. The modifier does not apply to bilateral procedures inclusive to one code.

80 **Assist-at-Surgery Allowed**

Services noted by this icon are allowed an assist at surgery with payment equal to 16 percent of the allowed amount for the global surgery for that procedure. No documentation is required.

80 **Assist-at-Surgery Allowed**

Services noted by this icon are allowed an assist at surgery with payment equal to 16 percent of the allowed amount for the global surgery for that procedure. Documentation is required.

+ **Add-on Codes**

This icon identifies procedures reported in addition to the primary procedure. The icon **+** denotes add-on codes. An add-on code is neither a stand-alone code nor subject to multiple procedure rules since it describes work in addition to the primary proceure.

⊘ **Modifier -51 Exempt**

Codes identified by this icon indicate that the procedure does not meet the definition of an add-on procedure and not subject to multiple procedure rules.

□ **Correct Coding Initiative (CCI)**

CPT Expert identifies those codes with a corresponding CCI edit in Version 7.3, effective October 1, 2001. The CCI edits define correct coding practices that now serve as the basis of the national Medicare policy for paying claims. The code noted is the comprehensive code.

X **CLIA Waived Test**

This icon identifies laboratory services which are not subject to the CLIA regulations.

❶❷❸❹❺❻❼❽ ASC Group

This icon identifies a service that is on the list of Medicare covered ASC procedures, and identifies the ASC group.

N **Newborn**

This icon identifies procedures that by definition should only be used for newborns, generally between 0 and 12 months of age.

P **Pediatric**

This icon identifies procedures that are by definition should only be used for pediatric patients between 1 and 17 years of age.

N/P **Newborn/Pediatric**

This icon identifies procedures to be used for patients between 0 and 18 years of age.

M **Maternity**

This icon identifies procedures that by definition should only be used for maternity patients generally between 12 and 55 years of age.

♀ **Female Only**

This icon identifies procedures that should only be reported for female patients.

♂ **Male Only**

This icon identifies procedures that should only be reported for male patients.

Coding Alert

Code **Commonly Miscoded Procedure**

Time and experience (and a comprehensive database) allows us to draw your attention to procedures that are commonly miscoded and, consequently, delay reimbursement.

Code **Not Covered by Medicare**

Services and procedures identified by this color bar are never a covered benefit under Medicare. Services and procedures that are not covered may be billed directly to the patient at the time of the service.

Code **Unlisted Procedure**

Unlisted CPT codes report procedures that have not been assigned a specific code number. An unlisted code delays payment due to the extra time necessary for review. When using an unlisted procedure code, include cover notes, documentation of medical necessity, and operative reports.

APPENDICES

CPT Expert contains the most current information regarding HCPCS Level I (CPT) and Level II (National) modifiers and the 2002 changes in CPT code descriptions (additions, deletions, and revisions). You will also find an extensive glossary that gives lay understanding to Medicare language and procedural terminology. Among the terms are the definitions Medicare applies to preventive procedures such as early detection of colorectal cancer (colorectal cancer screening tests), early detection of prostate cancer (prostate cancer screening tests), and early detection of breast cancer (screening mammography). You will also learn what Medicare considers "Medical and Other Health Services" and the finer points that distinguishes covered services offered through Hospice, Home Health Care, and Comprehensive Outpatient Rehabilitation Facilities (CORF), to name only a few. Also included in this edition, as an appendix, is a brief explanation of the codes identified as being commonly miscoded and how to avoid the pitfalls of coding these services.

A

A-II (Angiotensin II), 82163

A Vitamin
See Vitamin, A

Abbe-Estlander Procedure, 40527

Abdomen, Abdominal
Abdominal Wall
  Repair
    Hernia, 49491–49525, 49590
      by Laparoscopy, 49650, 49651
  Tumor
    Excision, 22900
  Unlisted Services and Procedures, 22999
Abscess
  Drainage, 49020, 49040
    Fluid, 49080, 49081
    Peritoneal
      Open, 49020
        Percutaneous, 49021
      Peritonitis, localized, 49020
    Retroperitoneal
      Open, 49060
        Percutaneous, 49061
    Skin and Subcutaneous Tissue
      Complicated, 10061
        Multiple, 10061
        Single, 10060
        Simple, 10060
    Subdiaphragmatic
      Open, 49040
        Percutaneous, 49041
    Subphrenic, 49040
  Incision and drainage
    Open, 49040
    Pancreatitis, 48000
    Peritoneal, 49020
    Peritonitis, Localized, 49020
    Retroperitoneal, 49060
    Skin and Subcutaneous Tissue
      Complicated, 10061
        Multiple, 10061
        Single, 10060
        Simple, 10060
    Subdiaphragmatic, 49040
    Subphrenic, 49040
Angiography, 74175, 75635
Artery
  Ligation, 37617
Biopsy
  Open, 49000
  Percutaneous, 49180
  Skin and Subcutaneous Tissue, 11100, 11101
Bypass Graft, 35907
Cannula
  Catheter
    Insertion, 49420, 49421
    Removal, 49422
CAT Scan, 74150–74175, 75635
Celiotomy
  for Staging, 49220
Cyst
  Destruction
    Excision, 49200, 49201
Drainage
  Fluid, 49080, 49081
Ectopic Pregnancy, 59130
Endometrioma
  Destruction
    Excision, 49200, 49201
Excision
  Excess Skin, 15831
  Tumor, Abdominal Wall, 22900
Exploration, 49000, 49002
  Blood Vessel, 35840
  Staging, 58960
Hernia Repair, 49495–49525, 49560–49587
Incision, 49000
  Staging, 58960
Incision and Drainage
  Pancreatitis, 48000

Abdomen — *continued*
Injection
  Air, 49400
  Contrast Material, 49400
Insertion
  Catheter, 49420, 49421
  Venous Shunt, 49425
Intraperitoneal
  Catheter Removal, 49422
  Shunt
    Ligation, 49428
    Removal, 49429
Laparotomy
  Staging, 49220
Magnetic Resonance Imaging (MRI), 74181–74183
Needle Biopsy
  Mass, 49180
Peritoneocentesis, 49080, 49081
Radical Resection, 51597
Repair
  Blood Vessel, 35221
    Vein Graft, 35251
    with Other Graft, 35281
  Hernia, 49491–49525, 49560–49587
  Suture, 49900
Revision
  Venous Shunt, 49426
Suture, 49900
Tumor
  Destruction/Excision, 49200, 49201
Ultrasound, 76700, 76705
Unlisted Services and Procedures, 49999
Wound Exploration
  Penetrating, 20102
X-ray, 74000–74022

Abdominal Aorta
See Aorta, Abdominal

Abdominal Aortic Aneurysm
See Aorta, Abdominal, Aneurysm

Abdominal Deliveries
See Cesarean Delivery

Abdominal Hysterectomy
See Hysterectomy, Abdominal

Abdominal Lymphangiogram
See Lymphangiography, Abdomen

Abdominal Paracentesis
See Abdomen, Drainage

Abdominal Radiographies
See Abdomen, X-Ray

Abdominohysterectomy
See Hysterectomy, Abdominal

Abdominopelvic Amputation
See Amputation, Interpelviabdominal

Abdominoplasty, 15831

AEP, 92585, 92586

ABG, 82803, 82805

Ablation
Anal
  Polyp, 46615
  Tumor, 46615
CAT Scan Guidance, 76362
Colon
  Tumor, 45339
Endometrial, 0009T, 58353, 58563
Endometrium
  Ultrasound Guidance, 0009T
Endoscopic, Tumors or Polyps, 43228
Heart
  Arrhythmogenic Focus, 93650–93652
  Intracardiac Pacing and Mapping, 93631
    follow-up Study, 93624
    Stimulation and Pacing, 93623
Liver
  Tumor, 47380–47383
    Laparoscopic, 47370, 47371
Magnetic Resonance Guidance, 76934
Prostate, 55873
Renal Cyst, 50541

Ablation — *continued*
Turbinate Mucosa, 30801, 30802
Ultrasound Guidance, 76490

ABO, 86900

Abortion
See Obstetrical Care
Incomplete, 59812
Induced by
  Amniocentesis Injection, 59850–59852
  Dilation and Curettage, 59840
  Dilation and Evacuation, 59841
  Saline, 59850, 59851
  Vaginal Suppositories, 59855, 59856
  with Hysterotomy, 59100, 59852, 59857
Missed, 59820, 59821
  First Trimester, 59820
  Second Trimester, 59821
Septic, 59830
Spontaneous, 59812
Therapeutic, 59840–59852
  by Saline, 59850
    with Dilatation and Curettage, 59851
    with Hysterotomy, 59852, 59857

Abrasion, Skin
Chemical Peel, 15788–15793
Dermabrasion, 15780–15783
Lesion, 15786, 15787
Salabrasion, 15810, 15811

ABS, 86255, 86403, 86850

Abscess
Abdomen, 49040, 49041
  Drainage, 49020, 49040
    Fluid, 49080, 49081
    Peritoneal
      Open, 49020
        Percutaneous, 49021
      Peritonitis, localized, 49020
    Retroperitoneal
      Open, 49060
        Percutaneous, 49061
    Skin and Subcutaneous Tissue
      Complicated, 10061
        Multiple, 10061
        Single, 10060
        Simple, 10060
    Subdiaphragmatic, 49040
      Open, 49040
        Percutaneous, 49041
    Subphrenic, 49040
Anal
  Incision and Drainage, 46045, 46050
Ankle
  Incision and Drainage, 27603
Appendix
  Incision and Drainage, 44900
    Open, 44900
    Percutaneous, 44901
Arm, Lower, 25028
  Excision, 25145
  Incision and Drainage, 25035
Arm, Upper
  Incision and Drainage, 23930–23935
Auditory Canal, External, 69020
Bartholin's Gland
  Incision and Drainage, 56420
Bladder
  Incision and Drainage, 51080
Brain
  Drainage by
    Burrhole, 61150, 61151
    Craniotomy/Craniectomy, 61320, 61321
    Excision, 61514–61522
Breast
  Incision and Drainage, 19020
Carpals
  Incision, Deep, 25035
Clavicle
  Sequestrectomy, 23170

Anus — Arm

          2002 Ingenix, Inc.

Burkitt Herpevirus
See Epstein-Barr Virus

Burns
Allograft, 15350, 15351
Anesthesia, 01953
Debridement, 15000, 15001, 16010–16030
Dressing, 16010–16030
Escharotomy, 16035, 16036
Excision, 15000, 15001
Initial Treatment, 16000
Tissue Culture Skin Grafts, 15100–15121, 15342, 15343
Xenograft, 15400, 15401

Burr Hole
Skull
Biopsy, Brain, 61140
Catheterization, 61210
Drainage
Abscess, 61150, 61151
Cyst, 61150, 61151
Hematoma, 61154, 61156
Exploration
Infratentorial, 61253
Supratentorial, 61250
for Implant of Neurostimulator Array, 61862
Insertion
Catheter, 61210
Reservoir, 61210
with Injection, 61120

Burrow's Operation, 14000–14350

Bursa
Ankle, 27604
Arm, Lower, 25031
Elbow
Excision, 24105
Incision and Drainage, 23931
Femur
Excision, 27062
Foot
Incision and Drainage, 28001
Hip
Incision and Drainage, 26991
Injection, 20600–20610
Ischial
Excision, 27060
Joint
Aspiration, 20600–20610
Drainage, 20600–20610
Injection, 20600–20610
Knee
Excision, 27340
Leg, Lower, 27604
Palm
Incision and Drainage, 26025, 26030
Pelvis
Incision and Drainage, 26991
Shoulder
Drainage, 23031
Wrist, 25031
Excision, 25115, 25116
Incision and Drainage, 25020
Infected Bursa, 25031

Bursectomy
of Hand, 26989

Bursitis, Radiohumeral
See Tennis Elbow

Bursocentesis
See Aspiration, Bursa

Buttock
Excision
Excess Skin, 15835

Button
Nasal Septal Prosthesis
Insertion, 30220

Butyrylcholine Esterase
See Cholinesterase

Bypass, Cardiopulmonary
See Cardiopulmonary Bypass

Bypass Graft
Axillary Artery, 35516–35521, 35533, 35616–35623, 35650, 35654
Carotid Artery, 35501–35509, 35526, 35601, 35606, 35626, 35642
Celiac Artery, 35331, 35631
Coronary Artery
Angiography, 93556
Arterial, 33533–33536
Venous Graft, 33510–33516
Excision
Abdomen, 35907
Extremity, 35903
Neck, 35901
Thorax, 35905
Femoral Artery, 35521, 35533, 35546, 35551, 35566, 35621, 35646, 35647, 35651–35661, 35666, 35700
Harvest
Upper Extremity Vein, 35500
Iliac Artery, 35541, 35563, 35641, 35663
Iliofemoral Artery, 35548, 35549, 35565, 35665
Mesenteric Artery, 35531, 35631
Peroneal Artery, 35566, 35571, 35666, 35671
Placement
Vein Patch, 35685
Popliteal Artery, 35551–35558, 35571, 35623, 35651, 35656, 35671
Renal Artery, 35536, 35560, 35631, 35636
Reoperation, 35700
Repair
Abdomen, 35907
Extremity, 35903
Lower Extremity
with Composite Graft, 35681–35683
Neck, 35901
Thorax, 35905
Revascularization
Extremity, 35903
Neck, 35901
Thorax, 35905
Revision
Lower Extremity
with Angioplasty, 35879
with Vein Interposition, 35881
Secondary Repair, 35870
Splenic Artery, 35536, 35636
Subclavian Artery, 35506, 35507, 35511–35516, 35526, 35606–35616, 35626, 35645, 35693
Thrombectomy, 35875, 35876
Tibial Artery, 35566, 35571, 35623, 35666, 35671
Vertebral Artery, 35508, 35515, 35642, 35645
with Composite Graft, 35681
with Composite Graft, 35681–35683
Autogenous
Three or More Segments
Two Locations, 35683
Two Segments
Two Locations, 35682

Bypass In Situ
Femoral Artery, 35582–35585
Peroneal Artery, 35585, 35587
Popliteal Artery, 35582, 35583, 35587
Tibial Artery, 35585, 35587

C

C-13
Urea Breath Test , 83013, 83014
Urease Activity, 83013, 83014

C-14
Urea Breath Test, 78267, 78268
Urease Activity, 83013, 83014

C-Peptide, 80432, 846811

C-Reactive Protein, 86140, 86141

C-Section 59510–59515, 59618–59622
See also Cesarean Delivery

CA, 82310–82340

CABG, 33503–33505, 33510–33536

Cadmium
Urine, 82300

Calcaneus
Craterization, 28120
Cyst
Excision, 28100–28103
Diaphysectomy, 28120
Excision, 28118–28120
Fracture
Open Treatment, 28415, 28420
Percutaneous Fixation, 28406
with Manipulation, 28405, 28406
without Manipulation, 28400
Repair
Osteotomy, 28300
Saucerization, 28120
Tumor
Excision, 27647, 28100–28103
X-ray, 73650

Calcareous Deposits
Subdeltoid
Removal, 23000

Calcifediol
Blood or Urine, 82306

Calcifediol Assay
See Calciferol

Calciferol
Blood or Urine, 82307

Calcification
See Calcium, Deposits

Calciol
See Calciferol

Calcitonin
Blood or Urine, 82308
Stimulation Panel, 80410

Calcium
Blood
Infusion Test, 82331
Deposits
Removal, Calculi-Stone
Bile Duct, 43264, 47420, 47425, 47554, 47630
Bladder, 51050, 52310–52318
Gallbladder, 47480
Hepatic Duct, 47400
Kidney, 50060–50081, 50130, 50561, 50580
Pancreas, 48020
Pancreatic Duct, 43264
Salivary Gland, 42330–42340
Ureter, 50610–50630, 50961, 50980, 51060, 51065, 52320–52330, 52336, 52337
Urethra, 52310, 52315
Ionized, 82330
Total, 82310
Urine, 82340

Calcium-Binding Protein, Vitamin K-Dependent
See Osteocalcin

Calcium-Pentagastrin Stimulation, 80410

Calculus
Analysis, 82355–82370
Destruction
Bile Duct, 43265
Pancreatic Duct, 43265
Removal
Bile Duct, 43264, 47554, 74327
Bladder, 51050, 52310–52318, 52352
Kidney, 50060–50081, 50130–50561, 50580, 52352
Pancreatic Duct, 43264
Ureter, 50610–50630, 50961, 50980, 51060, 51065, 52320, 52325, 52352
Urethra, 52310, 52315, 52352

INDEX

Cornea

  2002 Ingenix, Inc.

            2002 Ingenix, Inc.

Fistula — Foot

  2002 Ingenix, Inc.

Pancreatorrhaphy, 48545

Pancreatotomy
See Incision, Pancreas

Pancreozymin-Secretin Test, 82938

Panel
See Organ or Disease Oriented panel

Panniculectomy
See Lipectomy

PAP, 88141–88167

Pap Smears, 88141–88155, 88164–88167

Paper, Chromatography
See Chromatography, Paper

Paper Chromatographies
See Chromatography, Paper

Papilla, Interdental
See Gums

Papillectomy, 46220

Papilloma
Destruction, 54050–54065

Papillotomy, 43262

PAPP D
See Lactogen, Human Placental

Para-Tyrosine
See Tyrosine

Paracentesis
Eye
Anterior Chamber
with Diagnostic Aspiration of
Aqueous, 65800
with Removal of Blood, 65815
with Removal Vitreous and
or Discission of Anterior Hyaloid
Membrane, 65810
with Therapeutic Release of Aqueous,
65805

Paracentesis, Abdominal
See Abdomen, Drainage

Paracentesis, Thoracic
See Thoracentesis

Paracervical Nerve
Injection
Anesthetic, 64435

Paraffin Bath Therapy, 97018
See Physical
Medicine/Therapy/Occupational
Therapy

Paraganglioma, Medullary
See Pheochromocytoma

Parainfluenza Virus
Antigen Detection
Immunofluorescence, 87279

Paralysis, Facial Nerve
See Facial Nerve Paralysis

Paralysis, Infantile
See Polio

Paranasal Sinuses
See Sinus

Parasites
Blood, 87207
Concentration, 87015
Examination, 87169
Smear, 87177

Parasitic Worms
See Helminth

Parathormone, 83970

Parathyrin
See Parathormone

Parathyroid Autotransplantation, 60512

Parathyroid Gland
Autotransplant, 60512
Biopsy, 60699
Excision, 60500, 60502

Parathyroid Gland — *continued*
Exploration, 60500–60505
Nuclear Medicine
Imaging, 78070

Parathyroid Hormone, 83970

Parathyroid Hormone Measurement
See Parathormone

Parathyroid Transplantation
See Transplantation, Parathyroid

Parathyroidectomy, 60500–60505

Paraurethral Gland
Abscess
Incision and Drainage, 53060

Paravertebral Nerve
Destruction, 64622, 64623
Injection
Anesthetic, 64470–64484
Neurolytic, 64622, 64623

Parietal Cell Vagotomies
See Vagotomy, Highly Selective

Parietal Craniotomy, 61556

Paring
Skin Lesion
Benign Hyperkeratotic
More than Four Lesions, 11057
Single Lesion, 11055
Two to Four Lesions, 11056

Park Posterior Anal Repair, 46761

Paronychia
Incision and Drainage, 10060, 10061

Parotid Duct
Diversion, 42507–42510
Reconstruction, 42507–42510

Parotid Gland
Abscess
Incision and Drainage, 42300, 42305
Calculi (Stone)
Excision, 42330, 42340
Excision
Partial, 42410, 42415
Total, 42420–42426
Tumor
Excision, 42410–42426

Parotidectomy, 61590

Parotitides, Epidemic
See Mumps

Pars Abdominalis Aortae
See Aorta, Abdominal

Partial Colectomy
See Colectomy, Partial

Partial Cystectomy
See Cystectomy, Partial

Partial Esophagectomy
See Esophagectomy, Partial

Partial Gastrectomy
See Excision, Stomach, Partial

Partial Glossectomy
See Excision, Tongue, Partial

Partial Hepatectomy
See Excision, Liver, Partial

Partial Mastectomies
See Breast, Excision, Lesion

Partial Nephrectomy
See Excision, Kidney, Partial

Partial Pancreatectomy
See Pancreatectomy, Partial

Partial Splenectomy
See Splenectomy, Partial

Partial Thromboplastin Time
See Thromboplastin, Partial, Time

Partial Ureterectomy
See Ureterectomy, Partial

Particle Agglutination, 86403, 86406

Parvovirus
Antibody, 86747

Patch
Allergy Tests, 95044
See Allergy Tests

Patella
See Knee
Dislocation, 27560–27566
Excision, 27350
with Reconstruction, 27424
Fracture, 27520, 27524
Reconstruction, 27437, 27438
Repair
Chondromalacia, 27418
Instability, 27420–27424

Patella, Chondromalacia
See Chondromalacia Patella

Patellar Tendon Bearing (PTB) Cast, 29435

Patellectomy, 27350, 27524, 27566
with Reconstruction, 27424

Paternity Testing, 86910, 86911

Patey's Operation
Mastectomy, Radical, 19200, 19220

Pathologic Dilatation
See Dilation

Pathology
Clinical
Consultation, 80500, 80502
Surgical
Consultation, 88321–88325
Intraoperative, 88329–88332
Decalcification Procedure, 88311
Electron Microscopy, 88348
Electron Microscopy, 88349
Gross and Micro Exam
Level II, 88302
Level III, 88304
Level IV, 88305
Level V, 88307
Level VI, 88309
Gross Exam
Level I, 88300
Histochemistry, 88318, 88319
Immunocytochemistry, 88342
Immunofluorescent Study, 88346, 88347
Morphometry
Nerve, 88356
Skeletal Muscle, 88355
Tumor, 88358
Nerve Teasing, 88362
Special Stain, 88312–88314
Staining, 88312–88314
Tissue Hybridization, 88365
Unlisted Services and Procedures,
88399, 89399

Patient
Dialysis Training
Completed Course, 90989

Patterson's Test
Blood Urea Nitrogen, 84520, 84525

Paul-Bunnell Test
See Antibody; Antibody Identification;
Microsomal Antibody

PBG
See Porphobilinogen

PCL, 27407, 29889

PCP, 83992

PCR (Polymerase Chain Reaction),
83898–83902, 83904–83912

Peak Flow Rate, 94150

Pean's Operation
Amputation, Leg, Upper, at Hip, 27290

Pectoral Cavity
See Chest Cavity

      2002 Ingenix, Inc.

Tumor — *continued*
Femoral, 27355–27358
Excision, 27365
Femur, 27065–27067
Excision, 27365
Fibula, 27635–27638
Excision, 27646
Finger
Excision, 26115–26117
Foot, 28043, 28045, 28046
Forearm
Radical Resection, 25077
Gums
Excision, 41825–41827
Hand, 26115–26117
Heart
Excision, 33120, 33130
Hip, 27047–27049, 27065–27067
Excision, 27075, 27076
Humerus
with Allograft, 23156
with Autograft, 23155
Excision, 23150, 23220–23222, 24110
with Allograft, 23156, 24116
with Autograft, 23155, 24115
Ileum, 27065–27067
Immunoassay for Antigen, 86294, 86316
CA 125, 86304
CA 15-3, 86300
CA 19–9, 86301
Innominate
Excision, 27077
Intestines, Small
Destruction, 44369
Ischial
Excision, 27078, 27079
Kidney
Excision, 52355
Knee
Excision, 27327–27329, 27365
Lacrimal Gland
Excision
Frontal Approach, 68540
with Osteotomy, 68550
Larynx, 31540, 31541
Excision, 31300
Endoscopic, 31540, 31541, 31578
Incision, 31300
Leg, Lower, 27615–27619
Leg, Upper
Excision, 27327–27329
Localization
with Nuclear Medicine, 78800–78803
Mandible, 21040–21045
Maxillary Torus Palatinus, 21032
Mediastinal
Excision, 39220
Mediastinum, 32662
Meningioma, 6151
Excision, 615192
Metacarpal, 26200, 26205, 26250, 26255
Metatarsal, 28104–28107
Excision, 28173
Neck
Excision, 21555, 21556
Radical Resection, 21557
Olecranon Process
with Allograft, 24126
with Autograft, 24125
Excision, 24120
Ovary
Resection, 58950, 58952–58954
Pancreatic Duct
Destruction, 43272
Parotid Gland
Excision, 42410–42426
Pelvis, 27047–27049
Pericardial
Endoscopic, 32661
Excision, 33050
Peritoneum
Resection, 58950, 58952–58954

Tumor — *continued*
Phalanges
Finger, 26210, 26215, 26260–26262
Toe, 28108
Excision, 28175
Pituitary Gland
Excision, 61546, 61548
Positron Emission Tomography (PET),
78810
Pubis, 27065–27067
Radiation Therapy, 77295
Radius, 25120–25126, 25170
Excision, 24120
with Allograft, 24126
with Autograft, 24125
Rectum
Destruction, 45190, 45320, 46937,
46938
Excision, 45160, 45170
Resection
Face, 21015
Scalp, 21015
with Cystourethroscopy, 52355
Retroperitoneal
Destruction
Excision, 49200, 49201
Sacrum, 49215
Scapula, 23140
Excision, 23140, 23210
with Allograft, 23146
with Autograft, 23145
Shoulder
Excision, 23075–23077
Skull
Excision, 61500
Soft Tissue
Elbow
Excision, 24075
Finger
Excision, 26115
Forearm
Radical Resection, 25077
Hand
Excision, 26115
Spinal Cord
Excision, 63275–63290
Stomach
Excision, 43610, 43611
Talus, 28100–28103
Excision, 27647
Tarsal, 28104–28107
Excision, 28171
Temporal Bone
Removal, 69970
Testis
Excision, 54530, 54535
Thorax
Excision, 21555, 21556
Radical Resection, 21557
Thyroid
Excision, 60200
Tibia, 27635–27638
Excision, 27645
Torus Mandibularis, 21031
Trachea
Excision
Cervical, 31785
Thoracic, 31786
Ulna, 25120–25126, 25170
Excision, 24120
with Allograft
Excision, 24126
with Autograft
Excision, 24125
Ureter
Excision, 52355
Urethra, 52234–52240, 53220
Excision, 52355
Uterus
Excision, 58140, 58145
Vagina
Excision, 57135

Tumor — *continued*
Vertebra
Additional Segment
Excision, 22103, 22116
Cervical
Excision, 22100
Lumbar, 22102
Thoracic
Excision, 22101
Wrist, 25075–25077, 25135, 25136
Excision, 25075
Radical Resection, 25077

Tunica Vaginalis
Hydrocele
Aspiration, 55000
Excision, 55040, 55041
Repair, 55060

Turbinate
Excision, 30130, 30140
Fracture
Therapeutic, 30930
Injection, 30200
Submucous Resection
Nose
Excision, 30140

Turbinate Mucosa
Ablation, 30801, 30802
Cauterization, 30801, 30802

Turcica, Sella
See Sella Turcica

Turnbuckle Jacket, 29020, 29025
Removal, 29715

TURP, 52601, 52612–52630

Tylectomy
See Breast, Excision, Lesion

Tylenol
Urine, 82003

Tympanic Membrane
Create Stoma, 69433, 69436
Incision, 69420, 69421
Reconstruction, 69620
Repair, 69450, 69610

Tympanic Nerve
Excision, 69676

Tympanolysis, 69450

Tympanometry, 92567
See Audiologic Function Tests

Tympanoplasty
See Myringoplasty
Radical or Complete, 69645
with Ossicular Chain Reconstruction,
69646
with Antrotomy or Mastoidectomy, 69635
with Ossicular Chain Reconstruction,
69636
and Synthetic Prosthesis, 69637
with Mastoidectomy, 69641
and Ossicular Chain Reconstruction,
69644
with Intact or Reconstructed Wall
and Ossicular Chain Reconstruction,
69644
without Ossicular Chain
Reconstruction, 69643
without Mastoidectomy, 69631
with Ossicular Chain Reconstruction,
69632
and Synthetic Prosthesis, 69633

Tympanostomy, 69433, 69436

Tympanotomy
See Myringotomy

Typhoid Vaccine, 90690–90693
AKD, 90693
Oral, 90690
H-P, 90692
Polysaccharide, 90691

EVALUATION AND MANAGEMENT

The following information is taken directly from the AMA's *Current Procedural Terminology.*

CLASSIFICATION OF EVALUATION AND MANAGEMENT (E/M) SERVICES

The E/M section is divided into broad categories such as office visits, hospital visits, and consultations. Most of the categories are further divided into two or more subcategories of E/M services. For example, there are two subcategories of office visits (new patient and established patient) and there are two subcategories of hospital visits (initial and subsequent). The subcategories of E/M services are further classified into levels of E/M services that are identified by specific codes. This classification is important because the nature of physician work varies by type of service, place of service, and the patient's status.

The basic format of the levels of E/M services is the same for most categories. First, a unique code number is listed. Second, the place and/or type of service is specified, eg, office consultation. Third, the content of the service is defined, eg, comprehensive history and comprehensive examination. (See "Levels of E/M Services," page 2, for details on the content of E/M services.) Fourth, the nature of the presenting problem(s) usually associated with a given level is described. Fifth, the time typically required to provide the service is specified. (A detailed discussion of time begins on page 2.)

DEFINITIONS OF COMMONLY USED TERMS

Certain key words and phrases are used throughout the E/M section. The following definitions are intended to reduce the potential for differing interpretations and to increase the consistency of reporting by physicians in differing specialties.

NEW AND ESTABLISHED PATIENT

Solely for the purposes of distinguishing between new and established patients, professional services are those face-to-face services rendered by a physician and reported by a specific CPT code(s). A new patient is one who has not received any professional services from the physician, or another physician of the same specialty who belongs to the same group practice, within the past three years.

An established patient is one who has received professional services from the physician, or another physician of the same specialty who belongs to the same group practice, within the past three years.

In the instance where a physician is on call for or covering for another physician, the patient's encounter will be classified as it would have been by the physician who is not available.

No distinction is made between new and established patients in the emergency department. E/M services in the emergency department category may be reported for any new or established patient who presents for treatment in the emergency department.

CHIEF COMPLAINT

A concise statement describing the symptom, problem, condition, diagnosis or other factor that is the reason for the encounter, usually stated in the patient's words.

CONCURRENT CARE

Concurrent care is the provision of similar services, eg, hospital visits, to the same patient by more than one physician on the same day. When concurrent care is provided, no special reporting is required. Modifier '-75' has been deleted.

COUNSELING

Counseling is a discussion with a patient and/or family concerning one or more of the following areas:

- diagnostic results, impressions, and/or recommended diagnostic studies;

- prognosis;

- risks and benefits of management (treatment) options;

- instructions for management (treatment) and/or follow-up;

- importance of compliance with chosen management (treatment) options;

- risk factor reduction; and

- patient and family education.

(For psychotherapy, see 90804-90857)

FAMILY HISTORY

A review of medical events in the patient's family that includes significant information about:

- the health status or cause of death of parents, siblings, and children;

- specific diseases related to problems identified in the Chief Complaint or History of the Present Illness, and/or System Review;

- diseases of family members which may be hereditary or place the patient at risk.

HISTORY OF PRESENT ILLNESS

A chronological description of the development of the patient's present illness from the first sign and/or symptom to the present. This includes a description of location, quality, severity, timing, context, modifying factors and associated signs and symptoms significantly related to the presenting problem(s).

LEVELS OF E/M SERVICES

Within each category or subcategory of E/M service, there are three to five levels of E/M services available for reporting purposes. Levels of E/M services are not interchangeable among the different categories or subcategories of service. For example, the first level of E/M services in the subcategory of office visit, new patient, does not have the same definition as the first level of E/M services in the subcategory of office visit, established patient.

The levels of E/M services include examinations, evaluations, treatments, conferences with or concerning patients, preventive pediatric and adult health supervision, and similar medical services, such as the determination of the need and/or location for appropriate care. Medical screening includes the history, examination, and medical decision-making required to determine the need and/or location for appropriate care and treatment of the patient (eg, office and other outpatient setting, emergency department, nursing facility, etc.). The levels of E/M services encompass the wide variations in skill, effort, time, responsibility and medical knowledge required for the prevention or diagnosis and treatment of illness or injury and the promotion of optimal health. Each level of E/M services may be used by all physicians.

The descriptors for the levels of E/M services recognize seven components, six of which are used in defining the levels of E/M services. These components are:

- history;

- examination;

- medical decision making;

- counseling;

- coordination of care;

- nature of presenting problem; and

- time.

The first three of these components (history, examination, and medical decision making) are considered the key components in selecting a level of E/M services. (See "Determine the Extent of History Obtained," page 5.)

The next three components (counseling, coordination of care, and the nature of the presenting problem) are considered contributory factors in the majority of encounters. Although the first two of these contributory factors are important E/M services, it is not required that these services be provided at every patient encounter.

Coordination of care with other providers or agencies without a patient encounter on that day is reported using the case management codes.

The final component, time, is discussed in detail below.

Any specifically identifiable procedure (ie, identified with a specific CPT code) performed on or subsequent to the date of initial or subsequent E/M services should be reported separately.

The actual performance and/or interpretation of diagnostic tests/studies ordered during a patient encounter are not included in the levels of E/M services. Physician performance of diagnostic tests/studies for which specific CPT codes are available may be reported separately, in addition to the appropriate E/M code. The physician's interpretation of the results of diagnostic tests/studies (ie, professional component) with preparation of a separate distinctly identifiable signed written report may also be reported separately, using the appropriate CPT code with the modifier '-26' appended.

The physician may need to indicate that on the day a procedure or service identified by a CPT code was performed, the patient's condition required a significant separately identifiable E/M service above and beyond other services provided or beyond the usual preservice and postservice care associated with the procedure that was performed. The E/M service may be caused or prompted by the symptoms or condition for which the procedure and/or service was provided. This circumstance may be reported by adding the modifier '-25' to the appropriate level of E/M service. As such, different diagnoses are not required for reporting of the procedure and the E/M services on the same date.

NATURE OF PRESENTING PROBLEM

A presenting problem is a disease, condition, illness, injury, symptom, sign, finding, complaint, or other reason for encounter, with or without a diagnosis being established at the time of the encounter. The E/M codes recognize five types of presenting problems that are defined as follows:

Minimal: A problem that may not require the presence of the physician, but service is provided under the physician's supervision.

Self-limited or minor: A problem that runs a definite and prescribed course, is transient in nature, and is not likely to permanently alter health status OR has a good prognosis with management/compliance.

Low severity: A problem where the risk of morbidity without treatment is low; there is little to no risk of mortality without treatment; full recovery without functional impairment is expected.

Moderate severity: A problem where the risk of morbidity without treatment is moderate; there is moderate risk of mortality without treatment; uncertain prognosis OR increased probability of prolonged functional impairment.

High severity: A problem where the risk of morbidity without treatment is high to extreme; there is a moderate to high risk of mortality without treatment OR high probability of severe, prolonged functional impairment.

PAST HISTORY

A review of the patient's past experiences with illnesses, injuries, and treatments that includes significant information about:

- prior major illnesses and injuries;
- prior operations;
- prior hospitalizations;
- current medications;
- allergies (eg, drug, food);
- age appropriate immunization status;
- age appropriate feeding/dietary status.

SOCIAL HISTORY

An age appropriate review of past and current activities that includes significant information about:

- marital status and/or living arrangements;
- current employment;

- occupational history;
- use of drugs, alcohol, and tobacco;
- level of education;
- sexual history;
- other relevant social factors.

SYSTEM REVIEW (REVIEW OF SYSTEMS)

An inventory of body systems obtained through a series of questions seeking to identify signs and/or symptoms which the patient may be experiencing or has experienced. For the purposes of CPT the following elements of a system review have been identified:

- Constitutional symptoms (fever, weight loss, etc.)
- Eyes
- Ears, Nose, Mouth, Throat
- Cardiovascular
- Respiratory
- Gastrointestinal
- Genitourinary
- Musculoskeletal
- Integumentary (skin and/or breast)
- Neurological
- Psychiatric
- Endocrine
- Hematologic/Lymphatic
- Allergic/Immunologic

The review of systems helps define the problem, clarify the differential diagnosis, identify needed testing, or serves as baseline data on other systems that might be affected by any possible management options.

TIME

The inclusion of time in the definitions of levels of E/M services has been implicit in prior editions of CPT. The inclusion of time as an explicit factor beginning in CPT 1992 is done to assist physicians in selecting the most appropriate level of E/M services. It should be recognized that the specific times expressed in the visit code descriptors are averages, and therefore represent a range of times which may be higher or lower depending on actual clinical circumstances.

Time is not a descriptive component for the emergency department levels of E/M services because emergency department services are typically provided on a variable intensity basis, often involving multiple encounters with several patients over an extended period of time. Therefore, it is often difficult for physicians to provide accurate estimates of the time spent face-to-face with the patient.

Studies to establish levels of E/M services employed surveys of practicing physicians to obtain data on the amount of time and work associated with typical E/M services. Since "work" is not easily quantifiable, the codes must rely on other objective, verifiable measures that correlate with physicians' estimates of their "work". It has been demonstrated that physicians' estimations of intraservice time (as explained on the next page), both within and across specialties, is a variable that is predictive of the "work" of E/M services. This same research has shown there is a strong relationship between intra-service time and total time for E/M services. Intra-service time, rather than total time, was chosen for inclusion with the codes because of its relative ease of measurement and because of its direct correlation with measurements of the total amount of time and work associated with typical E/M services.

Intra-service times are defined as face-to-face time for office and other outpatient visits and as unit/floor time for hospital and other inpatient visits. This distinction is necessary because most of the work of typical office visits takes place during the face-to-face time with the patient, while most of the work of typical hospital visits takes place during the time spent on the patient's floor or unit.

EVALUATION AND MANAGEMENT

Face-to-face time (office and other outpatient visits and office consultations): For coding purposes, face-to-face time for these services is defined as only that time that the physician spends face-to-face with the patient and/or family. This includes the time in which the physician performs such tasks as obtaining a history, performing an examination, and counseling the patient.

Physicians also spend time doing work before or after the face-to-face time with the patient, performing such tasks as reviewing records and tests, arranging for further services, and communicating further with other professionals and the patient through written reports and telephone contact.

This non-face-to-face time for office services—also called pre- and post-encounter time—is not included in the time component described in the E/M codes. However, the pre- and post-face-to-face work associated with an encounter was included in calculating the total work of typical services in physician surveys.

Thus, the face-to-face time associated with the services described by any E/M code is a valid proxy for the total work done before, during, and after the visit.

Unit/floor time (hospital observation services, inpatient hospital care, initial and follow-up hospital consultations, nursing facility): For reporting purposes, intra-service time for these services is defined as unit/floor time, which includes the time that the physician is present on the patient's hospital unit and at the bedside rendering services for that patient. This includes the time in which the physician establishes and/or reviews the patient's chart, examines the patient, writes notes and communicates with other professionals and the patient's family.

In the hospital, pre- and post-time includes time spent off the patient's floor performing such tasks as reviewing pathology and radiology findings in another part of the hospital.

This pre- and post-visit time is not included in the time component described in these codes. However, the pre- and post-work performed during the time spent off the floor or unit was included in calculating the total work of typical services in physician surveys.

Thus, the unit/floor time associated with the services described by any code is a valid proxy for the total work done before, during, and after the visit.

UNLISTED SERVICE

An E/M service may be provided that is not listed in this section of CPT. When reporting such a service, the appropriate "Unlisted" code may be used to indicate the service, identifying it by "Special Report", as discussed in the following paragraph. The "Unlisted Services" and accompanying codes for the E/M section are as follows:

99429	**Unlisted preventive medicine service**
99499	**Unlisted evaluation and management service**
99539	**Unlisted home visit service or procedure**

SPECIAL REPORT

An unlisted service or one that is unusual, variable, or new may require a special report demonstrating the medical appropriateness of the service. Pertinent information should include an adequate definition or description of the nature, extent, and need for the procedure; and the time, effort, and equipment necessary to provide the service. Additional items which may be included are complexity of symptoms, final diagnosis, pertinent physical findings, diagnostic and therapeutic procedures, concurrent problems, and follow-up care.

CLINICAL EXAMPLES

Clinical examples of the codes for E/M services are provided to assist physicians in understanding the meaning of the descriptors and selecting the correct code. The clinical examples are listed in Appendix D (of CPT 2001). Each example was developed by physicians in the specialties shown.

The same problem, when seen by physicians in different specialties, may involve different amounts of work. Therefore, the appropriate level of encounter should be reported using the descriptors rather than the examples.

The examples have been tested for validity and approved by the CPT Editorial Panel. Physicians were given the examples and asked to assign a code or assess the amount of time and work involved. Only those examples that were rated consistently have been included in Appendix D.

INSTRUCTIONS FOR SELECTING A LEVEL OF E/M SERVICE

IDENTIFY THE CATEGORY AND SUBCATEGORY OF SERVICE

The categories and subcategories of codes available for reporting E/M services are shown in Table 1 on the following page.

REVIEW THE REPORTING INSTRUCTIONS FOR THE SELECTED CATEGORY OR SUBCATEGORY

Most of the categories and many of the subcategories of service have special guidelines or instructions unique to that category or subcategory. Where these are indicated, eg, "Inpatient Hospital Care," special instructions will be presented preceding the levels of E/M services.

TABLE 1

CATEGORIES AND SUBCATEGORIES OF SERVICE

CATEGORY/SUBCATEGORY	CODE NUMBERS
Office or Other Outpatient Services	
New Patient	99201-99205
Established Patient	99211-99215
Hospital Observation Discharge Services	99217
Hospital Observation Services	99218-99220
Hospital Observation or Inpatient Care Services (Including Admission and Discharge Services)	99234-99236
Hospital Inpatient Services	
Initial Hospital Care	99221-99223
Subsequent Hospital Care	99231-99233
Hospital Discharge Services	99238-99239
Consultations	
Office Consultations	99241-99245
Initial Inpatient Consultations	99251-99255
Follow-up Inpatient Consultations	99261-99263
Confirmatory Consultations	99271-99275
Emergency Department Services	99281-99288
Patient Transport	99289-99290
Critical Care Services	99291-99292
Neonatal Intensive Care	99295-99298
Nursing Facility Services	
Comprehensive Nursing Facility Assessments	99301-99303
Subsequent Nursing Facility Care	99311-99313
Nursing Facility Discharge Services	99315-99316

CATEGORY/SUBCATEGORY	CODE NUMBERS
Domiciliary, Rest Home or Custodial Care Services	
New Patient	99321-99323
Established Patient	99331-99333
Home Services	
New Patient	99341-99345
Established Patient	99347-99350
Prolonged Services	
With Direct Patient Contact	99354-99357
Without Direct Patient Contact	99358-99359
Standby Services	99360
Case Management Services	
Team Conferences	99361-99362
Telephone Calls	99371-99373
Care Plan Oversight Services	99374-99380
Preventive Medicine Services	
New Patient	99381-99387
Established Patient	99391-99397
Individual Counseling	99401-99404
Group Counseling	99411-99412
Other	99420-99429
Newborn Care	99431-99440
Special E/M Services	99450-99456
Other E/M Services	99499

REVIEW THE LEVEL OF E/M SERVICE DESCRIPTORS AND EXAMPLES IN THE SELECTED CATEGORY OR SUBCATEGORY

The descriptors for the levels of E/M services recognize seven components, six of which are used in defining the levels of E/M services. These components are:

- history;
- examination;
- medical decision making;
- counseling;
- coordination of care;
- nature of presenting problem; and
- time.

The first three of these components (ie, history, examination, and medical decision making) should be considered the key components in selecting the level of E/M services. An exception to this rule is in the case of visits which consist predominantly of counseling or coordination of care. (See numbered paragraph 3, page 5.)

The nature of the presenting problem and time are provided in some levels to assist the physician in determining the appropriate level of E/M service.

DETERMINE THE EXTENT OF HISTORY OBTAINED

The extent of the history is dependent upon clinical judgment and on the nature of the presenting problems(s). The levels of E/M services recognize four types of history that are defined as follows:

Problem focused: chief complaint; brief history of present illness or problem.

Expanded problem focused: chief complaint; brief history of present illness; problem pertinent system review.

Detailed: chief complaint; extended history of present illness; problem pertinent system review extended to include a review of a limited number of additional systems; pertinent past, family, and/or social history directly related to the patient's problems.

Comprehensive: chief complaint; extended history of present illness; review of systems which is directly related to the problem(s) identified in the history of the present illness plus a review of all additional body systems; complete past, family, and social history.

The comprehensive history obtained as part of the preventive medicine evaluation and management service is not problem-oriented and does not involve a chief complaint or present illness. It does, however, include a comprehensive system review and comprehensive or interval past, family, and social history as well as a comprehensive assessment/history of pertinent risk factors.

DETERMINE THE EXTENT OF EXAMINATION PERFORMED

The extent of the examination performed is dependent on clinical judgment and on the nature of the presenting problem(s). The levels of E/M services recognize four types of examination that are defined as follows:

Problem focused: a limited examination of the affected body area or organ system.

Expanded problem focused: a limited examination of the affected body area or organ system and other symptomatic or related organ system(s).

Detailed: an extended examination of the affected body area(s) and other symptomatic or related organ system(s).

EVALUATION AND MANAGEMENT

Comprehensive: a general multi-system examination or a complete examination of a single organ system. Note: The comprehensive examination performed as part of the preventive medicine evaluation and management service is multisystem, but its extent is based on age and risk factors identified.

For the purposes of these CPT definitions, the following body areas are recognized:

- Head, including the face
- Neck
- Chest, including breasts and axilla
- Abdomen
- Genitalia, groin, buttocks
- Back
- Each extremity

For the purposes of these CPT definitions, the following organ systems are recognized:

- Eyes
- Ears, Nose, Mouth, and Throat
- Cardiovascular
- Respiratory
- Gastrointestinal
- Genitourinary
- Musculoskeletal
- Skin
- Neurologic
- Psychiatric
- Hematologic/Lymphatic/Immunologic

DETERMINE THE COMPLEXITY OF MEDICAL DECISION MAKING

Medical decision making refers to the complexity of establishing a diagnosis and/or selecting a management option as measured by:

- the number of possible diagnoses and/or the number of management options that must be considered;

- the amount and/or complexity of medical records, diagnostic tests, and/or other information that must be obtained, reviewed, and analyzed; and

- the risk of significant complications, morbidity, and/or mortality, as well as comorbidities, associated with the patient's presenting problems(s), the diagnostic procedure(s) and/or the possible management options.

Four types of medical decision making are recognized: straightforward; low complexity; moderate complexity; and high complexity. To qualify for a given type of decision making, two of the three elements in Table 2 on the following page must be met or ex- ceeded.

Comorbidities/underlying diseases, in and of themselves, are not considered in selecting a level of E/M services unless their presence significantly increases the complexity of the medical decision making.

SELECT THE APPROPRIATE LEVEL OF E/M SERVICES BASED ON THE FOLLOWING

1. For the following categories/subcategories, all of the key components, ie, history, examination, and medical decision making, must meet or exceed the stated requirements to qualify for a particular level of E/M service: office, new patient; hospital observation services; initial hospital care; office consultations; initial inpatient consultations; confirmatory consultations; emergency department services; comprehensive nursing facility assessments; domiciliary care, new patient; and home, new patient.

2. For the following categories/subcategories, two of the three key components (ie, history, examination, and medical decision making) must meet or exceed the stated requirements to qualify for a particular level of E/M services: office, established patient; subsequent hospital care; follow-up inpatient consultations; subsequent nursing facility care; domiciliary care, established patient; and home, established patient.

3. When counseling and/or coordination of care dominates (more than 50%) the physician/patient and/or family encounter (face-to-face time in the office or other outpatient setting or floor/unit time in the hospital or nursing facility), then time may be considered the key or controlling factor to qualify for a particular level of E/M services. This includes time spent with parties who have assumed responsibility for the care of the patient or decision making whether or not they are family members (eg, foster parents, person acting in locum parentis, legal guardian). The extent of counseling and/or coordination of care must be documented in the medical record.

TABLE 2

COMPLEXITY OF MEDICAL DECISION MAKING

NUMBER OF DIAGNOSES OR MANAGEMENT OPTIONS	AMOUNT AND/OR COMPLEXITY OF DATA TO BE REVIEWED	RISK OF COMPLICATIONS AND/OR MORBIDITY OR MORTALITY	TYPE OF DECISION MAKING
minimal	minimal or none	minimal	straightforward
limited	limited	low	low complexity
multiple	moderate	moderate	moderate complexity
extensive	extensive	high	high complexity

DOCUMENTATION GUIDELINES

Originally jointly developed by the American Medical Association (AMA) and the Health Care Financing Administration (HCFA) in 1995, the documentation guidelines for E/M services have experienced substantial revision in 1997 and are again being revised due to their controversial nature. These documentation guidelines are not included in CPT guidelines and AMA policy does not endorse them. For the time being, physicians may use either the 1995 or 1997 guidelines for Medicare purposes.

COMPONENTS

HISTORY COMPONENT GUIDELINES

- The chief complaint, review of systems, and the past, family, and/or social history may be included as separate elements of the history. Or, this information may be included in the description of the history of the present illness.

- A review of systems and/or a past, family, and/or social history obtained during an earlier encounter does not need to be re-recorded if there is evidence that the physician reviewed and updated the previous information. This may occur when a physician updates his or her own record, or in an institutional setting or group practice where many physicians use a common record. The review and update may be documented by describing any new review of systems and/or past, family, and/or social history information or noting there has been no change in the information and indicating the date and location of the earlier review of systems and/or past, family, and/or social history.

- The review of systems and/or past, family, and/or social history may be recorded by ancillary staff or on a form completed by the patient. To document that the physician reviewed the information, there must be a notation supplementing or confirming the information recorded by others.

- If the physician cannot obtain a history from the patient or other source, the record should describe the patient's condition or other circumstance that precludes obtaining this information.

- The medical record should clearly reflect the chief complaint.

- To qualify for brief history of present illness, the medical record should describe one to three elements of the present illness.

- To qualify for extended history of present illness, the medical record should describe four or more elements of the present illness or associated comorbidities.

- To qualify for problem pertinent review of systems, the patient's positive responses and pertinent negatives for the system related to the problem should be documented.

- To qualify for extended review of systems, the patient's positive responses and pertinent negatives for two to nine systems should be documented.

- To qualify for complete review of systems, at least 10 organ systems must be reviewed. Those systems with positive or pertinent negative responses must be individually documented. For the remaining systems, a notation indicating all other systems are negative is permissible.

- At least one specific item from any of the three history areas must be documented for a pertinent past, family, and/or social history.

- At least one specific item from two of the three history areas must be documented for a complete past, family, and/or social history for the following categories of E/M services: office or other outpatient services, established patient; emergency department; subsequent nursing facility care; domiciliary care, established patient; and home care, established patient.

- At least one specific item from each of the three history areas must be documented for a complete past, family, and/or social history for the following categories of E/M services: office or other outpatient services, new patient; hospital observation services; hospital inpatient services, initial care; consultations; comprehensive nursing facility assessments; domiciliary care, new patient; and home care, new patient.

EXAMINATION COMPONENT GUIDELINES

- Specific abnormal findings and relevant negative findings of the examination of the affected or symptomatic body area(s) or organ system(s) should be documented. A notation of "abnormal" without elaboration is insufficient.

- Abnormal or unexpected findings of the examination of the unaffected or asymptomatic body area(s) or organ system(s) should be described.

- A brief statement or notation indicated "negative" or "normal" is sufficient to document normal findings related to unaffected area(s) or asymptomatic organ system(s).

- Examinations are divided into two different types, general multi-system examinations or single organ system examinations. Either type of examination can be performed by any physician in any specialty. The type is based upon clinical judgment, the patient's history, and the nature of presenting problems.

- Specific elements have been identified for each type of examination and for each specialty. The elements for each are not included in this book as the tables are too lengthy to be reproduced here. Obtain a copy of the complete Documentation guidelines for specific details about each type of examination.

MEDICAL DECISION MAKING COMPONENT GUIDELINES

Make sure the following components are documented:

Number of diagnoses or management options

- An assessment, clinical impression, or diagnosis for each encounter. This information may be explicitly stated or implied in documented decisions regarding management plans and/or further evaluation.

- The initiation of, or changes in, treatment. Treatment includes a wide range of management options including patient instructions, nursing instructions, therapies, and medications.

Amount/complexity of data reviewed

- In cases of referrals or consultations, who requests the advice, and to which provider the referral or consultation is made.

- If a diagnostic service is ordered, planned, scheduled, or performed at the time of the E/M encounter, the type of service (e.g., lab or x-ray).

- The review of lab, radiology, and/or other diagnostic tests. An entry in a progress note such as "WBC elevated" or "chest x-ray unremarkable" is acceptable.

- A decision to obtain old records or a decision to obtain additional history from the family, caretaker, or other source to supplement that obtained from the patient.

- Relevant findings from the review of old records, and/or the receipt of additional history from the family, caretaker, or other source. If there is no relevant information beyond that already obtained, that fact should be documented. A notation of "old records reviewed" or "additional history obtained from family" without elaboration is insufficient.

- The results of discussion of laboratory, radiology, or other diagnostic test with the physician who performed or interpreted the study.

- The direct visualization and independent interpretation of an image, tracing, or specimen previously or subsequently interpreted by another physician.

RISKS OF COMPLICATIONS, MORBIDITY, MORTALITY

- Comorbidities, underlying diseases, or other factors that increase the complexity of medical decision making by increasing the risk of complications, morbidity, and/or mortality.

- If a surgical or invasive diagnostic procedure is ordered, planned, or scheduled at the time of the E/M encounter, the type of procedure (e.g., laparoscopy).

- If a surgical or invasive diagnostic procedure is performed at the time of the E/M encounter, the specific procedure.

- The referral for, or decision to perform, a surgical or invasive diagnostic procedure on an urgent basis.

CONTRIBUTING FACTORS

If the physician elects to report the level of service based on counseling and/or coordination of care, the total length of time of the encounter (face-to-face or floor time, as appropriate) should be documented. The record should describe the counseling and/or activities to coordinate care.

SUMMARY

- Clarify that a code may be selected and documented based on counseling/coordination of care, without reference needed to any other dimension of code selection (i.e., history, exam, and medical decision making).

- Emphasize that for established patients, only two of the three key components need be performed (i.e., history, examination, complexity of medical decision making).

- Simplify history selection by allowing documentation of two of the three history areas (HPI, ROS, and PFSH) instead of requiring all three to be documented.

- Add a note that, when a history cannot be obtained due to the patient's condition (e.g., inability to communicate, urgent, emergent situation), the history is deemed "comprehensive" for coding and documentation purposes.

- Simplify examination criteria by eliminating confusing instructions, while enhancing clinical flexibility by eliminating rigid distinctions between general multi-system vs. single system examinations.

- Simplify the medical decision making component by eliminating one level of complexity (straightforward) — the proposed levels are: low, moderate, and high complexity.

- Simplify the medical decision making component by allowing the highest complexity element (i.e., the number of diagnoses/risk of complications, diagnostic procedures/tests and or data to be reviewed, or management options) to drive the level of medical decision making selection. In addition to the noted changes in the glossary, clarifications in the proposed guidelines also include the following:

  - These documentation guidelines are not applicable to the Preventive Medicine Services, Critical Care, or Neonatal Intensive Care codes

  - Any record format for documenting history (including preprinted history forms completed by the patient and reviewed by the physician) is acceptable

  - The chief complaint and reason for the encounter requirements are not applicable to subsequent inpatient hospital services

  - Definitions of chief complaint, reason for encounter, and brief/extended history of present illness have been added

PLACE OF SERVICE DISTINCTIONS

The E/M code section is divided into subsections by type and place of service. Keep the following in mind when coding each service setting:

- A patient is considered an outpatient at a health care facility until formal inpatient admission occurs.

- Physicians, regardless of specialty, may use 99281–99285 for reporting emergency department services within hospital-based emergency facilities. Other Emergency Services (99288) is reserved for physician directed emergency care provided by the physician in a hospital emergency or critical care department in two-way communication with ambulance or rescue personnel outside the hospital.

- Consultation codes are linked to location.

- Initial hospital inpatient and hospital observation codes as well as initial nursing facility visit codes include evaluation and management services provided elsewhere (office visit codes or emergency department) by the admitting physician on the same day.

DOCUMENTING THE PATIENT RECORD

Physicians and staff members have developed numerous methods to document professional services, and there is no single "right" way as long as all pertinent components of the codes are documented. Some physicians check off a CPT code on an encounter form, while others make clinical notations in the patient's chart for the coding personnel to translate into codes.

E/M SUBCATEGORIES

E/M codes are intended to standardize the way physicians, coders, and claims processors code patient visits. The varied choices presented by E/M codes result in more consistent billing patterns.

OFFICE OR OTHER OUTPATIENT SERVICES

Use the office or other outpatient services codes (99201–99215) to report the services for most patient encounters. CPT does not provide instructions for reporting multiple office or outpatient visits provided by the same physician on the same calendar date. The most common practice is to report a single visit code per day, evaluating all services provided during that day to arrive at the correct level of service. Prolonged service codes may be used to report services beyond the usual.

Modifier -27 was added in 2001 to describe multiple outpatient hospital E/M encounters on the same date. The new modifier gives physicians a means of reporting circumstances involving E/M services provided in multiple outpatient settings.

HOSPITAL OBSERVATION SERVICES

Codes 99217–99220 report E/M services provided to patients designated or admitted as "observation status" in a hospital. It is not necessary that the patient be located in an observation area designated by the hospital to use these codes; however, whenever a patient is placed in a separately designated observation area of the hospital or emergency department, these codes should be used.

INITIAL OBSERVATION CARE

When a patient is admitted to observation status in the course of an encounter in another site of service (e.g., hospital emergency department, physician's office, nursing facility). All related E/M services provided by that physician on the same day are included in the admission for hospital observation. Only one physician can report initial observation services. Do not use these observation codes for post-recovery of a procedure that is considered a global surgical service.

OBSERVATION CARE DISCHARGE SERVICES

Use 99217 only if discharge from observation status occurs on a date other than the initial date of observation status. The code includes final examination of the patient, discussion of the hospital stay, instructions for continuing care, and preparation of discharge records. If a patient is admitted to and subsequently discharged from observation status on the same date, report the service observation/inpatient hospital care codes 99234–99236.

HOSPITAL INPATIENT SERVICES

The codes for hospital inpatient services report admission to a hospital setting, follow-up care provided in a hospital setting, observation or inpatient care for same day admission and discharge, and hospital discharge day management. For inpatient care, the time component includes not only face-to-face time with the patient, but also any unit/floor time related to the patient's care. This time may include family counseling or discussing the patient's condition with the family, establishing and reviewing the patient's record, documenting within the chart, and communicating with other health care professionals, such as other physicians, nursing staff, and respiratory therapists.

Initial hospital care codes (99221–99223) are used by the admitting physician to report the first hospital inpatient encounter. All evaluation and management services provided by the admitting physician in conjunction with the admission regardless of the site of the encounter are included in the initial hospital care service. Services provided in the emergency room, observation room, physician's office, or nursing facility specifically related to the admission cannot be reported separately. Physicians, other than the admitting physician, should not use initial hospital care codes, but should report their services with the appropriate consultation or subsequent hospital care codes.

Codes 99238 and 99239 report hospital discharge day management, but exclude discharge of a patient from observation status. Discharge services for newborns or neonates may be reported with 99238 or 99239 for lengths of stay of more than one day. When concurrent care is provided on discharge day by a physician other than the attending physician, report these services using subsequent hospital care codes.

Observation or Inpatient Care Services, which include admission and discharge services for the same date of service, are reported with 99234–99236. These codes are reported once and include all care provided by the admitting physician whether initiated at another site, within the observation unit, or on an inpatient basis.

CONSULTATIONS

Consultations are provided at the request of another physician or other appropriate source for the purpose of rendering an opinion or advice regarding the evaluation and management of a specific problem. Consultations in CPT fall under four subcategories: office or other outpatient consultations, initial inpatient consultations, follow-up inpatient consultations, and confirmatory consultations. Again, if counseling dominates the encounter, time determines the correct code in three of the four subcategories. Confirmatory consultations have no times established.

The general rules and requirements of a consultation are:

- Requests for consultation must come from an attending physician or other appropriate source, and the necessity for this service must be documented in the patient's record.

- The consultant may initiate diagnostic and/or therapeutic services, such as writing orders or prescriptions and initiating treatment plans.

- The opinion rendered and services ordered or performed and the physician ID number must be documented in the patient's medical record and a report of this information communicated to the requesting provider.

- Report separately any identifiable procedure or service performed on, or subsequent to, the date of the initial consultation.

- When the consultant assumes responsibility for the management of any or all of the patient's care subsequent to the consultation encounter, consult codes are no longer appropriate. Depending on the location, identify the correct subsequent or established patient codes.

- Confirmatory consultations may be requested by the patient and/or family or may result from the second (or third) opinion required by another source, such as the patient's insurance company.

EMERGENCY DEPARTMENT SERVICES

Emergency department (ED) service codes do not differentiate between new and established patients and are used by hospital-based and nonhospital-based physicians.

Time is not a descriptive component for the emergency department levels of E/M services since services are on a variable basis and usually involve multiple encounters with several patients over extended periods of time.

Use 99217–99220 to report evaluation and management services provided in the observation area of a hospital. Use 99291 and 99292 to report critical care provided in the emergency department.

An E/M service can be billed by a physician in addition to a surgical procedure when a separately identifiable E/M service is rendered. For example, if a physician sutures a scalp wound and performs a full neurological exam for a patient with head trauma, it would be proper to bill the surgery and the E/M service. This circumstance would be reported by adding modifier -25 to the appropriate E/M code. It would not be correct, however, if the evaluation only required identifying the need for sutures and confirming immunization status.

Associated with ED services is 99288 *Physician direction of emergency medical systems (EMS) emergency care, advanced life support.* The physician must be located in the ED or critical care department; be in two-way voice communication with the ambulance or rescue personnel outside the hospital; and direct the performance of necessary medical procedures.

CRITICAL CARE SERVICES

Critical care is not specific to a location such as an ICU or CCU. Rather it is determined by the patient's critical condition requiring this type of physician care. Therefore, routine visits to a stabilized patient in an ICU are not necessarily critical care.

Any services performed that are not listed in the margin as a coding axiom can be reported in addition to critical care E/M. Services such as endotracheal intubation (31500) and the insertion and placement of a flow directed catheter (e.g., Swan-Ganz, 93503) may be reported separately. Append modifier -25 to the critical care code to indicate a separate service was performed if the procedure performed is not a starred procedure and has a global follow-up period associated with it.

CRITICAL CARE SERVICES GUIDELINES

- Critical care codes include evaluation and management of the critically ill or injured patient, requiring direct delivery of medical care.

- Care provided to a patient who is not critically ill but happens to be in a critical care unit should be identified using subsequent hospital care codes or inpatient consultation codes as appropriate.

- Critical care of less than 30 minutes should be reported using an appropriate E/M code.

- Critical care codes identify the duration of time spent by a physician on a given date, even if the time is not continuous. Code 99291 reports the first hour and is used only once per date. Code 99292 reports each additional 30 minutes of critical care per date.

- Critical care of less than 15 minutes beyond the first hour or less than 15 minutes beyond the final 30 minutes should not be reported.

- Report the care for patients who are not critically ill but in a critical care unit using other E/M codes.

NEONATAL INTENSIVE CARE

Codes 99295–99298 report services provided by a physician directing care of a critically ill neonate or infant usually in a neonatal intensive care unit (NICU). Use these codes for neonates who are admitted to an intensive care unit at 30 days of age or less.

Initial NICU care does not include physician standby services (99360), attendance at delivery and initial stabilization (99436), or newborn resuscitation (99440) when the physician's presence for the delivery and resuscitation is required prior to transfer of the infant to the NICU. In addition, codes for prolonged physician services (99356 and 99357) may be

EVALUATION AND MANAGEMENT

used if prolonged, face-to-face services are required, prior to admission to NICU.

Neonatal intensive care includes initiation and management of mechanical ventilation or CPAP (when indicated); umbilical, central, or peripheral vessel catheterization; oral or NG tube placement; endotracheal intubation; lumbar puncture; suprapubic bladder aspiration; bladder catheterization; surfactant administration; intravascular fluid administration; transfusion of blood components; vascular punctures; monitoring of vital signs; bedside pulmonary function tests; and monitoring and interpretation of blood gases or oxygen saturation. Parent counseling and personal direct supervision of the health care team in the performance of cognitive and procedural activities are also included. Also included are additional services referred to in the introductory matter to neonatal intensive care codes or in a parenthetical note following the code itself. Report separately any services provided that are not specifically mentioned with each code or in the instructional notes.

NURSING FACILITY SERVICES

Nursing facility E/M services can be provided in skilled (SNFs), intermediate (ICFs), or long-term (LTCFs) facilities. They have been grouped into three subcategories: comprehensive nursing facility assessments (99301–99303), subsequent nursing facility care (99311–99313) and nursing facility discharge services (99315–99316). Included in these codes are E/M services provided to patients in psychiatric residential treatment centers. Report other services, such as medical psychotherapy, separately when provided in addition to E/M services.

DOMICILIARY, REST HOME, OR CUSTODIAL CARE SERVICES

These codes (99321–99333) report care given to patients residing in a long-term care facility that provides room and board, as well as other personal assistance services. The facility's services do not include a medical component and typical times have not been established.

HOME SERVICES

Services and care provided at the patient's home or other private residence are reported from this subcategory. While not all payers will reimburse for physician home services, it is important to document home visits and submit a claim.

PROLONGED SERVICES

This section of E/M codes includes three service categories.

PROLONGED PHYSICIAN SERVICE WITH DIRECT PATIENT CONTACT

These codes report services involving direct patient contact beyond the usual service, with separate codes for office or outpatient encounters (99354 and 99355) and for inpatient encounters (99356 and 99357). Prolonged physician services are add-on services and should be listed separately in addition to the E/M service. The codes report the total duration of face-to-face time spent by the physician on a given date, even if the time is not continuous.

Code 99354 or 99356 reports the first hour of prolonged service on a given date, depending on the place of service, with 99355 or 99357 used to report each additional 30 minutes for that date. Services lasting less than 30 minutes are not reportable in this category, and the services must extend 15 minutes or more into the next time period to be reportable. For example, services lasting one hour and 12 minutes are reported by 99354 or 99356 alone. Services lasting one hour and 17 minutes are reported by the code for the first hour plus the code for an additional 30 minutes.

PROLONGED PHYSICIAN SERVICE WITHOUT DIRECT PATIENT CONTACT

These prolonged physician services without direct patient contact are used before and/or after face-to-face patient care and may include review of extensive records and tests, and communication (other than telephone calls, 99371–99373) with other professionals and/or the patient and family. These are beyond the usual services and include both inpatient and outpatient settings. Report these services in addition to other services provided, including any level of E/M service.

Use 99358 to report the first hour and 99359 for each additional 30 minutes. All aspects of time reporting are the same as explained above for direct patient contact services.

PHYSICIAN STANDBY SERVICE

Code 99360 reports when a physician is requested by another physician to be on standby, and the standby physician has no direct patient contact. The standby physician may not provide services to other patients or be proctoring another physician for the time to be reportable. Also, if the standby physician ultimately provides services subject to a surgical package, the standby is not separately reportable.

This code reports cumulative standby time by date of service. Less than 30 minutes is not reportable and a full 30 minutes must be spent for each unit of service reported. For example, 25 minutes is not reportable and 50 minutes is reported as one unit (99360 x 1).

CASE MANAGEMENT SERVICES

Physician case management is a process of involving direct patient care as well as coordinating and controlling access to the patient or initiating and/or supervising other necessary health care services. Case management services include team conferences (99361–99362) and telephone calls (99371–99373).

CARE PLAN OVERSIGHT SERVICES

Codes 99374–99380 report the services of a physician providing ongoing review and revision of a patient's care plan involving complex or multidisciplinary care modalities. Care plan oversight services are reported separately from any necessary office/outpatient, hospital, home, nursing facility, or domiciliary services. Only one physician may report these codes per patient per 30-day period. Also, low intensity and infrequent supervision services are not reported separately.

PREVENTIVE MEDICINE SERVICES

Preventive medicine evaluation and management codes (99381–99397) are the most frequently used codes in this subsection. They are used to report periodic preventive medicine evaluation and management of infants, children, adolescents, and adults. Examples of services reported with these codes include well-child exams, annual gynecologic exams, and other annual or periodic exams specifically focused on promoting health and preventing illness.

Preventive medicine evaluation and management services can be reported with problem-oriented evaluation and management services (99201–99215) if the abnormality encountered or the pre-existing condition addressed during the preventive medicine exam requires significant additional work. Report with modifier -25 to indicate that a separately identifiable evaluation and management service was provided.

Codes 99381–99397 include counseling, anticipatory guidance, and risk factor reduction provided at the time of the preventive medicine service. Use 99401–99429 only when reporting counseling and risk factor reduction provided at a separate encounter. Report all ancillary lab, x-ray, and other procedures additionally.

NEWBORN CARE

Codes 99431–99440 describe care provided to normal or high-risk newborns in several different settings. The codes identify specific locations, such as the hospital or birthing room, or other than hospital or birthing room.

Discharge services provided to newborns admitted and discharged on the same date should be reported with 99435. Discharge services to newborns discharged on a date subsequent to the admission date should be reported with 99238–99239.

SPECIAL EVALUATION AND MANAGEMENT SERVICES

This group of codes (99450–99456) covers any purely evaluative services provided by a physician when no active management of the patient's problem is undertaken during the encounter.

Use these codes to report evaluations for life or disability insurance eligibility certificates and work-related medical disability. These services can be performed in the office or other setting, and no distinction is made between new or established patient.

These codes should not be used to indicate any active management of problems or conditions. If other E/M services and/or procedures are performed on the same date, report them with the appropriate E/M code in addition to the special evaluation code.

Code 99450 is a basic life or disability examination that includes a medical history; height, weight, and blood pressure measurement; collecting blood and urine specimens; and filling out the necessary forms and reports.

Codes 99455 and 99456 are used for work-related or medical disability. Use 99455 for the treating physician and 99456 for other than the treating physician.

OTHER EVALUATION AND MANAGEMENT SERVICES

Code 99499 is an unlisted code to report other E/M services not specifically defined in CPT.

OFFICE OR OTHER OUTPATIENT SERVICES

NEW PATIENT

MCM 4277. EXTERNAL COUNTERPULSATION (ECP)

Daily evaluation and management service, e.g., 99201-99205, 99211-99215, 99217-99220, 99241-99245, cannot be billed with the ECP treatments. Any evaluation and management service must be justified with adequate documentation of the medical necessity of the visit. Deductible and coinsurance apply. Professional services of a physician must be billed on Form HCFA-1500 paper or electronic equivalent. (HCPCS code G0166 (External counterpulsation, per session) is used to report ECP services and replaces 93799 Unlisted cardiovascular service or procedure).

MCM 15502. PAYMENT FOR OFFICE/OUTPATIENT VISITS (CODES 99201-99215)

A. Definition of New Patient For Selection Of Visit Code.—Interpret the phrase "new patient" to mean a patient who has not received any professional services from the physician within the previous three years.

B. Office/Outpatient Visits Provided On Same Day For Unrelated Problems.- Do not pay two office visits billed by a physician for the same beneficiary on the same day unless the physician documents that the visits were for unrelated problems in the office or outpatient setting which could not be provided during the same encounter (e.g., office visit for blood pressure medication evaluation, followed five hours later by a visit for evaluation of leg pain following an accident).

C. Office/Outpatient or Emergency Department Visit On Day Of Admission To Nursing Facility.—Do not pay a physician for an emergency department visit or an office visit and a comprehensive nursing facility assessment on the same day. Bundle evaluation and management services on the same date provided in sites other than the nursing facility into the initial nursing facility care code when performed on the same date as the nursing facility admission by the same physician.

D. Injection and Evaluation and Management Code Billed Separately on Same Day of Service.— Advise physicians that CPT code 99211 cannot be used to report a visit solely for the purpose of receiving an injection which meets the definition of CPT codes 90782, 90783, 90784, or 90788. Do not pay CPT codes 90782, 90783, 90784, or 90788 if any other physician fee schedule service was rendered.

The drug is billed as a J code, whether the injection is separately billable or not.

If no evaluation and management service or other service is provided on the same day as the injection, the injection code is billed.

99201 Office or other outpatient visit for the evaluation and management of a new patient, which requires these three key components: a problem focused history; a problem focused examination; and straightforward medical decision making. Counseling and/or coordination of care with other providers or agencies are provided consistent with the nature of the problem(s) and the patient's and/or family's needs. Usually, the presenting problems are self limited or minor. Physicians typically spend 10 minutes face-to-face with the patient and/or family.

99202 Office or other outpatient visit for the evaluation and management of a new patient, which requires these three key components: an expanded problem focused history; an expanded problem focused examination; and straightforward medical decision making. Counseling and/or coordination of care with other providers or agencies are provided consistent with the nature of the problem(s) and the patient's and/or family's needs. Usually, the presenting problem(s) are of low to moderate severity. Physicians typically spend 20 minutes face-to-face with the patient and/or family.

99203 Office or other outpatient visit for the evaluation and management of a new patient, which requires these three key components: a detailed history; a detailed examination; and medical decision making of low complexity. Counseling and/or coordination of care with other providers or agencies are provided consistent with the nature of the problem(s) and the patient's and/or family's needs. Usually, the presenting problem(s) are of moderate severity. Physicians typically spend 30 minutes face-to-face with the patient and/or family.

99204 Office or other outpatient visit for the evaluation and management of a new patient, which requires these three key components: a comprehensive history; a comprehensive examination; and medical decision making of moderate complexity. Counseling and/or coordination of care with other providers or agencies are provided consistent with the nature of the problem(s) and the patient's and/or family's needs. Usually, the presenting problem(s) are of moderate to high severity. Physicians typically spend 45 minutes face-to-face with the patient and/or family.

99205 Office or other outpatient visit for the evaluation and management of a new patient, which requires these three key components: a comprehensive history; a comprehensive examination; and medical decision making of high complexity. Counseling and/or coordination of care with other providers or agencies are provided consistent with the nature of the problem(s) and the patient's and/or family's needs. Usually, the presenting problem(s) are of moderate to high severity. Physicians typically spend 60 minutes face-to-face with the patient and/or family.

ESTABLISHED PATIENT

99211 Office or other outpatient visit for the evaluation and management of an established patient, that may not require the presence of a physician. Usually, the presenting problem(s) are minimal. Typically, 5 minutes are spent performing or supervising these services.

99212 Office or other outpatient visit for the evaluation and management of an established patient, which requires at least two of these three key components: a problem focused history; a problem focused examination; straightforward medical decision making. Counseling and/or coordination of care with other providers or agencies are provided consistent with the nature of the problem(s) and the patient's and/or family's needs. Usually, the presenting problem(s) are self limited or minor. Physicians typically spend 10 minutes face-to-face with the patient and/or family.

99213 Office or other outpatient visit for the evaluation and management of an established patient, which requires at least two of these three key components: an expanded problem focused history; an expanded problem focused examination; medical decision making of low complexity. Counseling and coordination of care with other providers or agencies are provided consistent with the nature of the problem(s) and the patient's and/or family's needs. Usually, the presenting problem(s) are of low to moderate severity. Physicians typically spend 15 minutes face-to-face with the patient and/or family.

99214 Office or other outpatient visit for the evaluation and management of an established patient, which requires at least two of these three key components: a detailed history; a detailed examination; medical decision making of moderate complexity. Counseling and/or coordination of care with other providers or agencies are provided consistent with the nature of the problem(s) and the patient's and/or family's needs. Usually, the presenting problem(s) are of moderate to high severity. Physicians typically spend 25 minutes face-to-face with the patient and/or family. 80

99215 Office or other outpatient visit for the evaluation and management of an established patient, which requires at least two of these three key components: a comprehensive history; a comprehensive examination; medical decision making of high complexity. Counseling and/or coordination of care with other providers or agencies are provided consistent with the nature of the problem(s) and the patient's and/or family's needs. Usually, the presenting problem(s) are of moderate to high severity. Physicians typically spend 40 minutes face-to-face with the patient and/or family. 80

HOSPITAL OBSERVATION SERVICES

MCM 4277. EXTERNAL COUNTERPULSATION (ECP)

Daily evaluation and management service, e.g., 99201-99205, 99211-99215, 99217-99220, 99241-99245, cannot be billed with the ECP treatments. Any evaluation and management service must be justified with adequate documentation of the medical necessity of the visit. Deductible and coinsurance apply. Professional services of a physician must be billed on Form HCFA-1500 paper or electronic equivalent. (HCPCS code G0166 (External counterpulsation, per session) is used to report ECP services and replaces 93799 Unlisted cardiovascular service or procedure).

MCM 15504. PAYMENT FOR HOSPITAL OBSERVATION SERVICES (CODES 99217-99220)

A. Who May Bill Initial Observation Care.—Pay for initial observation care billed by only the physician who admitted the patient to hospital observation and was responsible for the patient during his/her stay in observation. A physician who does not have inpatient admitting privileges but who is authorized to admit a patient to observation status may bill these codes.

For a physician to bill the initial observation care codes, there must be a medical observation record for the patient which contains dated and timed physician's admitting orders regarding the care the patient is to receive while in observation, nursing notes, and progress notes prepared by the physician while the patient was in observation status. This record must be in addition to any record prepared as a result of an emergency department or outpatient clinic encounter.

Payment for an initial observation care code is for all the care rendered by the admitting physician on the date the patient was admitted to observation. All other physicians who see the patient while he or she is in observation must bill the office and other outpatient service codes or outpatient consultation codes as appropriate when they provide services to the patient.

OBSERVATION CARE DISCHARGE SERVICES

If the patient is admitted to the hospital on the same day as admission to the observation area, consult CPT codes for Hospital Admission (99221-99223).

Consult CPT codes 99234-99236 for admission and discharge to observation area on same date.

99217 Observation care discharge day management (This code is to be utilized by the physician to report all services provided to a patient on discharge from "observation status" if the discharge is on other than the initial date of "observation status." To report services to a patient designated as "observation status" or "inpatient status" and discharged on the same date, use the codes for Observation or Inpatient Care Services [including Admission and Discharge Services, 99234-99236 as appropriate.]) 80

INITIAL OBSERVATION CARE

99218 Initial observation care, per day, for the evaluation and management of a patient which requires these three key components: a detailed or comprehensive history; a detailed or comprehensive examination; and medical decision making that is straightforward or of low complexity. Counseling and/or coordination of care with other providers or agencies are provided consistent with the nature of the problem(s) and the patient's and/or family's needs. Usually, the problem(s) requiring admission to observation status are of low severity. 80

NEW OR ESTABLISHED PATIENT

99219 Initial observation care, per day, for the evaluation and management of a patient, which requires these three key components: a comprehensive history; a comprehensive examination; and medical decision making of moderate complexity. Counseling and/or coordination of care with other providers or agencies are provided consistent with the nature of the problem(s) and the patient's and/or family's needs. Usually, the problem(s) requiring admission to observation status are of moderate severity. 80

99220 Initial observation care, per day, for the evaluation and management of a patient, which requires these three key components: a comprehensive history; a comprehensive examination; and medical decision making of high complexity. Counseling and/or coordination of care with other providers or agencies are provided consistent with the nature of the problem(s) and the patient's and/or family's needs. Usually, the problem(s) requiring admission to observation status are of high severity. 80

HOSPITAL INPATIENT SERVICES

INITIAL HOSPITAL CARE

99221 Initial hospital care, per day, for the evaluation and management of a patient which requires these three key components: a detailed or comprehensive history; a detailed or comprehensive examination; and medical decision making that is straightforward or of low complexity. Counseling and/or coordination of care with other providers or agencies are provided consistent with the nature of the problem(s) and the patient's and/or family's needs. Usually, the problem(s) requiring admission are of low severity. Physicians typically spend 30 minutes at the bedside and on the patient's hospital floor or unit. 80

99222 Initial hospital care, per day, for the evaluation and management of a patient, which requires these three key components: a comprehensive history; a comprehensive examination; and medical decision making of moderate complexity. Counseling and/or coordination of care with other providers or agencies are provided consistent with the nature of the problem(s) and the patient's and/or family's needs. Usually, the problem(s) requiring admission are of moderate severity. Physicians typically spend 50 minutes at the bedside and on the patient's hospital floor or unit. 80

99223 Initial hospital care, per day, for the evaluation and management of a patient, which requires these three key components: a comprehensive history; a comprehensive examination; and medical decision making of high complexity. Counseling and/or coordination of care with other providers or agencies are provided consistent with the nature of the problem(s) and the patient's and/or family's needs. Usually, the problem(s) requiring admission are of high severity. Physicians typically spend 70 minutes at the bedside and on the patient's hospital floor or unit. [80] [↘]

SUBSEQUENT HOSPITAL CARE

MCM 15505.2 SUBSEQUENT HOSPITAL VISIT AND HOSPITAL DISCHARGE MANAGEMENT (Codes 99231-99239)
Subsequent Hospital Visit and Discharge Management on Same Day.—Pay only the hospital discharge management code on the day of discharge (unless it is also the day of admission, in which case, the admission service and not the discharge management service is billed). Do not pay both a subsequent hospital visit in addition to hospital discharge day management service on the same day by the same physician. Instruct physicians that they may not bill for both a hospital visit and hospital discharge management for the same date of service.

99231 Subsequent hospital care, per day, for the evaluation and management of a patient, which requires at least two of these three key components: a problem focused interval history; a problem focused examination; medical decision making that is straightforward or of low complexity. Counseling and/or coordination of care with other providers or agencies are provided consistent with the nature of the problem(s) and the patient's and/or family's needs. Usually, the patient is stable, recovering or improving. Physicians typically spend 15 minutes at the bedside and on the patient's hospital floor or unit. [80] [↘]

99232 Subsequent hospital care, per day, for the evaluation and management of a patient, which requires at least two of these three key components: an expanded problem focused interval history; an expanded problem focused examination; medical decision making of moderate complexity. Counseling and/or coordination of care with other providers or agencies are provided consistent with the nature of the problem(s) and the patient's and/or family's needs. Usually, the patient is responding inadequately to therapy or has developed a minor complication. Physicians typically spend 25 minutes at the bedside and on the patient's hospital floor or unit. [80] [↘]

99233 Subsequent hospital care, per day, for the evaluation and management of a patient, which requires at least two of these three key components: a detailed interval history; a detailed examination; medical decision making of high complexity. Counseling and/or coordination of care with other providers or agencies are provided consistent with the nature of the problem(s) and the patient's and/or family's needs. Usually, the patient is unstable or has developed a significant complication or a significant new problem. Physicians typically spend 35 minutes at the bedside and on the patient's hospital floor or unit. [80] [↘]

OBSERVATION OR INPATIENT CARE SERVICES (INCLUDING ADMISSION AND DISCHARGE SERVICES)

Consult CPT codes 99217-99220 for patients that are admitted and discharged from observation on different dates. Consult CPT codes 99221-99223 and 99238-99239 for patients admitted for inpatient care and discharged on different dates.

99234 Observation or inpatient hospital care, for the evaluation and management of a patient including admission and discharge on the same date which requires these three key components: a detailed or comprehensive history; a detailed or comprehensive examination; and medical decision making that is straightforward or of low complexity. Counseling and/or coordination of care with other providers or agencies are provided consistent with the nature of the problem(s) and the patient's and/or family's needs. Usually the presenting problem(s) requiring admission are of low severity. [80] [↘]

99235 Observation or inpatient hospital care, for the evaluation and management of a patient including admission and discharge on the same date which requires these three key components: a comprehensive history; a comprehensive examination; and medical decision making of moderate complexity. Counseling and/or coordination of care with other providers or agencies are provided consistent with the nature of the problem(s) and the patient's and/or family's needs. Usually the presenting problem(s) requiring admission are of moderate severity. [80] [↘]

99236 Observation or inpatient hospital care, for the evaluation and management of a patient including admission and discharge on the same date which requires these three key components: a comprehensive history; a comprehensive examination; and medical decision making of high complexity. Counseling and/or coordination of care with other providers or agencies are provided consistent with the nature of the problem(s) and the patient's and/or family's needs. Usually the presenting problem(s) requiring admission are of high severity. [80] [↘]

HOSPITAL DISCHARGE SERVICES

MCM 15505.2 SUBSEQUENT HOSPITAL VISIT AND HOSPITAL DISCHARGE MANAGEMENT (Codes 99231-99239).
Subsequent Hospital Visit and Discharge Management on Same Day.—Pay only the hospital discharge management code on the day of discharge (unless it is also the day of admission, in which case, the admission service and not the discharge management service is billed). Do not pay both a subsequent hospital visit in addition to hospital discharge day management service on the same day by the same physician. Instruct physicians that they may not bill for both a hospital visit and hospital discharge management for the same date of service.

Hospital Discharge Management (CPT Codes 99238 and 99239) and Nursing Facility Admission Code When Patient Is Discharged From Hospital and Admitted To Nursing Facility on Same Day.—Pay the hospital discharge code (codes 99238 or 99239) in addition to a nursing facility admission code when they are billed by the same physician with the same date of service.

99238 Hospital discharge day management; 30 minutes or less [80] [↘]

99239   more than 30 minutes   80 ▯

These codes are to be utilized by the physician to report all services provided to a patient on the date of discharge, if other than the initial date of inpatient status. To report services to a patient who is admitted as an inpatient, and discharged on the same date see codes 99234-99236 for observation or inpatient hospital care including the admission and discharge of the patient on the same date. To report concurrent care services provided by a physician(s) other than the attending physician, use subsequent hospital care codes (99231-99233) on the day of discharge. For Observation Care Discharge, consult CPT code 99217. For observation or inpatient hospital care including the admission and discharge of the patient on the same date, consult CPT codes 99234-99236. For Nursing Facility Care Discharge, consult CPT codes 99315 and 99316. If discharge services are provided to newborns admitted and discharged on the same date, consult CPT code 99435.

CONSULTATIONS

OFFICE OR OTHER OUTPATIENT CONSULTATIONS

NEW OR ESTABLISHED PATIENT

MCM 4277. EXTERNAL COUNTERPULSATION (ECP)

Daily evaluation and management service, e.g., 99201-99205, 99211-99215, 99217-99220, 99241-99245, cannot be billed with the ECP treatments. Any evaluation and management service must be justified with adequate documentation of the medical necessity of the visit. Deductible and coinsurance apply. Professional services of a physician must be billed on Form HCFA-1500 paper or electronic equivalent. (HCPCS code G0166 (External counterpulsation, per session) is used to report ECP services and replaces 93799 Unlisted cardiovascular service or procedure).

MCM 15506. CONSULTATIONS (Codes 99241 - 99275)

Consultation Versus Visit.—Pay for a consultation when all of the criteria for the use of a consultation code are met:

1. Specifically, a consultation is distinguished from a visit because it is provided by a physician whose opinion or advice regarding evaluation and/or management of a specific problem is requested by another physician or other appropriate source (unless it is a patient-generated confirmatory consultation).

2. A request for a consultation from an appropriate source and the need for consultation must be documented in the patient's medical record.

3. After the consultation is provided, the consultant prepares a written report of his/her findings which is provided to the referring physician.

99241 Office consultation for a new or established patient, which requires these three key components: a problem focused history; a problem focused examination; and straightforward medical decision making. Counseling and/or coordination of care with other providers or agencies are provided consistent with the nature of the problem(s) and the patient's and/or family's needs. Usually, the presenting problem(s) are self limited or minor. Physicians typically spend 15 minutes face-to-face with the patient and/or family.   80 ▯

99242 Office consultation for a new or established patient, which requires these three key components: an expanded problem focused history; an expanded problem focused examination; and straightforward medical decision making. Counseling and/or coordination of care with other providers or agencies are provided consistent with the nature of the problem(s) and the patient's and/or family's needs. Usually, the presenting problem(s) are of low severity. Physicians typically spend 30 minutes face-to-face with the patient and/or family.   80 ▯

99243 Office consultation for a new or established patient, which requires these three key components: a detailed history; a detailed examination; and medical decision making of low complexity. Counseling and/or coordination of care with other providers or agencies are provided consistent with the nature of the problem(s) and the patient's and/or family's needs. Usually, the presenting problem(s) are of moderate severity. Physicians typically spend 40 minutes face-to-face with the patient and/or family.   80 ▯

99244 Office consultation for a new or established patient, which requires these three key components: a comprehensive history; a comprehensive examination; and medical decision making of moderate complexity. Counseling and/or coordination of care with other providers or agencies are provided consistent with the nature of the problem(s) and the patient's and/or family's needs. Usually, the presenting problem(s) are of moderate to high severity. Physicians typically spend 60 minutes face-to-face with the patient and/or family.   80 ▯

99245 Office consultation for a new or established patient, which requires these three key components: a comprehensive history; a comprehensive examination; and medical decision making of high complexity. Counseling and/or coordination of care with other providers or agencies are provided consistent with the nature of the problem(s) and the patient's and/or family's needs. Usually, the presenting problem(s) are of moderate to high severity. Physicians typically spend 80 minutes face-to-face with the patient and/or family.   80 ▯

INITIAL INPATIENT CONSULTATIONS

CIM 50-8 CONSULTATION SERVICES RENDERED BY A PODIATRIST IN A SKILLED NURSING FACILITY

Consult services by a podiatrist in a skilled nursing facility are covered if reasonable and necessary and do not come within any of the specific statutory exclusions. Section 1862(a)(13) of the Act excludes payment for the treatment of flat foot conditions, the treatment of subluxations of the foot, and routine foot care. Routine physician exams exclude podiatric consults, except when a specific foot ailment is involved.

MCM 15506. CONSULTATIONS (Codes 99241 - 99275)

Consultation Versus Visit.—Pay for a consultation when all of the criteria for the use of a consultation code are met:

1. Specifically, a consultation is distinguished from a visit because it is provided by a physician whose opinion or advice regarding evaluation and/or management of a specific problem is requested by another physician or other appropriate source (unless it is a patient-generated confirmatory consultation).

2. A request for a consultation from an appropriate source and the need for consultation must be documented in the patient's medical record.

3. After the consultation is provided, the consultant prepares a written report of his/her findings which is provided to the referring physician.

99251 Initial inpatient consultation for a new or established patient, which requires these three key components: a problem focused history; a problem focused examination; and straightforward medical decision making. Counseling and/or coordination of care with other providers or agencies are provided consistent with the nature of the problem(s) and the patient's and/or family's needs. Usually, the presenting problem(s) are self limited or minor. Physicians typically spend 20 minutes at the bedside and on the patient's hospital floor or unit.   80 ▯

2G Professional Component Only   80/80 Assist-at-Surgery Allowed/With Documentation   Unlisted   Commonly Miscoded   Not Covered

TC Technical Component Only   **MCM & CIM** Medicare References   ❶❷❸❹❺❻❼❽ ASC Group   ♂ Male Only   ♀ Female Only

Evaluation and Management

99252 Initial inpatient consultation for a new or established patient, which requires these three key components: an expanded problem focused history; an expanded problem focused examination; and straightforward medical decision making. Counseling and/or coordination of care with other providers or agencies are provided consistent with the nature of the problem(s) and the patient's and/or family's needs. Usually, the presenting problem(s) are of low severity. Physicians typically spend 40 minutes at the bedside and on the patient's hospital floor or unit. 80 ⬑

99253 Initial inpatient consultation for a new or established patient, which requires these three key components: a detailed history; a detailed examination; and medical decision making of low complexity. Counseling and/or coordination of care with other providers or agencies are provided consistent with the nature of the problem(s) and the patient's and/or family's needs. Usually, the presenting problem(s) are of moderate severity. Physicians typically spend 55 minutes at the bedside and on the patient's hospital floor or unit. 80 ⬑

99254 Initial inpatient consultation for a new or established patient, which requires three key components: a comprehensive history; a comprehensive examination; and medical decision making of moderate complexity. Counseling and/or coordination of care with other providers or agencies are provided consistent with the nature of the problem(s) and the patient's and/or family's needs. Usually, the presenting problem(s) are of moderate to high severity. Physicians typically spend 80 minutes at the bedside and on the patient's hospital floor or unit. 80 ⬑

99255 Initial inpatient consultation for a new or established patient, which requires these three key components: a comprehensive history; a comprehensive examination; and medical decision making of high complexity. Counseling and/or coordination of care with other providers or agencies are provided consistent with the nature of the problem(s) and the patient's and/or family's needs. Usually, the presenting problem(s) are of moderate to high severity. Physicians typically spend 110 minutes at the bedside and on the patient's hospital floor or unit. 80 ⬑

FOLLOW-UP INPATIENT CONSULTATIONS

ESTABLISHED PATIENT

99261 Follow-up inpatient consultation for an established patient, which requires at least two of these three key components: a problem focused interval history; a problem focused examination; medical decision making that is straightforward or of low complexity. Counseling and/or coordination of care with other providers or agencies are provided consistent with nature of the problem(s) and the patient's and/or family's needs. Usually, the patient is stable, recovering or improving. Physicians typically spend 10 minutes at the bedside and on the patient's hospital floor or unit. 80 ⬑

99262 Follow-up inpatient consultation for an established patient which requires at least two of these three key components: an expanded problem focused interval history; an expanded problem focused examination; medical decision making of moderate complexity. Counseling and/or coordination of care with other providers or agencies are provided consistent with the nature of the problem(s) and the patient's and/or family's needs. Usually, the patient is responding inadequately to therapy or has developed a minor complication. Physicians typically spend 20 minutes at the bedside and on the patient's hospital floor or unit. 80 ⬑

99263 Follow-up inpatient consultation for an established patient which requires at least two of these three key components: a detailed interval history; a detailed examination; medical decision making of high complexity. Counseling and/or coordination of care with other providers or agencies are provided consistent with the nature of the problem(s) and the patient's and/or family's needs. Usually, the patient is unstable or has developed a significant complication or a significant new problem. Physicians typically spend 30 minutes at the bedside and on the patient's hospital floor or unit. 80 ⬑

CONFIRMATORY CONSULTATIONS

NEW OR ESTABLISHED PATIENT

<u>MCM 15506. CONSULTATIONS (Codes 99241 - 99275)</u>
Consultation Versus Visit.—Pay for a consultation when all of the criteria for the use of a consultation code are met:

1. Specifically, a consultation is distinguished from a visit because it is provided by a physician whose opinion or advice regarding evaluation and/or management of a specific problem is requested by another physician or other appropriate source (unless it is a patient-generated confirmatory consultation).

2. A request for a consultation from an appropriate source and the need for consultation must be documented in the patient's medical record.

3. After the consultation is provided, the consultant prepares a written report of his/her findings which is provided to the referring physician.

99271 Confirmatory consultation for a new or established patient, which requires these three key components: a problem focused history; a problem focused examination; and straightforward medical decision making. Counseling and/or coordination of care with other providers or agencies are provided consistent with the nature of the problem(s) and the patient's and/or family's needs. Usually, the presenting problem(s) are self limited or minor. 80 ⬑

99272 Confirmatory consultation for a new or established patient, which requires these three key components: an expanded problem focused history; an expanded problem focused examination; and straightforward medical decision making. Counseling and/or coordination of care with other providers or agencies are provided consistent with the nature of the problem(s) and the patient's and/or family's needs. Usually, the presenting problem(s) are of low severity. 80 ⬑

99273 Confirmatory consultation for a new or established patient, which requires these three key components: a detailed history; a detailed examination; and medical decision making of low complexity. Counseling and/or coordination of care with other providers or agencies are provided consistent with the nature of the problem(s) and the patient's and/or family's needs. Usually, the presenting problem(s) are of moderate severity. 80 ⬑

99274 Confirmatory consultation for a new or established patient, which requires these three key components: a comprehensive history; a comprehensive examination; and medical decision making of moderate complexity. Counseling and/or coordination of care with other providers or agencies are provided consistent with the nature of the problem(s) and the patient's and/or family's needs. Usually, the presenting problem(s) are of moderate to high severity. 80 ⬑

99252 — 99274

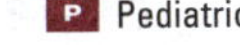

⬑ CCI Comprehensive Code   50 Bilateral Procedure   + CPT Add-on Code   ⊘ Modifier -51 Exempt Code   ● New Code   ▲ Revised Code

M Maternity   N Newborn   P Pediatric   N/P Newborn/Pediatric

99275 Confirmatory consultation for a new or established patient, which requires these three key components: a comprehensive history; a comprehensive examination; and medical decision making of high complexity. Counseling and/or coordination of care with other providers or agencies are provided consistent with the nature of the problem(s) and the patient's and/or family's needs. Usually, the presenting problem(s) are of moderate to high severity.　80 ☐

EMERGENCY DEPARTMENT SERVICES

MCM 15507. EMERGENCY DEPARTMENT VISITS (CODES 99281-99288)

Use Of Emergency Department Codes By Physicians Not Assigned To Emergency Department.—Pay the emergency department services codes regardless of whether the physician is assigned to the emergency department. Any physician seeing a patient registered in the emergency department may use these codes.

Use of Emergency Department Codes In Office.—Do not pay an emergency department code if the site of service is an office or outpatient setting or any sight of service other than an emergency department. The emergency department codes should only be used if the patient is seen in the emergency department. The emergency department is defined as an organized hospital-based facility for the provision of unscheduled or episodic services to patients who present for immediate medical attention.

Use of Emergency Department Codes To Bill Non-Emergency Services.—Pay emergency department codes regardless of whether the services were emergency services. The only requirement for using the emergency department codes is that the patient be seen in the emergency department for an unanticipated service. Normally a lower level emergency department code would be reported for such a non-emergency condition.

Advise physicians that if the physician asks the patient to meet him or her in the emergency department as an alternative to the physician's office and the patient is not registered as a patient in the emergency department, the physician should bill the appropriate office/outpatient visit codes.

99281 Emergency department visit for the evaluation and management of a patient, which requires these three key components: a problem focused history; a problem focused examination; and straightforward medical decision making. Counseling and/or coordination of care with other providers or agencies are provided consistent with the nature of the problem(s) and the patient's and/or family's needs. Usually, the presenting problem(s) are self limited or minor.　80 ☐

99282 Emergency department visit for the evaluation and management of a patient, which requires these three key components: an expanded problem focused history; an expanded problem focused examination; and medical decision making of low complexity. Counseling and/or coordination of care with other providers or agencies are provided consistent with the nature of the problem(s) and the patient's and/or family's needs. Usually, the presenting problem(s) are of low to moderate severity.　80 ☐

99283 Emergency department visit for the evaluation and management of a patient, which requires these three key components: an expanded problem focused history; an expanded problem focused examination; and medical decision making of moderate complexity. Counseling and/or coordination of care with other providers or agencies are provided consistent with the nature of the problem(s) and the patient's and/or family's needs. Usually, the presenting problem(s) are of moderate severity.　80 ☐

99284 Emergency department visit for the evaluation and management of a patient, which requires these three key components: a detailed history; a detailed examination; and medical decision making of moderate complexity. Counseling and/or coordination of care with other providers or agencies are provided consistent with the nature of the problem(s) and the patient's and/or family's needs. Usually, the presenting problem(s) are of high severity, and require urgent evaluation by the physician but do not pose an immediate significant threat to life or physiologic function.　80 ☐

99285 Emergency department visit for the evaluation and management of a patient, which requires these three key components within the constraints imposed by the urgency of the patient's clinical condition and/or mental status: a comprehensive history; a comprehensive examination; and medical decision making of high complexity. Counseling and/or coordination of care with other providers or agencies are provided consistent with the nature of the problem(s) and the patient's and/or family's needs. Usually, the presenting problem(s) are of high severity and pose an immediate significant threat to life or physiologic function.　80 ☐

OTHER EMERGENCY SERVICES

99288 Physician direction of emergency medical systems (EMS) emergency care, advanced life support

PATIENT TRANSPORT

● **99289** Physician constant attention of the critically ill or injured patient during an interfacility transport; first 30-74 minutes

● + **99290** each additional 30 minutes (List separately in addition to code for primary service)

Note that 99290 is an add-on code and must be used in conjunction with 99289.

Any time spent performing other services on the date of transfer, is not to be included in the time reported by these codes.

CRITICAL CARE SERVICES

The following CPT codes are considered part of critical care services and should not be separately reported: the interpretation of chest x-rays (71010-71020), cardiac output measurements (93561-93562), pulse oximetry (94760-94762), blood gases and other information stored in computers (e.g., blood pressures, hematologic date, ECG's (99090)), gastric intubation (43752 and 91105), ventilation management (94656-94662), temporary transcutaneous pacing (92953), and vascular procedures (36000, 36410, 36415, 36540, and 36600).

MCM 15508. CRITICAL CARE VISITS AND NEONATAL INTENSIVE CARE (CODES 99291-99292)

Use of Critical Care (Codes 99291 and 99292) in Cases Which Are Not Medical Emergencies.—Advise physicians that critical care includes the care of critically ill and unstable patients who require constant physician attention, whether the patient is in the course of a medical emergency or not. It involves decision making of high complexity to assess, manipulate, and support circulatory, respiratory, central nervous, metabolic, or other vital system function to prevent or treat single or multiple vital organ system failure. It often also requires extensive interpretation of multiple data bases and the application of advanced technology to manage the critically ill patient.

Critical care is usually, but not always, given in a critical care area such is the coronary care unit, intensive care unit, respiratory care unit, or the emergency department. However, payment may be made for critical care services provided in any location as long as the care provided meets the definition of critical care.

99291 Critical care, evaluation and management of the critically ill or critically injured patient; first 30-74 minutes ⃞80 ⃞↳

+ 99292 each additional 30 minutes (List separately in addition to code for primary service) ⃞80 ⃞↳

Note that 99292 is an add-on code and must be used in conjunction with 99291.

NEONATAL INTENSIVE CARE

99295 Initial neonatal intensive care, per day, for the evaluation and management of a critically ill neonate or infant This code is reserved for the date of admission for neonates who are critically ill. Critically ill neonates require cardiac and/or respiratory support (including ventilator or nasal CPAP when indicated), continuous or frequent vital sign monitoring, laboratory and blood gas interpretations, follow-up physician reevaluations, and constant observation by the health care team under direct physician supervision. Immediate preoperative evaluation and stabilization of neonates with life threatening surgical or cardiac conditions are included under this code. ⃞N ⃞80 ⃞↳

99296 Subsequent neonatal intensive care, per day, for the evaluation and management of a critically ill and unstable neonate or infant A critically ill and unstable neonate will require cardiac and/or respiratory support (including ventilator or nasal CPAP when indicated), continuous or frequent vital sign monitoring, laboratory and blood gas interpretations, follow-up physician re-evaluations throughout a 24-hour period, and constant observation by the health care team under direct physician supervision. In addition, most will require frequent ventilator changes, intravenous fluid alterations, and/or early initiation of parenteral nutrition. Neonates in the immediate post-operative period or those who become critically ill and unstable during the hospital stay will commonly qualify for this level of care. This code encompasses intensive care provided on dates subsequent to the admission date. ⃞N ⃞80 ⃞↳

99297 Subsequent neonatal intensive care, per day, for the evaluation and management of a critically ill though stable neonate or infant Critically ill though stable neonates require cardiac and/or respiratory support (including ventilator and nasal CPAP when indicated), continuous or frequent vital sign monitoring, laboratory and blood gas interpretations, follow-up physician re-evaluations throughout a 24 hour period, and constant observation by the health care team under direct physician supervision. Neonates at this level of care would be expected to require less frequent changes in respiratory, cardiovascular and fluid and electrolyte therapy as those included under code 99296. This code encompasses intensive care provided on dates subsequent to the admission date. ⃞N ⃞80 ⃞↳

99298 Subsequent neonatal intensive care, per day, for the evaluation and management of the recovering very low birth weight infant (less than 1500 grams) Very low birth weight neonates who are no longer critically ill continue to require intensive cardiac and respiratory monitoring, continuous and/or frequent vital sign monitoring, heat maintenance, enteral and/or parenteral nutritional adjustments, laboratory and oxygen monitoring and constant observation by the health care team under direct physician supervision. Neonates of this level of care would be expected to require infrequent changes in respiratory, cardiovascular and/or fluid and electrolyte therapy as those induced under 99296 or 99297. This code encompasses intensive care provided on days subsequent to the admission date. ⃞N ⃞80 ⃞↳

NURSING FACILITY SERVICES

COMPREHENSIVE NURSING FACILITY ASSESSMENTS

NEW OR ESTABLISHED PATIENT

MCM 15510. PHYSICIAN VISITS TO PATIENTS RESIDING IN VARIOUS PLACES OF SERVICE

Evaluation and Management services provided to patients residing in a Skilled Nursing Facility ((SNF) (CPT definition formerly identified as SNFs, intermediate care facilities (ICFs), or long term care facilities (LTCFs) must be reported using the appropriate level of service code within the range identified for Comprehensive Nursing Facility Assessments and Subsequent Nursing Facility Care services. Codes range from 99301 through 99303 for the former and 99311 through 99313 for the latter, and Nursing Facility Discharge Services codes 99315 - 99316. These codes are limited to the specific two digit POS 31 (SNF), 32 (Nursing Home/Nursing Facility), 54 (Intermediate Care Facility/Mentally Retarded) and 56 (Psychiatric Residential Treatment Center).

99301 Evaluation and management of a new or established patient involving an annual nursing facility assessment which requires these three key components: a detailed interval history; a comprehensive examination; and medical decision making that is straightforward or of low complexity. Counseling and/or coordination of care with other providers or agencies are provided consistent with the nature of the problem(s) and the patient's and/or family's needs. Usually, the patient is stable, recovering or improving. The review and affirmation of the medical plan of care is required. Physicians typically spend 30 minutes at the bedside and on the patient's facility floor or unit. ⃞80 ⃞↳

99302 Evaluation and management of a new or established patient involving a nursing facility assessment which requires these three key components: a detailed interval history; a comprehensive examination; and medical decision making of moderate to high complexity. Counseling and/or coordination of care with other providers or agencies are provided consistent with the nature of the problem(s) and the patient's and/or family's needs. Usually, the patient has developed a significant complication or a significant new problem and has had a major permanent change in status. The creation of a new medical plan of care is required. Physicians typically spend 40 minutes at the bedside and on the patient's facility floor or unit. ⃞80 ⃞↳

99303 Evaluation and management of a new or established patient involving a nursing facility assessment at the time of initial admission or readmission to the facility, which requires these three key components: a comprehensive history; a comprehensive examination; and medical decision making of moderate to high complexity. Counseling and/or coordination of care with other providers or agencies are provided consistent with the nature of the problem(s) and the patient's and/or family's needs. The creation of a medical plan of care is required. Physicians typically spend 50 minutes at the bedside and on the patient's facility floor or unit. ⃞80 ⃞↳

SUBSEQUENT NURSING FACILITY CARE

99311 Subsequent nursing facility care, per day, for the evaluation and management of a new or established patient, which requires at least two of these three key components: a problem focused interval history; a problem focused examination; medical decision making that is straightforward or of low complexity. Counseling and/or coordination of care with other providers or agencies are provided consistent with the nature of the problem(s) and the patient's and/or family's needs. Usually, the patient is stable, recovering or improving. Physicians typically spend 15 minutes at the bedside and on the patient's facility floor or unit. ⃞80 ⃞↳

99312   Subsequent nursing facility care, per day, for the evaluation and management of a new or established patient, which requires at least two of these three key components: an expanded problem focused interval history; an expanded problem focused examination; medical decision making of moderate complexity. Counseling and/or coordination of care with other providers or agencies are provided consistent with the nature of the problem(s) and the patient's and/or family's needs. Usually, the patient is responding inadequately to therapy or has developed a minor complication. Physicians typically spend 25 minutes at the bedside and on the patient's facility floor or unit.   80 ▣

99313   Subsequent nursing facility care, per day, for the evaluation and management of a new or established patient, which requires at least two of these three key components: a detailed interval history; a detailed examination; medical decision making of moderate to high complexity. Counseling and/or coordination of care with other providers or agencies are provided consistent with the nature of the problem(s) and the patient's and/or family's needs. Usually, the patient has developed a significant complication or a significant new problem. Physicians typically spend 35 minutes at the bedside and on the patient's facility floor or unit.   80 ▣

NURSING FACILITY DISCHARGE SERVICES

99315   Nursing facility discharge day management; 30 minutes or less   80 ▣

99316   more than 30 minutes   80 ▣

DOMICILIARY, REST HOME (EG, BOARDING HOME), OR CUSTODIAL CARE SERVICES

NEW PATIENT

MCM 15510. PHYSICIAN VISITS TO PATIENTS RESIDING IN VARIOUS PLACES OF SERVICE

CPT codes 99321 through 99333 are limited to the specific two digit places of service (POS) 33 (Custodial Care Facility) and 55 (Residential Substance Abuse Facility). These facilities are often referred to as adult living facilities or assisted living facilities.

99321   Domiciliary or rest home visit for the evaluation and management of a new patient which requires these three key components: a problem focused history; a problem focused examination; and medical decision making that is straightforward or of low complexity. Counseling and/or coordination of care with other providers or agencies are provided consistent with the nature of the problem(s) and the patient's and/or family's needs. Usually, the presenting problem(s) are of low severity.   80 ▣

99322   Domiciliary or rest home visit for the evaluation and management of a new patient, which requires these three key components: an expanded problem focused history; an expanded problem focused examination; and medical decision making of moderate complexity. Counseling and/or coordination of care with other providers or agencies are provided consistent with the nature of the problem(s) and the patient's and/or family's needs. Usually, the presenting problem(s) are of moderate severity.   80 ▣

99323   Domiciliary or rest home visit for the evaluation and management of a new patient, which requires these three key components: a detailed history; a detailed examination; and medical decision making of high complexity. Counseling and/or coordination of care with other providers or agencies are provided consistent with the nature of the problem(s) and the patient's and/or family's needs. Usually, the presenting problem(s) are of high complexity.   80 ▣

99331   Domiciliary or rest home visit for the evaluation and management of an established patient, which requires at least two of these three key components: a problem focused interval history; a problem focused examination; medical decision making that is straightforward or of low complexity. Counseling and/or coordination of care with other providers or agencies are provided consistent with the nature of the problem(s) and the patient's and/or family's needs. Usually, the patient is stable, recovering or improving.   80 ▣

99332   Domiciliary or rest home visit for the evaluation and management of an established patient, which requires at least two of these three key components: an expanded problem focused interval history; an expanded problem focused examination; medical decision making of moderate complexity. Counseling and/or coordination of care with other providers or agencies are provided consistent with the nature of the problem(s) and the patient's and/or family's needs. Usually, the patient is responding inadequately to therapy or has developed a minor complication.   80 ▣

99333   Domiciliary or rest home visit for the evaluation and management of an established patient, which requires at least two of these three key components: a detailed interval history; a detailed examination; medical decision making of high complexity. Counseling and/or coordination of care with other providers or agencies are provided consistent with the nature of the problem(s) and the patient's and/or family's needs. Usually, the patient is unstable or has developed a significant complication or a significant new problem.   80 ▣

HOME SERVICES

NEW PATIENT

MCM 15515. HOME SERVICES (CODES 99341 - 99350)

Requirement for Physician Presence.—Pay home services codes 99341-99350 when they are billed to report evaluation and management services provided in a private residence. A home visit cannot be billed by a physician unless the physician was actually present in the beneficiary's home.

Homebound Status.—Under the home health benefit the beneficiary must be confined to the home for services to be covered. For home services provided by a physician using these codes the beneficiary does not need to be confined to the home.

99341   Home visit for the evaluation and management of a new patient, which requires these three key components: a problem focused history; a problem focused examination; and straightforward medical decision making. Counseling and/or coordination of care with other providers or agencies are provided consistent with the nature of the problem(s) and the patient's and/or family's needs. Usually, the presenting problem(s) are of low severity. Physicians typically spend 20 minutes face-to-face with the patient and/or family.   80 ▣

99342   Home visit for the evaluation and management of a new patient, which requires these three key components: an expanded problem focused history; an expanded problem focused examination; and medical decision making of low complexity. Counseling and/or coordination of care with other providers or agencies are provided consistent with the nature of the problem(s) and the patient's and/or family's needs. Usually, the presenting problem(s) are of moderate severity. Physicians typically spend 30 minutes face-to-face with the patient and/or family.   80 ▣

99343   Home visit for the evaluation and management of a new patient, which requires these three key components: a detailed history; a detailed examination; and medical decision making of moderate complexity. Counseling and/or coordination of care with other providers or agencies are provided consistent with the nature of the problem(s) and the patient's and/or family's needs. Usually, the presenting problem(s) are of moderate to high severity. Physicians typically spend 45 minutes face-to-face with the patient and/or family. 〔80〕 ▣

99344   Home visit for the evaluation and management of a new patient, which requires these three key components: a comprehensive history; a comprehensive examination; and medical decision making of moderate complexity. Counseling and/or coordination of care with other providers or agencies are provided consistent with the nature of the problem(s) and the patient's and/or family's needs. Usually, the presenting problem(s) are of high severity. Physicians typically spend 60 minutes face-to-face with the patient and/or family. 〔80〕 ▣

99345   Home visit for the evaluation and management of a new patient, which requires these three key components: a comprehensive history; a comprehensive examination; and medical decision making of high complexity. Counseling and/or coordination of care with other providers or agencies are provided consistent with the nature of the problem(s) and the patient's and/or family's needs. Usually, the patient is unstable or has developed a significant new problem requiring immediate physician attention. Physicians typically spend 75 minutes face-to-face with the patient and/or family. 〔80〕 ▣

ESTABLISHED PATIENT

99347   Home visit for the evaluation and management of an established patient, which requires at least two of these three key components: a problem focused interval history; a problem focused examination; straightforward medical decision making. Counseling and/or coordination of care with other providers or agencies are provided consistent with the nature of the problem(s) and the patient's and/or family's needs. Usually, the presenting problem(s) are self-limited or minor. Physicians typically spend 15 minutes face-to-face with the patient and/or family. 〔80〕 ▣

99348   Home visit for the evaluation and management of an established patient, which requires at least two of these three components: an expanded problem focused interval history; an expanded problem focused examination; medical decision making of low complexity. Counseling and/or coordination of care with other providers or agencies are provided consistent with the nature of the problem(s) and the patient's and/or family's needs. Usually, the presenting problem(s) are of low to moderate severity. Physicians typically spend 25 minutes face-to-face with the patient and/or family. 〔80〕 ▣

99349   Home visit for the evaluation and management of an established patient, which requires at least two of these three key components: a detailed interval history; a detailed examination; medical decision making of moderate complexity. Counseling and/or coordination of care with other providers or agencies are provided consistent with the nature of the problem(s) and the patient's and/or family's needs. Usually, the presenting problem(s) are moderate to high severity. Physicians typically spend 40 minutes face-to-face with the patient and/or family. 〔80〕 ▣

99350   Home visit for the evaluation and management of an established patient, which requires at least two of these three key components: a comprehensive interval history; a comprehensive examination; medical decision making of moderate to high complexity. Counseling and/or coordination of care with other providers or agencies are provided consistent with the nature of the problem(s) and the patient's and/or family's needs. Usually, the presenting problem(s) are of moderate to high severity. The patient may be unstable or may have developed a significant new problem requiring immediate physician attention. Physicians typically spend 60 minutes face-to-face with the patient and/or family. 〔80〕 ▣

PROLONGED SERVICES

PROLONGED PHYSICIAN SERVICE WITH DIRECT (FACE-TO-FACE) PATIENT CONTACT

MCM 15511. PROLONGED SERVICES AND STANDBY SERVICES (CODES 99354-99360)

Pay prolonged services codes 99354-99355 when they are billed on the same day by the same physician as the companion evaluation and management codes and:

The companion codes for 99354 are 99201-99205, 99212-99215, or 99241-99245;

The companion codes for 99355 are 99354 and one of the evaluation and management codes required for 99354 to be used;

The companion codes for 99356 are 99221-99223, 99231-99233, 99251-99255, 99261-99263, 99301-99303, or 99311-99313; or

The companion codes for 99357 are 99356 and one of the evaluation and management codes required for 99357 to be used.

Do not pay prolonged services codes 99354-99358 unless they are accompanied by one of these companion codes.

\+   **99354**   Prolonged physician service in the office or other outpatient setting requiring direct (face-to-face) patient contact beyond the usual service (eg, prolonged care and treatment of an acute asthmatic patient in an outpatient setting); first hour (List separately in addition to code for office or other outpatient Evaluation and Management service) 〔80〕 ▣
     Note that 99354 is an add-on code and must be used in conjunction with 99201-99215, 99241-99245, and 99301-99350.

\+   **99355**   each additional 30 minutes (List separately in addition to code for prolonged physician service) 〔80〕 ▣
     Note that 99355 is an add-on code and must be used in conjunction with 99354.

\+   **99356**   Prolonged physician service in the inpatient setting, requiring direct (face-to-face) patient contact beyond the usual service (eg, maternal fetal monitoring for high risk delivery or other physiological monitoring, prolonged care of an acutely ill inpatient); first hour (List separately in addition to code for inpatient Evaluation and Management service) 〔80〕 ▣
     Note that 99356 is an add-on code and must be used in conjunction with 99221-99233, 99251-99255, and 99261-99263.

\+   **99357**   each additional 30 minutes (List separately in addition to code for prolonged physician service) 〔80〕 ▣

     Note that 99357 is an add-on code and must be used in conjunction with 99356.

▣ CCI Comprehensive Code   〔50〕 Bilateral Procedure   **+** CPT Add-on Code   ◊ Modifier -51 Exempt Code   ● New Code   ▲ Revised Code

〔M〕 Maternity   〔N〕 Newborn   〔P〕 Pediatric   〔N/P〕 Newborn/Pediatric

PROLONGED PHYSICIAN SERVICE WITHOUT DIRECT (FACE-TO-FACE) PATIENT CONTACT

MCM 15511. PROLONGED SERVICES AND STANDBY SERVICES (CODES 99354-99360)

Pay prolonged services codes 99354-99355 when they are billed on the same day by the same physician as the companion evaluation and management codes and:

The companion codes for 99354 are 99201-99205, 99212-99215, or 99241-99245;

The companion codes for 99355 are 99354 and one of the evaluation and management codes required for 99354 to be used;

The companion codes for 99356 are 99221-99223, 99231-99233, 99251-99255, 99261-99263, 99301-99303, or 99311-99313; or

The companion codes for 99357 are 99356 and one of the evaluation and management codes required for 99357 to be used.

Do not pay prolonged services codes 99354-99358 unless they are accompanied by one of these companion codes.

MCM 15511.2 PROLONGED SERVICES WITHOUT FACE-TO-FACE SERVICE (Codes 99358-99359).

Do not pay prolonged services codes 99358 and 99359, which do not require any direct patient contact. Payment for these services is included in the payment for direct face to face services that physicians bill. The physician cannot bill the patient for these services since they are Medicare covered services and payment is included in the payment for other billable services.

+ 99358 Prolonged evaluation and management service before and/or after direct (face-to-face) patient care (eg, review of extensive records and tests, communication with other professionals and/or the patient/family); first hour (List separately in addition to code(s) for other physician service(s) and/or inpatient or outpatient Evaluation and Management service)

   If telephone calls need to be reported, consult CPT codes 99371-99373.

+ 99359 each additional 30 minutes (List separately in addition to code for prolonged physician service)

   Note that 99359 is an add-on code and must be used in conjunction with 99358.

PHYSICIAN STANDBY SERVICES

MCM 2070 DIAGNOSTIC X-RAY, DIAGNOSTIC LABORATORY, AND OTHER DIAGNOSTIC TESTS

Medicare covers diagnostic x-ray, diagnostic laboratory, and other diagnostic tests, including materials and the services of technicians. Medicare covers diagnostic X-ray services performed in a facility directed by a physician or group of physicians if they are performed under the direct supervision of a physician. Certain diagnostic X-ray procedures are also covered when performed by technicians without direct personal physician supervision if the technicians' general supervision and training, as well as the maintenance of the necessary equipment and supplies, are the continuing responsibility of a physician. Covered diagnostic tests include:

Histopathology

Tissue Decalcification

Bone Marrow Biopsy

Tissue Pathology

Surgical pathology

Frozen sections

Autopsy and sections

MCM 15511.3 PHYSICIAN STANDBY SERVICE (CODE 99360)

Do not pay for physician standby services. They are covered as inpatient hospital services, not as physician's services since standing by is not a service to a patient. Physicians may not bill Medicare or beneficiaries for them since

payment for them is included in the payment made to the hospital for other general services necessary to provide quality care.

99360 Physician standby service, requiring prolonged physician attendance, each 30 minutes (eg, operative standby, standby for frozen section, for cesarean/high risk delivery, for monitoring EEG)

   Note that 99360 may be reported in addition to 99431 or 99440 as appropriate. However, 99360 cannot be reported in addition to 99436.

CASE MANAGEMENT SERVICES

TEAM CONFERENCES

MCM 15512 CASE MANAGEMENT SERVICES (CODES 99361-99373)

A. Team Conferences.—Do not pay for team conferences (codes 99361-99362). Payment for these services is included in the payment for the services to which they relate.

B. Telephone Calls.—Do not pay for telephone calls (codes 99371-99373) because payment for telephone calls is included in payment for billable services (e.g., visit, surgery, diagnostic procedure results).

99361 Medical conference by a physician with interdisciplinary team of health professionals or representatives of community agencies to coordinate activities of patient care (patient not present); approximately 30 minutes

99362 approximately 60 minutes

TELEPHONE CALLS

99371 Telephone call by a physician to patient or for consultation or medical management or for coordinating medical management with other health care professionals (eg, nurses, therapists, social workers, nutritionists, physicians, pharmacists); simple or brief (eg, to report on tests and/or laboratory results, to clarify or alter previous instructions, to integrate new information from other health professionals into the medical treatment plan, or to adjust therapy)

99372 intermediate (eg, to provide advice to an established patient on a new problem, to initiate therapy that can be handled by telephone, to discuss test results in detail, to coordinate medical management of a new problem in an established patient, to discuss and evaluate new information and details, or to initiate new plan of care)

99373 complex or lengthy (eg, lengthy counseling session with anxious or distraught patient, detailed or prolonged discussion with family members regarding seriously ill patient, lengthy communication necessary to coordinate complex services of several different health professionals working on different aspects of the total patient care plan)

CARE PLAN OVERSIGHT SERVICES

MCM 15513. CARE PLAN OVERSIGHT (CPO) SERVICES

Physicians may bill and be paid separately for CPT 99375 only if all of the following criteria are met:

1. The beneficiary must require complex or multi- disciplinary care modalities requiring ongoing physician involvement in the patient's plan of care;

2. The CPO services should be furnished during the period in which the beneficiary was receiving Medicare covered HHA or hospice services;

3. The physician who bills CPO must be the same physician who signed the home health or hospice plan of care;

4. The physician furnished at least 30 minutes of care plan oversight within the calendar month for which payment is claimed. Time spent by a

physician's nurse or the time spent consulting with one's nurse is not countable toward the 30 minute threshold. Low intensity services included as part of other evaluation and management services are not included as part of the 30 minutes required for coverage;

5. The work included in hospital discharge day management (codes 99238-99239) and discharge from observation (code 99217) is not countable toward the 30 minutes per month required for work on the same day as discharge but only for those services separately documented as occurring after the patient is actually physically discharged from the hospital;

6. The physician provided a covered physician service that required a face-to-face encounter with the beneficiary within the 6 months immediately preceding the first care plan oversight service. Only evaluation and management services in the ranges of codes 99201-99263 and codes 99281-99357 are acceptable prerequisite face-to-face encounters for CPO. EKG, lab, and surgical services are not sufficient face-to-face services for CPO;

7. The care plan oversight billed by the physician was not routine post-operative care provided in the global surgical period of a surgical procedure billed by the physician;

8. If the beneficiary is receiving home health agency services, the physician did not have a significant financial or contractual interest in the home health agency as defined in §15513. CPO services should not be billed by a physician who is an employee of a hospice, including a volunteer medical director. Payment for the services of a physician employed by the hospice are included in the payment to the hospice;

9. The care plan oversight services are personally furnished by the physician who bills them;

10. Services provided incident to a physician's service do not qualify as CPO and do not count toward the 30-minute requirement;

11. The physician is not billing for the Medicare ESRD capitation payment for the same beneficiary during the same month; and

12. The physician billing for CPO must document in the patient's record which services were furnished and the date and length of time associated with those services.

▲ **99374** Physician supervision of a patient under care of home health agency (patient not present) in home, domiciliary or equivalent environment (eg, Alzheimer's facility) requiring complex and multidisciplinary care modalities involving regular physician development and/or revision of care plans, review of subsequent reports of patient status, review of related laboratory and other studies, communication (including telephone calls) for purposes of assessment or care decisions with health care professional(s), family member(s), surrogate decision maker(s) (eg, legal guardian) and/or key caregiver(s) involved in patient's care, integration of new information into the medical treatment plan and/or adjustment of medical therapy, within a calendar month; 15-29 minutes

99375 30 minutes or more

▲ **99377** Physician supervision of a hospice patient (patient not present) requiring complex and multidisciplinary care modalities involving regular physician development and/or revision of care plans, review of subsequent reports of patient status, review of related laboratory and other studies, communication (including telephone calls) for purposes of assessment or care decisions with health care professional(s), family member(s), surrogate decision maker(s) (eg, legal guardian) and/or key caregiver(s) involved in patient's care, integration of new information into the medical treatment plan and/or adjustment of medical therapy, within a calendar month; 15-29 minutes

99378 30 minutes or more

▲ **99379** Physician supervision of a nursing facility patient (patient not present) requiring complex and multidisciplinary care modalities involving regular physician development and/or revision of care plans, review of subsequent reports of patient status, review of related laboratory and other studies, communication (including telephone calls) for purposes of assessment or care decisions with health care professional(s), family member(s), surrogate decision maker(s) (eg, legal guardian) and/or key caregiver(s) involved in patient's care, integration of new information into the medical treatment plan and/or adjustment of medical therapy, within a calendar month; 15-29 minutes

99380 30 minutes or more

PREVENTIVE MEDICINE SERVICES

MCM 15514. PREVENTIVE MEDICINE SERVICES (EXCLUDING IMMUNIZATIONS), NEWBORN SERVICES, AND OTHER EVALUATION AND MANAGEMENT SERVICES (CODES 99381-99499)

Preventive Medicine Services.—Do not pay for preventive medicine services (codes 99401- 99440) because Medicare law specifically excludes coverage of preventive medicine services.

Other Evaluation and Management Services.—Advise physicians to submit documentation when billing for unlisted evaluation and management services. If the services are covered, pay based upon the nature of the service. If you find that the service could or should have been billed using as existing code, base the payment upon the fee schedule payment for that code and advise the physician of how to correctly bill the service.

NEW PATIENT

Laboratory services, radiology services immunizations, other procedures, and screening tests, which are identified with their own CPT code, are separately reported. For immunizations, consult CPT codes 90471-90472 and 90476-90749.

▲ **99381** Initial comprehensive preventive medicine evaluation and management of an individual including an age and gender appropriate history, examination, counseling/anticipatory guidance/risk factor reduction interventions, and the ordering of appropriate immunization(s), laboratory/diagnostic procedures, new patient; infant (age under 1 year) **N**

If counseling/anticipatory guidance/risk factor reduction interventions are provided at an encounter separate from the preventive medicine examination, consult CPT codes 99401-99412.

99382 early childhood (age 1 through 4 years) **P**

99383 late childhood (age 5 through 11 years) **P**

99384 adolescent (age 12 through 17 years) **P**

99385 18-39 years

99386 40-64 years

99387 65 years and over

ESTABLISHED PATIENT

▲ **99391** Periodic comprehensive preventive medicine reevaluation and management of an individual including an age and gender appropriate history, examination, counseling/anticipatory guidance/risk factor reduction interventions, and the ordering of appropriate immunization(s), laboratory/diagnostic procedures, established patient; infant (age under 1 year) **N**

99392 early childhood (age 1 through 4 years) **P**

99393 late childhood (age 5 through 11 years) **P**

▢ CCI Comprehensive Code	50 Bilateral Procedure	✚ CPT Add-on Code	⊘ Modifier -51 Exempt Code	● New Code	▲ Revised Code
M Maternity	**N** Newborn	**P** Pediatric	**N/P** Newborn/Pediatric		

99394	adolescent (age 12 through 17 years)	P
99395	18-39 years	
99396	40-64 years	
99397	65 years and over	

COUNSELING AND/OR RISK FACTOR REDUCTION INTERVENTION

MCM 15514. PREVENTIVE MEDICINE SERVICES (EXCLUDING IMMUNIZATIONS), NEWBORN SERVICES, AND OTHER EVALUATION AND MANAGEMENT SERVICES (CODES 99381-99499)
Preventive Medicine Services.—Do not pay for preventive medicine services (codes 99401- 99440) because Medicare law specifically excludes coverage of preventive medicine services.

Other Evaluation and Management Services.—Advise physicians to submit documentation when billing for unlisted evaluation and management services. If the services are covered, pay based upon the nature of the service. If you find that the service could or should have been billed using as existing code, base the payment upon the fee schedule payment for that code and advise the physician of how to correctly bill the service.

PREVENTIVE MEDICINE, INDIVIDUAL COUNSELING

99401	Preventive medicine counseling and/or risk factor reduction intervention(s) provided to an individual (separate procedure); approximately 15 minutes
99402	approximately 30 minutes
99403	approximately 45 minutes
99404	approximately 60 minutes

PREVENTIVE MEDICINE, GROUP COUNSELING

99411	Preventive medicine counseling and/or risk factor reduction intervention(s) provided to individuals in a group setting (separate procedure); approximately 30 minutes
99412	approximately 60 minutes

OTHER PREVENTIVE MEDICINE SERVICES

99420	Administration and interpretation of health risk assessment instrument (eg, health hazard appraisal)
99429	Unlisted preventive medicine service

NEWBORN CARE

99431   History and examination of the normal newborn infant, initiation of diagnostic and treatment programs and preparation of hospital records. (This code should also be used for birthing room deliveries.) N 80

99432   Normal newborn care in other than hospital or birthing room setting, including physical examination of baby and conference(s) with parent(s) N 80

99433   Subsequent hospital care, for the evaluation and management of a normal newborn, per day N 80

99435   History and examination of the normal newborn infant, including the preparation of medical records (this code should only be used for newborns assessed and discharged from the hospital or birthing room on the same date) N 80

99436   Attendance at delivery (when requested by delivering physician) and initial stabilization of newborn N 80
Note that this procedure may be reported in addition to 99431. However, this procedure cannot be reported in addition to 99440.

99440   Newborn resuscitation: provision of positive pressure ventilation and/or chest compressions in the presence of acute inadequate ventilation and/or cardiac output N 80

SPECIAL EVALUATION AND MANAGEMENT SERVICES

BASIC LIFE AND/OR DISABILITY EVALUATION SERVICES

99450   Basic life and/or disability examination that includes: measurement of height, weight and blood pressure; completion of a medical history following a life insurance pro forma; collection of blood sample and/or urinalysis complying with "chain of custody" protocols; and completion of necessary documentation/certificates.

WORK RELATED OR MEDICAL DISABILITY EVALUATION SERVICES

99455   Work related or medical disability examination by the treating physician that includes: •completion of a medical history commensurate with the patient's condition; •performance of an examination commensurate with the patient's condition; •formulation of a diagnosis, assessment of capabilities and stability, and calculation of impairment; •development of future medical treatment plan; and •completion of necessary documentation/certificates and report. 80

99456   Work related or medical disability examination by other than the treating physician that includes: •completion of a medical history commensurate with the patient's condition; •performance of an examination commensurate with the patient's condition; •formulation of a diagnosis, assessment of capabilities and stability, and calculation of impairment; •development of future medical treatment plan; and •completion of necessary documentation/certificates and report. 80

OTHER EVALUATION AND MANAGEMENT SERVICES

99499   Unlisted evaluation and management service 80

ANESTHESIA

CPT Expert **is not intended to replace the AMA's CPT manual. It does not include the AMA's official rules and guidelines, and Ingenix recommends you use this in conjunction with the AMA's 2002 CPT book.**

CODING INFORMATION

Two organizations are responsible for developing anesthesia codes and guidelines. The American Medical Association (AMA) includes a section on anesthesia codes (00100-01999) in the CPT book immediately following the E/M section. In addition, the CPT book includes four codes (99100-99140) to report qualifying circumstances for anesthesia. Although categorized as medicine codes, the four codes can be found in the Anesthesia Section as part of the guidelines, as well as in the Medicine Section. The American Society of Anesthesiologists (ASA) publishes a Relative Value Guide (RVG) that contains codes from the anesthesia section of CPT but also includes: 1) codes to supplement those in the CPT anesthesia section and 2) codes from other sections of CPT for services frequently provided by anesthesiologists.

The CPT book and ASA guidelines are similar. Guidelines are as follows:

1. Both specify that reporting of anesthesia services is appropriate when provided by or under the medical supervision of a physician. The ASA further specifies that anesthesia services should be supervised by a physician anesthesiologist.

2. According to both sets of guidelines, anesthesia services include but are not limited to general, regional, supplementation of local anesthesia, and other supportive services required to afford the patient optimal anesthesia care. The ASA includes monitored anesthesia care in the service and also states that you report any professional anesthesia services as if an anesthetic was administered.

3. The ASA publication is a relative value guide. A relative value is a numeric ranking assigned to a procedure in relation to other procedures in terms of work and cost. Therefore, in addition to codes and descriptions, the ASA relative value guide provides information on the value of each anesthesia service. The ASA relative value guide is not a fee schedule, but only a guide intended to assist physicians in developing consistent and equitable fees for their services.

ORGANIZATION OF ANESTHESIA CODES

CPT

The anesthesia section of the CPT book is organized into 15 anatomical sites followed by four additional categories for radiological and other procedures, including a new section for obstetric anesthesia added in the CPT book of 2002. Codes are organized by type of procedure (open, closed, endoscopic, etc.), and each code relates to specific surgical procedures, though there is no direct one-to-one correspondence. One anesthesia code may be used to report several surgical procedures that share similar anesthesia requirements.

EXAMPLE 1

01202   **Anesthesia for arthroscopic procedures of hip joint**

This procedure code would be selected to report anesthesia services related to the following surgical procedures:

29860   **Arthroscopy, hip, diagnostic with or without synovial biopsy (separate procedure)**

29861   **Arthroscopy, hip, surgical; with removal of loose body or foreign body.**

29862   **with debridement/shaving of articular cartilage (chondroplasty), abrasion arthroplasty, and/or resection of labrum.**

29863   **with synovectomy**

ASA RELATIVE VALUE GUIDE

The codes in the main section of the ASA Relative Value Guide are the same as those in the CPT book with two exceptions: the ASA includes a few codes not found in CPT and excludes a few codes found in the CPT book. In addition, some of the narrative descriptions used by the ASA differ slightly from those found in the CPT book.

The ASA RVG also lists codes for other services frequently provided by anesthesiologists. These codes are CPT codes found in the Evaluation and Management, Medicine, and Surgery sections of the CPT book. The services include: pulmonary function testing, evaluation and management services, pain management and nerve blocks, and placement of venous catheters and monitoring devices. In all cases, the ASA provides a relative value designation for each code.

REPORTING ANESTHESIA SERVICES

Reporting anesthesia services differs from reporting other types of physician services. Reporting other physician services typically involves selecting the correct CPT code and submitting a specific fee for that CPT code. The fee is the same every time the service is provided. For example, a problem focused established patient exam and history is reported with code 99212 and the fee assigned to that procedure by a given physician is $30. The physician submits the fee of $30 every time he or she performs procedure 99212.

However, anesthesia billing is based on several variables specific to the particular anesthesia service. The fee submitted for a specific anesthesia code varies each time the code is reported.

The key terms described next are essential to the correct reporting of anesthesia services.

KEY TERMS

Basic Value or Base Unit. The basic value, also referred to as the base unit or relative value, has two components. One component reflects all usual services included in the anesthesia service. Usual services include: pre-operative and post-operative visits, administration of fluids and/or blood products incident to the procedure, and interpretation of non-invasive monitoring (ECG, temperature, blood pressure, oximetry, capnography, and mass spectrometry). The second component reflects the relative work or cost of the specific anesthesia service. Cost in this context refers to the physician's cost of doing business. For anesthesiologists, the majority of the cost goes to malpractice insurance. For example, the basic value for the anesthesia service related to a closed reduction of a radius fracture might be three, as it has a relatively low level of work or cost. The basic value for an anesthesia service associated with an intrathoracic coronary artery bypass graft procedure might be 20, reflecting a high level of work or cost.

The ASA lists two exceptions to using the basic value listed in the Relative Value Guide. A minimum basic value of five is allowed for all procedures of the head, neck or shoulder girdle, requiring field avoidance. In addition, any procedure performed in any position other than lithotomy or supine has a minimum basic value of five. If the anesthesia code associated with the surgical procedure carries a basic value greater than five the higher basic value is reported.

Base units for anesthesia listed in RVG are widely accepted across the United States by both physicians and payers. However, some payers, especially government agency payers, may use different relative value scales developed exclusively for their use. Other payers may use national relative value guides based on RVG, with some modification.

Time. Time is the actual time spent providing the anesthesia service. Time begins as the anesthesiologist prepares the patient for anesthesia care. Time ends when the personal attendance of the anesthesiologist is no longer required and the patient can be safely placed in post-anesthesia recovery under the supervision of nursing or other trained personnel.

Time is reported in units based on defined time increments. The most commonly used time increment is 15 minutes, with one unit being reported for each 15-minute increment. However, time units for anesthesia vary across the country. Both ASA and the CPT book suggest reporting time increments as customary in the geographic area.

The same holds for reporting fractions of time units. For example, a procedure requiring 65 minutes of anesthesia time, reported in 15-minute time increments, results in total time units of 4.33. In some areas, this is reported as the fractional amount 4.33; other areas might round to the nearest whole number four; or another geographical area might allow reporting of another full unit for any fractional amount to five.

For some anesthesia services, time is not reported additionally. The ASA RVG designates a +TM after the base unit for procedures requiring time reported separately. Do not list time separately for procedures without the designation.

Physical Status Modifiers. Physical status modifiers reflect the patient's state of health. Individuals undergoing surgery may be healthy or may have varying degrees of systemic disease. A patient's health status affects the work related to providing the anesthesia service. The CPT book states that physical status modifiers reflect the level of complexity associated with the anesthesia service.

Physical status modifiers in the CPT book and ASA RVG are represented with the letter P followed by a single digit (e.g., -P1, -P2). ASA RVG lists the number of additional anesthesia units allowed with each physical status modifier to the right in the column titled "units."

MODIFIER	DESCRIPTION	UNITS
-P1	Normal healthy patient	0
-P2	Patient with mild systemic disease	0
-P3	Patient with severe systemic disease	1
-P4	Patient with severe systemic disease that is a constant threat to life	2
-P5	Moribund patient who is not expected to survive without the operation	3
-P6	A declared brain-dead patient whose organs are being removed for donor purposes	0

Qualifying Circumstances. Many anesthesia services are provided under particularly difficult circumstances depending on factors such as extraordinary condition of patient, notable operative conditions, and unusual risk factors. The information provided by both the CPT book and the ASA RVG includes a list of important qualifying circumstances that significantly impact the character of the anesthesia service provided. These procedures are not be reported alone but as additional procedure numbers to qualify an anesthesia procedure or service. The ASA provides modifying units that may be added to the basic unit values, as follows:

CODE	DESCRIPTION	ASA RVG UNITS
99100	**Anesthesia for patient of extreme age, under one year and over seventy**	1
99116	**Anesthesia complicated by utilization of total body hypothermia**	5
99135	**Anesthesia complicated by utilization of controlled hypotension**	5
99140	**Anesthesia complicated by emergency conditions (specify)**	2

An emergency exists when a delay in treatment poses a significant increase in the threat to the patient's life or to a body part, as defined in both the CPT book and ASA RVG.

Conversion Factor. Anesthesia charges must be calculated by means of a conversion factor since the charges are not based on fixed amounts. A conversion factor is the dollar value associated with each unit of anesthesia. The dollar conversion factor is multiplied by the total number of anesthesia units for a given anesthesia service to arrive at the total charges for the anesthesia service.

The dollar conversion factor may vary significantly between geographical regions and to a lesser degree between physicians in a given geographic area. However, the standard formula to calculate total anesthesia units and anesthesia fees is basically the same both among regions and physicians as illustrated in the examples below.

Standard Formula. Now that the basic elements of the anesthesia service have been defined, total anesthesia units for a given anesthesia service can be determined. Using the total units and the conversion factor, the fee for a specific anesthesia service can then be calculated.

The total charge for a specific anesthesia service is calculated by means of the following formula:

Basic Value + Time Units + Modifying Units = Total Units

Total Units X Conversion Factor = Total Fee

A closed reduction of a distal radius fracture is accomplished under general anesthesia. The patient is a healthy 10-year-old. The procedure is not performed on an emergency basis. The anesthesiologist reports procedure 01820 that has a basic value of three. Total time for the procedure is 45 minutes. The anesthesiologist reports time units in 15-minute increments. The total units reported for the procedure are as follows:

Basic Value		3
Time Units (45 divided by 15)	+	3
Physical Status (P1)	+	0
Qualifying Circumstances (none)	+	0
Total Units	=	6

The anesthesiologist uses a conversion factor of $45 per unit of anesthesia.

Total Units		6
Conversion Factor	X	$45
Total Fee	=	$270

SPECIAL CODING SITUATIONS

MULTIPLE PROCEDURES

When multiple surgical procedures are performed during a single anesthetic administration, the ASA recommends reporting only the anesthesia procedure with the highest unit value. In other words, only one basic value is assigned per single surgical session.

ADDITIONAL PROCEDURES

Services not included in the usual anesthesia services may be reported separately. These services include unusual forms of monitoring, prolonged physician services, and provision of additional anesthesia services such as post-operative pain management. These additional services are reported in terms of units with the appropriate CPT or ASA codes under the designation "other procedures." They are calculated as an additional variable in the standard formula.

Unusual monitoring. Unusual forms of monitoring anesthesia are reported by most anesthesiologists and many payers allow benefits beyond the basic anesthesia service. Codes 36488-36491 for insertion of a central venous catheter; 36620-36625 for insertion of an intra-arterial catheter, and 93503 Swan-Ganz insertion, represent unusual forms of monitoring that may be rendered by an anesthesiologist.

Prolonged physician services. Extended pre- or post-operative care provided to a patient whose condition requires services beyond the usual may be reported additionally. These services would be billed with prolonged service codes (99354-99359).

Post-operative pain management. Normally post-operative pain management is provided or supervised by the surgeon by oral, intramuscular or intravenous medications. Post-operative pain management provided by the surgeon is included in the global fee for the surgical procedure. Some procedures and/or patients require more than the usual type of post-operative pain management, and this is frequently provided or supervised by an anesthesiologist. These services are additional procedures and are reported as follows:

Epidural or subarachnoid pain management is reported with procedure codes 62310-62319 for placement of the epidural or subarachnoid catheter that includes the initial day of pain management. Subsequent management is reported with 01996 and is reported per day.

Patient-controlled analgesia is reported with 01997 on a per day basis. Code 01997 is included only in the ASA Relative Value Guide not in CPT, but is recognized by most payers as a valid code for this anesthesia service.

Post-operative pain management services are not calculated based on time. These services are reported as a single, daily charge.

MONITORED (STAND-BY) ANESTHESIA

Monitored anesthesia care is defined in the ASA RVG as those instances when an anesthesiologist has been requested to provide specific services to a patient undergoing a planned procedure. The patient receives either local anesthesia or no anesthesia. However, the anesthesiologist is required to provide pre-operative assessment, to remain in attendance during the procedure to monitor the patient and to administer additional anesthetics should they be required, and to provide post-operative services as required.

Monitored care, as described above, is reported as is customary for any other anesthesia procedure. The procedure should be assigned the applicable anesthesia code with time and modifying units being added as is customary in the local area.

OBSTETRICAL ANESTHESIA

The formula for reporting of epidural analgesia for labor and delivery may differ from the standard formula in some geographical areas. When epidural analgesia is administered, an anesthesiologist may attend to more than one patient. The anesthesiologist may insert the epidural catheter, start the continuous anesthetic, and leave the patient's bedside. The anesthesiologist periodically returns to check on the patient or to increase the amount of anesthetic while attending to other patients who are also receiving epidurals for vaginal deliveries. For this reason epidural analgesia for labor and delivery may be reimbursed at a reduced rate.

The following are some variations in reporting anesthesia services when the anesthesiologist is not required to be in constant attendance.

1. Basic value and modifying units are reported as usual. The first hour of anesthesia is reported at the usual rate, but subsequent hours are reported at a reduced rate. For example, total units for the first hour would be reported in full, but units for the second hour would be reported at 50 percent and units for all subsequent hours at 25 percent. If 15-minute time increments were being used the first hour units would be reported as four units, the second hour as two, and third and subsequent hours as one unit each.

2. A flat rate may be established and reported regardless of the actual epidural time. Basic value units are included in the flat rate. For example, the anesthesiologist may bill $500 for anesthesia services provided at every vaginal delivery. Modifying units may or may not be reported separately.

3. Basic value and modifying units are reported as usual. Actual time spent in attendance of the patient may be used and reported at the usual rate. For example, a patient who received epidural analgesia for four hours might have required the anesthesiologist's presence for only two hours of the total time. If 15-minute time increments were used, the anesthesiologist would report eight units.

These are examples of possible variations and should not be adopted without evaluating current practices in the geographic area. Payers should be queried as to their rules for reporting anesthesia services related to obstetrical care.

REGIONAL ANESTHESIA

Disagreement regarding the correct method of reporting regional IV anesthesia centers on code 01995 that has been assigned for regional IV administration of local anesthetic agent (upper or lower extremity). This procedure has no time units associated with it. In practice, anesthesiologists rarely report this service, and instead report regional anesthesia with the anesthesia code that describes the surgical procedure performed. For example regional anesthesia for repair of a tendon injury of the hand is reported with 01810, not 01995. Applicable time and modifying units are also reported.

If the anesthesiologist performs regional anesthesia with the usual pre- and post-operative care and monitors the patient throughout the procedure, the anesthesia code that describes the surgical procedure should be reported along with time and modifying units. However, if the anesthesiologist provides no service other than the initial administration of regional anesthetic, it may be appropriate to report code 01995 instead.

UNUSUAL ANESTHESIA

CPT defines unusual anesthesia as follows:

-23 Unusual Anesthesia: Occasionally, a procedure, which usually requires either no anesthesia or local anesthesia, must be done under general anesthesia due to unusual circumstances. This circumstance may be reported by adding modifier -23 to the procedure code of the basic service or by use of the separate 5-digit modifier code 09923.

Although it is generally inappropriate to report anesthesia with some E/M, medicine, surgery, and radiology codes, there are situations where medical necessity requires anesthesia (e.g. a baby, small child, or hard-to-control patient needing dressings and/or debridement). Under these unusual circumstances, payers will usually allow the anesthesia charge. Submit an operative report and cover letter with the claim explaining the need for any unusual anesthesia.

CHRONIC PAIN MANAGEMENT SERVICES

Chronic pain management services are not anesthesia services. These are distinct services frequently performed by anesthesiologists who have additional training in pain management procedures. Pain management services are reported following the same rules as those for surgical procedures.

Pain management services include initial and subsequent evaluation and management (E/M) services, trigger point injections, spine and spinal cord injections, and nerve blocks.

E/M services may be reported with outpatient/office codes 99201-99215 or outpatient consultation codes 99241-99245 depending on the nature of the E/M service.

Trigger point injections are reported with code 20550. More than one trigger point may be injected per treatment. Use modifier -51 appended to second and subsequent injections on the same date of service.

Codes 62280-62284 and 62290-62319 report spine and spinal cord injections.

Nerve blocks are reported with codes 64400-64530. Nerve blocks are defined as the introduction or injection of an anesthetic agent into a nerve or nerve branch.

A new section in the CPT book of 2002 is the addition of Home Infusion Procedures (99551-99569). Two of these codes in the range report home infusion for pain therapy that, when reported, include the health care provider home visit and all supplies and equipment, excluding the drug, required to deliver the pain medication in a single 24-hour period.

Each code for pain management services should have a specific fee and the fee should be the same each time that specific code is reported. In other words, no adjustments are made based on time, physical status, or qualifying circumstances.

SPECIAL REPORT

A service that is rarely provided, unusual, variable, or new may require a special report to help the payer determine the medical appropriateness of the service. Pertinent information should include an adequate definition or description of the nature, extent, and need for the procedure; and the time, effort, and equipment necessary to provide the service.

COMMON BILLING ERRORS

Incorrect ICD-9-CM or CPT coding is a frequent problem encountered in anesthesia reporting. The code may be incorrect because it does not match the diagnosis or procedure reported by the surgeon. Claims must reflect the same diagnosis and procedure by the anesthesiologist and surgeon, with the exception of listing a global surgery code when only part of the service is provided.

There are codes in the surgery section of the CPT book designated as "add on" codes. These add-on codes, however, are not used for coding anesthesia services.

For example, 11001 is an "add on" code. The primary procedure code is 11000* *Debridement of extensive eczematous or infected skin; up to 10% of body surface.* Always report 11001 with or "in addition to" 11000* because its description states each additional 10 percent of the body surface. In this case, the appropriate CPT code for determining anesthesia base units and guidelines is 11000*.

HEAD

	00100	Anesthesia for procedures on salivary glands, including biopsy
	00102	Anesthesia for procedures on plastic repair of cleft lip
	00103	Anesthesia for reconstructive procedures of eyelid (eg, blepharoplasty, ptosis surgery)
	00104	Anesthesia for electroconvulsive therapy
	00120	Anesthesia for procedures on external, middle, and inner ear including biopsy; not otherwise specified
	00124	otoscopy
	00126	tympanotomy
	00140	Anesthesia for procedures on eye; not otherwise specified

CIM 35-44 USE OF VISUAL TESTS PRIOR TO AND GENERAL ANESTHESIA DURING CATARACT SURGERY

When the only diagnosis is cataract(s), Medicare does not cover testing other than one comprehensive eye exam (or a combination of a brief/intermediate exam not to exceed the charge of a comprehensive exam) and an A-scan or, if medically justifiable, a B-scan. Claims for additional tests are denied unless there is an additional diagnosis and the medical need is fully documented. Because cataract surgery is an elective procedure, the patient may decide not to have the surgery until later, or to have the surgery performed by a physician other than the diagnosing physician. The use of general anesthesia in cataract surgery may be considered reasonable and necessary if, for particular medical indications, it is the accepted procedure among ophthalmologists in the local community to use general anesthesia.

	00142	lens surgery
	00144	corneal transplant
	00145	vitreoretinal surgery
	00147	iridectomy
	00148	ophthalmoscopy
	00160	Anesthesia for procedures on nose and accessory sinuses; not otherwise specified
	00162	radical surgery
	00164	biopsy, soft tissue
	00170	Anesthesia for intraoral procedures, including biopsy; not otherwise specified
	00172	repair of cleft palate
	00174	excision of retropharyngeal tumor
	00176	radical surgery
	00190	Anesthesia for procedures on facial bones or skull; not otherwise specified
	00192	radical surgery (including prognathism)
	00210	Anesthesia for intracranial procedures; not otherwise specified
	00212	subdural taps
	00214	burr holes, including ventriculography
	00215	cranioplasty or elevation of depressed skull fracture, extradural (simple or compound)
	00216	vascular procedures
	00218	procedures in sitting position
▲	00220	cerebrospinal fluid shunting procedures
	00222	electrocoagulation of intracranial nerve

NECK

	00300	Anesthesia for all procedures on the integumentary system, muscles and nerves of head, neck, and posterior trunk, not otherwise specified
		If anesthesia is used for procedures on the cervical spine and cord, consult CPT codes 00600, 00604, and 00670.
	00320	Anesthesia for all procedures on esophagus, thyroid, larynx, trachea and lymphatic system of neck; not otherwise specified
	00322	needle biopsy of thyroid
	00350	Anesthesia for procedures on major vessels of neck; not otherwise specified
		If anesthesia is used for arteriograms, consult CPT code 01916.
	00352	simple ligation

THORAX (CHEST WALL AND SHOULDER GIRDLE)

	00400	Anesthesia for procedures on the integumentary system on the extremities, anterior trunk and perineum; not otherwise specified
	00402	reconstructive procedures on breast (eg, reduction or augmentation mammoplasty, muscle flaps)
	00404	radical or modified radical procedures on breast
	00406	radical or modified radical procedures on breast with internal mammary node dissection
	00410	electrical conversion of arrhythmias
	00450	Anesthesia for procedures on clavicle and scapula; not otherwise specified
	00452	radical surgery
	00454	biopsy of clavicle
	00470	Anesthesia for partial rib resection; not otherwise specified
	00472	thoracoplasty (any type)
	00474	radical procedures (eg, pectus excavatum)

INTRATHORACIC

	00500	Anesthesia for all procedures on esophagus
	00520	Anesthesia for closed chest procedures; (including bronchoscopy) not otherwise specified
	00522	needle biopsy of pleura
	00524	pneumocentesis
	00528	mediastinoscopy and diagnostic thoracoscopy

CIM 35-79 ANESTHESIA IN CARDIAC PACEMAKER SURGERY

The use of general or monitored anesthesia during transvenous cardiac pacemaker surgery may be covered under Medicare only if adequate documentation of medical necessity is provided on a case-by-case basis. A second type of pacemaker surgery that is sometimes performed involves the use of the thoracic method of implantation, which requires open surgery. Where the thoracic method is employed, general anesthesia is always used and should not require special medical documentation.

	00530	Anesthesia for permanent transvenous pacemaker insertion
	00532	Anesthesia for access to central venous circulation
	00534	Anesthesia for transvenous insertion or replacement of pacing cardioverter-defibrillator
		If anesthesia is used in a transthoracic approach, consult CPT code 00560.
	00537	Anesthesia for cardiac electrophysiologic procedures including radiofrequency ablation

	00540	Anesthesia for thoracotomy procedures involving lungs, pleura, diaphragm, and mediastinum (including surgical thoracoscopy); not otherwise specified
	00542	decortication
	00544	pleurectomy
	00546	pulmonary resection with thoracoplasty
	00548	intrathoracic procedures on the trachea and bronchi
	00550	Anesthesia for sternal debridement
▲	00560	Anesthesia for procedures on heart, pericardial sac, and great vessels of chest; without pump oxygenator
	00562	with pump oxygenator
	00563	with pump oxygenator with hypothermic circulatory arrest
	00566	Anesthesia for direct coronary artery bypass grafting without pump oxygenator
	00580	Anesthesia for heart transplant or heart/lung transplant

SPINE AND SPINAL CORD

00600 Anesthesia for procedures on cervical spine and cord; not otherwise specified

> If anesthesia is used in an injection procedure for myelography or diskography, consult CPT code 01905.

00604 procedures with patient in the sitting position

00620 Anesthesia for procedures on thoracic spine and cord; not otherwise specified

00622 thoracolumbar sympathectomy

00630 Anesthesia for procedures in lumbar region; not otherwise specified

> If anesthesia is used in an injection procedure for myelography or diskography, consult CPT code 01905.

00632 lumbar sympathectomy

00634 chemonucleolysis

00635 diagnostic or therapeutic lumbar puncture

00670 Anesthesia for extensive spine and spinal cord procedures (eg, spinal instrumentation or vascular procedures)

UPPER ABDOMEN

00700 Anesthesia for procedures on upper anterior abdominal wall; not otherwise specified

00702 percutaneous liver biopsy

00730 Anesthesia for procedures on upper posterior abdominal wall

00740 Anesthesia for upper gastrointestinal endoscopic procedures, endoscope introduced proximal to duodenum

00750 Anesthesia for hernia repairs in upper abdomen; not otherwise specified

00752 lumbar and ventral (incisional) hernias and/or wound dehiscence

00754 omphalocele

00756 transabdominal repair of diaphragmatic hernia

00770 Anesthesia for all procedures on major abdominal blood vessels

00790 Anesthesia for intraperitoneal procedures in upper abdomen including laparoscopy; not otherwise specified

00792 partial hepatectomy or management of liver hemorrhage (excluding liver biopsy)

00794 pancreatectomy, partial or total (eg, Whipple procedure)

CIM 45-22 LYMPHOCYTE IMMUNE GLOBULIN, ANTI-THYMOCYTE GLOBULIN (EQUINE)

The Food and Drug Administration (FDA) has approved one lymphocyte immune globulin preparation, anti-thymocyte globulin (equine). Medicare covers equine when used for managing allograft rejection episodes in renal transplantation.

00796 liver transplant (recipient)

> If this procedure is performed for harvesting the liver, consult CPT code 01990.

● **00797** gastric restrictive procedure for morbid obesity

LOWER ABDOMEN

00800 Anesthesia for procedures on lower anterior abdominal wall; not otherwise specified

00802 panniculectomy

00810 Anesthesia for lower intestinal endoscopic procedures, endoscope introduced distal to duodenum

00820 Anesthesia for procedures on lower posterior abdominal wall

00830 Anesthesia for hernia repairs in lower abdomen; not otherwise specified

00832 ventral and incisional hernias

00840 Anesthesia for intraperitoneal procedures in lower abdomen including laparoscopy; not otherwise specified

CIM 50-7 ULTRASOUND DIAGNOSTIC PROCEDURES

Medicare coverage is extended to the procedures listed in Category I. Techniques in Category II are considered experimental and should not be covered at this time.

Category I (covered, may be adjunct to radiologic and nuclear medicine diagnostic technique)

1. Echoencephalography, (Diencephalic Midline) (A-Mode)
2. Echoencephalography, Complete (Diencephalic Midline and Ventricular Size)
3. Ocular and Orbital Echography (A-Mode) (includes determining the suitability of aphakic patients for an artificial lens implant following cataract surgery)
4. Ocular and Orbital Sonography (B-Mode)
5. Echocardiography, Pericardial Effusion (M-Mode)
6. Pericardiocentesis, by Ultrasonic Guidance
7. Echocardiography, Cardiac Valve(s) (M-Mode)
8. Echocardiography, Complete (M-Mode)
9. Echocardiography, limited (e.g., follow-up or limited study) (M-Mode)
10. Pleural Effusion Echography
11. Thoracentesis, by Ultrasonic Guidance
12. Abdominal Sonography, complete survey study (B-Scan)
13. Abdominal Sonography, limited (e.g., follow-up or limited study) (B-Scan)
14. Renal Cyst Aspiration, by Ultrasonic Guidance
15. Renal Biopsy, by Ultrasonic Guidance
16. Pancreas Sonography (B-Scan)
17. Spleen Sonography (B-Scan)
18. Abdominal Aorta Echography (A-Mode)
19. Abdominal Aorta Sonography (B-Scan)
20. Retroperitoneal Sonography (B-Scan)
21. Retroperitoneal sonography does not include planning of fields for radiation therapy.
22. Urinary Bladder Sonography (B-Scan)
23. Urinary bladder sonography does not include staging of bladder tumors.
24. Pregnancy Diagnosis sonography (B-Scan)

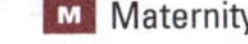 CCI Comprehensive Code　　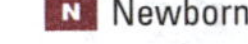 Bilateral Procedure　　✚ CPT Add-on Code　　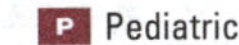 Modifier -51 Exempt Code　　● New Code　　▲ Revised Code

M Maternity　　**N** Newborn　　**P** Pediatric　　**N/P** Newborn/Pediatric

25. Fetal Age Determination (Biparietal Diameter) Sonography (B-Scan)

26. Fetal Growth Rate Sonography (B-Scan)

27. Placenta Localization Sonography (B-Scan)

28. Pregnancy Sonography, Complete (B-Scan)

29. Molar Pregnancy Diagnosis Sonography (B-Scan)

30. Ectopic Pregnancy Diagnosis sonography (B-Scan)

31. Passive Testing (Antepartum Monitoring of Fetal Heart Rate In the Resting Fetus)

32. Intrauterine Contraceptive Device Sonography (B-Scan)

33. Pelvic Mass Diagnosis Sonography (B-Scan)

34. Amniocentesis, by Ultrasonic Guidance

35. Arterial Flow Study, Peripheral (Doppler)

36. Venous Flow Study, Peripheral (Doppler)

37. Arterial Aneurysm, Peripheral (B-Scan)

38. Radiation Therapy Planning Sonography (B-Scan)

39. Thyroid Echography (A-Mode)

40. Thyroid Sonography (B-Scan)

41. Breast Echography (A-Mode)

42. Breast Sonography (B-Scan)

43. Hepatic Sonography (B-Scan)

44. Gallbladder Sonography

45. Renal Sonography

46. Two-Dimensional Echocardiography (B-Mode)

Category II (clinical reliability and efficacy not proven)

1. B-Scan for atherosclerotic narrowing of peripheral arteries

2. Monitoring of cardiac output (Doppler)

When appropriate, new uses for ultrasound diagnostic procedures should be forwarded to the Bureau of Eligibility, Reimbursement and Coverage, HCFA, so that revisions may be made in the coverage policy when appropriate.

00842	**amniocentesis**	M	♀
00844	**abdominoperineal resection**		
00846	**radical hysterectomy**		♀
00848	**pelvic exenteration**		
00850	~~Anesthesia for intraperitoneal procedures in lower abdomen including laparoscopy; cesarean section~~ **This code is deleted in 2002. See code 01961.**		
● 00851	**tubal ligation/transection**		♀
00855	~~Anesthesia for intraperitoneal procedures in lower abdomen including laparoscopy; cesarean hysterectomy~~ **This code is deleted in 2002. See code 01963.**		
00857	~~Neuraxial analgesia/anesthesia for labor ending in a cesarean delivery (includes any repeat subarachnoid needle placement and drug injection and/or any necessary replacement of an epidural catheter during labor)~~ **This code is deleted in 2002. See codes 01968, 01969.**		
00860	**Anesthesia for extraperitoneal procedures in lower abdomen, including urinary tract; not otherwise specified**		
00862	**renal procedures, including upper 1/3 of ureter, or donor nephrectomy**		
00864	**total cystectomy**		
00865	**radical prostatectomy (suprapubic, retropubic)**		♂
00866	**adrenalectomy**		

00868	**renal transplant (recipient)** If anesthesia is used for donor nephrectomy, consult CPT code 00862. If anesthesia is used for harvesting a kidney from a brain-dead patient, consult CPT code 01990.		
● 00869	**vasectomy, unilateral/bilateral**		♂
00870	**cystolithotomy**		
00872	**Anesthesia for lithotripsy, extracorporeal shock wave; with water bath**		
00873	**without water bath**		
00880	**Anesthesia for procedures on major lower abdominal vessels; not otherwise specified**		
00882	**inferior vena cava ligation**		
00884	~~Anesthesia for procedures on major lower abdominal vessels; transvenous umbrella insertion~~ **This code is deleted in 2002. See code 01930.**		

PERINEUM

00902	**Anesthesia for; anorectal procedure**		
00904	**radical perineal procedure**		
00906	**vulvectomy**		♀
00908	**perineal prostatectomy**		♂
00910	**Anesthesia for transurethral procedures (including urethrocystoscopy); not otherwise specified**		
00912	**transurethral resection of bladder tumor(s)**		
00914	**transurethral resection of prostate**		♂
00916	**post-transurethral resection bleeding**		
00918	**with fragmentation, manipulation and/or removal of ureteral calculus**		
00920	**Anesthesia for procedures on male genitalia (including open urethral procedures); not otherwise specified**		♂
00922	**seminal vesicles**		♂
00924	**undescended testis, unilateral or bilateral**		♂
00926	**radical orchiectomy, inguinal**		♂
00928	**radical orchiectomy, abdominal**		♂
00930	**orchiopexy, unilateral or bilateral**		♂
00932	**complete amputation of penis**		♂
00934	**radical amputation of penis with bilateral inguinal lymphadenectomy**		♂
00936	**radical amputation of penis with bilateral inguinal and iliac lymphadenectomy**		♂
00938	**insertion of penile prosthesis (perineal approach)**		♂

	00940	Anesthesia for vaginal procedures (including biopsy of labia, vagina, cervix or endometrium); not otherwise specified ♀
▲	00942	colpotomy, vaginectomy, colporrhaphy, and open urethral procedures ♀
	00944	vaginal hysterectomy ♀
	~~00946~~	~~Anesthesia for vaginal procedures (including biopsy of labia, vagina, cervix or endometrium); vaginal delivery~~ This code is deleted in 2002. See code 01960.
	00948	cervical cerclage ♀
	00950	culdoscopy ♀
	00952	hysteroscopy and/or hysterosalpingography ♀
	~~00955~~	~~Neuraxial analgesia/anesthesia for labor ending in a vaginal delivery (includes any repeat subarachnoid needle placement and drug injection and/or any necessary replacement of an epidural catheter during labor)~~ This code is deleted in 2002. See code 01967.

PELVIS (EXCEPT HIP)

MCM 2070 DIAGNOSTIC X-RAY, DIAGNOSTIC LABORATORY, AND OTHER DIAGNOSTIC TESTS

Medicare covers diagnostic x-ray, diagnostic laboratory, and other diagnostic tests, including materials and the services of technicians. Medicare covers diagnostic X-ray services performed in a facility directed by a physician or group of physicians if they are performed under the direct supervision of a physician. Certain diagnostic X-ray procedures are also covered when performed by technicians without direct personal physician supervision if the technicians' general supervision and training, as well as the maintenance of the necessary equipment and supplies, are the continuing responsibility of a physician. Covered diagnostic tests include:

Histopathology

Tissue Decalcification

Bone Marrow Biopsy

Tissue Pathology

Surgical pathology

Frozen sections

Autopsy and sections

	01112	Anesthesia for bone marrow aspiration and/or biopsy, anterior or posterior iliac crest
	01120	Anesthesia for procedures on bony pelvis
	01130	Anesthesia for body cast application or revision
	01140	Anesthesia for interpelviabdominal (hindquarter) amputation
	01150	Anesthesia for radical procedures for tumor of pelvis, except hindquarter amputation
	01160	Anesthesia for closed procedures involving symphysis pubis or sacroiliac joint
	01170	Anesthesia for open procedures involving symphysis pubis or sacroiliac joint
	01180	Anesthesia for obturator neurectomy; extrapelvic
	01190	intrapelvic

UPPER LEG (EXCEPT KNEE)

	01200	Anesthesia for all closed procedures involving hip joint
	01202	Anesthesia for arthroscopic procedures of hip joint
	01210	Anesthesia for open procedures involving hip joint; not otherwise specified
	01212	hip disarticulation
▲	01214	total hip arthroplasty
	01215	revision of total hip arthroplasty

	01220	Anesthesia for all closed procedures involving upper 2/3 of femur
	01230	Anesthesia for open procedures involving upper 2/3 of femur; not otherwise specified
	01232	amputation
	01234	radical resection
	01250	Anesthesia for all procedures on nerves, muscles, tendons, fascia, and bursa of upper leg
	01260	Anesthesia for all procedures involving veins of upper leg, including exploration
	01270	Anesthesia for procedures involving arteries of upper leg, including bypass graft; not otherwise specified
	01272	femoral artery ligation
	01274	femoral artery embolectomy

KNEE AND POPLITEAL AREA

	01320	Anesthesia for all procedures on nerves, muscles, tendons, fascia, and bursa of knee and/or popliteal area
	01340	Anesthesia for all closed procedures on lower 1/3 of femur
	01360	Anesthesia for all open procedures on lower 1/3 of femur
	01380	Anesthesia for all closed procedures on knee joint
	01382	Anesthesia for arthroscopic procedures of knee joint
	01390	Anesthesia for all closed procedures on upper ends of tibia, fibula, and/or patella
	01392	Anesthesia for all open procedures on upper ends of tibia, fibula, and/or patella
	01400	Anesthesia for open procedures on knee joint; not otherwise specified
▲	01402	total knee arthroplasty
	01404	disarticulation at knee
	01420	Anesthesia for all cast applications, removal, or repair involving knee joint
	01430	Anesthesia for procedures on veins of knee and popliteal area; not otherwise specified
	01432	arteriovenous fistula
	01440	Anesthesia for procedures on arteries of knee and popliteal area; not otherwise specified
	01442	popliteal thromboendarterectomy, with or without patch graft
	01444	popliteal excision and graft or repair for occlusion or aneurysm

LOWER LEG (BELOW KNEE, INCLUDES ANKLE AND FOOT)

	01462	Anesthesia for all closed procedures on lower leg, ankle, and foot
	01464	Anesthesia for arthroscopic procedures of ankle joint
	01470	Anesthesia for procedures on nerves, muscles, tendons, and fascia of lower leg, ankle, and foot; not otherwise specified
	01472	repair of ruptured Achilles tendon, with or without graft
	01474	gastrocnemius recession (eg, Strayer procedure)
	01480	Anesthesia for open procedures on bones of lower leg, ankle, and foot; not otherwise specified
	01482	radical resection (including below knee amputation)
	01484	osteotomy or osteoplasty of tibia and/or fibula

01486 — 01918

01486		total ankle replacement
01490		Anesthesia for lower leg cast application, removal, or repair
01500		Anesthesia for procedures on arteries of lower leg, including bypass graft; not otherwise specified
01502		embolectomy, direct or with catheter
01520		Anesthesia for procedures on veins of lower leg; not otherwise specified
01522		venous thrombectomy, direct or with catheter

SHOULDER AND AXILLA

These codes include procedures performed on the humeral head and neck, sternoclavicular, acromioclavicular and shoulder joints.

01610	Anesthesia for all procedures on nerves, muscles, tendons, fascia, and bursa of shoulder and axilla
01620	Anesthesia for all closed procedures on humeral head and neck, sternoclavicular joint, acromioclavicular joint, and shoulder joint
01622	Anesthesia for arthroscopic procedures of shoulder joint
01630	Anesthesia for open procedures on humeral head and neck, sternoclavicular joint, acromioclavicular joint, and shoulder joint; not otherwise specified
01632	radical resection
01634	shoulder disarticulation
01636	interthoracoscapular (forequarter) amputation
01638	total shoulder replacement
01650	Anesthesia for procedures on arteries of shoulder and axilla; not otherwise specified
01652	axillary-brachial aneurysm
01654	bypass graft
01656	axillary-femoral bypass graft
01670	Anesthesia for all procedures on veins of shoulder and axilla
01680	Anesthesia for shoulder cast application, removal or repair; not otherwise specified
01682	shoulder spica

UPPER ARM AND ELBOW

01710	Anesthesia for procedures on nerves, muscles, tendons, fascia, and bursa of upper arm and elbow; not otherwise specified
01712	tenotomy, elbow to shoulder, open
01714	tenoplasty, elbow to shoulder
01716	tenodesis, rupture of long tendon of biceps
01730	Anesthesia for all closed procedures on humerus and elbow
01732	Anesthesia for arthroscopic procedures of elbow joint
01740	Anesthesia for open procedures on humerus and elbow; not otherwise specified
01742	osteotomy of humerus
01744	repair of nonunion or malunion of humerus
01756	radical procedures
01758	excision of cyst or tumor of humerus
01760	total elbow replacement
01770	Anesthesia for procedures on arteries of upper arm and elbow; not otherwise specified
01772	embolectomy
01780	Anesthesia for procedures on veins of upper arm and elbow; not otherwise specified

01782	phleborrhaphy

FOREARM, WRIST, AND HAND

01810	Anesthesia for all procedures on nerves, muscles, tendons, fascia, and bursa of forearm, wrist, and hand
01820	Anesthesia for all closed procedures on radius, ulna, wrist, or hand bones
01830	Anesthesia for open procedures on radius, ulna, wrist, or hand bones; not otherwise specified
01832	total wrist replacement
01840	Anesthesia for procedures on arteries of forearm, wrist, and hand; not otherwise specified
01842	embolectomy
01844	Anesthesia for vascular shunt, or shunt revision, any type (eg, dialysis)
01850	Anesthesia for procedures on veins of forearm, wrist, and hand; not otherwise specified
01852	phleborrhaphy
01860	Anesthesia for forearm, wrist, or hand cast application, removal, or repair

RADIOLOGICAL PROCEDURES

~~01904~~		~~Anesthesia for injection procedure for pneumoencephalography~~ This code is deleted in 2002. See code 01905.
●	01905	Anesthesia for myelography, diskography, vertebroplasty
~~01906~~		~~Anesthesia for injection procedure for myelography; lumbar~~ This code is deleted in 2002. See code 01905.
~~01908~~		~~Anesthesia for injection procedure for myelography; cervical~~ This code is deleted in 2002. See code 01905.
~~01910~~		~~Anesthesia for injection procedure for myelography; posterior fossa~~ This code is deleted in 2002. See code 01905.
~~01912~~		~~Anesthesia for injection procedure for diskography; lumbar~~ This code is deleted in 2002. See code 01905.
~~01914~~		~~Anesthesia for injection procedure for diskography; cervical~~ This code is deleted in 2002. See code 01905.

CIM 50-37 NONINVASIVE TESTS OF CAROTID FUNCTION
Medicare covers the following tests, recognizing that this list is not inclusive and local medical consultants must make the determination:

DIRECT TESTS

- Carotid Phonoangiography
- Direct Bruit Analysis
- Spectral Bruit Analysis
- Doppler Flow Velocity
- Ultrasound Imaging including Real Time
- B-Scan and Doppler Devices

INDIRECT TESTS

- Periorbital Directional Doppler Ultrasonography
- Oculoplethysmography
- Ophthalmodynamometry

▲	01916	Anesthesia for diagnostic arteriography/venography Code 01916 cannot be used with therapeutic codes 01924–01926, 01930–01933.
	~~01918~~	~~Anesthesia for arteriograms, needle; retrograde, brachial or femoral~~ This code is deleted in 2002. See code 01916.

▲ **01920** **Anesthesia for cardiac catheterization including coronary angiography and ventriculography (not to include Swan-Ganz catheter)**

CIM 50-32 PERCUTANEOUS TRANSLUMINAL ANGIOPLASTY (PTA)

Percutaneous transluminal angioplasty (PTA) PTA is covered to treat the following indications:

- Atherosclerotic obstructive lesions
- In the lower extremities (upper extremities do not include head or neck vessels)
- Of a single coronary artery for patients who exhibit the following characteristics:

Angina refractory to optimal medical management

Objective evidence of myocardial ischemia

Lesions amenable to angioplasty

- Of the renal arteries for patients for whom surgery is the likely alternative (i.e., PTA for this group of patients is an alternative to surgery, not simply an addition to medical management.)
- Obstructive lesions of arteriovenous dialysis fistulas and grafts when performed through either a venous or arterial approach

Effective July 1, 2001, Medicare will cover PTA of the carotid artery concurrent with carotid stent placement when furnished in accordance with the Food and Drug Administration (FDA) approved protocols governing Category B Investigational Device Exemption (IDE) clinical trials.

01921 ~~Anesthesia for angioplasty~~ This code is deleted in 2002. See codes 01924–01926.

01922 **Anesthesia for non-invasive imaging or radiation therapy**

● **01924** **Anesthesia for therapeutic interventional radiologic procedures involving the arterial system; not otherwise specified**

● **01925** **carotid or coronary**

● **01926** **intracranial, intracardiac, or aortic**

● **01930** **Anesthesia for therapeutic interventional radiologic procedures involving the venous/lymphatic system (not to include access to the central circulation); not otherwise specified**

● **01931** **intrahepatic or portal circulation (eg, transcutaneous porto-caval shunt (TIPS))**

● **01932** **intrathoracic or jugular**

● **01933** **intracranial**

BURN EXCISIONS OR DEBRIDEMENT

CIM 45-12 PORCINE SKIN AND GRADIENT PRESSURE DRESSINGS

Porcine (pig) skin dressings are covered as an occlusive dressing for burns, donor sites of a homograft, and decubiti and other ulcers. Gradient pressure dressings are Jobst elasticized heavy-duty dressings used to reduce hypertrophic scarring and joint contractures following burn injury. They are covered when used for that purpose.

▲ **01951** **Anesthesia for second and third degree burn excision or debridement with or without skin grafting, any site, for total body surface area (TBSA) treated during anesthesia and surgery; less than four percent total body surface area**

▲ **01952** **between four and nine percent of total body surface area**

+ **01953** **each additional nine percent total body surface area or part thereof (List separately in addition to code for primary procedure)**
Note that 01953 is an add-on code and must be used in conjuction with code 01952.

OBSTETRIC

● **01960** Anesthesia for; vaginal delivery only M ♀

● **01961** cesarean delivery only M ♀

● **01962** urgent hysterectomy following delivery M ♀

● **01963** cesarean hysterectomy without any labor analgesia/anesthesia care M ♀

● **01964** abortion procedures M ♀

● **01967** Neuraxial labor analgesia/anesthesia for planned vaginal delivery (this includes any repeat subarachnoid needle placement and drug injection and/or any necessary replacement of an epidural catheter during labor) M ♀

● + **01968** Cesarean delivery following neuraxial labor analgesia/anesthesia (List separately in addition to code for primary procedure) M ♀
Note that 01968 is an add-on code and must be used in conjunction with code 01967.

● + **01969** Cesarean hysterectomy following neuraxial labor analgesia/anesthesia (List separately in addition to code for primary procedure) M ♀
Note that 01969 an add-on code and must be used in conjunction with code 01967.

OTHER PROCEDURES

01990 **Physiological support for harvesting of organ(s) from brain-dead patient**

▲ **01995** **Regional intravenous administration of local anesthetic agent or other medication (upper or lower extremity)**
For an intra-arterial or intravenous therapeutic prophylactic or diagnostic injection, consult CPT codes 90783 and 90784.

01996 **Daily management of epidural or subarachnoid drug administration**

01999 Unlisted anesthesia procedure(s)

□ CCI Comprehensive Code   50 Bilateral Procedure   + CPT Add-on Code   ⦸ Modifier -51 Exempt Code   ● New Code   ▲ Revised Code

M Maternity   N Newborn   P Pediatric   N/P Newborn/Pediatric

Surgery

SURGERY SERVICES

CPT Expert is not intended to replace the AMA's CPT manual. It does not include the AMA's official rules and guidelines, and Ingenix recommends you use this in conjunction with the AMA's 2002 CPT book.

CODING INFORMATION

ORGANIZATION

The surgery section (10021-69990) is the largest section of the CPT book. It is divided into 18 subsections by body system (eg., integumentary, endocrine), procedure site (eg., mediastinum and diaphragm), or type of service (eg., maternity care and delivery). The subsections are as follows:

- General
- Integumentary System
- Musculoskeletal System
- Respiratory System
- Cardiovascular System
- Hemic and Lymphatic Systems
- Mediastinum and Diaphragm
- Digestive System
- Urinary System
- Male Genital System
- Intersex Surgery
- Female Genital System
- Maternity Care and Delivery
- Endocrine System
- Nervous System
- Eye and Ocular Adnexa
- Auditory System
- Operating Microscope

Instructions that apply to all surgical codes are found at the beginning of the surgery section. In addition, information or notes, specific to subsections, groups of codes and single codes are found throughout the surgery section. Guidelines, including terms and concepts, important to all surgical codes will be explained first. Then guidelines and notes specific to subsections or codes will be reviewed.

FORMAT OF THE TERMINOLOGY

CPT guidelines state that some of the procedures are not printed in their entirety but refer back to a common portion of the procedure listed in a preceding entry. This space-saving format means that many "indented" codes within a code range repeat some common portion of a procedure's description.

While some procedures presented in this indented form are mutually exclusive (i.e., cannot be billed together), others are not. For procedures that are not mutually exclusive, payers may make special allowances. Knowing which procedures are mutually exclusive, however, is the key to avoiding unbundling.

GENERAL INFORMATION

Surgical procedures can generally be divided into two categories: diagnostic and therapeutic. Within those two broad categories, surgical procedures are either described as "package" services or "starred procedures." Understanding each of these terms and the special coding rules that apply to these different services is the key to correct coding.

SURGICAL PACKAGE

The majority of the CPT surgical codes are "package" services; they include the actual surgical procedure, local infiltration, metacarpal and digital block or topical anesthesia (when used), and the normal, uncomplicated postoperative care. When a patient is seen for a routine follow-up postoperative visit within the normal follow-up period, use 99024 for normal uncomplicated postoperative care for documentation purposes only.

Services *not* defined in the CPT book as part of the surgical package include preoperative care, care for postoperative complications, and care for unrelated conditions.

While preoperative care is not identified in CPT as included in the surgical package, many payers have strict guidelines related to reimbursement for preoperative services. Additional reimbursement for preoperative evaluation and management services is usually allowed prior to the decision for surgery or to establish the need for surgery. Reimbursement may be denied for any care provided after the decision for surgical intervention.

However, some payers may identify a specific preoperative period (24 hours to 3 days), during which no additional reimbursement will be made for evaluation and management services. Because of these differing payer policies, it is important for individual providers to establish a policy related to the reporting of preoperative services. Patients should be made aware of this policy. Review contractual arrangements with payers to verify that your policy is not in violation of those contracts.

Postoperative complications are not included in the surgical package and should be reported separately. Postoperative complications include conditions such as wound dehiscence, infection, and bleeding. A diagnosis code should be assigned to reflect the nature of the complication when billing for services rendered to treat the complication.

Unrelated care is always coded. Report services unrelated to the operative problem, such as care for other diseases or injuries, with an appropriate inpatient or outpatient level of service modifier and a corresponding diagnostic code that identifies a problem other than the surgical diagnosis.

FRAGMENTATION AND UNBUNDLING

Understanding unbundling and fragmentation can be accomplished by first defining the term, "bundle." A bundle is a defined set of items or services wrapped together in a group, bunch, or package. The items in the bundle can be related or unrelated, but all defined elements must be present to make a specific bundle. Unbundling or fragmentation occurs primarily two ways.

First, unbundling occurs when minor integral services are reported separately or in addition to a major procedure. Unfortunately, since all minor components of a procedure may not be listed explicitly, it is sometimes difficult to determine which services are integral to a given procedure. One way to approach this is to ask what services are normally performed with a given procedure. A simple example is an excision of a skin lesion. To excise the skin lesion, an incision must be made. An incision is always integral to an excision of a lesion and should not be billed separately. However, an incision is not described in the excision of skin lesion codes. It is implicit because it must be performed with every excision.

Second, unbundling occurs when a single procedure with two or more explicitly described components is broken into its component parts and reported with several CPT codes instead of the single CPT code for the combined service. A simple example of this type of unbundle can be illustrated with the procedure for a combined abdominal hysterectomy with colpo-urethrocystopexy. Because the two components of this procedure are frequently performed together, a combined code 58152 has been assigned to describe this service. However, it is also possible to perform each of the components separately (abdominal hysterectomy 58150 and colpo-urethrocystopexy 51840 or 51845). When the combined procedure is performed during a single surgical session, it must be reported with the bundled CPT code 58152. If it is reported with code 58150 in conjunction with 51840 or 58145, it is considered unbundled or fragmented.

Unbundling, whether intentional or not, is considered by payers to be a form of fraudulent or reckless billing. The rationale is simple. Unbundled services will frequently net more reimbursement than reporting the single bundled CPT code.

The Centers for Medicare and Medicaid Services or CMS (formerly the Health Care Financing Administration or HCFA) has adopted the Correct Coding Initiative (CCI) unbundling guidelines, an evolving list of codes that cannot be reported in combination with other codes for Medicare claims. The CPT book does not have a specific guideline for unbundling. Instead, payers and other interested parties have developed guidelines for bundled procedures from information that is listed in the CPT book. The most common areas of the CPT book used for these interpretations are the format of the terminology listed surgical procedures, separate procedures, and subsection information in the surgery guidelines.

SURGERY

PREVENTION TIPS

Your office can take some easy steps to avoid problems with fragmentation or unbundling.

- Use a current CPT book as well as the current rules, regulations, and provider manuals for Medicare and for the private payers with whom you have a contractual arrangement.

- Educate everyone on CPT guidelines as well as the rules and regulations of your payers. Educational sessions should occur any time changes are made.

- When using a preprinted charge ticket or routing sheet, specify the exact CPT code and description. Always have an area on the charge ticket for the physician to indicate that a service should be coded by hand and code from the operative report or medical record. Many providers feel reimbursement is better by coding directly from the record or operative report.

- Date the charge ticket and update codes annually: in January for CPT and HCPCS codes; in October for ICD-9-CM codes.

- Create your charge tickets or routing sheets to avoid fragmented billing. Adding the abbreviation "SP" to separate procedure codes alerts the coder that a separate procedure should not be reported when related to, or integral to, a major procedure.

- Make sure physicians provide coders with complete documentation and concise information. Query the physician if documentation is not adequate to support the codes selected.

- Use the correct modifiers as appropriate to clarify or append circumstances that can arise within global package time periods.

STARRED PROCEDURES

Certain relatively small surgical procedures are characterized by variable pre- and postoperative services. Because of these indefinite parameters, the usual package concept for surgical services cannot be applied. Such procedures are identified by a star (*) following the procedure code.

When a star follows a surgical procedure code, the service listed includes only the surgical procedure, not any associated pre- and postoperative services.

PREOPERATIVE SERVICES

Preoperative services are reported as follows:

- When a starred procedure is the major service provided to a new patient, procedure 99025 should be listed in lieu of the usual initial visit.

- When the starred procedure is carried out at the time of an initial or established patient visit involving significant identifiable services, the appropriate visit is listed with modifier -25 in addition to the starred procedure.

- When the starred procedure requires hospitalization, an appropriate hospital visit should be reported in addition to the starred procedure.

Postoperative care is reported on a service-by-service basis.

Complications requiring additional service should be reported additionally. Identify all complications with the correct ICD-9-CM diagnosis code.

DIAGNOSTIC PROCEDURES

Diagnostic procedures are performed to evaluate the patient's complaints or symptoms. These procedures help the physician establish the nature of the patient's disease or condition so that definitive care can be provided. Diagnostic procedures include endoscopy, arthroscopy, injection procedures, and biopsies. Follow-up care for diagnostic procedures includes only care directly related to recovery from the diagnostic procedure itself. Care of the condition identified by the diagnostic procedures or other concomitant conditions is not included and may be listed separately.

THERAPEUTIC SERVICES

Therapeutic services are performed for treatment of a specific diagnosis. These services include performance of the procedure, various incidental elements, and normal, related follow-up care, unless the therapeutic service is a starred procedure.

LISTED SURGICAL PROCEDURES

According to CPT guidelines, listed surgical procedures include the operation per se, local infiltration, metacarpal/digital block or topical anesthesia when used, and the normal, uncomplicated follow-up care. The concept is referred to as a "package" for surgical procedures. For example:

The physician performs a closed treatment of a phalangeal shaft fracture with manipulation after first performing a digital block.

INCORRECT REPORTING

26725   **Closed treatment of phalangeal shaft fracture, proximal or middle phalanx, finger or thumb; with manipulation, with or without skin or skeletal traction, each**

64450*   **Injection anesthetic agent; other peripheral nerve or branch**

The injection procedure (64450*) cannot be reported separately because all listed surgical procedures include metacarpal or digital block. Therefore, the digital block is an integral part of the fracture treatment.

CORRECT REPORTING

26725   **Closed treatment of phalangeal shaft fracture, proximal or middle phalanx, finger or thumb; with manipulation, with or without skin or skeletal traction, each**

SEPARATE PROCEDURES

Separate procedures are services that are commonly carried out as an integral part of a larger service, and as such do not warrant separate identification. These services are noted in the CPT book with the parenthetical phrase (separate procedure). When this phrase appears before the semicolon, all indented descriptions that follow are covered by it.

Separate procedures are often improperly reported as related procedures. Related procedures are performed for the same diagnosis and within the same operative area. Reporting a separate procedure in addition to the larger procedure to which it is related is improper. A separate procedure can be a component of, or incidental to, a larger, related procedure.

SEQUENCING

The highest dollar code is always sequenced first when reporting multiple procedures. The second and subsequent codes are ordered and listed in decreasing dollar values with the correct modifier appended. When reporting multiple procedures, do not reduce the amount of secondary codes. However, if overpaid, reimburse the payer for the overpayment. Set a ceiling on nonactionable overpayments in policy or contracts (e.g. up to $10 need not be refunded). Overpayments that are not returned to the payer may target an office for an audit.

MATERIALS SUPPLIED BY A PHYSICIAN

Many payers reimburse only for supplies that are excessive or extraordinarily expensive. Do not report supplies that are customarily included in surgical packages, such as gauze, sponges, applicators, or Steri-strips. Surgical services do not include the supply of medications and sterile trays, which may be coded and billed separately. Applicable CPT codes are the following:

- 99070 for supplies, including reusable and disposable items. Specify the supply or type of medication, and the amount that was provided.

- 96545 for the provision of chemotherapy agent.

- 92330 and 92335 for ocular prostheses. Additional supplies relating to the eye (including contact lenses and spectacles) are identified with 92390-92396. HCPCS Level II codes also can report ocular prostheses.

- 78990 and 79900 for radiopharmaceutical(s), diagnostic or therapeutic, respectively.

Surgery

- Many payers prefer or require the use of HCPCS Level II codes for reporting supplies as they provide greater specificity. When reporting supplies, attach a statement to the claim form, informing the payer of the physician's cost, including a reasonable charge for handling and provide a description of the supply used.

SURGICAL PROCEDURES

Several subsections of CPT contain guidelines, notes, definitions, and special instructions. Following is a list of some of the subsections:

Fine needle aspiration

Removal of skin tags

Shaving of epidermal/dermal lesions

Excision of benign and malignant lesions

Repair of wounds

Adjacent tissue transfers

Skin grafts and flaps

Destruction of lesions

Fracture care

Cast and splint application

Spine surgeries

Pacemaker/defibrillator care

Coronary artery bypass grafts

Vascular catheterization/injection

Gastrointestinal endoscopy

Hernia repair

Urodynamics

Cystoscopy, urethroscopy and cystourethroscopy

Vulvectomy

Maternity care and delivery

Surgery of skull base

GENERAL CODING RULES

BIOPSY SERVICES

Use biopsy codes to report the removal of a small amount of tissue to determine the extent of a disease or to determine or confirm a diagnosis. A single tissue sample may punched out with a needle, or a portion of the lesion may be biopsied by incising the lesion and repairing the incision with sutures. Biopsy codes are appropriate for needle aspiration, incisional biopsy, and partial excision, as well as for scraping, curetting, and using a skin punch. Examples include:

21920	**Biopsy, soft tissue of back or flank; superficial**
44025	**Colotomy, for exploration, biopsy(s), or foreign body removal**
58100*	**Endometrial sampling (biopsy) with or without endocervical sampling (biopsy), without cervical dilation, any method (separate procedure)**
67810*	**Biopsy of eyelid**

Use integumentary codes when the biopsy is of skin and subcutaneous tissue only. A biopsy code is reported when tissue is sampled; an excision code is reported when all suspect tissue is removed. If the biopsy and excision occur during the same surgical session, only the excision is reported. If the biopsy is performed on a different date, it is reported separately.

INTEGUMENTARY SYSTEM

REMOVAL OF SKIN TAGS (11200-11201)

Removal of skin tags may be accomplished by any single or combination of the following techniques: scissoring, sharp excision, ligature, strangulation, electrosurgical destruction. Administration of local anesthesia and any chemical or electrocautery is included.

SHAVING OF EPIDERMAL LESIONS (11300-11313)

Shaving is the removal of epidermal or dermal skin lesions without a full-thickness dermal excision by use of a transverse incision or horizontal slicing technique. Administration of local anesthesia and any chemical or electrocautery is included.

EXCISION BENIGN AND MALIGNANT LESIONS (11400-11646)

Excision is defined as a full-thickness removal of lesion including simple closure of the wound. Excision codes are selected on the basis of the type of lesion (benign or malignant), anatomic site, and lesion diameter. Benign lesions include those described as cicatricial, fibrous, inflammatory, congenital and cystic as well as any other lesion that is noninvasive or nonmalignant. Malignant lesions are typically invasive or have the potential to metastasize and include lesions such as basal cell carcinomas and melanomas of the skin.

Excision codes for malignant lesions are assigned according to the largest diameter of the lesion excised. Simple closure is included. When the excision of a malignancy results in a defect requiring complex closure, the closure of the defect (using intermediate or complex repair) is reported separately. Codes for adjacent tissue transfer or rearrangement include lesion excision. Lesion excision is not separately reportable with codes 14000-14350.

WOUND REPAIR (12001-13160)

Repair is the surgical closure of a wound. The wound may be a result of injury/trauma or it may be a surgically created defect. Repairs can be any of the following:

- Stand alone procedures

- Separately reportable services when performed with certain other procedures as in the case of excisions requiring intermediate or complex repair

- An integral part of a more complex procedure and not separately reportable

Repairs are divided into three categories: simple, intermediate, and complex. They are further described by anatomic site and wound size.

Simple repair is performed when the wound is superficial, e.g., involving partial or full-thickness damage to the skin and/or subcutaneous tissues. There is no significant involvement of deeper structures and only simple, one layer, primary suturing is required. This procedure includes local anesthetic and chemical or electrocauterization of wounds not closed.

Intermediate repair is performed for wounds and lacerations in which one or more of the deeper layers of subcutaneous tissue and non-muscle fascia are repaired in addition to the skin and subcutaneous tissue. Single-layer closure can also be coded as an intermediate repair if the wound is heavily contaminated and requires extensive cleaning or removal of particulate matter.

Complex repair includes repair of wounds requiring more than layered closure. Wounds coded from this category include those requiring revision, debridement, extensive undermining, and placement of stents or retention sutures. Complex repairs also include those requiring creation of a defect (e.g., extending excision) and special preparation of the site.

The following rules should be followed when reporting repairs:

1. Measure the length of the repaired wound or wounds and report in centimeters.

2. Add together the lengths of multiple wounds in the same classification and report as a single item.

   For example, a simple repair of a 2-centimeter scalp wound and a simple repair of a 1.5-centimeter wound of the forearm would be reported with a single code.

12002	**Simple repair of superficial wounds of scalp, neck, axillae, external genitalia, trunk and/or extremities (including hands and feet); 2.6 cm to 7.5 cm**

This procedure is coded with a single procedure code because both wounds are classified as simple and both are in the same group of simple repairs (12001-12007). Total length of the two wounds is 3.5 centimeters so 12002 is reported.

3. Wounds in more than one classification should be listed separately with the more complicated service listed as the primary procedure and the less complicated listed as the secondary procedure with modifier -51 appended.

4. Decontamination and debridement are considered integral to wound repair except when gross contamination requires prolonged cleansing or when appreciable amounts of devitalized contaminated tissue must be removed.

5. Repair of nerves, blood vessels, and tendons should be reported under the appropriate system. Repair of associated skin wounds is considered integral to the repair of nerves, blood vessels, and tendons and is not reported separately unless the wound repair qualifies as complex. In these instances report the complex repair code.

6. Simple exploration of nerves, blood vessels, and tendons exposed in an open wound is considered integral to the repair and should not be reported separately.

7. Wounds resulting from penetrating trauma that require exploration, enlargement, extension, dissection, removal of foreign body, and/or ligation or coagulation of minor blood vessels of subcutaneous tissue, muscle fascia, or muscle should be reported with 20100-20103 as indicated.

ADJACENT TISSUE TRANSFER/REARRANGEMENT (14000-14350)

Anatomic site and size of the defect defines adjacent tissue transfer or rearrangement. Adjacent tissue transfers include excision of the defect or lesion so excision codes should not be reported additionally. Terms used to describe transfer or rearrangement procedures include: Z-plasty, W-plasty, V-Y-plasty, rotation flap, advancement flap, double pedicle flap. When applied to primary traumatic wound closure, the configuration listed must be developed by the surgeon to accomplish the repair. Transfer and rearrangement codes should not be applied when traumatic wounds incidentally result in these configurations.

Tissue transfer or rearrangement codes describe moving normal tissue from the donor site to the recipient site. The donor site is adjacent or next to the affected area, allowing the tissue to remain attached to its original location and blood supply, ensuring survival of the graft.

FLAPS AND GRAFTS (15000-15776)

Flaps and grafts are procedures that involve moving normal tissue (skin, skin and deep tissues, muscle, composite tissue) from one site to another. The site where the tissue originates is referred to as the donor site, while the site where the tissue is being relocated is referred to as the recipient site. Surgical preparation of the recipient site should be reported separately with codes 15000-15001. Flap and grafts codes are divided into three sections.

Free skin grafts are defined by size, location of the defect (recipient site), and type of graft (pinch, split-thickness, full-thickness). Free skin grafts should be reported separately as a secondary procedure when done in conjunction with other procedures. Examples of procedures that might require skin grafts at the time of the primary procedure include musculoskeletal deep tumor removal, neck dissection, and radical mastectomy.

Flaps of skin and deep tissues are defined by type of graft (direct, tube, delayed, intermediate, muscle, myocutaneous, fasciocutaneous) and site. The site listed is the recipient site when the flap is being attached to the final site. However, when the flap is being formed for delayed transfer, the site refers to the donor site. Any extensive immobilization with casts or other devices is considered an additional procedure and should be reported separately. Repairs of the donor site with skin grafts or local flaps are reportable separately.

Other flaps and grafts include island pedicle, free muscle skin or fascial flaps requiring microvascular anastomosis and composite grafts.

DESTRUCTION OF LESIONS (17000-17380)

Destruction is defined as the ablation of benign, premalignant, or malignant tissue by any of the following methods used alone or in combination: electrosurgery, cryosurgery, laser, and chemical treatment. Lesions include condylomata, papillomata, molluscum contagiosum, herpetic lesions, warts, milia, actinic keratosis, or other benign, premalignant or malignant lesions. Destruction includes administration of local anesthesia. Codes from this section should not be used when a more specific destruction code is listed

under the specific anatomic site. For example, code 40820 should be used for destruction of lesions of the vestibule of the mouth.

Moh's micrographic surgery is listed in the destruction subsection. This is a special technique used to treat complex or ill-defined skin cancer and requires a single physician to provide two distinct services. The first service is surgical and involves the destruction of the lesion by a combination of chemosurgery and excision. The second service is that of a pathologist and includes mapping, color coding of specimens, microscopic examination of specimens, and complete histopathologic preparation.

MUSCULOSKELETAL SECTION

FRACTURE CARE

Fracture management codes are package services and include percutaneous pinning and open or closed treatment of the fracture, application and removal of the initial cast or splint, and normal, uncomplicated follow-up care.

Two types of fixation - internal and external - are described in CPT. Internal skeletal fixation involves wires, pins, screws, and/or plates placed through or within the fractured area to stabilize and immobilize the injury. This procedure is generally accomplished through an incision over the fracture site. It is commonly described as an open reduction with internal fixation (ORIF). Internal fixation may also be accomplished by percutaneous technique. Deep internal devices are usually left in place even after the fracture has healed. If the hardware is removed, report codes 20670* or 20680. Use modifier -78 return to the operating room for a related procedure or modifier -58 staged or related procedure by the same physician during the postoperative period, if removal is performed during the initial hospital care or during the postoperative follow-up period. If the removal is performed after the postoperative follow-up period, use 20670* or 20680. The ICD-9-CM code is assigned according to the reason for the removal (e.g., pain, infection). The codes describing internal fixation are placed throughout the fracture care codes according to anatomical site.

External fixation (20690-20694) is hardware passing through bone and skin and held rigid by cross-braces outside the body. External fixation is always removed after the fracture has healed and removal usually is considered part of the global service. However, if required to remain in place beyond the usual postoperative period, its removal should be reported (20694).

CASTS AND STRAPPING

Codes found in the application of casts and strapping section (29000-29799) should be reported separately when:

- The cast application or strapping is a replacement procedure used during or after the period of follow-up care

- The cast application or strapping is an initial service performed without restorative treatment or procedures to stabilize or protect a fracture, injury, or dislocation and/or to afford comfort to a patient

- An initial casting or strapping when no other treatment or procedure is performed or will be performed by the same physician

- A physician performs the initial application of a cast or strapping subsequent to another physician having performed a restorative treatment or procedure

- A physician who applies the initial cast, strap, or splint and also assumes all of the subsequent fracture, dislocation, or injury care cannot use the application of casts and strapping codes as an initial service. The first cast, splint, or strap application is included in the treatment of the fracture and/or dislocation codes.

ARTHROSCOPIC SURGICAL PROCEDURES

Surgical arthroscopy always includes a diagnostic arthroscopy. When a diagnostic arthroscopy of the temporomandibular joint (TMJ) is performed without a definitive surgical procedure, the following code applies:

29800 **Arthroscopy, temporomandibular joint, diagnostic, with or without synovial biopsy (separate procedure)**

However, when a surgical arthroscopy is performed in conjunction with the diagnostic arthroscopy, it would be reported as follows:

29804   **Arthroscopy temporomandibular joint, surgical**

Do not report 29800 separately as it is part of 29804.

When the arthroscopy is performed with an arthrotomy, modifier -51 or 09951 should be reported. In this case, do not report the primary and secondary procedures with a single code. Instead, report both codes, listing first the service with the highest value. List the secondary procedures (performed during the same operative session) as subsequent line items with their assigned fees and append modifier -51 to indicate a multiple procedure.

29877   **Arthroscopy, knee, surgical; debridement/shaving of articular cartilage (chondroplasty)**

27425-51   **Lateral retinacular release (any method) - Multiple procedure**

SPINAL SURGERY

Procedure codes for reporting spine surgeries are found in two sections of the CPT book. Fracture/dislocation, spinal fusion/instrumentation, and treatment of scoliosis/kyphosis are reported with codes from the musculoskeletal section. Procedures of the spine with spinal cord involvement are reported with codes from the nervous system section (62268-63746). It is not unusual for procedures to require a procedure from the musculoskeletal section (arthrodesis, instrumentation) with a procedure from the nervous system section (laminectomy, hemilaminectomy, diskectomy), and it is appropriate to report both procedures separately.

Arthrodesis is a joint fusion and spinal arthrodesis is reported with 22548-22632. These codes are assigned based on technique (anterior/anterolateral, posterior/posterolateral, or lateral). Codes 22548-22558, 22590-22612, 22630 are for single interspace arthrodesis - two adjacent vertebral segments. When the surgery is performed on more than one interspace, each additional interspace is reported with 22585, 22614, or 22632. These procedures are considered "add on" services and are not reported with modifier -51.

Procedures for scoliosis and kyphosis (22800-22819) also include arthrodesis procedures. The arthrodesis procedures in this section differ since they involve multiple vertebral segments, and the code is assigned based on the number of segments treated.

Spinal instrumentation (22840-22855) involves placement of rods, hooks, and/or wires to stabilize the fusion or fracture. Instrumentation codes are assigned based on the type of instrumentation (segmental, non-segmental), the approach (anterior, posterior) and the number of vertebral segments involved. Instrumentation codes are exempt from modifier -51 and are reported in addition to the definitive procedure.

Bone allografts and autografts should be reported separately with codes 20930-20938. These codes are also modifier -51 exempt and are reported in addition to the definitive procedure. Only one code from this section can be reported per operative session.

Procedures of the spine with spinal cord are found in the nervous system section (62268-63746) and include diskectomy, laminectomy, hemilaminectomy, and laminotomy.

Diskectomy is the excision of intervertebral disk material. Codes 63075-63078 are specific to this surgery; however, many other codes from this section of the nervous system include diskectomies as a component of the procedure. Laminectomy is the removal of the entire lamina on both sides, inclusive of the spinous process. Hemilaminectomy is the excision of the right or left lamina, the posterior bony covering of the spinal cord. Laminotomy is the process of creating a hole in the lamina to achieve the required result, for example, excising a herniated intervertebral disk.

CARDIOVASCULAR SYSTEM

PACEMAKER/DEFIBRILLATOR CARE (33200-33249)

Pacemaker and defibrillator systems include a pulse generator. The pulse generator is placed in a subcutaneous pocket. Electrodes are inserted through a vein (transvenous) or on the surface of the heart (epicardial). Pacemaker systems are either single or dual chamber systems. In a single chamber system a single electrode is placed in either the atrium or ventricle. In a dual chamber system two electrodes are placed, one into the atrium and one into the ventricle.

Repositioning or replacement procedures performed during the first 14 days after the initial insertion or reportable replacement are included in the code for the initial procedure and should not be reported separately. Repositioning and replacement procedures performed after 14 days are considered new, not repeat, services and modifiers -76 and -77 should not be used.

Replacement of a pulse generator requires assignment of two codes, one for the removal and another for the insertion.

CORONARY ARTERY BYPASS GRAFTS (33510-33536)

Coronary artery bypass grafts (CABG) are coded by type of graft. Venous grafting alone is reported with 33510-33516. Arterial grafting alone is reported with 33533-33545. Combined arterial-venous grafting is reported with 33517-33523 in combination with 33533-33535. Codes 33517-33523 cannot be reported alone.

Procurement of vein and artery grafts is included in CABG procedures and should not be reported separately. If a second surgeon procures the graft, report the services as assistant surgeon services with modifier -80 appended to the applicable CABG code.

VASCULAR CATHETERIZATION/INJECTION (36000-36299)

Vascular catheterization/injection services include local anesthesia, introduction of needle or catheter, injection of contrast media, and use of power injections. Since these are diagnostic procedures, only the pre-injection and post-injection care directly related to the procedure is included. Catheters, drugs, and contrast media should be reported separately.

Selective vascular catheterization codes include introduction and all lesser order vessels catheterized used in the approach. Selective catheterization of the right middle cerebral artery includes the introduction and placement catheterization of the right common and internal carotid arteries. Only code 36217 for the third order branch would be reported. Additional second or third order vessels supplied by the same first order branch are reported with "add on" procedure codes 36012, 36218, and 36248.

These procedures are reported by vascular family and, as such, any procedure performed on more than one vascular family is reported separately using the conventions described above. Bilateral procedures are reported as separate vascular families.

DIGESTIVE SYSTEM

GASTROINTESTINAL ENDOSCOPY

Gastrointestinal endoscopy codes are reported by site and are listed as follows: esophagus (43200-43232), upper gastrointestinal (43234-43259), endoscopic retrograde cholangiopancreatography (ERCP) (43260-43272), other small intestine or stomal (44360-44397), and large intestine (45300-45387).

Endoscopic procedures may be diagnostic or surgical. The procedure is considered diagnostic when performed to visualize an abnormality or determine the extent of disease. When anything more than visualization is performed, the procedure is considered to be a surgical procedure. A surgical endoscopy always includes a diagnostic endoscopy.

For example, if the patient is to have a diagnostic flexible sigmoidoscopy with biopsy of a lesion during the same surgical session, the diagnostic portion of the procedure (45330) would not be reported separately. Only the surgical portion of the procedure (45331) would be reported.

Diagnostic endoscopic procedures can be reported with open or incisional procedures.

HERNIA REPAIR (49495-49611)

Hernia repair codes are categorized primarily by type of hernia (inguinal, femoral, incisional/ventral, epigastric, umbilical, spigelian). Some hernias are further categorized based on whether there has been a previous hernia repair (initial, recurrent). Additional variables include patient age and clinical presentation (reducible, strangulated/incarcerated).

Implantation of mesh or prosthesis may be performed with hernia repairs. However, the implantation should be reported separately only when used for repair of incisional and ventral hernias (49560-49566). When used for repair of other types of hernias, it is not considered a separately reportable procedure. For laparoscopic repair of inguinal and other hernias, see codes 49650-49659.

Repair of strangulated organs or structures should be reported in addition to the hernia repair. Structures most often involved include intestine (44120), testicles (54520), and ovaries (58940).

URINARY SYSTEM

URODYNAMICS (51725-51797)
Urodynamics is a diagnostic service performed to evaluate the storage of urine and urine flow through the urinary tract. All procedures in this section represent complete procedures (both the professional and technical components). Physicians reporting these services as complete procedures are expected to supply all instruments/equipment, supplies, and technician services. A physician performing only the operation of the equipment and interpretation of the report should report only the professional component by appending modifier -26 to the procedure codes.

CYSTOSCOPY, URETHROSCOPY, AND CYSTOURETHROSCOPY (52000-52700)
Cystoscopy, urethroscopy, and cystourethroscopy are listed so that the main procedure can be identified without listing all minor related procedures performed. For example, a cystourethroscopy with dilation of a urethral stricture (52281) includes calibration, meatotomy, and the injection procedure for cystography, which are all explicitly described in the procedure.

Secondary endoscopic procedures performed on the same site which are not explicitly included and involve significant additional time and work may be reported either of two ways. The secondary procedure should not be reported additionally, but reported instead by modifier -22 appended to the primary procedure. However, many physicians report secondary procedures with a separate code and append modifier -51. When billing for the secondary procedure either with modifier -22 or with the actual procedure code, verify that it can be justified based on the additional time and work required. Documentation may need to be submitted with the claim.

Many procedures on the ureter require placement of a temporary stent. Placement and removal of temporary stents are not reported separately. However, placement of more permanent, self-retaining, indwelling stents (52332) should be reported with the code for the primary procedure.

FEMALE GENITAL SYSTEM

VULVECTOMY (56620-56640)
The following definitions would be employed when selecting a vulvectomy code:

- Simple - Removal of skin and superficial subcutaneous tissues
- Radical - Removal of skin and deep subcutaneous tissues
- Partial - Removal of less than 80 percent of the vulvar area
- Complete - Removal of 80 percent or more of the vulvar area

MATERNITY CARE AND DELIVERY
Maternity care is outlined in the maternity care and delivery section. The codes for normal, uncomplicated care to the maternity patient (59400, 59510, 59610, 59618) include antepartum care, delivery, and postpartum care by the same physician.

Antepartum care includes the initial and routine subsequent history and physical exams, patient's weight, blood pressure, fetal heart tones, and routine urinalysis.

Delivery includes admission to the hospital, including the admitting history and exam, the management of uncomplicated labor, and either a vaginal or cesarean delivery.

Postpartum care includes the inpatient hospital care and any office visits following vaginal or cesarean delivery.

Six delivery codes deserve some additional explanation. These codes report delivery after a previous cesarean delivery when an attempt is made to accomplish the delivery vaginally, also referred to as a VBAC. Codes 59610-59614 report a successful vaginal delivery after a previous cesarean delivery (VBAC). Codes 59618-59622 are reported if a vaginal birth attempt is unsuccessful and another cesarean delivery is carried out. These codes for global care are reported on claims following the delivery.

When different physicians provide components of the total obstetric service, report the services separately using the codes designated for each component. Codes 59425 and 59426 identify a different physician providing four or more antepartum care visits. Use the appropriate E/M codes when a different physician provides one to three antepartum care visits. Use 59409, 59514, 59612, or 59620 when the physician performs vaginal or cesarean delivery only. Use 59410, 59515, 59614, or 59622 when the physician performs vaginal or cesarean delivery with postpartum care.

Services unrelated to the pregnancy should be reported with Evaluation and Management codes or the procedure codes for the service. For example, a patient seen for a sore throat with a throat culture should have both the throat culture and E/M service reported separately. Clearly identify the reasons for the services as pharyngitis, not pregnancy.

Services directly related to the pregnancy, but not included in the global service, should be reported separately. Examples include ultrasound examination of pregnant uterus (76805-76816), glucose tolerance test (82951-82953), and Pap smear (88150). New to the CPT book of 2002 is the addition of anesthesia code for obstetrical procedures (01960-01969), which includes anesthesia for vaginal and cesarean deliveries and neuraxial labor analgesia/anesthesia following vaginal and cesarean deliveries. The neuraxial codes are reported in addition to the primary procedures.

Normal maternity care includes monthly visits up to 28 weeks gestation, biweekly visits to 36 weeks gestation, and weekly visits until delivery. For the patient at risk who is seen more frequently or for other medical/surgical intervention, code the additional services with a code representing the appropriate level of E/M service. The documentation must reflect the necessity of these visits as well as any additional laboratory or radiologic tests performed.

When the physician monitors the patient for a prolonged period, document the time spent in actual attendance and use prolonged services codes as appropriate. Codes 99356 and 99357 describe maternal-fetal monitoring, which is reported in addition to the delivery. Always include documentation to substantiate medical necessity.

NERVOUS SYSTEM

SURGERY OF SKULL BASE (61580-61619)
Neurosurgical procedures of lesions involving the skull base often require the skills of several surgeons of different surgical specialties. These procedures have been broken into their component parts, categorized by the approach, definitive procedure, and repair/reconstruction of surgical defects following the definitive procedure.

The approach is defined as the portion of the procedure necessary to obtain adequate exposure of the lesion. It is described by anatomical area involved that includes anterior, middle, or posterior cranial fossa; brain stem; and upper spinal cord.

The definitive portion includes biopsy, excision, resection or repair of the lesion, and primary closure of the dura, mucous membrane and skin.

Repair/reconstruction is reported separately only when extensive dural grafting, cranioplasty, myocutaneous flaps, or extensive skin grafts are employed to close the surgical defect.

When different surgeons perform the component parts of skull base procedures, each reports only the code for the specific portion the physician has performed.

If one surgeon performs both the approach and definitive procedure, both codes should be reported, appending modifier -51 to the secondary procedure.

Integumentary System

10021 — 11201

GENERAL

If one physician only interprets the results and/or operates the equipment, modifier -26 should be appended.

- **10021**   **Fine needle aspiration; without imaging guidance**
- **10022**   **with imaging guidance**

    If radiological supervision and interpretation is performed, consult CPT codes 76003, 76360, 76942.

    If percutaneous needle biopsy is performed, consult CPT code 32405 for lung, 47000, 47001 for liver, 48102 for pancreas, 29180 for abdominal or retroperitoneal mass.

    If evaluation of fine needle aspirate is performed, consult CPT codes 88172, 88173.

INTEGUMENTARY SYSTEM

SKIN, SUBCUTANEOUS AND ACCESSORY STRUCTURES

INCISION AND DRAINAGE

- **10040*** **Acne surgery (eg, marsupialization, opening or removal of multiple milia, comedones, cysts, pustules)**

- **10060*** **Incision and drainage of abscess (eg, carbuncle, suppurative hidradenitis, cutaneous or subcutaneous abscess, cyst, furuncle, or paronychia); simple or single**

- **10061**   **complicated or multiple**
- **10080*** **Incision and drainage of pilonidal cyst; simple**
- **10081**   **complicated**

    If an excision of a pilonidal cyst or sinus is performed, consult CPT codes 11770-11772.

- **10120*** **Incision and removal of foreign body, subcutaneous tissues; simple**
- **10121**   **complicated**

    If exploration of a penetrating wound, not requiring thoracotomy or laparotomy, is performed, consult CPT codes 20100-20103. If debridement related to an open fracture(s) and/or dislocation(s) is performed, consult CPT codes 11010-11012.

- **10140*** **Incision and drainage of hematoma, seroma or fluid collection**

    To report imaging guidance, consult CPT codes 76030, 76393, 76942.

- **10160*** **Puncture aspiration of abscess, hematoma, bulla, or cyst**

    To report imaging guidance consult CPT codes 76360, 76393, 76942.

- **10180**   **Incision and drainage, complex, postoperative wound infection**

    If secondary closure of surgical wound is performed, consult CPT codes 12020-12021 and 13160.

EXCISION-DEBRIDEMENT

If dermabrasions are performed, consult CPT codes 15780-15791. If nail debridement is performed, consult CPT codes 11720-11721. If burns are being treated, consult CPT codes 16000-16035.

- **11000*** **Debridement of extensive eczematous or infected skin; up to 10% of body surface**

- + **11001**   **each additional 10% of the body surface (List separately in addition to code for primary procedure)**

    Note that 11001 is an add-on code and must be used in conjunction with 11000.

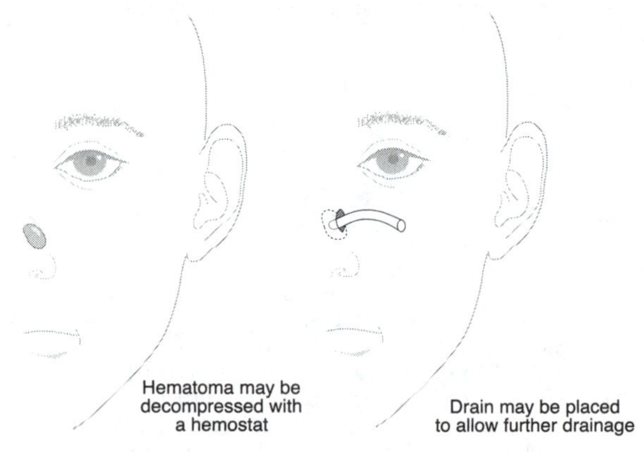

- **11010**   **Debridement including removal of foreign material associated with open fracture(s) and/or dislocation(s); skin and subcutaneous tissues**

- **11011**   **skin, subcutaneous tissue, muscle fascia, and muscle**
- **11012**   **skin, subcutaneous tissue, muscle fascia, muscle, and bone**
- **11040**   **Debridement; skin, partial thickness**

    For active wound care management see 97601-97602. Do not report 11040-11044 with 97601, 97602.

- **11041**   **skin, full thickness**
- **11042**   **skin, and subcutaneous tissue**
- **11043**   **skin, subcutaneous tissue, and muscle**
- **11044**   **subcutaneous tissue, muscle, and bone**

PARING OR CUTTING

- **11055**   **Paring or cutting of benign hyperkeratotic lesion (eg, corn or callus); single lesion**
- **11056**   **two to four lesions**
- **11057**   **more than four lesions**

BIOPSY

- **11100**   **Biopsy of skin, subcutaneous tissue and/or mucous membrane (including simple closure), unless otherwise listed (separate procedure); single lesion**

    If the conjunctiva is biopsied, consult CPT code 68100; if the eyelid is biopsied, consult CPT code 67810.

- + **11101**   **each separate/additional lesion (List separately in addition to code for primary procedure)**

    Note that 11101 is an add-on code and must be used in conjunction with 11100.

REMOVAL OF SKIN TAGS

CPT codes 11200 and 11201 identify the use of scissors or other sharp methods, ligature strangulation, electrosurgical destruction or any combination of treatment methods including electrosurgical techniques or the use of chemicals. Local anesthesia is included in these services.

- **11200*** **Removal of skin tags, multiple fibrocutaneous tags, any area; up to and including 15 lesions**

- + **11201**   **each additional ten lesions (List separately in addition to code for primary procedure)**

    Note that 11201 is an add-on code and must be used in conjunction with 11200.

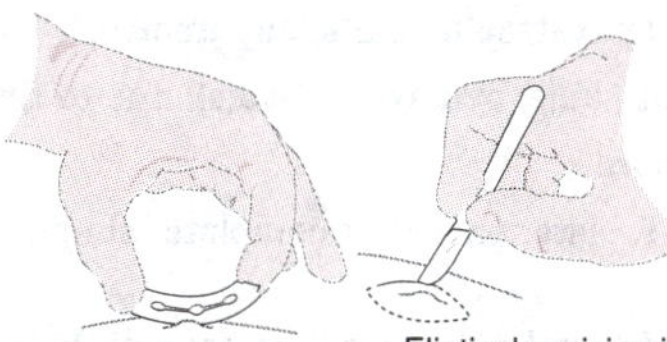

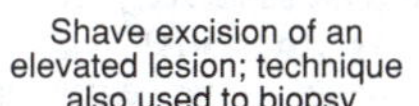

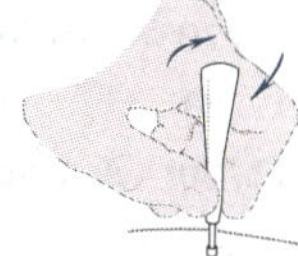

Shave excision of an elevated lesion; technique also used to biopsy

Eliptical excision is often used when tissue removal is larger than 4 mm or when deep pathology is suspected

A punch biopsy cuts a core of tissue as the tool is twisted downward

The skin is the largest organ of the human body and accounts for about 20 percent of total body weight. It serves mainly as a protective barrier, a temperature regulator, and as a sensory device. The epidermis is outermost and is the thinnest of the skin layers; the major part of the dermis is high in collagen and is notable for its great elasticity and strength; the major blood and nerve network is found in the middermis. Adnexal structures are the hair follicles, sebaceous glands, sweat glands, and the follicles that produce fingernails and toenails. Lesions are small areas of skin disease and may be solitary or multiple

SHAVING OF EPIDERMAL OR DERMAL LESIONS

Shaving of lesions is defined as the sharp removal by horizontal slicing or by transverse incision of epidermal or dermal lesions.

CPT codes 11300-11313, include local anesthesia, chemical or electrocauterization of the wound. These wounds do not require suture closure.

11300* Shaving of epidermal or dermal lesion, single lesion, trunk, arms or legs; lesion diameter 0.5 cm or less

11301 lesion diameter 0.6 to 1.0 cm

11302 lesion diameter 1.1 to 2.0 cm

11303 lesion diameter over 2.0 cm

11305* Shaving of epidermal or dermal lesion, single lesion, scalp, neck, hands, feet, genitalia; lesion diameter 0.5 cm or less

11306 lesion diameter 0.6 to 1.0 cm

11307 lesion diameter 1.1 to 2.0 cm

11308 lesion diameter over 2.0 cm

11310* Shaving of epidermal or dermal lesion, single lesion, face, ears, eyelids, nose, lips, mucous membrane; lesion diameter 0.5 cm or less

11311 lesion diameter 0.6 to 1.0 cm

11312 lesion diameter 1.1 to 2.0 cm

11313 lesion diameter over 2.0 cm

EXCISION-BENIGN LESIONS

In CPT excision of benign lesions is defined as a full thickness removal of the lesion. Benign lesions may include cysts and growths caused by inflammation, fibrous tissue, and tissues present since birth. The lesions may occur in the skin or tissues below the skin. Non-layered closure and local anesthesia are included.

Layered, intermediate or complex closure of the defect created by the excision of the lesion is separately reported.

If an excision of a benign lesion(s) requiring more than simple closure (e.g., requiring intermediate, or complex closure) is performed, report the appropriate closure CPT codes (12031-12057 for intermediate, 13100-13160 for complex) in addition to appropriate lesion removal code (11400-11446). For reconstructive closure report CPT codes 14000-14300, 15000-15261, and 15570-15770 in addition to appropriate lesion removal code. If electrosurgery, cryosurgery, laser, or chemical treatment is used, consult CPT code 17000 and subsequent codes.

If the excision is unusual or complicated, append modifier -22 or 09922.

11400 Excision, benign lesion, except skin tag (unless listed elsewhere), trunk, arms or legs; lesion diameter 0.5 cm or less

11401 lesion diameter 0.6 to 1.0 cm

11402 lesion diameter 1.1 to 2.0 cm

11403 lesion diameter 2.1 to 3.0 cm

11404 lesion diameter 3.1 to 4.0 cm

11406 lesion diameter over 4.0 cm

11420 Excision, benign lesion, except skin tag (unless listed elsewhere), scalp, neck, hands, feet, genitalia; lesion diameter 0.5 cm or less

11421 lesion diameter 0.6 to 1.0 cm

11422 lesion diameter 1.1 to 2.0 cm

11423 lesion diameter 2.1 to 3.0 cm

11424 lesion diameter 3.1 to 4.0 cm

11426 lesion diameter over 4.0 cm

11440 Excision, other benign lesion (unless listed elsewhere), face, ears, eyelids, nose, lips, mucous membrane; lesion diameter 0.5 cm or less

If the excision on the eyelids involves more than skin, consult CPT codes 67800 and subsequent codes.

11441 lesion diameter 0.6 to 1.0 cm

11442 lesion diameter 1.1 to 2.0 cm

11443 lesion diameter 2.1 to 3.0 cm

11444 lesion diameter 3.1 to 4.0 cm

11446 lesion diameter over 4.0 cm

If codes 11450-11471 are performed bilaterally, append modifier -50 or 09950.

11450 Excision of skin and subcutaneous tissue for hidradenitis, axillary; with simple or intermediate repair

11451 with complex repair

If a skin graft or flap is used for closure, consult the appropriate CPT code and use in addition to 11451.

11462 Excision of skin and subcutaneous tissue for hidradenitis, inguinal; with simple or intermediate repair

11463 with complex repair

If a skin graft or flap is used for closure, consult the appropriate CPT code and use in addition to 11463.

11470 Excision of skin and subcutaneous tissue for hidradenitis, perianal, perineal, or umbilical; with simple or intermediate repair

11471 with complex repair

If a skin graft or flap is used for closure, consult the appropriate CPT code and use in addition to 11471.

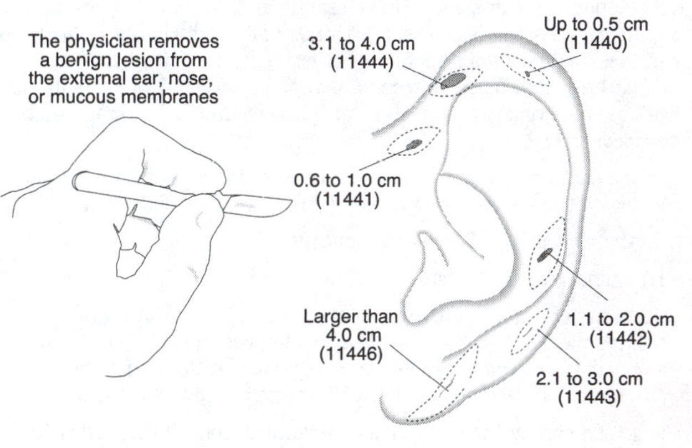

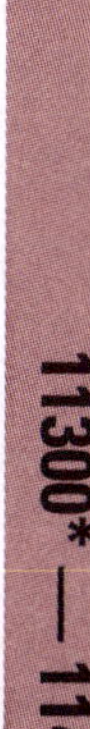

Integumentary System

11600 — 11976

EXCISION-MALIGNANT LESIONS

In CPT, excision of malignant lesions is defined as a full thickness removal of the lesion. Non-layered closure and local anesthesia are included.

Layered, intermediate or complex closure of the defect created by the excision of the lesion is separately reported.

If an excision of a malignant lesion(s) requiring more than simple closure (e.g., requiring intermediate, or complex closure) is performed, report the appropriate closure CPT codes (12031-12057 for intermediate, 13100-13160 for complex) in addition to appropriate lesion removal code (11600-11646). For reconstructive closure report CPT codes 14000-14300, 15000-15261, and 15570-15770 in addition to appropriate lesion removal code.

11600	Excision, malignant lesion, trunk, arms, or legs; lesion diameter 0.5 cm or less
11601	lesion diameter 0.6 to 1.0 cm
11602	lesion diameter 1.1 to 2.0 cm
11603	lesion diameter 2.1 to 3.0 cm
11604	lesion diameter 3.1 to 4.0 cm
11606	lesion diameter over 4.0 cm
11620	Excision, malignant lesion, scalp, neck, hands, feet, genitalia; lesion diameter 0.5 cm or less
11621	lesion diameter 0.6 to 1.0 cm
11622	lesion diameter 1.1 to 2.0 cm
11623	lesion diameter 2.1 to 3.0 cm
11624	lesion diameter 3.1 to 4.0 cm
11626	lesion diameter over 4.0 cm
11640	Excision, malignant lesion, face, ears, eyelids, nose, lips; lesion diameter 0.5 cm or less
11641	lesion diameter 0.6 to 1.0 cm
11642	lesion diameter 1.1 to 2.0 cm
11643	lesion diameter 2.1 to 3.0 cm
11644	lesion diameter 3.1 to 4.0 cm
11646	lesion diameter over 4.0 cm

NAILS

MCM 2323. FOOT CARE AND SUPPORTIVE DEVICES FOR FEET

The following foot care services generally are not covered under both Part A and Part B:

1. Services or devices directed toward the care or correction of flat foot (flattening of the arches), including the prescription of supportive devices, are not covered.

2. Surgical or nonsurgical treatments undertaken for the sole purpose of correcting a subluxated structure in the foot as an isolated entity are not covered. This exclusion does not apply to medical or surgical treatment of subluxation of the ankle joint (talo- crural joint). Medicare covers medical or surgical services, diagnosis, or treatment for conditions associated with partial displacement of structures. For example, if a patient has osteoarthritis that has resulted in a partial displacement of joints in the foot, and the primary treatment is for the osteoarthritis, coverage is provided.

3. Routine foot care is excluded from coverage. Services that normally are considered routine and not covered by Medicare include the following:

- Cutting or removal of corns and calluses

- Trimming, cutting, clipping, or debriding nails

- Other hygienic and preventive maintenance care, such as cleaning and soaking the feet, the use of skin creams to maintain skin tone of either ambulatory or bedfast patients, and any other service performed in the absence of localized illness, injury, or symptoms involving the foot.

If drainage of a paronychia or onychia is performed, consult CPT codes 10060 and 10061.

11719	Trimming of nondystrophic nails, any number
11720	Debridement of nail(s) by any method(s); one to five
11721	six or more
11730*	Avulsion of nail plate, partial or complete, simple; single
+ 11732	each additional nail plate (List separately in addition to code for primary procedure)

Note that 11732 is an add-on code and must be used in conjunction with 11730.

11740	Evacuation of subungual hematoma
11750	Excision of nail and nail matrix, partial or complete, (eg, ingrown or deformed nail) for permanent removal;
11752	with amputation of tuft of distal phalanx

If a skin graft is performed, consult CPT code 15050.

▲ 11755	Biopsy of nail unit (eg, plate, bed, matrix, hyponychium, proximal and lateral nail folds) (separate procedure)
11760	Repair of nail bed
11762	Reconstruction of nail bed with graft
11765	Wedge excision of skin of nail fold (eg, for ingrown toenail)

Cotting's operation

11770	Excision of pilonidal cyst or sinus; simple

If a pilonidal cyst is incised, consult CPT codes 10080 and 10081.

11771	extensive
11772	complicated

INTRODUCTION

If the injection of sclerosing solution is for a vein, consult CPT codes 36470-36471. If intralesional chemotherapy is administered, consult CPT codes 96405-96406.

Do not report 11900, 11901 for preoperative local anesthetic injections.

11900*	Injection, intralesional; up to and including seven lesions
11901*	more than seven lesions
11920	Tattooing, intradermal introduction of insoluble opaque pigments to correct color defects of skin, including micropigmentation; 6.0 sq cm or less
11921	6.1 to 20.0 sq cm
+ 11922	each additional 20.0 sq cm (List separately in addition to code for primary procedure)

Note that 11922 is an add-on code and must be used in conjunction with 11921.

11950	Subcutaneous injection of filling material (eg, collagen); 1 cc or less
11951	1.1 to 5.0 cc
11952	5.1 to 10.0 cc
11954	over 10.0 cc
11960	Insertion of tissue expander(s) for other than breast, including subsequent expansion

If the breast is reconstructed with a tissue expander(s), consult CPT code 19357.

11970	Replacement of tissue expander with permanent prosthesis
11971	Removal of tissue expander(s) without insertion of prosthesis
11975	Insertion, implantable contraceptive capsules
11976	Removal, implantable contraceptive capsules

11977	Removal with reinsertion, implantable contraceptive capsules	♀
11980	Subcutaneous hormone pellet implantation (implantation of estradiol and/or testosterone pellets beneath the skin)	⊡
● 11981	Insertion, non-biodegradable drug delivery implant	
● 11982	Removal, non-biodegradable drug delivery implant	
● 11983	Removal with reinsertion, non-biodegradable drug delivery implant	

REPAIR (CLOSURE)

Record wound lengths in centimeters. If multiple wounds are repaired from the same classification (e.g., simple, intermediate, complex) and anatomic grouping, add together the lengths of multiple repairs and code as one wound.

Debridement is included in the initial wound repair unless gross contamination necessitates extended cleaning and/or removal of substantial amounts of devitalized/contaminated tissue. Simple exploration of exposed nerves, tendons, or blood vessels in the open wound is included in wound repair.

Within an anatomic grouping, add together the lengths of multiple repairs and code as one repair.

REPAIR - SIMPLE

12001*	Simple repair of superficial wounds of scalp, neck, axillae, external genitalia, trunk and/or extremities (including hands and feet); 2.5 cm or less	⊡
12002*	2.6 cm to 7.5 cm	⊡
12004*	7.6 cm to 12.5 cm	⊡
12005	12.6 cm to 20.0 cm	②⊡
12006	20.1 cm to 30.0 cm	②⊡
12007	over 30.0 cm	②⊡
12011*	Simple repair of superficial wounds of face, ears, eyelids, nose, lips and/or mucous membranes; 2.5 cm or less	⊡
12013*	2.6 cm to 5.0 cm	⊡
12014	5.1 cm to 7.5 cm	⊡
12015	7.6 cm to 12.5 cm	⊡
12016	12.6 cm to 20.0 cm	②⊡
12017	20.1 cm to 30.0 cm	②⑧⊡
12018	over 30.0 cm	②⑧⊡
12020	Treatment of superficial wound dehiscence; simple closure	❶⊡

If the secondary wound closure is extensive or complicated, consult CPT code 13160.

12021	with packing	❶⊡

REPAIR - INTERMEDIATE

12031*	Layer closure of wounds of scalp, axillae, trunk and/or extremities (excluding hands and feet); 2.5 cm or less	⊡
12032*	2.6 cm to 7.5 cm	⊡
12034	7.6 cm to 12.5 cm	②⊡
12035	12.6 cm to 20.0 cm	②⊡
12036	20.1 cm to 30.0 cm	②⊡
12037	over 30.0 cm	②⑧⊡
12041*	Layer closure of wounds of neck, hands, feet and/or external genitalia; 2.5 cm or less	⊡
12042	2.6 cm to 7.5 cm	⊡
12044	7.6 cm to 12.5 cm	②⊡
12045	12.6 cm to 20.0 cm	②⊡
12046	20.1 cm to 30.0 cm	②⑧⊡

12047	over 30.0 cm	②⑧⊡
12051*	Layer closure of wounds of face, ears, eyelids, nose, lips and/or mucous membranes; 2.5 cm or less	⊡
12052	2.6 cm to 5.0 cm	⊡
12053	5.1 cm to 7.5 cm	⊡
12054	7.6 cm to 12.5 cm	②⊡
12055	12.6 cm to 20.0 cm	②⊡
12056	20.1 cm to 30.0 cm	②⑧⊡
12057	over 30.0 cm	②⑧⊡

REPAIR - COMPLEX

13100	Repair, complex, trunk; 1.1 cm to 2.5 cm	②⊡

If the repair is 1.0 cm or less, see simple or intermediate repairs.

13101	2.6 cm to 7.5 cm	❸⊡
+ 13102	each additional 5 cm or less (List separately in addition to code for primary procedure)	⊡

Note that 13102 is an add-on code and must be used in conjunction with 13101.

13120	Repair, complex, scalp, arms, and/or legs; 1.1 cm to 2.5 cm	②⊡

If the repair is 1.0 cm or less, see simple or intermediate repairs.

13121	2.6 cm to 7.5 cm	❸⊡
+ 13122	each additional 5 cm or less (List separately in addition to code for primary procedure)	⊡

Note that 13122 is an add-on code and must be used in conjunction with 13121.

13131	Repair, complex, forehead, cheeks, chin, mouth, neck, axillae, genitalia, hands and/or feet; 1.1 cm to 2.5 cm	②⊡

If the repair is 1.0 cm or less, see simple or intermediate repairs.

13132	2.6 cm to 7.5 cm	❸⊡
+ 13133	each additional 5 cm or less (List separately in addition to code for primary procedure)	⊡

Note that 13133 is an add-on code and must be used in conjunction with 13132.

13150	Repair, complex, eyelids, nose, ears and/or lips; 1.0 cm or less	❸⊡

If full thickness repair of the lip or the eyelid is required, consult relevant anatomical subsections.

13151	1.1 cm to 2.5 cm	❸⊡
13152	2.6 cm to 7.5 cm	❸⊡
+ 13153	each additional 5 cm or less (List separately in addition to code for primary procedure)	⊡

Note that 13153 is an add-on code and must be used in conjunction with 13152.

13160	Secondary closure of surgical wound or dehiscence, extensive or complicated	②⊡

ADJACENT TISSUE TRANSFER OR REARRANGEMENT

Adjacent tissue transfer is the technique of moving skin near a wound to close the wound These codes are used when the physician intentionally alters skin adjacent to the wound using flaps or a Z-plasty, for example, to repair the wound. Do not use these codes if the physician's repair of the wound results in a similar shape.

A skin graft that is needed to close a secondary defect is coded as an additional procedure.

Consult the glossary for additional definitions and guidelines.

Integumentary System

14000 — 15261

14000	Adjacent tissue transfer or rearrangement, trunk; defect 10 sq cm or less	❷ ⬚
	Burrow's operation	
14001	defect 10.1 sq cm to 30.0 sq cm	❸ ⬚
14020	Adjacent tissue transfer or rearrangement, scalp, arms and/or legs; defect 10 sq cm or less	❸ ⬚
14021	defect 10.1 sq cm to 30.0 sq cm	❸ ⬚
14040	Adjacent tissue transfer or rearrangement, forehead, cheeks, chin, mouth, neck, axillae, genitalia, hands and/or feet; defect 10 sq cm or less	❷ ⬚
	Krimer's palatoplasty	
14041	defect 10.1 sq cm to 30.0 sq cm	❸ ⬚
14060	Adjacent tissue transfer or rearrangement, eyelids, nose, ears and/or lips; defect 10 sq cm or less	❸ ⬚
	Denonvillier's operation	
14061	defect 10.1 sq cm to 30.0 sq cm	❸ ⬚
14300	Adjacent tissue transfer or rearrangement, more than 30 sq cm, unusual or complicated, any area	❹ ⬚
14350	Filleted finger or toe flap, including preparation of recipient site	❸ 80 ⬚

FREE SKIN GRAFTS

Free skin grafts are the use of skin from another site, tissue-cultured skin, or a substitute for skin to close a wound. Choose the code by identifying the size and location of the defect along with the type of graft. CPT says this group of codes includes simple debridement. Report the repair of the donor site separately.

Allografts are grafts from the same species either from the patient or a cadaver donor. With skin, this means whole or meshed skin.

Xenografts are the application of grafts that are not directly from a human, and can be meshed skin or skin taken from a pig donor.

CIM 45-12 PORCINE SKIN AND GRADIENT PRESSURE DRESSINGS

Porcine (pig) skin dressings are covered as an occlusive dressing for burns, donor sites of a homograft, and decubiti and other ulcers. Gradient pressure dressings are Jobst elasticized heavy-duty dressings used to reduce hypertrophic scarring and joint contractures following burn injury. They are covered when used for that purpose.

15000	Surgical preparation or creation of recipient site by excision of open wounds, burn eschar, or scar (including subcutaneous tissues); first 100 sq cm or one percent of body area of infants and children	❷ ⬚

For appropriate skin grafts, see 15050-15261; list the free graft separately by its procedure number when the graft, immediate or delayed, is applied.

+ 15001	each additional 100 sq cm or each additional one percent of body area of infants and children (List separately in addition to code for primary procedure)	80

Note that 15001 is an add-on code and must be used in conjunction with 15000.

15050	Pinch graft, single or multiple, to cover small ulcer, tip of digit, or other minimal open area (except on face), up to defect size 2 cm diameter	❷ ⬚

If the flap is microvascular, consult CPT codes 15756-15758.

If tissue-cultured skin grafts are performed, consult CPT codes 15100-15121. These codes include harvesting of keratinocytes and/or application of skin substitute/neodermis. Procedures are coded by recipient site.

15100	Split graft, trunk, arms, legs; first 100 sq cm or less, or one percent of body area of infants and children (except 15050)	❷ ⬚

If the flap is microvascular, consult CPT codes 15756-15758.

+ 15101	each additional 100 sq cm, or each additional one percent of body area of infants and children, or part thereof (List separately in addition to code for primary procedure)	❸

Note that 15101 is an add-on code and must be used in conjunction with 15100.

15120	Split graft, face, scalp, eyelids, mouth, neck, ears, orbits, genitalia, hands, feet and/or multiple digits; first 100 sq cm or less, or one percent of body area of infants and children (except 15050)	

If the flap is microvascular, consult CPT codes 15756-15758.

+ 15121	each additional 100 sq cm, or each additional one percent of body area of infants and children, or part thereof (List separately in addition to code for primary procedure)	❸

Note that 15121 is an add-on code and must be used in conjunction with 15120. If the split graft is performed on the eyelids, consult also CPT code 67961 and subsequent codes.

15200	Full thickness graft, free, including direct closure of donor site, trunk; 20 sq cm or less	❸ ⬚

If the flap is microvascular, consult CPT codes 15756-15758.

+ 15201	each additional 20 sq cm (List separately in addition to code for primary procedure)	❷ 80

Note that 15201 is an add-on code and must be used in conjunction with 15200.

15220	Full thickness graft, free, including direct closure of donor site, scalp, arms, and/or legs; 20 sq cm or less	❷ ⬚

If the flap is microvascular, consult CPT codes 15756-15758.

+ 15221	each additional 20 sq cm (List separately in addition to code for primary procedure)	❷

Note that 15221 is an add-on code and must be used in conjunction with 15220.

15240	Full thickness graft, free, including direct closure of donor site, forehead, cheeks, chin, mouth, neck, axillae, genitalia, hands, and/or feet; 20 sq cm or less	❸ ⬚

If the flap is microvascular, consult CPT codes 15756-15758.

If the graft is performed on the fingertip, consult CPT code 15050. If the repair is performed on a web finger (syndactyly), consult CPT codes 26560-26562.

+ 15241	each additional 20 sq cm (List separately in addition to code for primary procedure)	❸

Note that 15241 is an add-on code and must be used in conjunction with 15240.

15260	Full thickness graft, free, including direct closure of donor site, nose, ears, eyelids, and/or lips; 20 sq cm or less	❷ ⬚
+ 15261	each additional 20 sq cm (List separately in addition to code for primary procedure)	❷

Note that 15261 is an add-on code and must be used in conjunction with 15260. If a full-thickness graft is performed on the eyelids, consult also 67961 and subsequent codes. If the donor site repair requires a skin graft or local flaps, the procedure is to be added as an additional separate procedure.

15342   **Application of bilaminate skin substitute/neodermis; 25 sq cm**
> Consult CPT code 15000 for initial wound preparation for these procedures.

+ 15343   **each additional 25 sq cm (List separately in addition to code for primary procedure)**
> Note that 15343 is an add-on code and must be used in conjunction with 15342.

15350   **Application of allograft, skin; 100 sq cm or less**
> If a staged tissue graft is implanted, append modifier -58 or 09958.

+ 15351   **each additional 100 sq cm (List separately in addition to code for primary procedure)**
> Note that 15351 is an add-on code and must be used in conjunction with 15350.

15400   **Application of xenograft, skin; 100 sq cm or less**
> If the flap is microvascular, consult CPT codes 15756-15758.

+ 15401   **each additional 100 sq cm (List separately in addition to code for primary procedure)**
> Note that 15401 is an add-on code and must be used in conjunction with 15400.

FLAPS (SKIN AND/OR DEEP TISSUES)

If your physician is attaching the flap in transfer or to a final site, select these codes by recipient site. If the physician is forming a tube for later or there will be a delay of the flap, report these codes by donor site.

If repair of the donor site requires skin grafts or local flaps, code as an additional procedure.

If the flap is microvascular, consult CPT codes 15756-15758.

15570   **Formation of direct or tubed pedicle, with or without transfer; trunk**

15572   **scalp, arms, or legs**

15574   **forehead, cheeks, chin, mouth, neck, axillae, genitalia, hands or feet**

15576   **eyelids, nose, ears, lips, or intraoral**

15600   **Delay of flap or sectioning of flap (division and inset); at trunk**

15610   **at scalp, arms, or legs**

15620   **at forehead, cheeks, chin, neck, axillae, genitalia, hands (except 15625), or feet**

15630   **at eyelids, nose, ears, or lips**

15650   **Transfer, intermediate, of any pedicle flap (eg, abdomen to wrist, Walking tube), any location**
> If the transfer is performed on the eyelids, nose, ears, or lips, consult also the anatomical area.
>
> If a pedical flap or skin graft is revised, defatted, or rearranged, consult CPT codes 13100-14300.

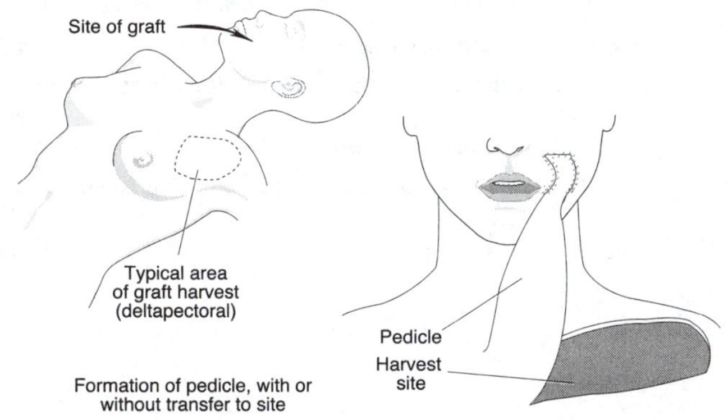

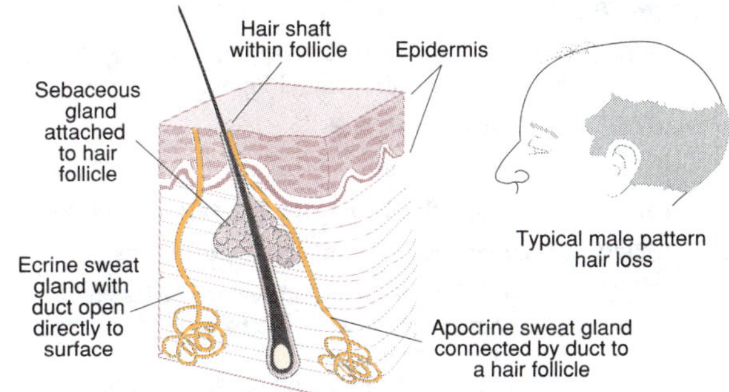

Alopecia means hair loss and the condition is separated into two major categories: that which occurs with associated, visable scalp disease, and that which occurs in the absence of visible disease. Male and female pattern hair loss is of the latter category. Hirsutism is excess hair growth, particularly in women, and is often a sign of a systemic medical syndrome

▲ **15732**   **Muscle, myocutaneous, or fasciocutaneous flap; head and neck (eg, temporalis, masseter muscle, sternocleidomastoid, levator scapulae)**
> If the flap is microvascular, consult CPT codes 15756-15758.
>
> These procedures are described by the donor site of the muscle, myocutaneous, or fasciocutaneous flap.

15734   **trunk**
> If the flap is microvascular, consult CPT codes 15756-15758.
>
> These procedures are described by the donor site of the muscle, myocutaneous, or fasciocutaneous flap.

15736   **upper extremity**
> If the flap is microvascular, consult CPT codes 15756-15758.
>
> These procedures are described by the donor site of the muscle, myocutaneous, or fasciocutaneous flap.

15738   **lower extremity**
> If the flap is microvascular, consult CPT codes 15756-15758.
>
> These procedures are described by the donor site of the muscle, myocutaneous, or fasciocutaneous flap.

OTHER FLAPS AND GRAFTS

If repair of the donor site requires skin grafts or local flaps, code as an additional procedure.

15740   **Flap; island pedicle**

15750   **neurovascular pedicle**

15756   **Free muscle flap with or without skin with microvascular anastomosis**
> Do not report 69990 in addition to code 15756 as the operating microscope is considered an inclusive component of the surgery.

15757   **Free skin flap with microvascular anastomosis**
> Do not report 69990 in addition to code 15757 as the operating microscope is considered an inclusive component of the surgery.

15758   **Free fascial flap with microvascular anastomosis**
> Do not report 69990 in addition to code 15758 as the operating microscope is considered an inclusive component of the surgery.

15760   **Graft; composite (eg, full thickness of external ear or nasal ala), including primary closure, donor area**

15770   **derma-fat-fascia**

15775   **Punch graft for hair transplant; 1 to 15 punch grafts**

15776   **more than 15 punch grafts**
> If the procedure is a strip transplant, consult CPT code 15220.

Integumentary System

15780 — 15935

OTHER PROCEDURES

15780   **Dermabrasion; total face (eg, for acne scarring, fine wrinkling, rhytids, general keratosis)**   80

15781   **segmental, face**

15782   **regional, other than face**   80

15783   **superficial, any site, (eg, tattoo removal)**   80

15786*   **Abrasion; single lesion (eg, keratosis, scar)**

+ 15787   **each additional four lesions or less (List separately in addition to code for primary procedure)**
Note that 15787 is an add-on code and must be used in conjunction with 15786.

15788   **Chemical peel, facial; epidermal**

15789   **dermal**

15792   **Chemical peel, nonfacial; epidermal**   80

15793   **dermal**   80

15810   **Salabrasion; 20 sq cm or less**   80

15811   **over 20 sq cm**   80

15819   **Cervicoplasty**   80

15820   **Blepharoplasty, lower eyelid;**   80   50

15821   **with extensive herniated fat pad**   80   50

15822   **Blepharoplasty, upper eyelid;**   50
Consult also CPT codes 67916, 67917, 67923, and 67924.

15823   **with excessive skin weighting down lid**   50

15824   **Rhytidectomy; forehead**   80   50
If the brow ptosis is repaired, consult CPT code 67900.

15825   **neck with platysmal tightening (platysmal flap, P-flap)**   80   50

15826   **glabellar frown lines**   80   50

15828   **cheek, chin, and neck**   80   50

15829   **superficial musculoaponeurotic system (SMAS) flap**   80   50

15831   **Excision, excessive skin and subcutaneous tissue (including lipectomy); abdomen (abdominoplasty)**   80

15832   **thigh**   80

15833   **leg**   80

15834   **hip**   80

15835   **buttock**   80

15836   **arm**   80

15837   **forearm or hand**   80

15838   **submental fat pad**   80

15839   **other area**   80

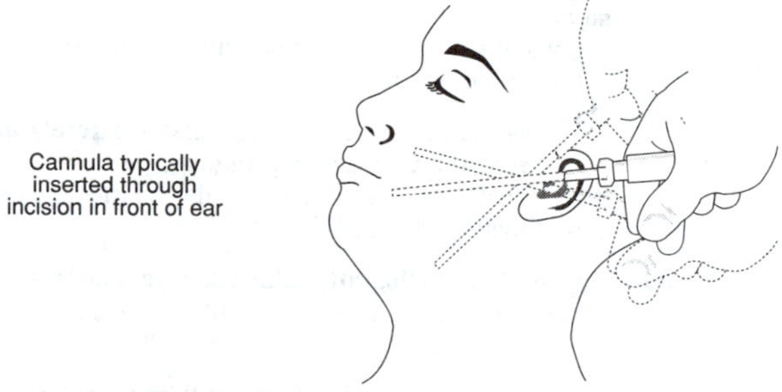

In 15876, a liposuction cannula is inserted through fat deposits creating tunnels and removing excess deposits

15840   **Graft for facial nerve paralysis; free fascia graft (including obtaining fascia)**   ❶
If an intravenous fluorescein examination of blood flow is part of the procedure, consult CPT code 15860. If a nerve is transferred, decompressed, or repaired, consult CPT codes 64831-64876, 64905, 64907, 69720, 69725, 69740, 69745, 69955

15841   **free muscle graft (including obtaining graft)**   ❹ 80

15842   **free muscle flap by microsurgical technique**   ❹ 80
Do not report CPT code 69990 together with 15842.

15845   **regional muscle transfer**   ❹ 80

15850   **Removal of sutures under anesthesia (other than local), same surgeon**

15851   **Removal of sutures under anesthesia (other than local), other surgeon**

15852   **Dressing change (for other than burns) under anesthesia (other than local)**

CIM 45-11 AUTOGENOUS EPIDURAL BLOOD GRAFT

Medicare covers autogenous epidural blood grafts as a remedy for severe headaches that may occur after spinal anesthesia, spinal taps, or myelograms. In the procedure, blood is removed from the patient's vein and injected into the epidural space to seal the leak and stop the pain.

▲ **15860**   **Intravenous injection of agent (eg, fluorescein) to test vascular flow in flap or graft**   80

15876   **Suction assisted lipectomy; head and neck**   80

15877   **trunk**   80

15878   **upper extremity**   80

15879   **lower extremity**   80

PRESSURE ULCERS (DECUBITUS ULCERS)

15920   **Excision, coccygeal pressure ulcer, with coccygectomy; with primary suture**   ❸ 80
If a free skin graft is used to close an ulcer or the donor site, consult CPT code 15000 and subsequent codes.

15922   **with flap closure**   ❹ 80

15931   **Excision, sacral pressure ulcer, with primary suture;**   ❸

15933   **with ostectomy**   ❸ 80

15934   **Excision, sacral pressure ulcer, with skin flap closure;**   ❸

15935   **with ostectomy**   ❹ 80

15936   Excision, sacral pressure ulcer, in preparation for muscle or myocutaneous flap or skin graft closure; ❹☒
> If a defect is repaired using a muscle or a myocutaneous flap, consult CPT code(s) 15734 and/or 15738 in addition to 15936. If a defect is repaired using a split skin graft, consult CPT code(s) 15100 and/or 15101 in addition to 15936.

15937   with ostectomy ❹80☒
> If a defect is repaired using a muscle or a myocutaneous flap, consult CPT code(s) 15734 and/or 15738 in addition to 15937. If a defect is repaired using a split skin graft, consult CPT code(s) 15100 and/or 15101 in addition to 15937.

15940   Excision, ischial pressure ulcer, with primary suture; ❸☒

15941   with ostectomy (ischiectomy) ❸80☒

15944   Excision, ischial pressure ulcer, with skin flap closure; ❸80☒

15945   with ostectomy ❹80☒

15946   Excision, ischial pressure ulcer, with ostectomy, in preparation for muscle or myocutaneous flap or skin graft closure ❹80☒
> If a defect is repaired using a muscle or a myocutaneous flap, consult CPT code(s) 15734 and/or 15738 in addition to 15946. If a defect is repaired using a split skin graft, consult CPT code(s) 15100 and/or 15101 in addition to 15946.

15950   Excision, trochanteric pressure ulcer, with primary suture; ❸☒

15951   with ostectomy ❹80☒

15952   Excision, trochanteric pressure ulcer, with skin flap closure; ❸80☒

15953   with ostectomy ❹☒

15956   Excision, trochanteric pressure ulcer, in preparation for muscle or myocutaneous flap or skin graft closure; ❸☒
> If a defect is repaired using a muscle or a myocutaneous flap, consult CPT code(s) 15734 and/or 15738 in addition to 15956. If a defect is repaired using a split skin graft, consult CPT code(s) 15100 and/or 15101 in addition to 15956.

15958   with ostectomy ❹80☒
> If a defect is repaired using a muscle or a myocutaneous flap, consult CPT code(s) 15734 and/or 15738 in addition to 15958. If a defect is repaired using a split skin graft, consult CPT code(s) 15100 and/or 15101 in addition to 15958.
>
> If a free skin graft is used to close an ulcer or the donor site, consult CPT code 15000 and subsequent codes.

15999   Unlisted procedure, excision pressure ulcer 80
> If a free skin graft is used to close an ulcer or the donor site, consult CPT code 15000 and subsequent codes.

BURNS, LOCAL TREATMENT

CPT codes 16000-16036 identify local treatment of burned surface only. For management of burn patients (e.g., prolonged detention, hospital visits) and related medical services, consult appropriate services in the Medicine or Evaluation and Management Chapters.

CIM 45-12 PORCINE SKIN AND GRADIENT PRESSURE DRESSINGS

Porcine (pig) skin dressings are covered as an occlusive dressing for burns, donor sites of a homograft, and decubiti and other ulcers. Gradient pressure dressings are Jobst elasticized heavy-duty dressings used to reduce hypertrophic scarring and joint contractures following burn injury. They are covered when used for that purpose.

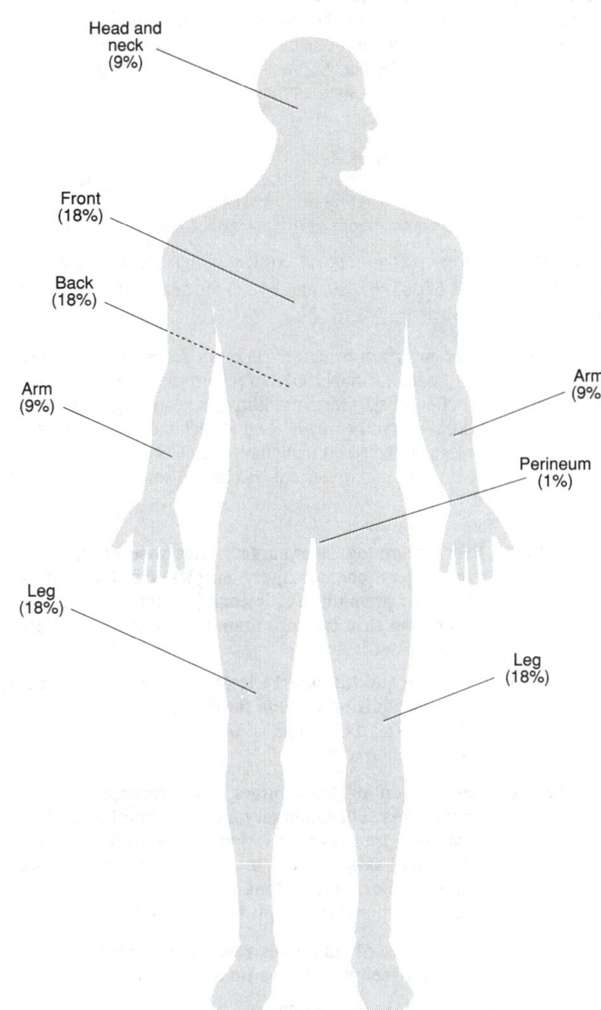

Rule of Nines for Burns

16000   Initial treatment, first degree burn, when no more than local treatment is required ☒
> If a skin graft is performed, consult CPT codes 15100-15650.

16010   Dressings and/or debridement, initial or subsequent; under anesthesia, small ☒

16015   under anesthesia, medium or large, or with major debridement ❷☒

16020*   without anesthesia, office or hospital, small ☒

16025*   without anesthesia, medium (eg, whole face or whole extremity) ☒

16030   without anesthesia, large (eg, more than one extremity) ❶☒

16035   Escharotomy; initial incision ❷☒
> If a debridement, curettement of burn wound is performed, consult CPT codes 16010-16030.

+ 16036   each additional incision (List separately in addition to code for primary procedure)
> If a skin graft is performed, consult CPT codes 15100-15650.
>
> If a debridement, curettement of burn wound is performed, consult CPT codes 16010-16030.
>
> Note that 16036 is an add-on code and must be used in conjunction with 16035.

☒ CCI Comprehensive Code   50 Bilateral Procedure   + CPT Add-on Code   ⊘ Modifier -51 Exempt Code   ● New Code   ▲ Revised Code

M Maternity   N Newborn   P Pediatric   N/P Newborn/Pediatric

Integumentary System

17000* — 17999

DESTRUCTION

BENIGN OR PREMALIGNANT LESIONS

Lesion destruction is performed by the use of chemicals, cryotherapy, laser and other methods, including curettement. These procedures usually do not require closure. Lesions can be benign, such as warts, premalignant, such as actinic kerartoses, or malignant, such as melanoma.

CIM 35-52 LASER PROCEDURES

Coverage is determined on the basis that the use of lasers to alter, revise, or destroy tissue is a surgical procedure and restricted to practitioners with training in the surgical management of the disease or condition being treated.

Consult CPT codes 40820, 46900-46917, 46924, 54050-54057, 54065, 56501, 56515, 57061, 57065, 67850, and 68135 for destruction of lesion(s) of specified anatomical sites.

To report the paring or cutting of benign hyperkeratotic lesions (e.g., corns or calluses), consult CPT codes 11055-11057. To report sharp removal or electrosurgical destruction of skin tags and fibrocutaneous tags, consult CPT codes 11200 and 11201. If cryotherapy is used for acne, consult CPT code 17340. If destruction is performed on malignant skin lesions, consult CPT codes 17260-17286. If epidermal or dermal lesions are shaved, consult CPT codes 11300-11313.

▲ **17000*** **Destruction (eg, laser surgery, electrosurgery, cryosurgery, chemosurgery, surgical curettement), all benign or premalignant lesions (eg, actinic keratoses) other than skin tags or cutaneous vascular proliferative lesions; first lesion**

+ **17003** **second through 14 lesions, each (List separately in addition to code for first lesion)**
Note that 17003 is and add-on code and must be used in conjunction with 17000.

▲ ⃠ **17004** **Destruction (eg, laser surgery, electrosurgery, cryosurgery, chemosurgery, surgical curettement), all benign or premalignant lesions (eg, actinic keratoses) other than skin tags or cutaneous vascular proliferative lesions; 15 or more lesions**
Do not report 17004 with 17000-17003.

17106 **Destruction of cutaneous vascular proliferative lesions (eg, laser technique); less than 10 sq cm**

17107 **10.0 - 50.0 sq cm**

17108 **over 50.0 sq cm**

▲ **17110*** **Destruction (eg, laser surgery, electrosurgery, cryosurgery, chemosurgery, surgical curettement), of flat warts, molluscum contagiosum, or milia; up to 14 lesions**

17111 **15 or more lesions**
For the destruction of common or plantar warts, consult CPT codes 17000, 17003, and 17004.

17250* **Chemical cauterization of granulation tissue (proud flesh, sinus or fistula)**

MALIGNANT LESIONS, ANY METHOD

CIM 35-52 LASER PROCEDURES

Coverage is determined on the basis that the use of lasers to alter, revise, or destroy tissue is a surgical procedure and restricted to practitioners with training in the surgical management of the disease or condition being treated.

Consult CPT codes 40820, 46900-46917, 46924, 54050-54057, 54065, 56501, 56515, 57061, 57065, 67850, and 68135 for destruction of lesion(s) of specified anatomical sites.

To report the paring or cutting of benign hyperkeratotic lesions (e.g., corns or calluses), consult CPT codes 11055-11057. To report sharp removal or electrosurgical destruction of skin tags and fibrocutaneous tags, consult CPT codes 11200 and 11201. If cryotherapy is used for acne, consult CPT code 17340. If destruction is performed on malignant skin lesions, consult CPT codes 17260-17286. If epidermal or dermal lesions are shaved, consult CPT codes 11300-11313.

▲ **17260*** **Destruction, malignant lesion (eg, laser surgery, electrosurgery, cryosurgery, chemosurgery, surgical curettement), trunk, arms or legs; lesion diameter 0.5 cm or less**

17261 **lesion diameter 0.6 to 1.0 cm**

17262 **lesion diameter 1.1 to 2.0 cm**

17263 **lesion diameter 2.1 to 3.0 cm**

17264 **lesion diameter 3.1 to 4.0 cm**

17266 **lesion diameter over 4.0 cm**

▲ **17270*** **Destruction, malignant lesion (eg, laser surgery, electrosurgery, cryosurgery, chemosurgery, surgical curettement), scalp, neck, hands, feet, genitalia; lesion diameter 0.5 cm or less**

17271 **lesion diameter 0.6 to 1.0 cm**

17272 **lesion diameter 1.1 to 2.0 cm**

17273 **lesion diameter 2.1 to 3.0 cm**

17274 **lesion diameter 3.1 to 4.0 cm**

17276 **lesion diameter over 4.0 cm**

▲ **17280*** **Destruction, malignant lesion (eg, laser surgery, electrosurgery, cryosurgery, chemosurgery, surgical curettement), face, ears, eyelids, nose, lips, mucous membrane; lesion diameter 0.5 cm or less**

17281 **lesion diameter 0.6 to 1.0 cm**

17282 **lesion diameter 1.1 to 2.0 cm**

17283 **lesion diameter 2.1 to 3.0 cm**

17284 **lesion diameter 3.1 to 4.0 cm**

17286 **lesion diameter over 4.0 cm**

MOHS' MICROGRAPHIC SURGERY

If a single physician is not acting as both the surgeon and the pathologist for these procedures, this group of CPT codes should not be used. When repair is performed, consult appropriate CPT codes for the type of repair (e.g., graft, wound repair). If this is an initiation or a follow-up care of topical chemotherapy (eg, 5-FU or similar agents), consult appropriate office visits.

⃠ **17304** **Chemosurgery (Mohs' micrographic technique), including removal of all gross tumor, surgical excision of tissue specimens, mapping, color coding of speci-mens, microscopic examination of specimens by the surgeon, and complete histopathologic preparation; first stage, fresh tissue technique, up to 5 specimens**

⃠ **17305** **second stage, fixed or fresh tissue, up to 5 specimens**

⃠ **17306** **third stage, fixed or fresh tissue, up to 5 specimens**

⃠ **17307** **additional stage(s), up to 5 specimens, each stage**

⃠ **17310** **more than 5 specimens, fixed or fresh tissue, any stage**

OTHER PROCEDURES

17340* **Cryotherapy (CO2 slush, liquid N2) for acne**

17360* **Chemical exfoliation for acne (eg, acne paste, acid)**

17380* **Electrolysis epilation, each 1/2 hour**
If this procedure includes actinotherapy, consult CPT code 96900.

17999 **Unlisted procedure, skin, mucous membrane and subcutaneous tissue**

BREAST

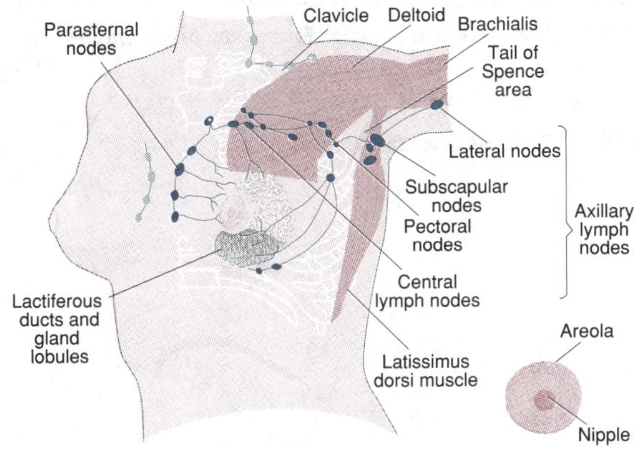

INCISION

19000*   **Puncture aspiration of cyst of breast;**   ⊡ 50

+ 19001   **each additional cyst (List separately in addition to code for primary procedure)**   50

Note that 19001 is an add-on code and must be used in conjunction with 19000.

To report imaging guidance, consult CPT codes76095, 76096, 76393, 76942.

19020   **Mastotomy with exploration or drainage of abscess, deep**   ❷ ⊡ 50

19030   **Injection procedure only for mammary ductogram or galactogram**   ⊡ 50

If radiological supervision and interpretation is performed, consult CPT codes 76086 and 76088.

EXCISION

19100   **Biopsy of breast; percutaneous, needle core, not using imaging guidance (separate procedure)**   ❶ ⊡ 50

To report fine needle aspiration, consult CPT code 10021.

To report image guided breast biopsy, consult CPT codes 19102, 19103, 10022.

19101   **open, incisional**   ❷ ⊡ 50

19102   **percutaneous, needle core, using imaging guidance**   50

For placement of percutaneous localization clip, report 19295 in conjunction with 19102.

To report the radiologic guidance in conjunction with a breast biopsy, consult CPT codes 76095, 76096, 76360, 76393, and 76942.

19103   **percutaneous, automated vacuum assisted or rotating biopsy device, using imaging guidance**   50

To report the radiologic guidance in conjunction with a breast biopsy, consult CPT codes 76095, 76096, 76360, 76393, and 76942.

For placement of percutaneous localization clip, report 19295 in conjunction with 19103.

19110   **Nipple exploration, with or without excision of a solitary lactiferous duct or a papilloma lactiferous duct**   ❷ ⊡ 50

19112   **Excision of lactiferous duct fistula**   ❸ 80 ⊡ 50

19120   **Excision of cyst, fibroadenoma, or other benign or malignant tumor aberrant breast tissue, duct lesion, nipple or areolar lesion (except 19140), open, male or female, one or more lesions**   ❸ ⊡ 50

19125   **Excision of breast lesion identified by preoperative placement of radiological marker, open; single lesion**   ❸ ⊡ 50

+ 19126   **each additional lesion separately identified by a preoperative radiological marker (List separately in addition to code for primary procedure)**   ❸

Note that 19126 is an add-on code and must be used in conjunction with 19125.

19140   **Mastectomy for gynecomastia**   ♂ ❹ ⊡ 50

19160   **Mastectomy, partial;**   ❸ 80 ⊡ 50

19162   **with axillary lymphadenectomy**   ❼ 80 ⊡ 50

19180   **Mastectomy, simple, complete**   ❹ 80 ⊡ 50

For immediate or delayed implant insertion, consult CPT code 19340 or 19342. If the mastectomy is for gynecomastia, consult CPT code 19140.

19182   **Mastectomy, subcutaneous**   ❹ 80 ⊡ 50

19200   **Mastectomy, radical, including pectoral muscles, axillary lymph nodes**   80 ⊡ 50

Halsted mastectomy

19220   **Mastectomy, radical, including pectoral muscles, axillary and internal mammary lymph nodes (Urban type operation)**   80 ⊡ 50

19240   **Mastectomy, modified radical, including axillary lymph nodes, with or without pectoralis minor muscle, but excluding pectoralis major muscle**   80 ⊡ 50

Patey's mastectomy

19260   **Excision of chest wall tumor including ribs**   ❻ 80 ⊡

19271   **Excision of chest wall tumor involving ribs, with plastic reconstruction; without mediastinal lymphadenectomy**   80 ⊡

19272   **with mediastinal lymphadenectomy**   80 ⊡

INTRODUCTION

19290   **Preoperative placement of needle localization wire, breast;**   ❶ ⊡ 50

For radiological supervision and interpretation, consult CPT codes 76095, 76096, 76942.

+ 19291   **each additional lesion (List separately in addition to code for primary procedure)**   ❶ 80

Note that 19291 is an add-on code and must be used in conjunction with 19290.

For radiological supervision and interpretation, consult CPT codes 76095, 76096, 76942.

+ 19295   **Image guided placement, metallic localization clip, percutaneous, during breast biopsy (List separately in addition to code for primary procedure)**   80

Code 19102 or 19103 for biopsy in addition to 19295.

⊡ CCI Comprehensive Code   50 Bilateral Procedure   + CPT Add-on Code   ⊘ Modifier -51 Exempt Code   ● New Code   ▲ Revised Code

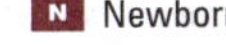 M Maternity   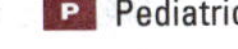 N Newborn   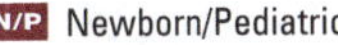 P Pediatric   N/P Newborn/Pediatric

Integumentary System

19316 — 19499

REPAIR AND/OR RECONSTRUCTION

19316	**Mastopexy**	80 ↩ 50
19318	**Reduction mammaplasty**	④ 80 ↩ 50
	Aries-Pitanguy mammaplasty	

19324   **Mammaplasty, augmentation; without prosthetic implant**   80 ↩ 50

> If a flap or graft is needed, consult also appropriate number.

19325   **with prosthetic implant**   80 ↩ 50

> Consult CPT code 99070 for supply of implant.
> If a flap or graft is needed, consult also appropriate number.

19328	**Removal of intact mammary implant**	❶ ↩ 50
19330	**Removal of mammary implant material**	❶ ↩ 50

<u>CIM 35-47 BREAST RECONSTRUCTION FOLLOWING MASTECTOMY</u>

(Cosmetic surgery is excluded from coverage under §1862(a)(l0) of the Social Security Act.)

Reconstruction of the affected and the contralateral unaffected breast following a medically necessary mastectomy is considered a relatively safe and effective noncosmetic procedure. Accordingly, program payment may be made for breast reconstruction surgery following removal of a breast for any medical reason. Program payment may not be made for breast reconstruction for cosmetic reasons.

19340   **Immediate insertion of breast prosthesis following mastopexy, mastectomy or in reconstruction**   ❷ 50

> Consult CPT code 99070 for supply of implant. If a custom breast implant is prepared, consult CPT code 19396.

19342   **Delayed insertion of breast prosthesis following mastopexy, mastectomy or in reconstruction**   ❸ 80 ↩ 50

> Consult CPT code 99070 for supply of implant. If a custom breast implant is prepared, consult CPT code 19396.

19350	**Nipple/areola reconstruction**	④ ↩ 50
19355	**Correction of inverted nipples**	80 ↩ 50

19357   **Breast reconstruction, immediate or delayed, with tissue expander, including subsequent expansion**   ❺ 80 ↩ 50

19361   **Breast reconstruction with latissimus dorsi flap, with or without prosthetic implant**   80 ↩ 50

19364   **Breast reconstruction with free flap**   ❺ 80 ↩ 50

> Do not report 69990 in addition to code 19364 as the operating microscope is considered an inclusive component of the surgery. Note that 19364 includes harvesting of the flap, microvascular transfer, closure of the donor site, and inset shaping the flap into a breast.

19366   **Breast reconstruction with other technique**   ❺ 80 ↩ 50

> If an operating microscope is used, consult CPT code 69990. If a prostheses is inserted, consult also CPT code 19340 or 19342.

19367   **Breast reconstruction with transverse rectus abdominis myocutaneous flap (TRAM), single pedicle, including closure of donor site;**   80 ↩ 50

19368   **with microvascular anastomosis (supercharging)**   80 ↩ 50

> Do not report 69990 in addition to code 19368 as the operating microscope is considered an inclusive component of the surgery.

19369   **Breast reconstruction with transverse rectus abdominis myocutaneous flap (TRAM), double pedicle, including closure of donor site**   80 ↩ 50

19370   **Open periprosthetic capsulotomy, breast**   ④ ↩ 50

19371	**Periprosthetic capsulectomy, breast**	④ ↩ 50
19380	**Revision of reconstructed breast**	❺ ↩ 50
19396	**Preparation of moulage for custom breast implant**	
		80 ↩ 50

OTHER PROCEDURES

19499   **Unlisted procedure, breast**   80 50

MUSCULOSKELETAL SYSTEM

Codes listed in the Musculoskeletal chapter include the application and removal of the first cast or traction device. Replacement of casts and/or traction devices subsequent to the first should be reported separately. CPT codes for other additional procedures, such as obtaining grafts and external fixation, should only be used if the procedure is not already listed as included as part of the basic procedure. Consult the glossary for additional terms and guidelines.

GENERAL

INCISION

20000* Incision of soft tissue abscess (eg, secondary to osteomyelitis); superficial

20005   deep or complicated

WOUND EXPLORATION - TRAUMA (EG, PENETRATING GUNSHOT, STAB WOUND)

Use these codes to describe the physician's surgical treatment of a traumatic penetrating wound resulting from knives, guns, or other sources. The physician may explore or enlarge the wound, dissect the wound to determine penetration, remove foreign bodies, debridement, and repair minor blood vessels. When a thoracotomy or laparotomy is necessary to repair major structures or blood vessels, the code for that procedure is used instead of the 20100-20103 series.

20100 Exploration of penetrating wound (separate procedure); neck

20101   chest

20102   abdomen/flank/back

20103   extremity

EXCISION

20150 Excision of epiphyseal bar, with or without autogenous soft tissue graft obtained through same fascial incision

     If bone marrow is aspirated, consult CPT code 38220.

20200 Biopsy, muscle; superficial

     If excision of a muscle tumor, deep, is included, consult specific anatomical section.

20205   deep

20206* Biopsy, muscle, percutaneous needle

     To report imaging guidance, consult CPT codes 76360, 76393, 76942.

     To report fine needle aspiration, consult CPT codes 10021 or 10022.

     To report evaluation of fine needle aspirate, consult CPT codes 88172-88173.

CIM 50-44 BONE (MINERAL) DENSITY STUDIES

Medicare covers the following bone (mineral) density studies

1. Single Photon Absorptiometry - A non-invasive radiological technique that provides a quantitative measurement of the bone mineral of cortical and trabecular bone, and is used in assessing an individual's treatment response at appropriate intervals. Medicare covers when used in assessing changes in bone density of patients with osteodystrophy or osteoporosis performed on the same individual at intervals of 6 to 12 months.

2. Bone Biopsy - A physiologic test used in ascertaining a differential diagnosis of bone disorders and is used primarily to differentiate osteomalacia from osteoporosis. Bone biopsy is covered under Medicare when used for the qualitative evaluation of bone no more than four times per patient, unless there is special justification given.

3. Photodensitometry (radiographic absorptiometry) - A noninvasive radiological procedure that provides a quantitative measurement of the bone mineral of cortical bone, and is used for monitoring gross bone change.

20220 Biopsy, bone, trocar, or needle; superficial (eg, ilium, sternum, spinous process, ribs)

▲ **20225**   deep (eg, vertebral body, femur)

     If bone marrow is biopsied, consult CPT code 38221.

     To report radiologic supervision and interpretation, consult CPT codes 76003, 76360, 76393.

20240 Biopsy, bone, excisional; superficial (eg, ilium, sternum, spinous process, ribs, trochanter of femur)

     If sequestrectomy, osteomyelitis, or drainage of a bone abscess is needed, consult appropriate anatomical area.

20245   deep (eg, humerus, ischium, femur)

20250 Biopsy, vertebral body, open; thoracic

20251   lumbar or cervical

INTRODUCTION OR REMOVAL

If an injection procedure for arthrography is performed, consult appropriate anatomical area.

20500* Injection of sinus tract; therapeutic (separate procedure)

20501*   diagnostic (sinogram)

     To report radiologic supervision and interpretation, consult CPT code 76080.

20520* Removal of foreign body in muscle or tendon sheath; simple

20525   deep or complicated

● **20526** Injection, therapeutic (eg, local anesthetic, corticosteroid), carpal tunnel

▲ **20550*** Injection; tendon sheath, ligament, ganglion cyst

     To report imaging guidance, consult CPT codes 76003, 76393, 76942.

● **20551**   tendon origin/insertion

● **20552**   single or multiple trigger point(s), one or two muscle group(s)

● **20553**   single or multiple trigger point(s), three or more muscle groups

20600* Arthrocentesis, aspiration and/or injection; small joint, bursa or ganglion cyst (eg, fingers, toes)

20605*   intermediate joint, bursa or ganglion cyst (eg, temporomandibular, acromioclavicular, wrist, elbow or ankle, olecranon bursa)

20610*   major joint or bursa (eg, shoulder, hip, knee joint, subacromial bursa)

     To report imaging guidance, consult CPT codes 76003, 76350, 76393, 76942.

20615 Aspiration and injection for treatment of bone cyst

20650* Insertion of wire or pin with application of skeletal traction, including removal (separate procedure)

⊘ **20660** Application of cranial tongs, caliper, or stereotactic frame, including removal (separate procedure)

20661 Application of halo, including removal; cranial

20662   pelvic

20663   femoral

20664 Application of halo, including removal, cranial, 6 or more pins placed, for thin skull osteology (eg, pediatric patients, hydrocephalus, osteogenesis imperfecta), requiring general anesthesia

20665* Removal of tongs or halo applied by another physician

Musculoskeletal System

20670* — 20973

	20670*	Removal of implant; superficial, (eg, buried wire, pin or rod) (separate procedure)
	20680	deep (eg, buried wire, pin, screw, metal band, nail, rod or plate)
⊘	**20690**	Application of a uniplane (pins or wires in one plane), unilateral, external fixation system
⊘	**20692**	Application of a multiplane (pins or wires in more than one plane), unilateral, external fixation system (eg, Ilizarov, Monticelli type)
	20693	Adjustment or revision of external fixation system requiring anesthesia (eg, new pin(s) or wire(s) and/or new ring(s) or bar(s))
	20694	Removal, under anesthesia, of external fixation system

REPLANTATION

	20802	Replantation, arm (includes surgical neck of humerus through elbow joint), complete amputation
	20805	Replantation, forearm (includes radius and ulna to radial carpal joint), complete amputation
	20808	Replantation, hand (includes hand through metacarpophalangeal joints), complete amputation
	20816	Replantation, digit, excluding thumb (includes metacarpophalangeal joint to insertion of flexor sublimis tendon), complete amputation
	20822	Replantation, digit, excluding thumb (includes distal tip to sublimis tendon insertion), complete amputation
	20824	Replantation, thumb (includes carpometacarpal joint to MP joint), complete amputation
	20827	Replantation, thumb (includes distal tip to MP joint), complete amputation
	20838	Replantation, foot, complete amputation

GRAFTS (OR IMPLANTS)

If spinal surgery bone graft(s) is needed, consult CPT codes 20930-20938. If needle aspiration of bone marrow for the purpose of bone grafting is needed, consult CPT code 38220. Do not report modifier -62 with any codes in range 20900-20938.

⊘	**20900**	Bone graft, any donor area; minor or small (eg, dowel or button)
⊘	**20902**	major or large
⊘	**20910**	Cartilage graft; costochondral
⊘	**20912**	nasal septum
⊘	**20920**	Fascia lata graft; by stripper
⊘	**20922**	by incision and area exposure, complex or sheet
⊘	**20924**	Tendon graft, from a distance (eg, palmaris, toe extensor, plantaris)
⊘	**20926**	Tissue grafts, other (eg, paratenon, fat, dermis)
⊘	**20930**	Allograft for spine surgery only; morselized
		Note that 20930-20938 are reported in addition to the code for the definitive procedure(s) without modifier -51. Only one bone graft procedure can be reported per operative session.
⊘	**20931**	structural
⊘	**20936**	Autograft for spine surgery only (includes harvesting the graft); local (eg, ribs, spinous process, or laminar fragments) obtained from same incision

⊘	**20937**	morselized (through separate skin or fascial incision)
		If bone marrow needle aspiration is needed for the purpose of bone grafting, consult CPT code 38220.
⊘	**20938**	structural, bicortical or tricortical (through separate skin or fascial incision)
		If bone marrow needle aspiration is needed for the purpose of bone grafting, consult CPT code 38220.

OTHER PROCEDURES

	20950	Monitoring of interstitial fluid pressure (includes insertion of device, eg, wick catheter technique, needle manometer technique) in detection of muscle compartment syndrome
	20955	Bone graft with microvascular anastomosis; fibula
		Do not report 69990 in addition to codes 20955-20962 as the operating microscope is considered an inclusive component of these procedures.
	20956	iliac crest
	20957	metatarsal
	20962	other than fibula, iliac crest, or metatarsal
	20969	Free osteocutaneous flap with microvascular anastomosis; other than iliac crest, metatarsal, or great toe
		Do not report 69990 in addition to codes 20969-20973 as the operating microscope is considered an inclusive component of these procedures.
	20970	iliac crest
	20972	metatarsal
	20973	great toe with web space
		If a great toe wrap-around procedure is completed, consult CPT code 26551.

CIM 35-48 OSTEOGENIC STIMULATION

Electrical stimulation to augment bone repair can be either invasive or noninvasive. Invasive devices provide electrical stimulation directly at the fracture site either through percutaneously placed cathodes or by implanting a coiled cathode wire into the fracture site.

The noninvasive stimulator device is covered only for the following indications:

- Nonunion of long bone fractures

- Failed fusion, where a minimum of nine months has elapsed since the last surgery

- Congenital pseudarthroses

- As an adjunct to spinal fusion surgery for patients at high risk of pseudarthrosis due to previously failed spinal fusion at the same site or for those undergoing multiple level fusion. A multiple level fusion involves three or more vertebrae (e.g., L3-L5, L4-S1, etc)

The invasive stimulator device is covered only for the following indications:

- Nonunion of long bone fractures

- As an adjunct to spinal fusion surgery for patients at high risk of pseudarthrosis due to previously failed spinal fusion at the same site or for those undergoing multiple level fusion

Effective for services performed on or after April 1, 2000, nonunion of long bone fractures, for both noninvasive and invasive devices, is considered to exist only when serial radiographs have confirmed that fracture healing has ceased for three or more months prior to starting treatment with the electrical osteogenic stimulator. Serial radiographs must include a minimum of two sets of radiographs, each including multiple views of the fracture site, separated by a minimum of 90 days.

Medicare does not cover ultrasonic osteogenic stimulators.

| ⊘ | **20974** | **Electrical stimulation to aid bone healing; noninvasive (nonoperative)** | ▣ |
| ⊘ | **20975** | **invasive (operative)** | ❷ 80 ▣ |

CIM 50-7 ULTRASOUND DIAGNOSTIC PROCEDURES

Medicare coverage is extended to the procedures listed in Category I. Techniques in Category II are considered experimental and should not be covered at this time.

Category I (covered, may be adjunct to radiologic and nuclear medicine diagnostic technique)

1. Echoencephalography, (Diencephalic Midline) (A-Mode)
2. Echoencephalography, Complete (Diencephalic Midline and Ventricular Size)
3. Ocular and Orbital Echography (A-Mode) (includes determining the suitability of aphakic patients for an artificial lens implant following cataract surgery)
4. Ocular and Orbital Sonography (B-Mode)
5. Echocardiography, Pericardial Effusion (M-Mode)
6. Pericardiocentesis, by Ultrasonic Guidance
7. Echocardiography, Cardiac Valve(s) (M-Mode)
8. Echocardiography, Complete (M-Mode)
9. Echocardiography, limited (e.g., follow-up or limited study) (M-Mode)
10. Pleural Effusion Echography
11. Thoracentesis, by Ultrasonic Guidance
12. Abdominal Sonography, complete survey study (B-Scan)
13. Abdominal Sonography, limited (e.g., follow-up or limited study) (B-Scan)
14. Renal Cyst Aspiration, by Ultrasonic Guidance
15. Renal Biopsy, by Ultrasonic Guidance
16. Pancreas Sonography (B-Scan)
17. Spleen Sonography (B-Scan)
18. Abdominal Aorta Echography (A-Mode)
19. Abdominal Aorta Sonography (B-Scan)
20. Retroperitoneal Sonography (B-Scan)
21. Retroperitoneal sonography does not include planning of fields for radiation therapy.
22. Urinary Bladder Sonography (B-Scan)
23. Urinary bladder sonography does not include staging of bladder tumors.
24. Pregnancy Diagnosis sonography (B-Scan)
25. Fetal Age Determination (Biparietal Diameter) Sonography (B-Scan)
26. Fetal Growth Rate Sonography (B-Scan)
27. Placenta Localization Sonography (B-Scan)
28. Pregnancy Sonography, Complete (B-Scan)
29. Molar Pregnancy Diagnosis Sonography (B-Scan)
30. Ectopic Pregnancy Diagnosis sonography (B-Scan)
31. Passive Testing (Antepartum Monitoring of Fetal Heart Rate In the Resting Fetus)
32. Intrauterine Contraceptive Device Sonography (B-Scan)
33. Pelvic Mass Diagnosis Sonography (B-Scan)
34. Amniocentesis, by Ultrasonic Guidance
35. Arterial Flow Study, Peripheral (Doppler)
36. Venous Flow Study, Peripheral (Doppler)
37. Arterial Aneurysm, Peripheral (B-Scan)
38. Radiation Therapy Planning Sonography (B-Scan)
39. Thyroid Echography (A-Mode)
40. Thyroid Sonography (B-Scan)
41. Breast Echography (A-Mode)
42. Breast Sonography (B-Scan)
43. Hepatic Sonography (B-Scan)
44. Gallbladder Sonography
45. Renal Sonography
46. Two-Dimensional Echocardiography (B-Mode)

Category II (clinical reliability and efficacy not proven)

1. B-Scan for atherosclerotic narrowing of peripheral arteries
2. Monitoring of cardiac output (Doppler)

When appropriate, new uses for ultrasound diagnostic procedures should be forwarded to the Bureau of Eligibility, Reimbursement and Coverage, HCFA, so that revisions may be made in the coverage policy when appropriate.

| | **20979** | **Low intensity ultrasound stimulation to aid bone healing, noninvasive (nonoperative)** | |
| | **20999** | **Unlisted procedure, musculoskeletal system, general** | 80 |

HEAD

Codes listed in the Musculoskeletal chapter include the application and removal of the first cast or traction device. Replacement of casts and/or traction devices subsequent to the first should be reported separately. CPT codes for other additional procedures, such as obtaining grafts and external fixation, should only be used if the procedure is not already listed as included as part of the basic procedure. Consult the glossary for additional terms and guidelines.

This section includes the skull, facial bones and the temporomandibular joint.

INCISION

21010   **Arthrotomy, temporomandibular joint**   ❷ 80 ▣ 50
If a superficial abscess and hematoma is drained, consult CPT code 20000. If an embedded foreign body is removed from the dentoalveolar structure, consult CPT codes 41805 and 41806.

EXCISION

21015   **Radical resection of tumor (eg, malignant neoplasm), soft tissue of face or scalp**   ▣
If only a biopsy is done, consult CPT codes 20220 and 20240.

21025   **Excision of bone (eg, for osteomyelitis or bone abscess); mandible**   ❷ ▣

21026   **facial bone(s)**   ❷ ▣

21029   **Removal by contouring of benign tumor of facial bone (eg, fibrous dysplasia)**   80 ▣

21030   **Excision of benign tumor or cyst of facial bone other than mandible**   ▣

21031   **Excision of torus mandibularis**   ▣

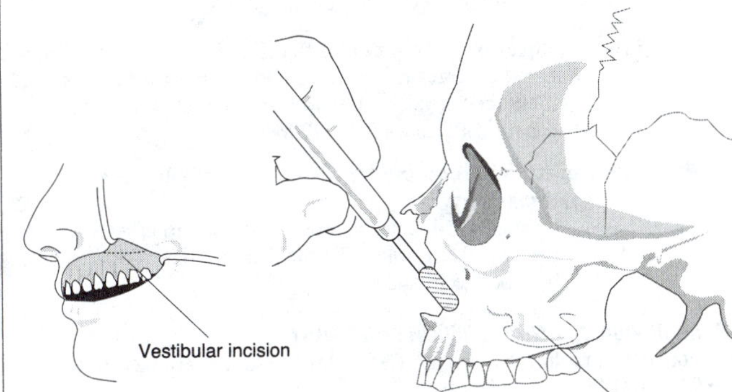

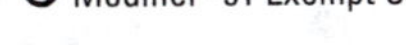

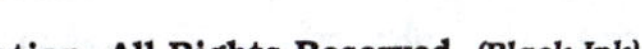

| ▣ CCI Comprehensive Code | 50 Bilateral Procedure | ✚ CPT Add-on Code | ⊘ Modifier -51 Exempt Code | ● New Code | ▲ Revised Code |
| M Maternity | | N Newborn | | P Pediatric | N/P Newborn/Pediatric |

21032	**Excision of maxillary torus palatinus**	
21034	**Excision of malignant tumor of facial bone other than mandible**	③ 80
21040	**Excision of benign cyst or tumor of mandible; simple**	❷
21041	**complex**	❷
21044	**Excision of malignant tumor of mandible;**	❷ 80
21045	**radical resection**	80

If a bone graft is done, consult CPT code 21215.

| 21050 | **Condylectomy, temporomandibular joint (separate procedure)** | ③ 80 50 |

If only a biopsy is done, consult CPT codes 20220 and 20240.

| 21060 | **Meniscectomy, partial or complete, temporomandibular joint (separate procedure)** | ❷ 80 50 |
| 21070 | **Coronoidectomy (separate procedure)** | ③ 80 50 |

INTRODUCTION OR REMOVAL

Codes listed in the Musculoskeletal chapter include the application and removal of the first cast or traction device. Replacement of casts and/or traction devices subsequent to the first should be reported separately. CPT codes for other additional procedures, such as obtaining grafts and external fixation, should only be used if the procedure is not already listed as included as part of the basic procedure. Consult the glossary for additional terms and guidelines.

CPT codes 21076-21089 are reported only if the physician (not an outside lab) actually designs, prepares, and supplies the prosthesis.

21076	**Impression and custom preparation; surgical obturator prosthesis**	80
21077	**orbital prosthesis**	80 50
21079	**interim obturator prosthesis**	
21080	**definitive obturator prosthesis**	
21081	**mandibular resection prosthesis**	80
21082	**palatal augmentation prosthesis**	80
21083	**palatal lift prosthesis**	80
21084	**speech aid prosthesis**	80
21085	**oral surgical splint**	80
21086	**auricular prosthesis**	80 50
21087	**nasal prosthesis**	80
21088	**facial prosthesis**	80
21089	**Unlisted maxillofacial prosthetic procedure**	
21100*	**Application of halo type appliance for maxillofacial fixation, includes removal (separate procedure)**	❷ 80

If application or removal of caliper or tongs is performed, consult CPT codes 20660 and 20665.

| 21110 | **Application of interdental fixation device for conditions other than fracture or dislocation, includes removal** | |

If another physician removes an interdental fixation, consult CPT codes 20670-20680.

| 21116 | **Injection procedure for temporomandibular joint arthrography** | |

If radiological supervision and interpretation is performed, consult CPT code 70332. Code 76003 cannot be reported in addition to 70332.

REPAIR, REVISION, AND/OR RECONSTRUCTION

If cranioplasty is performed, consult CPT codes 21179, 21180, 62116, 62120, and 62140-62147.

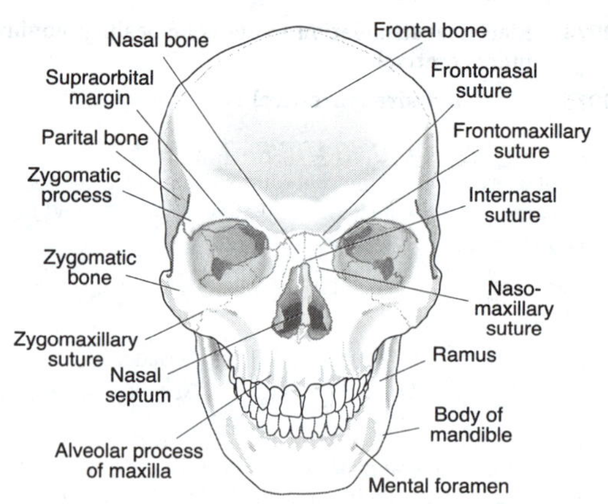

21120	**Genioplasty; augmentation (autograft, allograft, prosthetic material)**	
21121	**sliding osteotomy, single piece**	80
21122	**sliding osteotomies, two or more osteotomies (eg, wedge excision or bone wedge reversal for asymmetrical chin)**	80
21123	**sliding, augmentation with interpositional bone grafts (includes obtaining autografts)**	80
21125	**Augmentation, mandibular body or angle; prosthetic material**	80
21127	**with bone graft, onlay or interpositional (includes obtaining autograft)**	80
21137	**Reduction forehead; contouring only**	80
21138	**contouring and application of prosthetic material or bone graft (includes obtaining autograft)**	80
21139	**contouring and setback of anterior frontal sinus wall**	80
21141	**Reconstruction midface, LeFort 1; single piece, segment movement in any direction (eg, for Long Face Syndrome), without bone graft**	80
21142	**two pieces, segment movement in any direction, without bone graft**	80
21143	**three or more pieces, segment movement in any direction, without bone graft**	80
21145	**single piece, segment movement in any direction, requiring bone grafts (includes obtaining autografts)**	80
21146	**two pieces, segment movement in any direction, requiring bone grafts (includes obtaining autografts) (eg, ungrafted unilateral alveolar cleft)**	80

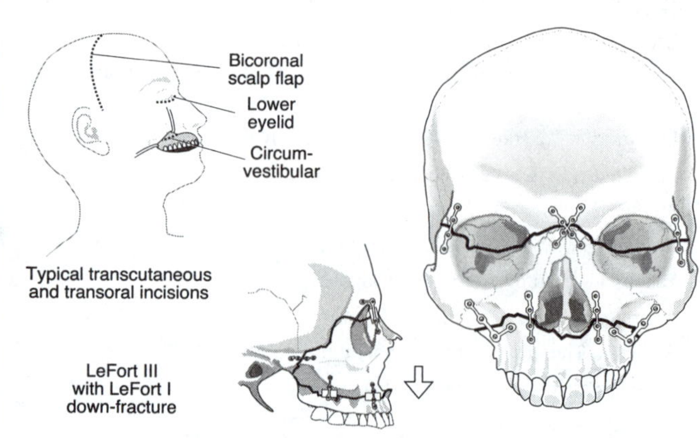

| 26 Professional Component Only | 80/80 Assist-at-Surgery Allowed/With Documentation | **Unlisted** | Commonly Miscoded | Not Covered |
| TC Technical Component Only | **MCM & CIM** Medicare References | ❶❷❸❹❺❻❼❽ ASC Group | ♂ Male Only | ♀ Female Only |

21147	three or more pieces, segment movement in any direction, requiring bone grafts (includes obtaining autografts) (eg, ungrafted bilateral alveolar cleft or multiple osteotomies) 80
21150	Reconstruction midface, LeFort II; anterior intrusion (eg, Treacher-Collins Syndrome) 80
21151	any direction, requiring bone grafts (includes obtaining autografts) 80
21154	Reconstruction midface, LeFort III (extracranial), any type, requiring bone grafts (includes obtaining autografts); without LeFort I 80
21155	with LeFort I 80
21159	Reconstruction midface, LeFort III (extra and intracranial) with forehead advancement (eg, mono bloc), requiring bone grafts (includes obtaining autografts); without LeFort I 80
21160	with LeFort I 80
21172	Reconstruction superior-lateral orbital rim and lower forehead, advancement or alteration, with or without grafts (includes obtaining autografts) 80

If frontal or parietal craniotomy is performed for craniosynostosis, consult CPT code 61556.

21175	Reconstruction, bifrontal, superior-lateral orbital rims and lower forehead, advancement or alteration (eg, plagiocephaly, trigonocephaly, brachycephaly), with or without grafts (includes obtaining autografts) 80

If bifrontal craniotomy is performed for craniosynostosis, consult CPT code 61557.

21179	Reconstruction, entire or majority of forehead and/or supraorbital rims; with grafts (allograft or prosthetic material) 80
21180	with autograft (includes obtaining grafts) 80

If an extensive craniectomy for multiple suture craniosynostosis is performed, consult CPT code 61558 or 61559.

21181	Reconstruction by contouring of benign tumor of cranial bones (eg, fibrous dysplasia), extracranial 80
▲ 21182	Reconstruction of orbital walls, rims, forehead, nasoethmoid complex following intra- and extracranial excision of benign tumor of cranial bone (eg, fibrous dysplasia), with multiple autografts (includes obtaining grafts); total area of bone grafting less than 40 sq cm 80
▲ 21183	total area of bone grafting greater than 40 sq cm but less than 80 sq cm 80
▲ 21184	total area of bone grafting greater than 80 sq cm 80

If a benign tumor of the cranial bones is excised, consult CPT codes 61563 and 61564.

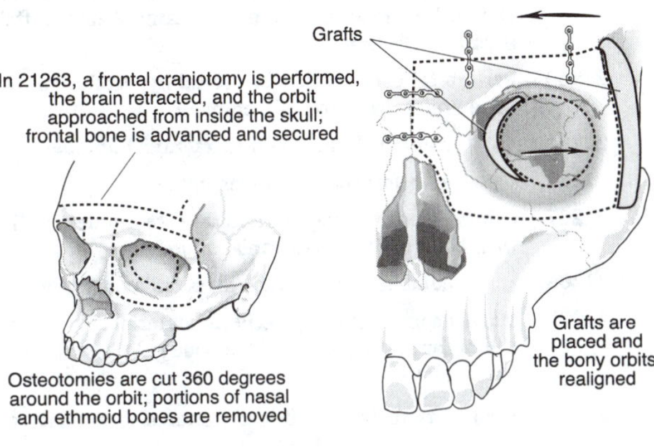

21188	Reconstruction midface, osteotomies (other than LeFort type) and bone grafts (includes obtaining autografts) 80
21193	Reconstruction of mandibular rami, horizontal, vertical, C, or L osteotomy; without bone graft 80
21194	with bone graft (includes obtaining graft) 80
21195	Reconstruction of mandibular rami and/or body, sagittal split; without internal rigid fixation 80
21196	with internal rigid fixation 80
21198	Osteotomy, mandible, segmental; 80
21199	with genioglossus advancement 80
21206	Osteotomy, maxilla, segmental (eg, Wassmund or Schuchard) 5 80
21208	Osteoplasty, facial bones; augmentation (autograft, allograft, or prosthetic implant) 7 80
21209	reduction 5 80
21210	Graft, bone; nasal, maxillary or malar areas (includes obtaining graft) 7

If the cleft palate is repaired, consult CPT codes 42200-42225.

21215	mandible (includes obtaining graft) 7
21230	Graft; rib cartilage, autogenous, to face, chin, nose or ear (includes obtaining graft) 7 80
21235	ear cartilage, autogenous, to nose or ear (includes obtaining graft) 7
21240	Arthroplasty, temporomandibular joint, with or without autograft (includes obtaining graft) 4 80 50
21242	Arthroplasty, temporomandibular joint, with allograft 5 80 50
21243	Arthroplasty, temporomandibular joint, with prosthetic joint replacement 5 80 50
21244	Reconstruction of mandible, extraoral, with transosteal bone plate (eg, mandibular staple bone plate) 7 80
21245	Reconstruction of mandible or maxilla, subperiosteal implant; partial 7 80
21246	complete 7 80
21247	Reconstruction of mandibular condyle with bone and cartilage autografts (includes obtaining grafts) (eg, for hemifacial microsomia) 80
21248	Reconstruction of mandible or maxilla, endosteal implant (eg, blade, cylinder); partial 7
21249	complete 7 80
21255	Reconstruction of zygomatic arch and glenoid fossa with bone and cartilage (includes obtaining autografts) 80

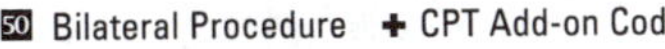

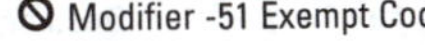

Musculoskeletal System

21256 — 21436

21256	Reconstruction of orbit with osteotomies (extracranial) and with bone grafts (includes obtaining autografts) (eg, micro-ophthalmia)
21260	Periorbital osteotomies for orbital hypertelorism, with bone grafts; extracranial approach
21261	combined intra- and extracranial approach
21263	with forehead advancement
21267	Orbital repositioning, periorbital osteotomies, unilateral, with bone grafts; extracranial approach
21268	combined intra- and extracranial approach
21270	Malar augmentation, prosthetic material

If malar augmentation with a bone graft is performed, consult CPT code 21210.

21275	Secondary revision of orbitocraniofacial reconstruction
21280	Medial canthopexy (separate procedure)

If medial canthoplasty is performed, consult CPT code 67950.

21282	Lateral canthopexy
21295	Reduction of masseter muscle and bone (eg, for treatment of benign masseteric hypertrophy); extraoral approach
21296	intraoral approach

OTHER PROCEDURES

21299	Unlisted craniofacial and maxillofacial procedure

FRACTURE AND/OR DISLOCATION

21300	Closed treatment of skull fracture without operation

If operative repair is needed, consult CPT codes 62000-62010.

21310	Closed treatment of nasal bone fracture without manipulation
21315*	Closed treatment of nasal bone fracture; without stabilization
21320	with stabilization
21325	Open treatment of nasal fracture; uncomplicated
21330	complicated, with internal and/or external skeletal fixation
21335	with concomitant open treatment of fractured septum
21336	Open treatment of nasal septal fracture, with or without stabilization
21337	Closed treatment of nasal septal fracture, with or without stabilization
21338	Open treatment of nasoethmoid fracture; without external fixation
21339	with external fixation
21340	Percutaneous treatment of nasoethmoid complex fracture, with splint, wire or headcap fixation, including repair of canthal ligaments and/or the nasolacrimal apparatus
21343	Open treatment of depressed frontal sinus fracture
21344	Open treatment of complicated (eg, comminuted or involving posterior wall) frontal sinus fracture, via coronal or multiple approaches
21345	Closed treatment of nasomaxillary complex fracture (LeFort II type), with interdental wire fixation or fixation of denture or splint
21346	Open treatment of nasomaxillary complex fracture (LeFort II type); with wiring and/or local fixation
21347	requiring multiple open approaches
21348	with bone grafting (includes obtaining graft)
21355*	Percutaneous treatment of fracture of malar area, including zygomatic arch and malar tripod, with manipulation
21356	Open treatment of depressed zygomatic arch fracture (eg, Gilles approach)
21360	Open treatment of depressed malar fracture, including zygomatic arch and malar tripod
21365	Open treatment of complicated (eg, comminuted or involving cranial nerve foramina) fracture(s) of malar area, including zygomatic arch and malar tripod; with internal fixation and multiple surgical approaches
21366	with bone grafting (includes obtaining graft)
21385	Open treatment of orbital floor blowout fracture; transantral approach (Caldwell-Luc type operation)
21386	periorbital approach
21387	combined approach
21390	periorbital approach, with alloplastic or other implant
21395	periorbital approach with bone graft (includes obtaining graft)
21400	Closed treatment of fracture of orbit, except blowout; without manipulation
21401	with manipulation
21406	Open treatment of fracture of orbit, except blowout; without implant
21407	with implant
21408	with bone grafting (includes obtaining graft)
21421	Closed treatment of palatal or maxillary fracture (LeFort I type), with interdental wire fixation or fixation of denture or splint
21422	Open treatment of palatal or maxillary fracture (LeFort I type);
21423	complicated (comminuted or involving cranial nerve foramina), multiple approaches
21431	Closed treatment of craniofacial separation (LeFort III type) using interdental wire fixation of denture or splint
21432	Open treatment of craniofacial separation (LeFort III type); with wiring and/or internal fixation
21433	complicated (eg, comminuted or involving cranial nerve foramina), multiple surgical approaches
21435	complicated, utilizing internal and/or external fixation techniques (eg, head cap, halo device, and/or intermaxillary fixation)

If an internal or an external fixation device is removed, consult CPT code 20670.

21436	complicated, multiple surgical approaches, internal fixation, with bone grafting (includes obtaining graft)

---

26 Professional Component Only	**80**/**80** Assist-at-Surgery Allowed/With Documentation	Unlisted
TC Technical Component Only	**MCM & CIM** Medicare References **❶❷❸❹❺❻❼❽** ASC Group	Commonly Miscoded Not Covered

♂ Male Only   ♀ Female Only

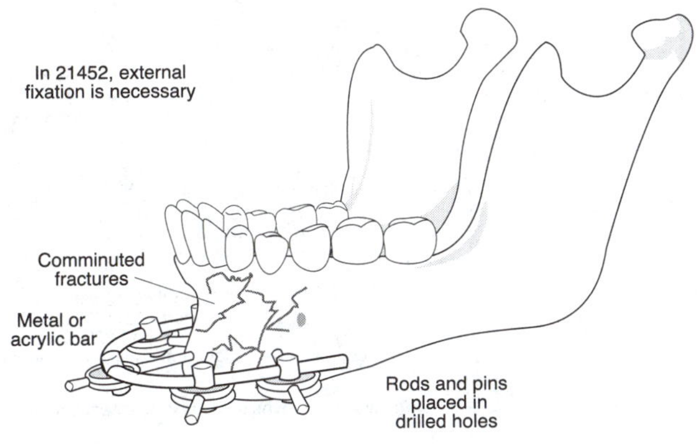

21440 Closed treatment of mandibular or maxillary alveolar ridge fracture (separate procedure)

21445 Open treatment of mandibular or maxillary alveolar ridge fracture (separate procedure

21450 Closed treatment of mandibular fracture; without manipulation

21451   with manipulation

21452 Percutaneous treatment of mandibular fracture, with external fixation

21453 Closed treatment of mandibular fracture with interdental fixation

21454 Open treatment of mandibular fracture with external fixation

21461 Open treatment of mandibular fracture; without interdental fixation

21462   with interdental fixation

21465 Open treatment of mandibular condylar fracture

21470 Open treatment of complicated mandibular fracture by multiple surgical approaches including internal fixation, interdental fixation, and/or wiring of dentures or splints

21480 Closed treatment of temporomandibular dislocation; initial or subsequent

21485   complicated (eg, recurrent requiring intermaxillary fixation or splinting), initial or subsequent

21490 Open treatment of temporomandibular dislocation

If interdental wire is fixated, consult CPT code 21497.

21493 Closed treatment of hyoid fracture; without manipulation

21494   with manipulation

21495 Open treatment of hyoid fracture
If the larynx is fractured, consult CPT codes 31584-31586.

21497 Interdental wiring, for condition other than fracture

OTHER PROCEDURES

21499 Unlisted musculoskeletal procedure, head
If a craniofacial or a maxillofacial procedure is unlisted, consult CPT code 21299.

NECK (SOFT TISSUES) AND THORAX

If these procedures are being performed on the cervical spine and back, consult CPT codes 21920. If an injection is needed at the fracture site or trigger point, consult CPT code 20550.

INCISION

If a superficial abscess or hematoma is incised and drained, consult CPT codes 10060 and 10140.

21501 Incision and drainage, deep abscess or hematoma, soft tissues of neck or thorax;

21502   with partial rib ostectomy

21510 Incision, deep, with opening of bone cortex (eg, for osteomyelitis or bone abscess), thorax

EXCISION

If a needle biopsy of soft tissue is performed, consult CPT code 20206.

If bone biopsy is performed, consult CPT codes 20220-20251.

21550 Biopsy, soft tissue of neck or thorax

21555 Excision tumor, soft tissue of neck or thorax; subcutaneous

21556   deep, subfascial, intramuscular

21557 Radical resection of tumor (eg, malignant neoplasm), soft tissue of neck or thorax

21600 Excision of rib, partial
If a radical resection for a tumor is performed, consult CPT code 19260.
If a radical debridement due to injury is performed, consult CPT codes 11040-11044.

21610 Costotransversectomy (separate procedure)

21615 Excision first and/or cervical rib;

21616   with sympathectomy

21620 Ostectomy of sternum, partial

21627 Sternal debridement
If both debridement and closure are performed, consult CPT code 21750.

21630 Radical resection of sternum;

21632   with mediastinal lymphadenectomy

REPAIR, REVISION, AND/OR RECONSTRUCTION

If the wound is superficial, consult the Integumentary System section under Repair, Simple.

21700 Division of scalenus anticus; without resection of cervical rib

21705   with resection of cervical rib

21720 Division of sternocleidomastoid for torticollis, open operation; without cast application
If nerve transection is performed consult CPT codes 63191, 64722.

21725   with cast application

21740 Reconstructive repair of pectus excavatum or carinatum

▲ **21750** Closure of median sternotomy separation with or without debridement (separate procedure)

FRACTURE AND/OR DISLOCATION

21800 Closed treatment of rib fracture, uncomplicated, each

21805 Open treatment of rib fracture without fixation, each

Musculoskeletal System

21810 — 22328

21810	Treatment of rib fracture requiring external fixation (flail chest)	❷ 80 ↴
21820	Closed treatment of sternum fracture	❶ ↴
21825	Open treatment of sternum fracture with or without skeletal fixation	80 ↴

If the sternoclavicular is dislocated, consult CPT codes 23520-23532.

OTHER PROCEDURES

| 21899 | Unlisted procedure, neck or thorax | 80 |

BACK AND FLANK, EXCISION

| 21920 | Biopsy, soft tissue of back or flank; superficial | ❶ ↴ |
| 21925 | deep | ❷ ↴ |

If the soft tissue is in need of a needle biopsy, consult CPT code 20206.

| 21930 | Excision, tumor, soft tissue of back or flank | ❷ ↴ |
| 21935 | Radical resection of tumor (eg, malignant neoplasm), soft tissue of back or flank | ❸ ↴ |

SPINE (VERTEBRAL COLUMN)

EXCISION

For the injection procedure of a myelography, consult CPT code 62284. For the injection procedure of a diskography, consult CPT codes 62290 and 62291. For the injection procedure for chemonucleolysis, single or multiple levels, consult CPT code 62292. For the injection procedure of facet joints, consult CPT codes 64470-64476 and 64622-64627.

22100	Partial excision of posterior vertebral component (eg, spinous process, lamina or facet) for intrinsic bony lesion, single vertebral segment; cervical	❸ 80 ↴
22101	thoracic	❸ 80 ↴
22102	lumbar	❸ 80 ↴
+ 22103	each additional segment (List separately in addition to code for primary procedure)	❸ 80

Note that 22103 is an add-on code and must be used in conjunction with 22100, 22101, 22102.

22110	Partial excision of vertebral body for intrinsic bony lesion, without decompression of spinal cord or nerve root(s), single vertebral segment; cervical	80 ↴
22112	thoracic	80 ↴
22114	lumbar	80 ↴
+ 22116	each additional vertebral segment (List separately in addition to code for primary procedure)	80

Note that 22116 is an add-on code and must be used in conjunction with 22110, 22112 and 22114.

OSTEOTOMY

Codes listed in the Musculoskeletal chapter include the application and removal of the first cast or traction device. Replacement of casts and/or traction devices subsequent to the first should be reported separately. CPT codes for other additional procedures, such as obtaining grafts and external fixation, should only be used if the procedure is not already listed as included as part of the basic procedure. Consult the glossary for additional terms and guidelines.

Additional procedures, such as arthrodesis (CPT codes 22590-22632), bone grafting (CPT codes 20930-20938), and instrumentation (CPT codes 22840-22855), are reported in addition to the CPT codes for the definitive procedure. Do not append modifier -51.

22210	Osteotomy of spine, posterior or posterolateral approach, one vertebral segment; cervical	80 ↴
22212	thoracic	80 ↴
22214	lumbar	80 ↴

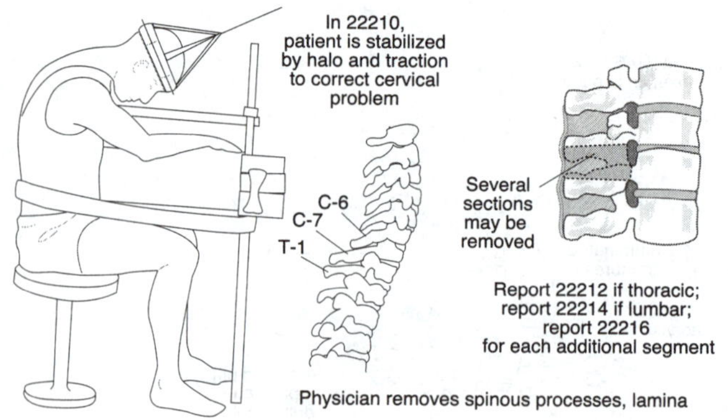

| + 22216 | each additional vertebral segment (List separately in addition to primary procedure) | 80 50 |

Note that 22216 is an add-on code and must be used in conjunction with 22210, 22212, and 22214.

22220	Osteotomy of spine, including diskectomy, anterior approach, single vertebral segment; cervical	80 ↴
22222	thoracic	80 ↴
22224	lumbar	80 ↴
+ 22226	each additional vertebral segment (List separately in addition to code for primary procedure)	80 50

Note that 22226 is an add-on code and must be used in conjunction with 22220, 22222, and 22224.

FRACTURE AND/OR DISLOCATION

For the injection procedure of a myelography, consult CPT code 62284. For the injection procedure of a diskography, consult CPT codes 62290 and 62291. For the injection procedure for chemonucleolysis, single or multiple levels, consult CPT code 62292. For the injection procedure of facet joints, consult CPT codes 64470-64476 and 64622-64627.

22305	Closed treatment of vertebral process fracture(s)	❶ ↴
22310	Closed treatment of vertebral body fracture(s), without manipulation, requiring and including casting or bracing	❶ ↴
22315	Closed treatment of vertebral fracture(s) and/or dislocations(s) requiring casting or bracing, with and including casting and/or bracing, with or without anesthesia, by manipulation or traction	❷ ↴

If spinal subluxation is performed, consult CPT code 97140.

22318	Open treatment and/or reduction of odontoid fracture(s) and or dislocation(s) (including os odontoideum), anterior approach, including placement of internal fixation; without grafting	80 ↴
22319	with grafting	80 ↴
22325	Open treatment and/or reduction of vertebral fracture(s) and/or dislocation(s); posterior approach, one fractured vertebrae or dislocated segment; lumbar	❸ 80 ↴
22326	cervical	❸ 80 ↴
22327	thoracic	❸ 80 ↴
+ 22328	each additional fractured vertebrae or dislocated segment (List separately in addition to code for primary procedure)	❸ 80

Note that 22328 is an add-on code and must be used in conjunction with 22325, 22326, and 22327.

    CPT only © 2001 American Medical Association. All Rights Reserved. *(Black Ink)*   ©**2001 INGENIX, Inc.** *(Blue Ink)*

MANIPULATION

Codes listed in the Musculoskeletal chapter include the application and removal of the first cast or traction device. Replacement of casts and/or traction devices subsequent to the first should be reported separately. CPT codes for other additional procedures, such as obtaining grafts and external fixation, should only be used if the procedure is not already listed as included as part of the basic procedure. Consult the glossary for additional terms and guidelines.

22505 Manipulation of spine requiring anesthesia, any region

VERTEBRAL BODY, EMBOLIZATION OR INJECTION

Codes listed in the Musculoskeletal chapter include the application and removal of the first cast or traction device. Replacement of casts and/or traction devices subsequent to the first should be reported separately. CPT codes for other additional procedures, such as obtaining grafts and external fixation, should only be used if the procedure is not already listed as included as part of the basic procedure. Consult the glossary for additional terms and guidelines.

These CPT codes describe the injection of a fixative into the vertebral body to bond bone fragments.

For radiological supervision and interpretation, consult codes 76012, 76013.

22520 Percutaneous vertebroplasty, one vertebral body, unilateral or bilateral injection; thoracic

22521 lumbar

+ 22522 each additional thoracic or lumbar vertebral body (List separately in addition to code for primary procedure)
> Note that 22522 is an add-on code and must be used in conjunction with 22520 and 22521.

ARTHRODESIS—ANTERIOR OR ANTEROLATERAL APPROACH TECHNIQUE

Codes listed in the Musculoskeletal chapter include the application and removal of the first cast or traction device. Replacement of casts and/or traction devices subsequent to the first should be reported separately. CPT codes for other additional procedures, such as obtaining grafts and external fixation, should only be used if the procedure is not already listed as included as part of the basic procedure. Consult the glossary for additional terms and guidelines.

These codes address surgical approaches to the spine from the front or to the side of the front. CPT codes 22554-22558 are used to report arthrodesis of a single vertebral interspace. Consult CPT code 22585 for additional interspaces. The non-bony compartment between two adjacent vertebral bodies that contain the intervertebral disk, the nucleus pulposus, annulus fibrosus and two cartilagenous endplates is considered the vertebral interspace.

Additional procedures, such as bone grafting (CPT codes 20930-20938) and instrumentation (CPT codes 22840-22855), are reported in addition to the CPT codes for the definitive procedure. Do not append modifier -51.

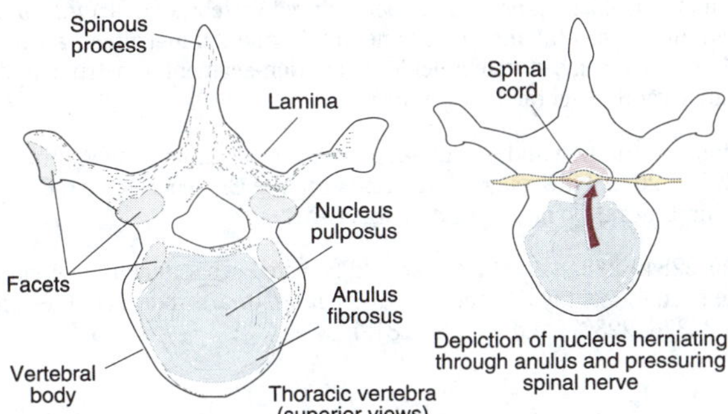

Intervertebral disc displacement and prolapse are major causes of disability among working people. When a disc prolapses, nuclear material bursts through the anulus fibrosus damaging ligaments, nerve roots, and other structures. The herniated matter usually fibroses and shrinks over time

CIM 35-48 OSTEOGENIC STIMULATION

Electrical stimulation to augment bone repair can be either invasive or noninvasive. Invasive devices provide electrical stimulation directly at the fracture site either through percutaneously placed cathodes or by implanting a coiled cathode wire into the fracture site.

The noninvasive stimulator device is covered only for the following indications:

- Nonunion of long bone fractures
- Failed fusion, where a minimum of nine months has elapsed since the last surgery
- Congenital pseudarthroses
- As an adjunct to spinal fusion surgery for patients at high risk of pseudarthrosis due to previously failed spinal fusion at the same site or for those undergoing multiple level fusion. A multiple level fusion involves three or more vertebrae (e.g., L3-L5, L4-S1, etc)

The invasive stimulator device is covered only for the following indications:

- Nonunion of long bone fractures
- As an adjunct to spinal fusion surgery for patients at high risk of pseudarthrosis due to previously failed spinal fusion at the same site or for those undergoing multiple level fusion

Effective for services performed on or after April 1, 2000, nonunion of long bone fractures, for both noninvasive and invasive devices, is considered to exist only when serial radiographs have confirmed that fracture healing has ceased for three or more months prior to starting treatment with the electrical osteogenic stimulator. Serial radiographs must include a minimum of two sets of radiographs, each including multiple views of the fracture site, separated by a minimum of 90 days.

Medicare does not cover ultrasonic osteogenic stimulators.

22548 Arthrodesis, anterior transoral or extraoral technique, clivus-C1-C2 (atlas-axis), with or without excision of odontoid process
> For the injection procedure of a myelography, consult CPT code 62284. For the injection procedure of a diskography, consult CPT codes 62290 and 62291. For the injection procedure for chemonucleolysis, single or multiple levels, consult CPT code 62292. For the injection procedure of facet joints, consult CPT codes 64470-64476 and 64622-64627.

22554 Arthrodesis, anterior interbody technique, including minimal diskectomy to prepare interspace (other than for decompression); cervical below C2

22556 thoracic

22558 lumbar

+ 22585 each additional interspace (List separately in addition to code for primary procedure)
> Note that 22585 is an add-on code and must be used in conjunction with 22554, 22556, and 22558.

ARTHRODESIS—POSTERIOR, POSTEROLATERAL OR LATERAL TRANSVERSE PROCESS TECHNIQUE

Codes listed in the Musculoskeletal chapter include the application and removal of the first cast or traction device. Replacement of casts and/or traction devices subsequent to the first should be reported separately. CPT codes for other additional procedures, such as obtaining grafts and external fixation, should only be used if the procedure is not already listed as included as part of the basic procedure. Consult the glossary for additional terms and guidelines.

These codes address surgical approaches to the spine from the back and side. The non-bony compartment between two adjacent vertebral bodies that contain the intervertebral disk, the nucleus pulposus, annulus fibrosus and two cartilagenous endplates is considered the vertebral interspace.

Additional procedures, such as bone grafting (CPT codes 20930-20938) and instrumentation (CPT codes 22840-22855), are reported in addition to the CPT codes for the definitive procedure. Do not append modifier -51.

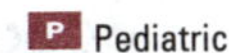

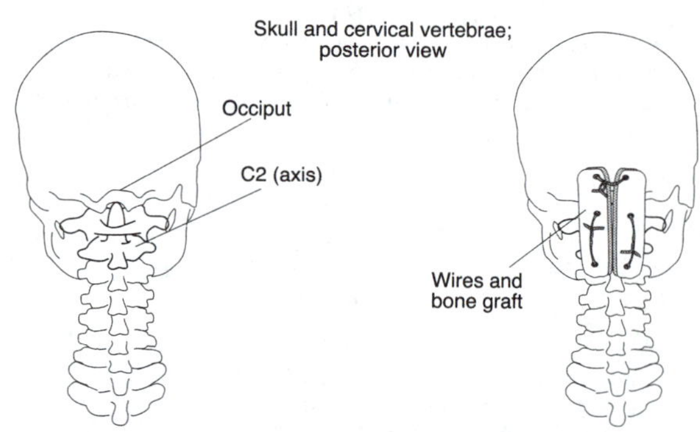

In 22590, the physician fuses skull to C2 (axis) to stabilize cervical vertebrae; anchor holes are drilled in the occiput of the skull

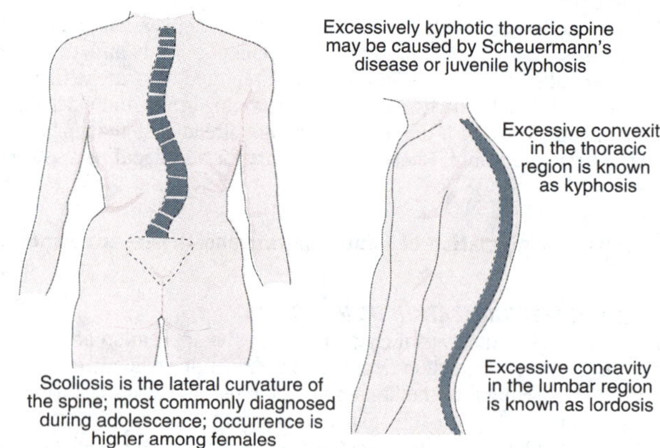

22590   **Arthrodesis, posterior technique, craniocervical (occiput-C2)**   80 ▣

> For the injection procedure of a myelography, consult CPT code 62284. For the injection procedure of a diskography, consult CPT codes 62290 and 62291. For the injection procedure for chemonucleolysis, single or multiple levels, consult CPT code 62292. For the injection procedure of facet joints, consult CPT codes 64470-64476 and 64622-64627.

22595   **Arthrodesis, posterior technique, atlas-axis (C1-C2)**   80 ▣

22600   **Arthrodesis, posterior or posterolateral technique, single level; cervical below C2 segment**   80 ▣

22610   **thoracic (with or without lateral transverse technique)**   80 ▣

22612   **lumbar (with or without lateral transverse technique)**   80 ▣

+ 22614   **each additional vertebral segment (List separately in addition to code for primary procedure)**   80

> Note that 22614 is an add-on code and must be used in conjunction with 22600, 22610, and 22612.

22630   **Arthrodesis, posterior interbody technique, including laminectomy and/or diskectomy to prepare interspace (other than for decompression), single interspace; lumbar**   80 ▣

+ 22632   **each additional interspace (List separately in addition to code for primary procedure)**   80

> Note that 22632 is an add-on code and must be used in conjunction with 22630.

SPINE DEFORMITY (EG, SCOLIOSIS, KYPHOSIS)

Codes listed in the Musculoskeletal chapter include the application and removal of the first cast or traction device. Replacement of casts and/or traction devices subsequent to the first should be reported separately. CPT codes for other additional procedures, such as obtaining grafts and external fixation, should only be used if the procedure is not already listed as included as part of the basic procedure. Consult the glossary for additional terms and guidelines.

Additional procedures, such as bone grafting (CPT codes 20930-20938) and instrumentation (CPT codes 22840-22855), are reported in addition to the CPT codes for the definitive procedure. Do not append modifier -51.

Consult the glossary for additional terms and guidelines.

22800   **Arthrodesis, posterior, for spinal deformity, with or without cast; up to 6 vertebral segments**   80 ▣

22802   **7 to 12 vertebral segments**   80 ▣

22804   **13 or more vertebral segments**   80 ▣

22808   **Arthrodesis, anterior, for spinal deformity, with or without cast; 2 to 3 vertebral segments**   80 ▣

> *Smith-Robinson arthrodesis*

22810   **4 to 7 vertebral segments**   80 ▣

22812   **8 or more vertebral segments**   80 ▣

22818   **Kyphectomy, circumferential exposure of spine and resection of vertebral segment(s) (including body and posterior elements); single or 2 segments**   80 ▣

22819   **3 or more segments**   80 ▣

> If arthrodesis is performed, consult CPT codes 22800-22804 and append modifier -51.

EXPLORATION

22830   **Exploration of spinal fusion**   80 ▣

> For the injection procedure of a myelography, consult CPT code 62284. For the injection procedure of a diskography, consult CPT codes 62290 and 62291. For the injection procedure for chemonucleolysis, single or multiple levels, consult CPT code 62292. For the injection procedure of facet joints, consult CPT codes 64470-64476 and 64622-64627.

SPINAL INSTRUMENTATION

Codes listed in the Musculoskeletal chapter include the application and removal of the first cast or traction device. Replacement of casts and/or traction devices subsequent to the first should be reported separately. CPT codes for other additional procedures, such as obtaining grafts and external fixation, should only be used if the procedure is not already listed as included as part of the basic procedure. Consult the glossary for additional terms and guidelines.

This section describes the instruments affixed to the spine to correct defects resulting from injury or deformity. The instrumentation may correct the spine's anatomic position or help support injured vertebrae. Instrumentation is divided into segmental and non-segmental. Segmental instrumentation connects to each or most vertebra(e) it spans. Non-segmental instrumentation may span several vertebrae between fixation.

Spinal instrumentation and additional procedures, such as bone grafting (CPT codes 20930-20938) are reported in addition to the CPT code(s) for the primary procedure. Do not append modifier -51.

Note that 22840-22848 and 22851 should be listed separately in addition to the code used to identify the fracture, dislocation, or arthrodesis of the spine (22325, 22326, 22327, and 22548-22812).

⊘ **22840** Posterior non-segmental instrumentation (eg, Harrington rod technique, pedicle fixation across one interspace, atlantoaxial transarticular screw fixation, sublaminar wiring at C1, facet screw fixation) 80 ▣

⊘ **22841** Internal spinal fixation by wiring of spinous processes
    Hibb's fusion

⊘ **22842** Posterior segmental instrumentation (eg, pedicle fixation, dual rods with multiple hooks and sublaminal wires); 3 to 6 vertebral segments 80 ▣

⊘ **22843**   7 to 12 vertebral segments 80 ▣

⊘ **22844**   13 or more vertebral segments 80 ▣

⊘ **22845** Anterior instrumentation; 2 to 3 vertebral segments 80 ▣
    Dwyer instrumentation technique

⊘ **22846**   4 to 7 vertebral segments 80 ▣

⊘ **22847**   8 or more vertebral segments 80 ▣
    Dwyer instrumentation technique

⊘ **22848** Pelvic fixation (attachment of caudal end of instrumentation to pelvic bony structures) other than sacrum 80 ▣

22849 Reinsertion of spinal fixation device 80 ▣

22850 Removal of posterior nonsegmental instrumentation (eg, Harrington rod) 80 ▣

⊘ **22851** Application of intervertebral biomechanical device(s) (eg, synthetic cage(s), threaded bone dowel(s), methylmethacrylate) to vertebral defect or interspace 80 ▣

22852 Removal of posterior segmental instrumentation 80 ▣

22855 Removal of anterior instrumentation 80 ▣

OTHER PROCEDURES

22899 Unlisted procedure, spine
80

ABDOMEN

Codes listed in the Musculoskeletal chapter include the application and removal of the first cast or traction device. Replacement of casts and/or traction devices subsequent to the first should be reported separately. CPT codes for other additional procedures, such as obtaining grafts and external fixation, should only be used if the procedure is not already listed as included as part of the basic procedure. Consult the glossary for additional terms and guidelines.

EXCISION

22900 Excision, abdominal wall tumor, subfascial (eg, desmoid) ❹ 80 ▣

OTHER PROCEDURES

22999 Unlisted procedure, abdomen, musculoskeletal system 80

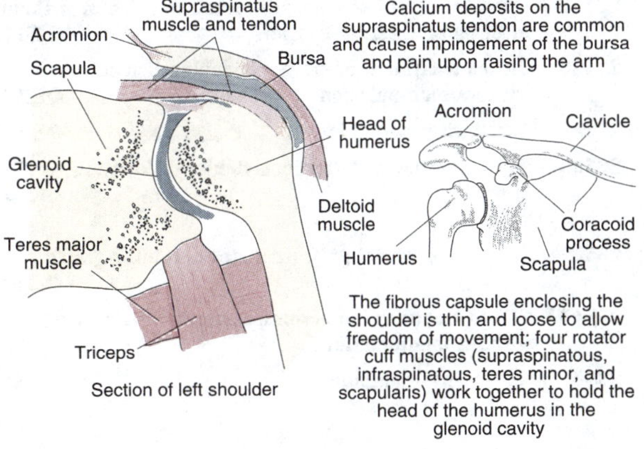

SHOULDER

Codes listed in the Musculoskeletal chapter include the application and removal of the first cast or traction device. Replacement of casts and/or traction devices subsequent to the first should be reported separately. CPT codes for other additional procedures, such as obtaining grafts and external fixation, should only be used if the procedure is not already listed as included as part of the basic procedure. Consult the glossary for additional terms and guidelines.

This section includes the acromioclavicular joint, clavicle, head and neck of the humerus, shoulder joint, and sternoclavicular joint.

INCISION

▲ **23000** Removal of subdeltoid calcareous deposits, open ❷ 80 ▣

23020 Capsular contracture release (eg, Sever type procedure) ❷ 80 ▣ 50
    If superficial incision and drainage is performed, consult CPT codes 10040-10160.

23030 Incision and drainage, shoulder area; deep abscess or hematoma ❶ ▣

23031   infected bursa ▣ 50

23035 Incision, bone cortex (eg, osteomyelitis or bone abscess), shoulder area ❸ 80 ▣ 50

23040 Arthrotomy, glenohumeral joint, including exploration, drainage, or removal of foreign body ❸ 80 ▣ 50

23044 Arthrotomy, acromioclavicular, sternoclavicular joint, including exploration, drainage, or removal of foreign body ❶ ▣ 50

EXCISION

23065 Biopsy, soft tissue of shoulder area; superficial ❶ ▣ 50

23066   deep ❷ ▣ 50
    If a needle biopsy of soft tissue is performed, consult CPT code 20206.

23075 Excision, soft tissue tumor, shoulder area; subcutaneous ❷ ▣ 50

23076   deep, subfascial or intramuscular ❷ ▣ 50

23077 Radical resection of tumor (eg, malignant neoplasm), soft tissue of shoulder area ❸ 80 ▣ 50

23100 Arthrotomy, glenohumeral joint, including biopsy ❷ 80 ▣ 50

23101 Arthrotomy, acromioclavicular joint or sternoclavicular joint, including biopsy and/or excision of torn cartilage ❼ ▣ 50

23105 Arthrotomy; glenohumeral joint, with synovectomy, with or without biopsy ❹ 80 ▣ 50

23106   sternoclavicular joint, with synovectomy, with or without biopsy ❶ ▣ 50

23107 Arthrotomy, glenohumeral joint, with joint exploration, with or without removal of loose or foreign body ❹ 80 ▣ 50

23120 Claviculectomy; partial ❺ 80 ▣
    If performed arthroscopically consult CPT code 29824.
    Mumford claviculectomy

23125   total ❺ 80 ▣ 50

23130 Acromioplasty or acromionectomy, partial, with or without coracoacromial ligament release ❺ ▣ 50

23140 Excision or curettage of bone cyst or benign tumor of clavicle or scapula; ❹ ▣ 50

23145   with autograft (includes obtaining graft) ❺ 80 ▣ 50

23146   with allograft ❺ 80 ▣ 50

Musculoskeletal System

23150 — 23545

23150	Excision or curettage of bone cyst or benign tumor of proximal humerus;	❹ 80 ↔ 50
23155	with autograft (includes obtaining graft)	❻ 80 ↔ 50
23156	with allograft	❻ 80 ↔ 50
23170	Sequestrectomy (eg, for osteomyelitis or bone abscess), clavicle	❷ ↔ 50
23172	Sequestrectomy (eg, for osteomyelitis or bone abscess), scapula	❷ 80 ↔ 50
23174	Sequestrectomy (eg, for osteomyelitis or bone abscess), humeral head to surgical neck	❷ 80 ↔ 50
23180	Partial excision (craterization, saucerization, or diaphysectomy) bone (eg, osteomyelitis), clavicle	❹ ↔ 50
23182	Partial excision (craterization, saucerization, or diaphysectomy) bone (eg, osteomyelitis), scapula	❹ 80 ↔ 50
23184	Partial excision (craterization, saucerization, or diaphysectomy) bone (eg, osteomyelitis), proximal humerus	❹ 80 ↔ 50
23190	Ostectomy of scapula, partial (eg, superior medial angle)	❹ 80 ↔ 50
23195	Resection humeral head	❻ 80 ↔ 50

If replacement is performed with an implant, consult CPT code 23470.

23200	Radical resection for tumor; clavicle	80 ↔ 50
23210	scapula	80 ↔ 50
23220	Radical resection of bone tumor, proximal humerus;	80 ↔ 50
23221	with autograft (includes obtaining graft)	80 ↔ 50
23222	with prosthetic replacement	80 ↔ 50

INTRODUCTION OR REMOVAL

If arthrocentesis or needling of bursa is performed, consult CPT code 20610. If a K-wire or a pin is inserted or removed, consult CPT codes 20650, 20670, and 20680.

If radiological supervision and interpretation is performed, consult CPT code 73040.

Fluoroscopy (76003) is included in 73040, and not reported separately.

If fluoroscopic guided injection is performed for enhanced CT arthrography, use codes 23350, 76003, and 73201 or 73202, for enhanced MR arthrography, use codes 23350, 76003, and 73222 or 73223.

23330	Removal of foreign body, shoulder; subcutaneous	❶ 80 ↔ 50
23331	deep (eg, Neer hemiarthroplasty removal)	❶ 80 ↔ 50
23332	complicated (eg, total shoulder)	80 ↔ 50
▲ 23350	Injection procedure for shoulder arthrography or enhanced CT/MRI shoulder arthrography	↔ 50

REPAIR, REVISION, AND/OR RECONSTRUCTION

23395	Muscle transfer, any type, shoulder or upper arm; single	❻ 80 ↔
23397	multiple	❼ 80 ↔
23400	Scapulopexy (eg, Sprengel's deformity or for paralysis)	❼ 80 ↔ 50
23405	Tenotomy, shoulder area; single tendon	❷ 80 ↔
23406	multiple tendons through same incision	❷ 80 ↔
23410	Repair of ruptured musculotendinous cuff (eg, rotator cuff); acute	❻ 80 ↔
23412	chronic	❼ 80 ↔ 50

| 23415 | Coracoacromial ligament release, with or without acromioplasty | ❻ ↔ 50 |

If performed arthroscopically, consult CPT code 29826.

23420	Reconstruction of complete shoulder (rotator) cuff avulsion, chronic (includes acromioplasty)	❼ 80 ↔ 50
23430	Tenodesis of long tendon of biceps	❹ 80 ↔ 50
23440	Resection or transplantation of long tendon of biceps	❹ 80 ↔ 50
23450	Capsulorrhaphy, anterior; Putti-Platt procedure or Magnuson type operation	❻ 80 ↔ 50

If arthroscopic thermal capsulorrhaphy is performed, use 29999.

| 23455 | with labral repair (eg, Bankart procedure) | ❼ 80 ↔ 50 |

If performed arthroscopically, consult CPT code 29807.

| 23460 | Capsulorrhaphy, anterior, any type; with bone block | ❻ 80 ↔ 50 |

If open thermal capsulorrhaphy is performed, use 23929.

Bristow procedure

| 23462 | with coracoid process transfer | ❼ 80 ↔ 50 |
| 23465 | Capsulorrhaphy, glenohumeral joint, posterior, with or without bone block | ❻ 80 ↔ 50 |

If the sternoclavicular and acromioclavicular are reconstructed, consult CPT codes 23530 and 23550.

23466	Capsulorrhaphy, glenohumeral joint, any type multi-directional instability	❼ 80 ↔ 50
23470	Arthroplasty, glenohumeral joint; hemiarthroplasty	80 ↔ 50
23472	total shoulder (glenoid and proximal humeral replacement (eg, total shoulder))	80 ↔ 50

If the total shoulder implant is removed, consult CPT codes 23331 and 23332. If an osteotomy on the proximal humerus is performed, consult CPT code 24400.

23480	Osteotomy, clavicle, with or without internal fixation;	❹ ↔ 50
23485	with bone graft for nonunion or malunion (includes obtaining graft and/or necessary fixation)	❼ 80 ↔ 50
23490	Prophylactic treatment (nailing, pinning, plating or wiring) with or without methylmethacrylate; clavicle	❸ 80 ↔ 50
23491	proximal humerus	❸ 80 ↔ 50

FRACTURE AND/OR DISLOCATION

23500	Closed treatment of clavicular fracture; without manipulation	❶ ↔ 50
23505	with manipulation	❶ ↔ 50
23515	Open treatment of clavicular fracture, with or without internal or external fixation	❸ 80 ↔ 50
23520	Closed treatment of sternoclavicular dislocation; without manipulation	❶ 80 ↔ 50
23525	with manipulation	❶ 80 ↔ 50
23530	Open treatment of sternoclavicular dislocation, acute or chronic;	❸ 80 ↔ 50
23532	with fascial graft (includes obtaining graft)	❹ 80 ↔ 50
23540	Closed treatment of acromioclavicular dislocation; without manipulation	❶ ↔ 50
23545	with manipulation	❶ 80 ↔ 50

23550	Open treatment of acromioclavicular dislocation, acute or chronic; **③ 80 ■ 50**
23552	with fascial graft (includes obtaining graft) **④ 80 ■ 50**
23570	Closed treatment of scapular fracture; without manipulation **❶ ■ 50**
23575	with manipulation, with or without skeletal traction (with or without shoulder joint involvement) **❶ 86 ■ 50**
23585	Open treatment of scapular fracture (body, glenoid or acromion) with or without internal fixation **③ 80 ■ 50**
23600	Closed treatment of proximal humeral (surgical or anatomical neck) fracture; without manipulation **❶ ■ 50**
23605	with manipulation, with or without skeletal traction **❷ ■ 50**
23615	Open treatment of proximal humeral (surgical or anatomical neck) fracture, with or without internal or external fixation, with or without repair of tuberosity(s); **④ 80 ■ 50**
23616	with proximal humeral prosthetic replacement **④ 80 ■ 50**
23620	Closed treatment of greater humeral tuberosity fracture; without manipulation **❶ ■ 50**
23625	with manipulation **❷ ■ 50**
23630	Open treatment of greater humeral tuberosity fracture, with or without internal or external fixation **❺ 80 ■ 50**
23650	Closed treatment of shoulder dislocation, with manipulation; without anesthesia **❶ ■ 50**
23655	requiring anesthesia **❶ ■ 50**
23660	Open treatment of acute shoulder dislocation **③ 80 ■ 50**
	If recurrent dislocations are repaired, consult CPT codes 23450-23466.
23665	Closed treatment of shoulder dislocation, with fracture of greater humeral tuberosity, with manipulation **❷ ■ 50**
23670	Open treatment of shoulder dislocation, with fracture of greater humeral tuberosity, with or without internal or external fixation **③ 80 ■ 50**
23675	Closed treatment of shoulder dislocation, with surgical or anatomical neck fracture, with manipulation **❷ ■ 50**
23680	Open treatment of shoulder dislocation, with surgical or anatomical neck fracture, with or without internal or external fixation **③ 80 ■ 50**

MANIPULATION

23700*	Manipulation under anesthesia, shoulder joint, including application of fixation apparatus (dislocation excluded) **❶ ■**

ARTHRODESIS

23800	Arthrodesis, glenohumeral joint; **④ 80 ■ 50**
23802	with autogenous graft (includes obtaining graft) **❼ 80 ■**

AMPUTATION

23900	Interthoracoscapular amputation (forequarter) **80 ■**
23920	Disarticulation of shoulder; **80 ■**
23921	secondary closure or scar revision **③ ■**

OTHER PROCEDURES

23929	Unlisted procedure, shoulder **80**

HUMERUS (UPPER ARM) AND ELBOW

Codes listed in the Musculoskeletal chapter include the application and removal of the first cast or traction device. Replacement of casts and/or traction devices subsequent to the first should be reported separately. CPT codes for other additional procedures, such as obtaining grafts and external fixation, should only be used if the procedure is not already listed as included as part of the basic procedure. Consult the glossary for additional terms and guidelines.

The elbow is considered to include the olecranon process and the radius's head and neck.

If superficial incision and drainage procedures are performed, consult CPT codes 10040-10160.

INCISION

23930	Incision and drainage, upper arm or elbow area; deep abscess or hematoma **❶ ■ 50**
23931	bursa **❷ ■ 50**
23935	Incision, deep, with opening of bone cortex (eg, for osteomyelitis or bone abscess), humerus or elbow **❷ 80 ■ 50**
24000	Arthrotomy, elbow, including exploration, drainage, or removal of foreign body **④ 80 ■ 50**
24006	Arthrotomy of the elbow, with capsular excision for capsular release (separate procedure) **80 ■ 50**

EXCISION

24065	Biopsy, soft tissue of upper arm or elbow area; superficial **❶ ■ 50**
24066	deep (subfascial or intramuscular) **❷ ■ 50**
	If needle biopsy of soft tissue is performed, consult CPT code 20206.
▲ 24075	Excision, tumor, soft tissue of upper arm or elbow area; subcutaneous **❷ ■ 50**
24076	deep, subfascial or intramuscula **❷ ■ 50**
24077	Radical resection of tumor (eg, malignant neoplasm), soft tissue of upper arm or elbow area **③ 80 ■ 50**
24100	Arthrotomy, elbow; with synovial biopsy only **❶ 80 ■ 50**
24101	with joint exploration, with or without biopsy, with or without removal of loose or foreign body **④ 80 ■ 50**
24102	with synovectomy **④ 80 ■ 50**
24105	Excision, olecranon bursa **③ ■ 50**
24110	Excision or curettage of bone cyst or benign tumor, humerus; **❷ ■ 50**
24115	with autograft (includes obtaining graft) **③ 80 ■ 50**
24116	with allograft **③ 80 ■ 50**
24120	Excision or curettage of bone cyst or benign tumor of head or neck of radius or olecranon process; **③ 80 ■ 50**
24125	with autograft (includes obtaining graft) **③ 80 ■ 50**
24126	with allograft **③ 80 ■ 50**
24130	Excision, radial head **③ ■ 50**
	If replacement is performed with an implant, consult CPT code 24366.
24134	Sequestrectomy (eg, for osteomyelitis or bone abscess), shaft or distal humerus **❷ 80 ■ 50**
24136	Sequestrectomy (eg, for osteomyelitis or bone abscess), radial head or neck **❷ ■ 50**
24138	Sequestrectomy (eg, for osteomyelitis or bone abscess), olecranon process **❷ 80 ■ 50**
24140	Partial excision (craterization, saucerization, or diaphysectomy) bone (eg, osteomyelitis), humerus **③ 80 ■ 50**

24145	Partial excision (craterization, saucerization, or diaphysectomy) bone (eg, osteomyelitis), radial head or neck	❸ 80 ⬚ 50
24147	Partial excision (craterization, saucerization, or diaphysectomy) bone (eg, osteomyelitis), olecranon process	❷ ⬚ 50
24149	Radical resection of capsule, soft tissue, and heterotopic bone, elbow, with contracture release (separate procedure)	80 ⬚ 50

If capsular and soft tissue is released only, consult CPT code 24006.

24150	Radical resection for tumor, shaft or distal humerus;	❸ 80 ⬚ 50
24151	with autograft (includes obtaining graft)	❹ 80 ⬚ 50
24152	Radical resection for tumor, radial head or neck;	❸ 80 ⬚ 50
24153	with autograft (includes obtaining graft)	❹ 80 ⬚ 50
24155	Resection of elbow joint (arthrectomy)	❸ 80 ⬚ 50

INTRODUCTION OR REMOVAL

If a K-wire or a pin is inserted or removed, consult CPT codes 20650, 20670, and 20680. If arthrocentesis or needling of a bursa or a joint is performed, consult CPT code 20605.

24160	Implant removal; elbow joint	❷ ⬚ 50
24164	radial head	❸ ⬚ 50
24200	Removal of foreign body, upper arm or elbow area; subcutaneous	80 ⬚ 50
24201	deep (subfascial or intramuscular)	❷ ⬚ 50
24220	Injection procedure for elbow arthrography	80 ⬚ 50

If radiological supervision and interpretation is performed, consult CPT code 73085. Do not report 76003 in addition to 73085.

If an injection is performed for tennis elbow, consult CPT code 20550.

REPAIR, REVISION, AND/OR RECONSTRUCTION

| ● 24300 | Manipulation, elbow, under anesthesia |

If external fixation is applied, consult CPT codes 20690 or 20692.

24301	Muscle or tendon transfer, any type, upper arm or elbow, single (excluding 24320-24331)	❹ 80 ⬚
24305	Tendon lengthening, upper arm or elbow, each tendon	80 ⬚
24310	Tenotomy, open, elbow to shoulder, each tendon	❸ 80 ⬚
24320	Tenoplasty, with muscle transfer, with or without free graft, elbow to shoulder, single (Seddon-Brookes type procedure)	❸ 80 ⬚
24330	Flexor-plasty, elbow (eg, Steindler type advancement);	❸ 80 ⬚ 50
24331	with extensor advancement	❸ 80 ⬚ 50
● 24332	Tenolysis, triceps	
24340	Tenodesis of biceps tendon at elbow (separate procedure)	❸ 80 ⬚ 50
24341	Repair, tendon or muscle, upper arm or elbow, each tendon or muscle, primary or secondary (excludes rotator cuff)	80 ⬚ 50
24342	Reinsertion of ruptured biceps or triceps tendon, distal, with or without tendon graft	❸ 80 ⬚ 50

● 24343	Repair lateral collateral ligament, elbow, with local tissue	
● 24344	Reconstruction lateral collateral ligament, elbow, with tendon graft (includes harvesting of graft)	
● 24345	Repair medial collateral ligament, elbow, with local tissue	
● 24346	Reconstruction medial collateral ligament, elbow, with tendon graft (includes harvesting of graft)	
24350	Fasciotomy, lateral or medial (eg, tennis elbow or epicondylitis);	❸ 80 ⬚ 50
24351	with extensor origin detachment	❸ 80 ⬚ 50
24352	with annular ligament resection	❸ 80 ⬚ 50
24354	with stripping	❸ ⬚ 50
24356	with partial ostectomy	❸ 80 ⬚ 50
24360	Arthroplasty, elbow; with membrane (eg, fascial)	❺ 80 ⬚ 50
24361	with distal humeral prosthetic replacement	❻ 80 ⬚ 50
24362	with implant and fascia lata ligament reconstruction	❻ 80 ⬚ 50
24363	with distal humerus and proximal ulnar prosthetic replacement (eg, total elbow)	❼ 80 ⬚ 50
24365	Arthroplasty, radial head;	❺ 80 ⬚ 50
24366	with implant	❺ 80 ⬚ 50
24400	Osteotomy, humerus, with or without internal fixation	❹ 80 ⬚ 50
24410	Multiple osteotomies with realignment on intramedullary rod, humeral shaft (Sofield type procedure)	❹ 80 ⬚ 50
24420	Osteoplasty, humerus (eg, shortening or lengthening) (excluding 64876)	❸ 80 ⬚ 50
24430	Repair of nonunion or malunion, humerus; without graft (eg, compression technique)	❸ 80 ⬚ 50
24435	with iliac or other autograft (includes obtaining graft)	❹ 80 ⬚ 50

If a nonunion or malunion repair of the radius and/or ulna is performed, consult CPT codes 25400-25420.

24470	Hemiepiphyseal arrest (eg, cubitus varus or valgus, distal humerus)	❸ 80 ⬚ 50
24495	Decompression fasciotomy, forearm, with brachial artery exploration	❷ 80 ⬚ 50
24498	Prophylactic treatment (nailing, pinning, plating or wiring), with or without methylmethacrylate, humeral shaft	❸ 80 ⬚ 50

FRACTURE AND/OR DISLOCATION

24500	Closed treatment of humeral shaft fracture; without manipulation	❶ ⬚ 50
24505	with manipulation, with or without skeletal traction	❶ ⬚ 50
24515	Open treatment of humeral shaft fracture with plate/screws, with or without cerclage	❹ 80 ⬚ 50
24516	Open treatment of humeral shaft fracture, with insertion of intramedullary implant, with or without cerclage and/or locking screws	❹ 80 ⬚ 50
24530	Closed treatment of supracondylar or transcondylar humeral fracture, with or without intercondylar extension; without manipulation	❶ ⬚ 50
24535	with manipulation, with or without skin or skeletal traction	❶ ⬚ 50

24538	Percutaneous skeletal fixation of supracondylar or transcondylar humeral fracture, with or without intercondylar extension	② ▣ 50
24545	Open treatment of humeral supracondylar or trans-condylar fracture, with or without internal or external fixation; without intercondylar extension	④ 80 ▣ 50
24546	with intercondylar extension	⑤ 80 ▣ 50
24560	Closed treatment of humeral epicondylar fracture, medial or lateral; without manipulation	① ▣ 50
24565	with manipulation	② ▣ 50
24566	Percutaneous skeletal fixation of humeral epicondylar fracture, medial or lateral, with manipulation	② ▣ 50
24575	Open treatment of humeral epicondylar fracture, medial or lateral, with or without internal or external fixation	③ 80 ▣ 50
24576	Closed treatment of humeral condylar fracture, medial or lateral; without manipulation	① ▣ 50
24577	with manipulation	① ▣ 50
24579	Open treatment of humeral condylar fracture, medial or lateral, with or without internal or external fixation	③ 80 ▣ 50
24582	Percutaneous skeletal fixation of humeral condylar fracture, medial or lateral, with manipulation	② ▣ 50
24586	Open treatment of periarticular fracture and/or dislocation of the elbow (fracture distal humerus and proximal ulna and/or proximal radius);	④ 80 ▣ 50
24587	with implant arthroplasty Consult also CPT code 24361.	⑤ 80 ▣ 50
24600	Treatment of closed elbow dislocation; without anesthesia	① ▣ 50
24605	requiring anesthesia	② ▣ 50
24615	Open treatment of acute or chronic elbow dislocation	③ 80 ▣ 50
24620	Closed treatment of Monteggia type of fracture dislo-cation at elbow (fracture proximal end of ulna with dis-location of radial head), with manipulation	② 80 ▣ 50
24635	Open treatment of Monteggia type of fracture dislocation at elbow (fracture proximal end of ulna with dislocation of radial head), with or without internal or external fixation	③ 80 ▣ 50
24640*	Closed treatment of radial head subluxation in child, nursemaid elbow, with manipulation	P 80 ▣ 50
24650	Closed treatment of radial head or neck fracture; without manipulation	▣ 50
24655	with manipulation	① ▣ 50
24665	Open treatment of radial head or neck fracture, with or without internal fixation or radial head excision;	④ 80 ▣ 50
24666	with radial head prosthetic replacement	④ 80 ▣ 50
24670	Closed treatment of ulnar fracture, proximal end (olecranon process); without manipulation	① ▣ 50
24675	with manipulation	① ▣ 50
24685	Open treatment of ulnar fracture proximal end (olecranon process), with or without internal or external fixation	③ 80 ▣ 50

ARTHRODESIS

24800	Arthrodesis, elbow joint; local	④ 80 ▣ 50
24802	with autogenous graft (includes obtaining graft)	⑤ 80 ▣ 50

AMPUTATION

24900	Amputation, arm through humerus; with primary closure	80 ▣ 50
24920	open, circular (guillotine)	80 ▣ 50
24925	secondary closure or scar revision	③ 80 ▣ 50
24930	re-amputation	80 ▣ 50
24931	with implant	80 ▣ 50
24935	Stump elongation, upper extremity	80 ▣ 50
24940	Cineplasty, upper extremity, complete procedure	80 ▣ 50

OTHER PROCEDURES

24999	Unlisted procedure, humerus or elbow	80 50

FOREARM AND WRIST

Codes listed in the Musculoskeletal chapter include the application and removal of the first cast or traction device. Replacement of casts and/or traction devices subsequent to the first should be reported separately. CPT codes for other additional procedures, such as obtaining grafts and external fixation, should only be used if the procedure is not already listed as included as part of the basic procedure. Consult the glossary for additional terms and guidelines.

INCISION

	25000	Incision, extensor tendon sheath, wrist (eg, deQuervain's disease)	③ ▣ 50
		If decompression of a median nerve is performed or for carpal tunnel syndrome, consult CPT code 64721.	
●	25001	Incision, flexor tendon sheath, wrist (eg, flexor carpi radialis)	
▲	25020	Decompression fasciotomy, forearm and/or wrist, flexor OR extensor compartment; without debridement of nonviable muscle and/or nerve	③ ▣ 50
	25023	with debridement of nonviable muscle and/or nerve	③ 80 ▣ 50
		If debridement is performed, consult also CPT codes 11000-11044.	
		If decompression fasciotomy with brachial artery exploration is performed, consult CPT code 24495.	
●	25024	Decompression fasciotomy, forearm and/or wrist, flexor AND extensor compartment; without debridement of nonviable muscle and/or nerve	③
●	25025	with debridement of nonviable muscle and/or nerve	
	25028	Incision and drainage, forearm and/or wrist; deep abscess or hematoma	① ▣ 50
		If superficial incision and drainage procedures are performed, consult CPT codes 10040-10160.	
	25031	bursa	② 80 ▣ 50
	25035	Incision, deep, bone cortex, forearm and/or wrist (eg, osteomyelitis or bone abscess)	② 80 ▣ 50
	25040	Arthrotomy, radiocarpal or midcarpal joint, with exploration, drainage, or removal of foreign body	⑤ 80 ▣ 50

EXCISION

	25065	Biopsy, soft tissue of forearm and/or wrist; superficial	① ▣ 50
		If a needle biopsy of soft tissue is performed, consult CPT code 20206.	
	25066	deep (subfascial or intramuscular)	② ▣ 50

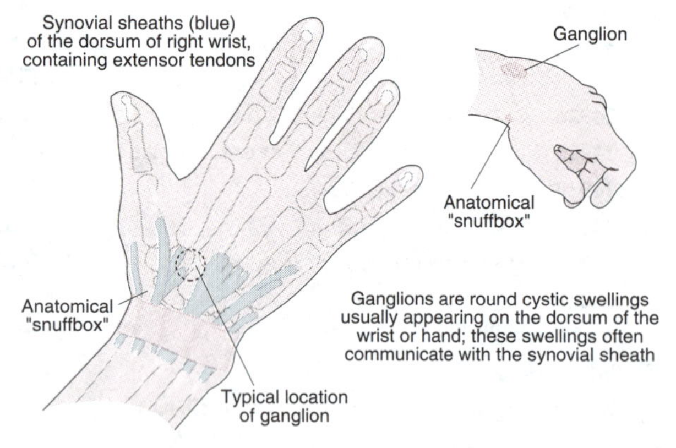

▲ **25075** Excision, tumor, soft tissue of forearm and/or wrist area; subcutaneous ❷ ↻ 50

25076 deep, subfascial or intramuscular ❸ ↻ 50

25077 Radical resection of tumor (eg, malignant neoplasm), soft tissue of forearm and/or wrist area ❸ ↻ 50

25085 Capsulotomy, wrist (eg, contracture) ❸ 80 ↻ 50

25100 Arthrotomy, wrist joint; with biopsy ❷ 80 ↻ 50

25101 with joint exploration, with or without biopsy, with or without removal of loose or foreign body ❸ 80 ↻ 50

25105 with synovectomy ❹ 80 ↻ 50

25107 Arthrotomy, distal radioulnar joint including repair of triangular cartilage, complex ❸ 80 ↻ 50

25110 Excision, lesion of tendon sheath, forearm and/or wrist ❸ ↻ 50

25111 Excision of ganglion, wrist (dorsal or volar); primary ❸ ↻ 50
If this procedure involves the hand or finger, consult CPT code 26160.

25112 recurrent ❹ ↻ 50

25115 Radical excision of bursa, synovia of wrist, or forearm tendon sheaths (eg, tenosynovitis, fungus, Tbc, or other granulomas, rheumatoid arthritis); flexors ❹ ↻ 50
If finger synovectomies are performed, consult CPT code 26145.

25116 extensors, with or without transposition of dorsal retinaculum ❹ 80 ↻ 50

25118 Synovectomy, extensor tendon sheath, wrist, single compartment; ❷ ↻ 50

25119 with resection of distal ulna ❸ 80 ↻ 50

25120 Excision or curettage of bone cyst or benign tumor of radius or ulna (excluding head or neck of radius and olecranon process); ❸ 80 ↻ 50
If this procedure involves the head or the neck of the radius or the olecranon process, consult CPT codes 24120-24126.

25125 with autograft (includes obtaining graft) ❸ 80 ↻ 50

25126 with allograft ❸ 80 ↻ 50

25130 Excision or curettage of bone cyst or benign tumor of carpal bones; ❸ 80 ↻ 50

25135 with autograft (includes obtaining graft) ❸ 80 ↻ 50

25136 with allograft ❸ 80 ↻ 50

25145 Sequestrectomy (eg, for osteomyelitis or bone abscess), forearm and/or wrist ❷ 80 ↻ 50

25150 Partial excision (craterization, saucerization or diaphysectomy) of bone (eg, for osteomyelitis); ulna ❷ 50

25151 radius ❷ 80 ↻ 50
If this procedure involves the head or the neck of the radius or the olecranon process, consult CPT codes 24145 and 24147.

25170 Radical resection for tumor, radius or ulna ❸ 80 ↻ 50

25210 Carpectomy; one bone ❸ 80 ↻
If carpectomy is performed with an implant, consult CPT codes 25441-25445.

25215 all bones of proximal row ❹ 80 ↻

25230 Radial styloidectomy (separate procedure) ❹ ↻ 50

25240 Excision distal ulna partial or complete (eg, Darrach type or matched resection) ❹ 80 ↻ 50
If an implant replacement is performed for the distal ulna, consult CPT code 25442. If obtaining fascia for interposition, consult CPT codes 20920 and 20922.

INTRODUCTION OR REMOVAL

If a K-wire, a pin, or a rod is inserted or removed, consult CPT codes 20650, 20670, and 20680.

25246 Injection procedure for wrist arthrography ↻ 50
If radiological supervision and interpretation is needed, consult CPT code 73115. Code 76003 cannot be reported in addition to 73115.

25248 Exploration with removal of deep foreign body, forearm or wrist ❷ ↻ 50
If a superficial foreign body is removed, consult CPT code 20520.

25250 Removal of wrist prosthesis; (separate procedure) ❶ 80 ↻ 50

25251 complicated, including total wrist ❶ 80 ↻

● **25259** Manipulation, wrist, under anesthesia
If external fixation is applied, consult CPT codes 20690 or 20692.

REPAIR, REVISION, AND/OR RECONSTRUCTION

25260 Repair, tendon or muscle, flexor, forearm and/or wrist; primary, single, each tendon or muscle ❹ ↻

25263 secondary, single, each tendon or muscle ❷ 80 ↻

25265 secondary, with free graft (includes obtaining graft), each tendon or muscle ❸ 80 ↻

25270 Repair, tendon or muscle, extensor, forearm and/or wrist; primary, single, each tendon or muscle ❹ 80 ↻

25272 secondary, single, each tendon or muscle ❸ 80 ↻

▲ **25274** secondary, with free graft (includes obtaining graft), each tendon or muscle ❹ 80 ↻

● **25275** Repair, tendon sheath, extensor, forearm and/or wrist, with free graft (includes obtaining graft) (eg, for extensor carpi ulnaris subluxation) ❹

25280 Lengthening or shortening of flexor or extensor tendon, forearm and/or wrist, single, each tendon ❹ 80 ↻

25290 Tenotomy, open, flexor or extensor tendon, forearm and/or wrist, single, each tendon ❸ ↻

25295 Tenolysis, flexor or extensor tendon, forearm and/or wrist, single, each tendon ❸ ↻

25300 Tenodesis at wrist; flexors of fingers ❸ 80 ↻ 50

25301 extensors of fingers ❸ 80 ↻ 50

25310 Tendon transplantation or transfer, flexor or extensor, forearm and/or wrist, single; each tendon ❸ 80 ↻

25312 with tendon graft(s) (includes obtaining graft), each tendon ❹ 80 ↻

25315	Flexor origin slide (eg, for cerebral palsy, Volkmann contracture), forearm and/or wrist;	
25316	with tendon(s) transfer	
25320	Capsulorrhaphy or reconstruction, wrist, any method (eg, capsulodesis, ligament repair, tendon transfer or graft) (includes synovectomy, capsulotomy and open reduction) for carpal instability	
25332	Arthroplasty, wrist, with or without interposition, with or without external or internal fixation	

25332 — If obtaining fascia for interposition, consult CPT codes 20920 and 20992. If arthroplasty with a prosthetic replacement is performed, consult CPT codes 25441-25446.

25335	Centralization of wrist on ulna (eg, radial club hand)	
25337	Reconstruction for stabilization of unstable distal ulna or distal radioulnar joint, secondary by soft tissue stabilization (eg, tendon transfer, tendon graft or weave, or tenodesis) with or without open reduction of distal radioulnar joint	

25337 — If a fascia lata graft is harvested, consult CPT codes 20920 and 20922.

25350	Osteotomy, radius; distal third	
25355	middle or proximal third	
25360	Osteotomy; ulna	
25365	radius AND ulna	
25370	Multiple osteotomies, with realignment on intramedullary rod (Sofield type procedure); radius OR ulna	
25375	radius AND ulna	
25390	Osteoplasty, radius OR ulna; shortening	
25391	lengthening with autograft	
25392	Osteoplasty, radius AND ulna; shortening (excluding 64876)	
25393	lengthening with autograft	
● 25394	Osteoplasty, carpal bone, shortening	
25400	Repair of nonunion or malunion, radius OR ulna; without graft (eg, compression technique)	
▲ 25405	with autograft (includes obtaining graft)	
25415	Repair of nonunion or malunion, radius AND ulna; without graft (eg, compression technique)	
▲ 25420	with autograft (includes obtaining graft)	
25425	Repair of defect with autograft; radius OR ulna	
25426	radius AND ulna	
● 25430	Insertion of vascular pedicle into carpal bone (eg, Harii procedure)	
● 25431	Repair of nonunion of carpal bone (excluding carpal scaphoid (navicular)) (includes obtaining graft and necessary fixation), each bone	
▲ 25440	Repair of nonunion, scaphoid carpal (navicular) bone, with or without radial styloidectomy (includes obtaining graft and necessary fixation)	
25441	Arthroplasty with prosthetic replacement; distal radius	
25442	distal ulna	
▲ 25443	scaphoid carpal (navicular)	
25444	lunate	
25445	trapezium	
25446	distal radius and partial or entire carpus (total wrist)	

25447	Arthroplasty, interposition, intercarpal or carpometacarpal joints	

25447 — If wrist arthroplasty is performed, consult CPT code 25332.

25449	Revision of arthroplasty, including removal of implant, wrist joint	
25450	Epiphyseal arrest by epiphysiodesis or stapling; distal radius OR ulna	
25455	distal radius AND ulna	
25490	Prophylactic treatment (nailing, pinning, plating or wiring) with or without methylmethacrylate; radius	
25491	ulna	
25492	radius AND ulna	

FRACTURE AND/OR DISLOCATION

25500	Closed treatment of radial shaft fracture; without manipulation	
25505	with manipulation	
25515	Open treatment of radial shaft fracture, with or without internal or external fixation	
▲ 25520	Closed treatment of radial shaft fracture and closed treatment of dislocation of distal radioulnar joint (Galeazzi fracture/dislocation)	
25525	Open treatment of radial shaft fracture, with internal and/or external fixation and closed treatment of dislocation of distal radioulnar joint (Galeazzi fracture/dislocation), with or without percutaneous skeletal fixation	
▲ 25526	Open treatment of radial shaft fracture, with internal and/or external fixation and open treatment, with or without internal or external fixation of distal radioulnar joint (Galeazzi fracture/dislocation), includes repair of triangular fibrocartilage complex	
25530	Closed treatment of ulnar shaft fracture; without manipulation	
25535	with manipulation	
25545	Open treatment of ulnar shaft fracture, with or without internal or external fixation	
25560	Closed treatment of radial and ulnar shaft fractures; without manipulation	
25565	with manipulation	
25574	Open treatment of radial AND ulnar shaft fractures, with internal or external fixation; of radius OR ulna	
25575	of radius AND ulna	
25600	Closed treatment of distal radial fracture (eg, Colles or Smith type) or epiphyseal separation, with or without fracture of ulnar styloid; without manipulation	
25605	with manipulation	
25611	Percutaneous skeletal fixation of distal radial fracture (eg, Colles or Smith type) or epiphyseal separation, with or without fracture of ulnar styloid, requiring manipulation, with or without external fixation	
25620	Open treatment of distal radial fracture (eg, Colles or Smith type) or epiphyseal separation, with or without fracture of ulnar styloid, with or without internal or external fixation	
25622	Closed treatment of carpal scaphoid (navicular) fracture; without manipulation	
25624	with manipulation	

Musculoskeletal System

25628 — 26117

	25628	Open treatment of carpal scaphoid (navicular) fracture, with or without internal or external fixation ❸🔟 🔲 50
	25630	Closed treatment of carpal bone fracture (excluding carpal scaphoid (navicular)); without manipulation, each bone 🔲 50
	25635	with manipulation, each bone ❶🔟 🔲 50
▲	25645	Open treatment of carpal bone fracture (other than carpal scaphoid (navicular)), each bone ❸🔟 🔲 50
	25650	Closed treatment of ulnar styloid fracture 🔲 50
●	25651	Percutaneous skeletal fixation of ulnar styloid fracture
●	25652	Open treatment of ulnar styloid fracture
	25660	Closed treatment of radiocarpal or intercarpal dislocation, one or more bones, with manipulation ❶🔟 🔲 50
	25670	Open treatment of radiocarpal or intercarpal dislocation, one or more bones ❸🔟 🔲 50
●	25671	Percutaneous skeletal fixation of distal radioulnar dislocation ❶
	25675	Closed treatment of distal radioulnar dislocation with manipulation ❶🔟 🔲 50
	25676	Open treatment of distal radioulnar dislocation, acute or chronic ❷🔟 🔲 50
	25680	Closed treatment of trans-scaphoperilunar type of fracture dislocation, with manipulation ❷🔟 🔲 50
	25685	Open treatment of trans-scaphoperilunar type of fracture dislocation ❸🔟 🔲 50
	25690	Closed treatment of lunate dislocation, with manipulation ❶🔟 🔲 50
	25695	Open treatment of lunate dislocation ❷🔟 🔲 50

ARTHRODESIS

25800	Arthrodesis, wrist; complete, without bone graft (includes radiocarpal and/or intercarpal and/or carpometacarpal joints) ❹🔟 🔲 50
25805	with sliding graft ❺🔟 🔲 50
25810	with iliac or other autograft (includes obtaining graft) ❺🔟 🔲 50
25820	Arthrodesis, wrist; limited, without bone graft (eg, intercarpal or radiocarpal) ❹🔟 🔲 50
25825	with autograft (includes obtaining graft) ❺🔟 🔲 50
25830	Arthrodesis, distal radioulnar joint with segmental resection of ulna, with or without bone graft (eg, Sauve-Kapandji procedure) 🔟 🔲 50

AMPUTATION

25900	Amputation, forearm, through radius and ulna; 🔟 🔲 50
25905	open, circular (guillotine) 🔟 🔲 50
25907	secondary closure or scar revision ❸🔟 🔲 50
25909	re-amputation 🔟 🔲 50
25915	Krukenberg procedure 🔟 🔲 50
25920	Disarticulation through wrist; 🔟 🔲 50
25922	secondary closure or scar revision ❸🔟 🔲 50
25924	re-amputation 🔟 🔲 50
25927	Transmetacarpal amputation; 🔟 🔲 50
25929	secondary closure or scar revision ❸🔟 🔲 50
25931	re-amputation 🔟 50

OTHER PROCEDURES

25999	Unlisted procedure, forearm or wrist 🔟 50

HAND AND FINGERS

Codes listed in the Musculoskeletal chapter include the application and removal of the first cast or traction device. Replacement of casts and/or traction devices subsequent to the first should be reported separately. CPT codes for other additional procedures, such as obtaining grafts and external fixation, should only be used if the procedure is not already listed as included as part of the basic procedure. Consult the glossary for additional terms and guidelines.

INCISION

26010*	Drainage of finger abscess; simple 🔲
26011*	complicated (eg, felon) ❶🔲
26020	Drainage of tendon sheath, digit and/or palm, each ❷🔲
26025	Drainage of palmar bursa; single, bursa ❶🔟🔲
26030	multiple bursa ❷🔟🔲
26034	Incision, bone cortex, hand or finger (eg, osteomyelitis or bone abscess) ❷🔲
26035	Decompression fingers and/or hand, injection injury (eg, grease gun) ❹🔟🔲
26037	Decompressive fasciotomy, hand (excludes 26035) ❹🔟🔲
	If decompression of the fingers and/or hand for an injection injury is performed, consult CPT code 26035.
26040	Fasciotomy, palmar (eg, Dupuytrens contracture); percutaneous ❹🔲 50
26045	open, partial ❸🔲 50
	If a fasciectomy is performed, consult CPT codes 26121-26125.
26055	Tendon sheath incision (eg, for trigger finger) ❷🔲
26060	Tenotomy, percutaneous, single, each digit ❷🔟🔲
26070	Arthrotomy, with exploration, drainage, or removal of loose or foreign body; carpometacarpal joint ❷🔲 50
26075	metacarpophalangeal joint, each ❹🔲 50
26080	interphalangeal joint, each ❹🔲

EXCISION

26100	Arthrotomy with biopsy; carpometacarpal joint, each ❷🔟 🔲 50
26105	metacarpophalangeal joint, each ❶🔟 🔲 50
26110	interphalangeal joint, each ❶🔲
▲ 26115	Excision, tumor or vascular malformation, soft tissue of hand or finger; subcutaneous ❷🔲
▲ 26116	deep (subfascial or intramuscular) ❷🔲
26117	Radical resection of tumor (eg, malignant neoplasm), soft tissue of hand or finger ❸🔲

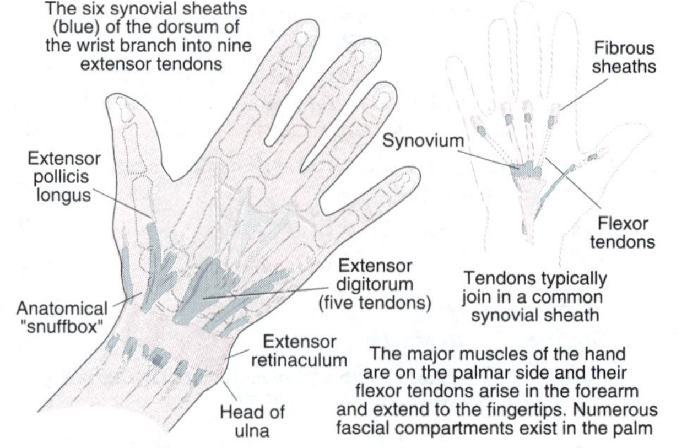

26121	Fasciectomy, palm only, with or without Z-plasty, other local tissue rearrangement, or skin grafting (includes obtaining graft)	❹ ⬛ 50

If a fasciotomy is performed, consult CPT codes 26040 and 26045.

26123	Fasciectomy, partial palmar with release of single digit including proximal interphalangeal joint, with or without Z-plasty, other local tissue rearrangement, or skin grafting (includes obtaining graft);	❹ ⬛ 50
+ 26125	each additional digit (List separately in addition to code for primary procedure)	❹

Note that 26125 is an add-on code and must be used in conjunction with 26123.

26130	Synovectomy, carpometacarpal joint	❸ ⬛ 50
26135	Synovectomy, metacarpophalangeal joint including intrinsic release and extensor hood reconstruction, each digit	❹ 80 ⬛
26140	Synovectomy, proximal interphalangeal joint, including extensor reconstruction, each interphalangeal joint	❷ ⬛
26145	Synovectomy, tendon sheath, radical (tenosynovectomy), flexor tendon, palm and/or finger, each tendon	❸ ⬛

If a tendon sheath synovectomy is performed at the wrist, consult CPT codes 25115 and 25116.

▲ 26160	Excision of lesion of tendon sheath or joint capsule (eg, cyst, mucous cyst, or ganglion), hand or finger	❸ ⬛

If dealing with a wrist ganglion, consult CPT codes 25111 and 25112. If this procedure is performed on a trigger digit, consult CPT code 26055.

26170	Excision of tendon, palm, flexor, single (separate procedure), each	❸ 80 ⬛
26180	Excision of tendon, finger, flexor (separate procedure), each tendon	❸ 80 ⬛
26185	Sesamoidectomy, thumb or finger (separate procedure)	80 ⬛ 50
26200	Excision or curettage of bone cyst or benign tumor of metacarpal;	❷ 80 ⬛
26205	with autograft (includes obtaining graft)	❸ ⬛
26210	Excision or curettage of bone cyst or benign tumor of proximal, middle or distal phalanx of finger;	❷ ⬛
26215	with autograft (includes obtaining graft)	❸ ⬛
26230	Partial excision (craterization, saucerization, or diaphysectomy) bone (eg, osteomyelitis); metacarpal	❼ 80 ⬛
26235	proximal or middle phalanx of finger	❸ 80 ⬛
26236	distal phalanx of finger	❸ ⬛
26250	Radical resection, metacarpal (eg, tumor);	❸ 80 ⬛
26255	with autograft (includes obtaining graft)	❸ 80 ⬛
26260	Radical resection, proximal or middle phalanx of finger (eg, tumor);	❸ 80 ⬛
26261	with autograft (includes obtaining graft)	❸ 80 ⬛
26262	Radical resection, distal phalanx of finger (eg, tumor)	❷ 80 ⬛

INTRODUCTION OR REMOVAL

26320	Removal of implant from finger or hand	❷ ⬛

If a foreign body is removed in the hand or the finger, consult CPT codes 20520 and 20525

REPAIR, REVISION, AND/OR RECONSTRUCTION

● 26340	Manipulation, finger joint, under anesthesia, each joint	

If external fixation is applied, consult CPT codes 20690 or 20692.

▲ 26350	Repair or advancement, flexor tendon, not in zone 2 digital flexor tendon sheath (eg, no man's land); primary or secondary without free graft, each tendon	❶ ⬛
26352	secondary with free graft (includes obtaining graft), each tendon	❹ 80 ⬛
▲ 26356	Repair or advancement, flexor tendon, in zone 2 digital flexor tendon sheath (eg, no man's land); primary or secondary without free graft, each tendon	❹ ⬛
26357	secondary, each tendon	❹ 80 ⬛
26358	secondary with free graft (includes obtaining graft), each tendon	❹ 80 ⬛
26370	Repair or advancement of profundus tendon, with intact superficialis tendon; primary, each tendon	❹ 80 ⬛
26372	secondary with free graft (includes obtaining graft), each tendon	❹ 80 ⬛
26373	secondary without free graft, each tendon	❸ 80 ⬛
▲ 26390	Excision flexor tendon, with implantation of synthetic rod for delayed tendon graft, hand or finger, each rod	❹ 80 ⬛
▲ 26392	Removal of synthetic rod and insertion of flexor tendon graft, hand or finger (includes obtaining graft), each rod	❸ 80 ⬛
26410	Repair, extensor tendon, hand, primary or secondary; without free graft, each tendon	❸ ⬛
26412	with free graft (includes obtaining graft), each tendon	❸ 80 ⬛
▲ 26415	Excision of extensor tendon, with implantation of synthetic rod for delayed tendon graft, hand or finger, each rod	❹ 80 ⬛
▲ 26416	Removal of synthetic rod and insertion of extensor tendon graft (includes obtaining graft), hand or finger, each rod	❸ ⬛
26418	Repair, extensor tendon, finger, primary or secondary; without free graft, each tendon	❹ ⬛
26420	with free graft (includes obtaining graft) each tendon	❹ 80 ⬛
▲ 26426	Repair of extensor tendon, central slip, secondary (eg, boutonniere deformity); using local tissue(s), including lateral band(s), each finger	❸ ⬛
▲ 26428	with free graft (includes obtaining graft), each finger	❸ 80 ⬛
26432	Closed treatment of distal extensor tendon insertion, with or without percutaneous pinning (eg, mallet finger)	❸ ⬛
26433	Repair of extensor tendon, distal insertion, primary or secondary; without graft (eg, mallet finger)	❸ ⬛
26434	with free graft (includes obtaining graft)	❸ 80 ⬛

If a tenovaginotomy is performed on the trigger finger, consult CPT code 26055.

26437	Realignment of extensor tendon, hand, each tendon	❸ ⬛
26440	Tenolysis, flexor tendon; palm OR finger; each tendon	❸ ⬛
26442	palm AND finger, each tendon	❸ ⬛
▲ 26445	Tenolysis, extensor tendon, hand OR finger; each tendon	❸ ⬛
26449	Tenolysis, complex, extensor tendon, finger, including forearm, each tendon	❸ 80 ⬛
26450	Tenotomy, flexor, palm, open, each tendon	❸ 80 ⬛
26455	Tenotomy, flexor, finger, open, each tendon	❸ 80 ⬛

26460	Tenotomy, extensor, hand or finger, open, each tendon	③ TC
26471	Tenodesis; of proximal interphalangeal joint, each joint	② 80 TC
26474	of distal joint, each joint	② 80 TC
26476	Lengthening of tendon, extensor, hand or finger, each tendon	① TC
26477	Shortening of tendon, extensor, hand or finger, each tendon	① TC
26478	Lengthening of tendon, flexor, hand or finger, each tendon	① 80 TC
26479	Shortening of tendon, flexor, hand or finger, each tendon	① 80 TC
26480	Transfer or transplant of tendon, carpometacarpal area or dorsum of hand; without free graft, each tendon	③ 80 TC
26483	with free tendon graft (includes obtaining graft), each tendon	③ 80 TC
26485	Transfer or transplant of tendon, palmar; without free tendon graft, each tendon	② 80 TC
26489	with free tendon graft (includes obtaining graft), each tendon	③ 80 TC
26490	Opponensplasty; superficialis tendon transfer type, each tendon	③ 80 TC
26492	tendon transfer with graft (includes obtaining graft), each tendon	③ 80 TC
26494	hypothenar muscle transfer	③ 80 TC
26496	other methods	③ 80 TC

If thumb fusion in opposition is performed, consult CPT code 26820.

26497	Transfer of tendon to restore intrinsic function; ring and small finger	③ 80 TC
26498	all four fingers	④ 80 TC
26499	Correction claw finger, other methods	③ 80 TC
26500	Reconstruction of tendon pulley, each tendon; with local tissues (separate procedure)	④ 80 TC
26502	with tendon or fascial graft (includes obtaining graft) (separate procedure)	④ 80 TC
26504	with tendon prosthesis (separate procedure)	④ 80 TC
26508	Release of thenar muscle(s) (eg, thumb contracture)	③ 80 TC
▲ 26510	Cross intrinsic transfer, each tendon	③ 80 TC
26516	Capsulodesis, metacarpophalangeal joint; single digit	① 80 TC
26517	two digits	③ 80 TC
26518	three or four digits	③ 80 TC
26520	Capsulectomy or capsulotomy; metacarpophalangeal joint, each joint	③ TC
26525	interphalangeal joint, each joint	③ TC
26530	Arthroplasty, metacarpophalangeal joint; each joint	③ 80 TC
26531	with prosthetic implant, each joint	⑦ 80 TC
26535	Arthroplasty, interphalangeal joint; each joint	⑤ TC
26536	with prosthetic implant, each joint	⑤ 80 TC
26540	Repair of collateral ligament, metacarpophalangeal or interphalangeal join	④ 80 TC
26541	Reconstruction, collateral ligament, metacarpophalangeal joint, single, with tendon or fascial graft (includes obtaining graft)	⑦ 80 TC
26542	with local tissue (eg, adductor advancement)	④ 80 TC
26545	Reconstruction, collateral ligament, interphalangeal joint, single, including graft, each joint	④ 80 TC
26546	Repair non-union, metacarpal or phalanx, (includes obtaining bone graft with or without external or internal fixation)	80 TC 50
26548	Repair and reconstruction, finger, volar plate, interphalangeal joint	④ 80 TC
26550	Pollicization of a digit	② 80 TC
26551	Transfer, toe-to-hand with microvascular anastomosis; great toe wrap-around with bone graft	④ 80 TC

Do not report 69990 in addition to 26551-26554 as the operating microscope is considered an inclusive component of these procedures.

If a free osteocutaneous flap with microvascular anastomosis is performed on the great toe with web space, consult CPT code 20973.

26553	other than great toe, single	② 80 TC
26554	other than great toe, double	② 80 TC
26555	Transfer, finger to another position without microvascular anastomosis	③ 80 TC
26556	Transfer, free toe joint, with microvascular anastomosis	80 TC

Do not report 69990 in addition to 26556 as the operating microscope is considered an inclusive component of the surgery.

26560	Repair of syndactyly (web finger) each web space; with skin flaps	② 80 TC
26561	with skin flaps and grafts	③ 80 TC
26562	complex (eg, involving bone, nails)	④ 80 TC
26565	Osteotomy; metacarpal, each	⑤ 80 TC
26567	phalanx of finger, each	⑤ 80 TC
26568	Osteoplasty, lengthening, metacarpal or phalanx	③ 80 TC
26580	Repair cleft hand	⑤ 80 TC

Barsky's procedure

~~26585~~	~~Repair bifid digit~~ This code is deleted in 2002. See code 26587.	⑤ 80 TC
▲ 26587	Reconstruction of polydactylous digit, soft tissue and bone	⑤ 80 TC

If an excision is performed on the supernumerary digit, soft tissue only, consult CPT code 11200.

▲ 26590	Repair macrodactylia, each digit	⑤ 80 TC
26591	Repair, intrinsic muscles of hand, each muscle	③ 80 TC
26593	Release, intrinsic muscles of hand, each muscle	③ TC
26596	Excision of constricting ring of finger, with multiple Z-plasties	② 80 TC
~~26597~~	~~Release of scar contracture, flexor or extensor, with skin grafts, rearrangement flaps, or Z-plasties, hand and/or finger~~ This code is deleted in 2002. See codes 11041–11042, 14040–14041, 15120, or 15240.	③ 80 TC

FRACTURE AND/OR DISLOCATION

26600	Closed treatment of metacarpal fracture, single; without manipulation, each bone	TC
26605	with manipulation, each bone	② TC

▲	26607	Closed treatment of metacarpal fracture, with manipulation, with external fixation, each bone ❷80▣
	26608	Percutaneous skeletal fixation of metacarpal fracture, each bone 80▣
	26615	Open treatment of metacarpal fracture, single, with or without internal or external fixation, each bone ❹▣
	26641	Closed treatment of carpometacarpal dislocation, thumb, with manipulation 80▣
	26645	Closed treatment of carpometacarpal fracture dislocation, thumb (Bennett fracture), with manipulation ❶80▣
	26650	Percutaneous skeletal fixation of carpometacarpal fracture dislocation, thumb (Bennett fracture), with manipulation, with or without external fixation ❷▣
	26665	Open treatment of carpometacarpal fracture dislocation, thumb (Bennett fracture), with or without internal or external fixation ❹▣
▲	26670	Closed treatment of carpometacarpal dislocation, other than thumb, with manipulation, each joint; without anesthesia 80▣
	26675	requiring anesthesia ❷80▣
▲	26676	Percutaneous skeletal fixation of carpometacarpal dislocation, other than thumb, with manipulation, each joint ❷▣
▲	26685	Open treatment of carpometacarpal dislocation, other than thumb; with or without internal or external fixation, each joint ❸▣
	26686	complex, multiple or delayed reduction ❸80▣
	26700	Closed treatment of metacarpophalangeal dislocation, single, with manipulation; without anesthesia ▣
	26705	requiring anesthesia ❷80▣
	26706	Percutaneous skeletal fixation of metacarpophalangeal dislocation, single, with manipulation ❷▣
	26715	Open treatment of metacarpophalangeal dislocation, single, with or without internal or external fixation ❹80▣
	26720	Closed treatment of phalangeal shaft fracture, proximal or middle phalanx, finger or thumb; without manipulation, each ▣
	26725	with manipulation, with or without skin or skeletal traction, each ▣
	26727	Percutaneous skeletal fixation of unstable phalangeal shaft fracture, proximal or middle phalanx, finger or thumb, with manipulation, each ❼▣
	26735	Open treatment of phalangeal shaft fracture, proximal or middle phalanx, finger or thumb, with or without internal or external fixation, each ❹▣
	26740	Closed treatment of articular fracture, involving metacarpophalangeal or interphalangeal joint; without manipulation, each ▣
	26742	with manipulation, each ❷▣
	26746	Open treatment of articular fracture, involving metacarpophalangeal or interphalangeal joint, with or without internal or external fixation, each ❺▣
	26750	Closed treatment of distal phalangeal fracture, finger or thumb; without manipulation, each ▣
	26755	with manipulation, each ▣
	26756	Percutaneous skeletal fixation of distal phalangeal fracture, finger or thumb, each ❷80▣
	26765	Open treatment of distal phalangeal fracture, finger or thumb, with or without internal or external fixation, each ❹▣

	26770	Closed treatment of interphalangeal joint dislocation, single, with manipulation; without anesthesia ▣
	26775	requiring anesthesia ▣
	26776	Percutaneous skeletal fixation of interphalangeal joint dislocation, single, with manipulation ❷▣
	26785	Open treatment of interphalangeal joint dislocation, with or without internal or external fixation, single ❷▣

ARTHRODESIS

	26820	Fusion in opposition, thumb, with autogenous graft (includes obtaining graft) ❻80▣
	26841	Arthrodesis, carpometacarpal joint, thumb, with or without internal fixation; ❹80▣
	26842	with autograft (includes obtaining graft) ❹80▣
▲	26843	Arthrodesis, carpometacarpal joint, digit, other than thumb, each; ❸80▣
	26844	with autograft (includes obtaining graft) ❸80▣
	26850	Arthrodesis, metacarpophalangeal joint, with or without internal fixation; ❹80▣
	26852	with autograft (includes obtaining graft) ❹80▣
	26860	Arthrodesis, interphalangeal joint, with or without internal fixation; ❸▣
+	26861	each additional interphalangeal joint (List separately in addition to code for primary procedure) ❷

Note that 26861 is an add-on code and must be used in conjunction with 26860.

	26862	with autograft (includes obtaining graft) ❹80▣
+	26863	with autograft (includes obtaining graft), each additional joint (List separately in addition to code for primary procedure) ❸80

Note that 26863 is an add-on code and must be used in conjunction with 26862.

AMPUTATION

If the amputation is on the hand through metacarpal bones, consult CPT code 25927

	26910	Amputation, metacarpal, with finger or thumb (ray amputation), single, with or without interosseous transfer ❸▣

If repositioning is performed, consult CPT codes 26550 and 26555.

	26951	Amputation, finger or thumb, primary or secondary, any joint or phalanx, single, including neurectomies; with direct closure ❷▣
	26952	with local advancement flaps (V-Y, hood) ❹▣

If repair of a soft tissue defect requiring a split or a full thickness graft or other pedicle flaps is performed, consult CPT codes 15050-15755.

OTHER PROCEDURES

	26989	Unlisted procedure, hands or fingers

▣ CCI Comprehensive Code	50 Bilateral Procedure + CPT Add-on Code ⃠ Modifier -51 Exempt Code ● New Code ▲ Revised Code

M Maternity   N Newborn   P Pediatric   N/P Newborn/Pediatric

PELVIS AND HIP JOINT

Codes listed in the Musculoskeletal chapter include the application and removal of the first cast or traction device. Replacement of casts and/or traction devices subsequent to the first should be reported separately. CPT codes for other additional procedures, such as obtaining grafts and external fixation, should only be used if the procedure is not already listed as included as part of the basic procedure. Consult the glossary for additional terms and guidelines.

INCISION

26990 Incision and drainage, pelvis or hip joint area; deep abscess or hematoma [①][TC]

    If superficial incision and drainage procedures are performed, consult CPT codes 10040-10160.

26991 infected bursa [①][80][TC]

26992 Incision, bone cortex, pelvis and/or hip joint (eg, osteomyelitis or bone abscess) [②][80][TC]

27000 Tenotomy, adductor of hip, percutaneous (separate procedure) [②][TC][50]

27001 Tenotomy, adductor of hip, open [③][80][TC][50]

27003 Tenotomy, adductor, subcutaneous, open, with obturator neurectomy [③][80][TC][50]

27005 Tenotomy, hip flexor(s), open (separate procedure) [80][TC][50]

27006 Tenotomy, abductors and/or extensor(s) of hip, open (separate procedure) [80][TC][50]

27025 Fasciotomy, hip or thigh, any type [80][TC][50]

27030 Arthrotomy, hip, with drainage (eg, infection) [③][80][TC][50]

27033 Arthrotomy, hip, including exploration or removal of loose or foreign body [③][80][TC][50]

CIM 35-17 INDUCED LESIONS OF NERVE TRACTS

Surgically induced lesions of nerve tracts, which involve destroying nerve tissue, control the chronic or acute pain arising from conditions such as terminal cancer or lumbar degenerative arthritis. Induced lesions of nerve tracts may be produced by surgical cutting of the nerve (rhizolysis), chemical destruction of the nerve, or by creation of a radio-frequency lesion (electrocautery). Accordingly, program payment may be made for these denervation procedures when used in selected cases (concurred in by contractor's medical staff) to treat chronic pain.

27035 Denervation, hip joint, intrapelvic or extrapelvic intra-articular branches of sciatic, femoral, or obturator nerves [④][80][TC][50]

    If an obturator neurectomy is performed, consult CPT codes 64763 and 64766.

27036 Capsulectomy or capsulotomy, hip, with or without excision of heterotopic bone, with release of hip flexor muscles (ie, gluteus medius, gluteus minimus, tensor fascia latae, rectus femoris, sartorius, iliopsoas) [80][TC][50]

EXCISION

27040 Biopsy, soft tissue of pelvis and hip area; superficial [①][TC][50]

    If a needle biopsy of the soft tissue is performed, consult CPT code 20206.

27041 deep, subfascial or intramuscular [②][TC][50]

27047 Excision, tumor, pelvis and hip area; subcutaneous tissue [②][TC][50]

27048 deep, subfascial, intramuscular [③][80][TC][50]

27049 Radical resection of tumor, soft tissue of pelvis and hip area (eg, malignant neoplasm) [③][80][TC][50]

27050 Arthrotomy, with biopsy; sacroiliac joint [③][80][TC][50]

27052 hip joint [③][80][TC][50]

27054 Arthrotomy with synovectomy, hip joint [80][TC][50]

27060 Excision; ischial bursa [⑤][TC][50]

    If arthrocentesis or needling of the bursa is performed, consult CPT code 20610.

27062 trochanteric bursa or calcification [⑤][TC][50]

27065 Excision of bone cyst or benign tumor; superficial (wing of ilium, symphysis pubis, or greater trochanter of femur) with or without autograft [⑤][80][TC][50]

27066 deep, with or without autograft [⑤][80][TC][50]

27067 with autograft requiring separate incision [80][TC][50]

27070 Partial excision (craterization, saucerization) (eg, osteomyelitis or bone abscess); superficial (eg, wing of ilium, symphysis pubis, or greater trochanter of femur) [80][TC][50]

27071 deep (subfascial or intramuscular) [80][TC][50]

27075 Radical resection of tumor or infection; wing of ilium, one pubic or ischial ramus or symphysis pubis [80][TC][50]

27076 ilium, including acetabulum, both pubic rami, or ischium and acetabulum [80][TC]

27077 innominate bone, total [80][TC]

27078 ischial tuberosity and greater trochanter of femur [80][TC]

27079 ischial tuberosity and greater trochanter of femur, with skin flaps [80][TC]

27080 Coccygectomy, primary [②][80][TC]

    If this procedure involves a pressure (decubitus) ulcer, consult CPT codes 15920, 15922, and 15931-15958.

INTRODUCTION OR REMOVAL

27086* Removal of foreign body, pelvis or hip; subcutaneous tissue [①][80][TC][50]

27087 deep (subfascial or intramuscular) [③][80][TC][50]

27090 Removal of hip prosthesis; (separate procedure) [80][TC][50]

27091 complicated, including total hip prosthesis, methylmethacrylate with or without insertion of spacer [80][TC][50]

27093 Injection procedure for hip arthrography; without anesthesia [TC][50]

    For radiological supervision and interpretation of procedure, consult CPT code 73525. Do not report 76003 in addition to 73525.

27095 with anesthesia [TC][50]

    For radiological supervision and interpretation of procedure, consult CPT code 73525. Do not report 76003 in addition to 73525.

27096 Injection procedure for sacroiliac joint, arthrography and/or anesthetic/steroid [TC][50]

    Report 27096 only with imaging confirmation of intra-articular needle positioning.

    To report radiological supervision and interpretation of sacroiliac joint arthrography, consult CPT code 73542.

    To report fluoroscopic guidance without formal arthrography, use 76005.

REPAIR, REVISION, AND/OR RECONSTRUCTION

27097 Release or recession, hamstring, proximal [③][80][TC][50]

27098 Transfer, adductor to ischium [③][80][TC][50]

27100 Transfer external oblique muscle to greater trochanter including fascial or tendon extension (graft) [④][80][TC][50]

    Eggers procedure

27105	Transfer paraspinal muscle to hip (includes fascial or tendon extension graft)	④ 80 ↔ 50
▲ 27110	Transfer iliopsoas; to greater trochanter of femur	④ 80 ↔ 50
27111	to femoral neck	④ 80 ↔ 50
27120	Acetabuloplasty; (eg, Whitman, Colonna, Haygroves, or cup type)	80 ↔ 50
27122	resection, femoral head (eg, Girdlestone procedure)	80 ↔ 50
27125	Hemiarthroplasty, hip, partial (eg, femoral stem prosthesis, bipolar arthroplasty)	80 ↔ 50

If prosthetic replacement follows a fracture of the hip, consult CPT code 27236.

▲ 27130	Arthroplasty, acetabular and proximal femoral prosthetic replacement (total hip arthroplasty), with or without autograft or allograft	80 ↔ 50
▲ 27132	Conversion of previous hip surgery to total hip arthroplasty, with or without autograft or allograft	80 ↔ 50
27134	Revision of total hip arthroplasty; both components, with or without autograft or allograft	80 ↔ 50
27137	acetabular component only, with or without autograft or allograft	80 ↔ 50
27138	femoral component only, with or without allograft	80 ↔ 50
▲ 27140	Osteotomy and transfer of greater trochanter of femur (separate procedure)	80 ↔ 50
27146	Osteotomy, iliac, acetabular or innominate bone;	80 ↔ 50
	Salter osteotomy	
27147	with open reduction of hip	80 ↔ 50
	Pemberton osteotomy	
27151	with femoral osteotomy	80 ↔ 50
27156	with femoral osteotomy and with open reduction of hip	80 ↔ 50
	Chiari osteotomy	
27158	Osteotomy, pelvis, bilateral (eg, congenital malformation)	80 ↔
27161	Osteotomy, femoral neck (separate procedure)	80 ↔ 50
27165	Osteotomy, intertrochanteric or subtrochanteric including internal or external fixation and/or cast	80 ↔
27170	Bone graft, femoral head, neck, intertrochanteric or subtrochanteric area (includes obtaining bone graft)	80 ↔ 50
27175	Treatment of slipped femoral epiphysis; by traction, without reduction	80 ↔ 50
27176	by single or multiple pinning, in situ	80 ↔ 50
27177	Open treatment of slipped femoral epiphysis; single or multiple pinning or bone graft (includes obtaining graft)	80 ↔ 50
27178	closed manipulation with single or multiple pinning	80 ↔ 50
27179	osteoplasty of femoral neck (Heyman type procedure)	80 ↔ 50
27181	osteotomy and internal fixation	80 ↔ 50
▲ 27185	Epiphyseal arrest by epiphysiodesis or stapling, greater trochanter of femur	↔ 50
27187	Prophylactic treatment (nailing, pinning, plating or wiring) with or without methylmethacrylate, femoral neck and proximal femur	80 ↔ 50

FRACTURE AND/OR DISLOCATION

27193	Closed treatment of pelvic ring fracture, dislocation, diastasis or subluxation; without manipulation	① ↔ 50
27194	with manipulation, requiring more than local anesthesia	② 80 ↔
27200	Closed treatment of coccygeal fracture	↔
27202	Open treatment of coccygeal fracture	② 80 ↔
27215	Open treatment of iliac spine(s), tuberosity avulsion, or iliac wing fracture(s) (eg, pelvic fracture(s) which do not disrupt the pelvic ring), with internal fixation	80 ↔
27216	Percutaneous skeletal fixation of posterior pelvic ring fracture and/or dislocation (includes ilium, sacroiliac joint and/or sacrum)	80 ↔
27217	Open treatment of anterior ring fracture and/or dislocation with internal fixation, (includes pubic symphysis and/or rami)	80 ↔
27218	Open treatment of posterior ring fracture and/or dislocation with internal fixation (includes ilium, sacroiliac joint and/or sacrum)	80 ↔
27220	Closed treatment of acetabulum (hip socket) fracture(s); without manipulation	↔ 50
27222	with manipulation, with or without skeletal traction	↔ 50
27226	Open treatment of posterior or anterior acetabular wall fracture, with internal fixation	80 ↔ 50
27227	Open treatment of acetabular fracture(s) involving anterior or posterior (one) column, or a fracture running transversely across the acetabulum, with internal fixation	80 ↔ 50
27228	Open treatment of acetabular fracture(s) involving anterior and posterior (two) columns, includes T-fracture and both column fracture with complete articular detachment, or single column or transverse fracture with associated acetabular wall fracture, with internal fixation	80 ↔ 50
27230	Closed treatment of femoral fracture, proximal end, neck; without manipulation	① ↔ 50
27232	with manipulation, with or without skeletal traction	↔ 50
27235	Percutaneous skeletal fixation of femoral fracture, proximal end, neck, undisplaced, mildly displaced, or impacted fracture	↔ 50
27236	Open treatment of femoral fracture, proximal end, neck, internal fixation or prosthetic replacement	80 ↔ 50
27238	Closed treatment of intertrochanteric, pertrochanteric, or subtrochanteric femoral fracture; without manipulation	① ↔ 50
27240	with manipulation, with or without skin or skeletal traction	↔ 50
27244	Open treatment of intertrochanteric, pertrochanteric or subtrochanteric femoral fracture; with plate/screw type implant, with or without cerclage	80 ↔ 50
27245	with intramedullary implant, with or without interlocking screws and/or cerclage	80 ↔ 50
27246	Closed treatment of greater trochanteric fracture, without manipulation	① ↔ 50
27248	Open treatment of greater trochanteric fracture, with or without internal or external fixation	80 ↔ 50
27250	Closed treatment of hip dislocation, traumatic; without anesthesia	① ↔ 50
27252	requiring anesthesia	② ↔ 50

Musculoskeletal System

27253 — 27360

27253	Open treatment of hip dislocation, traumatic, without internal fixation	80 ↔ 50
27254	Open treatment of hip dislocation, traumatic, with acetabular wall and femoral head fracture, with or without internal or external fixation	80 ↔ 50
27256*	Treatment of spontaneous hip dislocation (developmental, including congenital or pathological), by abduction, splint or traction; without anesthesia, without manipulation	80 ↔ 50
27257*	with manipulation, requiring anesthesia	80 ↔ 50
27258	Open treatment of spontaneous hip dislocation (developmental, including congenital or pathological), replacement of femoral head in acetabulum (including tenotomy, etc);	80 ↔ 50
	Lorenz's operation	
27259	with femoral shaft shortening	80 ↔ 50
27265	Closed treatment of post hip arthroplasty dislocation; without anesthesia	❶ ↔ 50
27266	requiring regional or general anesthesia	❷ ↔ 50

MANIPULATION

| 27275* | Manipulation, hip joint, requiring general anesthesia | ❷ ↔ |

ARTHRODESIS

27280	Arthrodesis, sacroiliac joint (including obtaining graft)	80 ↔ 50
27282	Arthrodesis, symphysis pubis (including obtaining graft)	80 ↔
27284	Arthrodesis, hip joint (including obtaining graft);	80 ↔ 50
27286	with subtrochanteric osteotomy	80 ↔ 50

AMPUTATION

27290	Interpelviabdominal amputation (hindquarter amputation)	80 ↔
	Pean's amputation	
27295	Disarticulation of hip	80 ↔

OTHER PROCEDURES

| 27299 | Unlisted procedure, pelvis or hip joint | 80 50 |

FEMUR (THIGH REGION) AND KNEE JOINT

Codes listed in the Musculoskeletal chapter include the application and removal of the first cast or traction device. Replacement of casts and/or traction devices subsequent to the first should be reported separately. CPT codes for other additional procedures, such as obtaining grafts and external fixation, should only be used if the procedure is not already listed as included as part of the basic procedure. Consult the glossary for additional terms and guidelines.

INCISION

27301	Incision and drainage, deep abscess, bursa, or hematoma, thigh or knee region	❸ ↔ 50
	If a superficial abscess or hematoma is incised and drained, consult CPT codes 10040-10160.	
27303	Incision, deep, with opening of bone cortex, femur or knee (eg, osteomyelitis or bone abscess)	❷ 80 ↔ 50
27305	Fasciotomy, iliotibial (tenotomy), open	❷ 80 ↔ 50
	If a combined Ober-Yount fasciotomy is performed, consult CPT code 27025.	
27306	Tenotomy, percutaneous, adductor or hamstring; single tendon (separate procedure)	❸ 80 ↔ 50
27307	multiple tendons	❸ 80 ↔ 50

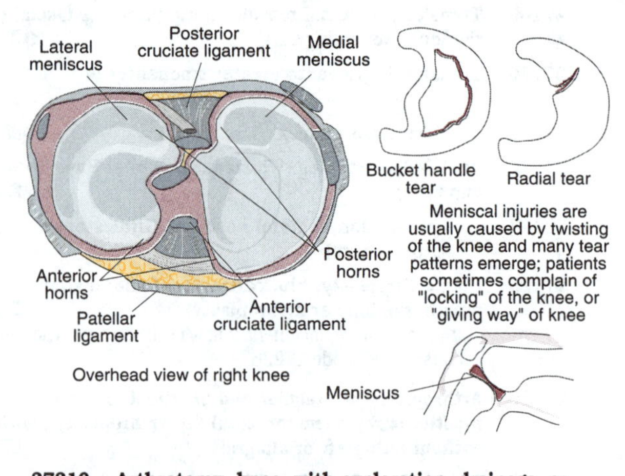

27310	Arthrotomy, knee, with exploration, drainage, or removal of foreign body (eg, infection)	❹ 80 ↔ 50
27315	Neurectomy, hamstring muscle	❷ 80 ↔ 50
27320	Neurectomy, popliteal (gastrocnemius)	❷ 80 ↔ 50

EXCISION

27323	Biopsy, soft tissue of thigh or knee area; superficial	❶ ↔ 50
	If a needle biopsy of soft tissue is performed, consult CPT code 20206.	
27324	deep (subfascial or intramuscular)	❶ ↔ 50
27327	Excision, tumor, thigh or knee area; subcutaneous	❷ ↔ 50
27328	deep, subfascial, or intramuscular	❸ ↔ 50
27329	Radical resection of tumor (eg, malignant neoplasm), soft tissue of thigh or knee area	80 ↔ 50
27330	Arthrotomy, knee; with synovial biopsy only	❹ ↔ 50
27331	including joint exploration, biopsy, or removal of loose or foreign bodies	❹ 80 ↔ 50
27332	Arthrotomy, with excision of semilunar cartilage (meniscectomy) knee; medial OR lateral	❹ 80 ↔ 50
27333	medial AND lateral	❹ 80 ↔ 50
27334	Arthrotomy, with synovectomy, knee; anterior OR posterior	❹ 80 ↔ 50
27335	anterior AND posterior including popliteal area	❹ 80 ↔ 50
27340	Excision, prepatellar bursa	❸ ↔ 50
27345	Excision of synovial cyst of popliteal space (eg, Bakers cyst)	❹ 80 ↔ 50
27347	Excision of lesion of meniscus or capsule (eg, cyst, ganglion), knee	80 ↔ 50
27350	Patellectomy or hemipatellectomy	❹ 80 ↔ 50
27355	Excision or curettage of bone cyst or benign tumor of femur;	❸ 80 ↔ 50
27356	with allograft	❹ 80 ↔ 50
27357	with autograft (includes obtaining graft)	80 ↔ 50
+ 27358	Excision or curettage of bone cyst or benign tumor of femur; with internal fixation (List in addition to code for primary procedure)	80 ↔ 50
	Note that 27358 is an add-on code and must be used in conjunction with 27355, 27356, or 27357.	
27360	Partial excision (craterization, saucerization, or diaphysectomy) bone, femur, proximal tibia and/or fibula (eg, osteomyelitis or bone abscess)	❺ 80 ↔ 50

27365 Radical resection of tumor, bone, femur or knee 80 50
    If a radical resection of a tumor, soft tissue, is performed, consult CPT code 27329.

INTRODUCTION OR REMOVAL

27370 Injection procedure for knee arthrography 50
    If radiological supervision and interpretation is performed, consult CPT code 73580. Code 76003 cannot be reported in addition to 73580.

27372 Removal of foreign body, deep, thigh region or knee area 7 80 50
    If a knee prosthesis, including "total knee," is removed, consult CPT code 27488.

REPAIR, REVISION, AND/OR RECONSTRUCTION

27380 Suture of infrapatellar tendon; primary 1 80 50

27381   secondary reconstruction, including fascial or tendon graft 3 80 50

27385 Suture of quadriceps or hamstring muscle rupture; primary 3 80 50

27386   secondary reconstruction, including fascial or tendon graft 3 80 50

27390 Tenotomy, open, hamstring, knee to hip; single tendon 1 80

27391   multiple tendons, one leg 2 80

27392   multiple tendons, bilateral 3 80

27393 Lengthening of hamstring tendon; single tendon 2 80

27394   multiple tendons, one leg 3 80

27395   multiple tendons, bilateral 3 80

27396 Transplant, hamstring tendon to patella; single tendon 3 80

27397   multiple tendons 3 80

27400 Transfer, tendon or muscle, hamstrings to femur (eg, Egger's type procedure) 3 80

27403 Arthrotomy with meniscus repair, knee 4 80 50
    If arthroscopic repair is performed, consult CPT code 29882.

27405 Repair, primary, torn ligament and/or capsule, knee; collateral 4 80 50

27407   cruciate 4 80 50

27409   collateral and cruciate ligaments 4 80 50

27418 Anterior tibial tubercleplasty (eg, Maquet type procedure) 3 80 50

27420 Reconstruction of dislocating patella; (eg, Hauser type procedure) 3 80 50

27422   with extensor realignment and/or muscle advancement or release (eg, Campbell, Goldwaite type procedure) 7 80 50

27424   with patellectomy 3 80 50

27425 Lateral retinacular release (any method) 7 50

27427 Ligamentous reconstruction (augmentation), knee; extra-articular 3 80 50
    If a primary repair of ligament(s) is performed in addition to reconstruction, report CPT code 27405, 27407, or 27409 in addition to 27427, 27428, or 27429.

27428   intra-articular (open) 4 80 50

27429   intra-articular (open) and extra-articular 4 80 50

27430 Quadricepsplasty (eg, Bennett or Thompson type) 4 80 50

27435 Capsulotomy, posterior capsular release, knee 4 80 50

27437 Arthroplasty, patella; without prosthesis 4 50

27438   with prosthesis 5 80 50

27440 Arthroplasty, knee, tibial plateau; 6 80 50

27441   with debridement and partial synovectomy 5 80 50

27442 Arthroplasty, femoral condyles or tibial plateau(s), knee; 5 80 50

27443   with debridement and partial synovectomy 5 80 50

27445 Arthroplasty, knee, hinge prosthesis (eg, Walldius type) 80 50

27446 Arthroplasty, knee, condyle and plateau; medial OR lateral compartment 80 50

▲ 27447   medial AND lateral compartments with or without patella resurfacing (total knee arthroplasty) 80 50
    If a total knee arthroplasty is revised, consult CPT code 27487. If a total knee prosthesis is removed, consult CPT code 27488.

27448 Osteotomy, femur, shaft or supracondylar; without fixation 80 50

27450   with fixation 80 50

27454 Osteotomy, multiple, with realignment on intramedullary rod, femoral shaft (eg, Sofield type procedure) 80 50

27455 Osteotomy, proximal tibia, including fibular excision or osteotomy (includes correction of genu varus (bowleg) or genu valgus (knock-knee)); before epiphyseal closure 80 50

27457   after epiphyseal closure 80 50

27465 Osteoplasty, femur; shortening (excluding 64876) 80 50

27466   lengthening 80 50

27468   combined, lengthening and shortening with femoral segment transfer 80 50

27470 Repair, nonunion or malunion, femur, distal to head and neck; without graft (eg, compression technique) 80 50

27472   with iliac or other autogenous bone graft (includes obtaining graft) 80 50

27475 Arrest, epiphyseal, any method (eg, epiphysiodesis); distal femur 50

27477   tibia and fibula, proximal 50

27479   combined distal femur, proximal tibia and fibula 80 50

27485 Arrest, hemiepiphyseal, distal femur or proximal tibia or fibula (eg, genu varus or valgus) 50

27486 Revision of total knee arthroplasty, with or without allograft; one component 80 50

27487   femoral and entire tibial component 80 50

27488 Removal of prosthesis, including total knee prosthesis, methylmethacrylate with or without insertion of spacer, knee 80 50

27495 Prophylactic treatment (nailing, pinning, plating or wiring) with or without methylmethacrylate, femur 80 50

27496 Decompression fasciotomy, thigh and/or knee, one compartment (flexor or extensor or adductor); 50

27497	with debridement of nonviable muscle and/or nerve	80 ↕ 50
27498	Decompression fasciotomy, thigh and/or knee, multiple compartments;	80 ↕ 50
27499	with debridement of nonviable muscle and/or nerve	80 ↕ 50

FRACTURE AND/OR DISLOCATION

If an arthroscopic treatment of the intercondylar spine(s) and tuberosity fracture(s) of the knee is performed, consult CPT codes 29850 and 29851.

27500	Closed treatment of femoral shaft fracture, without manipulation	❶ ↕ 50
27501	Closed treatment of supracondylar or transcondylar femoral fracture with or without intercondylar extension, without manipulation	❷ 80 ↕ 50
27502	Closed treatment of femoral shaft fracture, with manipulation, with or without skin or skeletal traction	❷ ↕ 50
27503	Closed treatment of supracondylar or transcondylar femoral fracture with or without intercondylar extension, with manipulation, with or without skin or skeletal traction	❸ 80 ↕ 50
27506	Open treatment of femoral shaft fracture, with or without external fixation, with insertion of intramedullary implant, with or without cerclage and/or locking screws	80 ↕ 50
27507	Open treatment of femoral shaft fracture with plate/screws, with or without cerclage	❹ 80 ↕ 50
27508	Closed treatment of femoral fracture, distal end, medial or lateral condyle, without manipulation	❶ ↕ 50
27509	Percutaneous skeletal fixation of femoral fracture, distal end, medial or lateral condyle, or supracondylar or transcondylar, with or without intercondylar extension, or distal femoral epiphyseal separation	❸ 80 ↕ 50
27510	Closed treatment of femoral fracture, distal end, medial or lateral condyle, with manipulation	❶ ↕ 50
27511	Open treatment of femoral supracondylar or transcondylar fracture without intercondylar extension, with or without internal or external fixation	❹ 80 ↕ 50
27513	Open treatment of femoral supracondylar or transcondylar fracture with intercondylar extension, with or without internal or external fixation	❺ 80 ↕ 50
27514	Open treatment of femoral fracture, distal end, medial or lateral condyle, with or without internal or external fixation	80 ↕ 50
27516	Closed treatment of distal femoral epiphyseal separation; without manipulation	❶ ↕ 50
27517	with manipulation, with or without skin or skeletal traction	❶ 80 ↕ 50
27519	Open treatment of distal femoral epiphyseal separation, with or without internal or external fixation	80 ↕ 50
27520	Closed treatment of patellar fracture, without manipulation	❶ ↕ 50
27524	Open treatment of patellar fracture, with internal fixation and/or partial or complete patellectomy and soft tissue repair	❸ 80 ↕ 50
27530	Closed treatment of tibial fracture, proximal (plateau); without manipulation	❶ ↕ 50
	If arthroscopic treatment of a tibial fracture is performed, consult CPT codes 29855 and 29856.	
27532	with or without manipulation, with skeletal traction	❶ ↕ 50

27535	Open treatment of tibial fracture, proximal (plateau); unicondylar, with or without internal or external fixation	❸ 80 ↕ 50
27536	bicondylar, with or without internal fixation	80 ↕ 50
27538	Closed treatment of intercondylar spine(s) and/or tuberosity fracture(s) of knee, with or without manipulation	❶ 80 ↕ 50
	If treated arthroscopically, consult CPT codes 29850, 29851.	
27540	Open treatment of intercondylar spine(s) and/or tuberosity fracture(s) of the knee, with or without internal or external fixation	80 ↕ 50
27550	Closed treatment of knee dislocation; without anesthesia	❶ 80 ↕ 50
27552	requiring anesthesia	❶ 80 ↕ 50
27556	Open treatment of knee dislocation, with or without internal or external fixation; without primary ligamentous repair or augmentation/reconstruction	80 ↕ 50
27557	with primary ligamentous repair	80 ↕ 50
27558	with primary ligamentous repair, with augmentation/reconstruction	80 ↕ 50
27560	Closed treatment of patellar dislocation; without anesthesia	❶ ↕ 50
	If this is a recurrent dislocation, consult CPT codes 27420-27424.	
27562	requiring anesthesia	❶ 80 ↕ 50
27566	Open treatment of patellar dislocation, with or without partial or total patellectomy	❷ 80 ↕ 50

MANIPULATION

27570*	Manipulation of knee joint under general anesthesia (includes application of traction or other fixation devices)	❶ ↕

ARTHRODESIS

27580	Arthrodesis, knee, any technique	80 ↕ 50
	Albert's operation	

AMPUTATION

27590	Amputation, thigh, through femur, any level;	80 ↕ 50
27591	immediate fitting technique including first cast	80 ↕ 50
27592	open, circular (guillotine)	80 ↕ 50
27594	secondary closure or scar revision	↕ 50
27596	re-amputation	50
27598	Disarticulation at knee	80 ↕ 50
	Batch-Spittler-McFaddin operation	

OTHER PROCEDURES

27599	Unlisted procedure, femur or knee	80 50

LEG (TIBIA AND FIBULA) AND ANKLE JOINT

Codes listed in the Musculoskeletal chapter include the application and removal of the first cast or traction device. Replacement of casts and/or traction devices subsequent to the first should be reported separately. CPT codes for other additional procedures, such as obtaining grafts and external fixation, should only be used if the procedure is not already listed as included as part of the basic procedure. Consult the glossary for additional terms and guidelines.

INCISION

27600 Decompression fasciotomy, leg; anterior and/or lateral compartments only

If a decompression fasciotomy is performed with debridement, consult CPT codes 27892-27894.

27601 posterior compartment(s) only

27602 anterior and/or lateral, and posterior compartment(s)

27603 Incision and drainage, leg or ankle; deep abscess or hematoma

If superficial incision and drainage is performed, consult CPT codes 10040-10160.

27604 infected bursa

27605* Tenotomy, percutaneous, Achilles tendon (separate procedure); local anesthesia

27606 general anesthesia

27607 Incision (eg, osteomyelitis or bone abscess), leg or ankle

27610 Arthrotomy, ankle, including exploration, drainage, or removal of foreign body

27612 Arthrotomy, posterior capsular release, ankle, with or without Achilles tendon lengthening

Consult also CPT code 27685.

EXCISION

27613 Biopsy, soft tissue of leg or ankle area; superficial

If a needle biopsy is performed on soft tissue, consult CPT code 20206.

27614 deep (subfascial or intramuscular)

27615 Radical resection of tumor (eg, malignant neoplasm), soft tissue of leg or ankle area

27618 Excision, tumor, leg or ankle area; subcutaneous tissue

27619 deep (subfascial or intramuscular)

27620 Arthrotomy, ankle, with joint exploration, with or without biopsy, with or without removal of loose or foreign body

27625 Arthrotomy, with synovectomy, ankle;

27626 including tenosynovectomy

27630 Excision of lesion of tendon sheath or capsule (eg, cyst or ganglion), leg and/or ankle

27635 Excision or curettage of bone cyst or benign tumor, tibia or fibula;

27637 with autograft (includes obtaining graft)

27638 with allograft

27640 Partial excision (craterization, saucerization, or diaphysectomy) bone (eg, osteomyelitis or exostosis); tibia

27641 fibula

27645 Radical resection of tumor, bone; tibia

27646 fibula

27647 talus or calcaneus

INTRODUCTION OR REMOVAL

27648 Injection procedure for ankle arthrography

If radiological supervision and interpretation is performed, consult CPT code 73615. Do not report 76003 in addition to 73615.

If ankle arthroscopy is performed, consult CPT codes 29894-29898.

REPAIR, REVISION, AND/OR RECONSTRUCTION

27650 Repair, primary, open or percutaneous, ruptured Achilles tendon;

27652 with graft (includes obtaining graft)

27654 Repair, secondary, Achilles tendon, with or without graft

27656 Repair, fascial defect of leg

27658 Repair, flexor tendon, leg; primary, without graft, each tendon

27659 secondary, with or without graft, each tendon

27664 Repair, extensor tendon, leg; primary, without graft, each tendon

27665 secondary, with or without graft, each tendon

27675 Repair, dislocating peroneal tendons; without fibular osteotomy

27676 with fibular osteotomy

27680 Tenolysis, flexor or extensor tendon, leg and/or ankle; single, each tendon

27681 multiple tendons (through separate incision(s))

27685 Lengthening or shortening of tendon, leg or ankle; single tendon (separate procedure)

27686 multiple tendons (through same incision), each

27687 Gastrocnemius recession (eg, Strayer procedure)

27690 Transfer or transplant of single tendon (with muscle redirection or rerouting); superficial (eg, anterior tibial extensors into midfoot)

Toe extensors as a group are considered a single tendon when transplanted into midfoot.

27691 deep (eg, anterior tibial or posterior tibial through interosseous space, flexor digitorum longus, flexor hallicus longus, or peroneal tendon to midfoot or hindfoot)

Barr procedure

+ 27692 each additional tendon (List in addition to code for primary procedure)

Note that 27692 is an add-on code and must be used in conjunction with 27690 and 27691.

27695 Repair, primary, disrupted ligament, ankle; collateral

27696 both collateral ligaments

27698 Repair, secondary, disrupted ligament, ankle, collateral (eg, Watson-Jones procedure)

27700 Arthroplasty, ankle;

27702 with implant (total ankle)

27703 revision, total ankle

27704 Removal of ankle implant

Musculoskeletal System

27705 — 27884

27705	Osteotomy; tibia	② 80 ⟷ 50
27707	fibula	② ⟷ 50
27709	tibia and fibula	② 80 ⟷ 50
27712	multiple, with realignment on intramedullary rod (eg, Sofield type procedure)	80 ⟷ 50

If an osteotomy is performed to correct genu varus (bowleg) or genu valgus (knock-knee), consult CPT codes 27455-27457.

27715	Osteoplasty, tibia and fibula, lengthening or shortening	④ 80 ⟷ 50

Anderson tibial lengthening

27720	Repair of nonunion or malunion, tibia; without graft, (eg, compression technique)	80 ⟷ 50
27722	with sliding graft	80 ⟷ 50
27724	with iliac or other autograft (includes obtaining graft)	80 ⟷ 50
27725	by synostosis, with fibula, any method	80 ⟷ 50
27727	Repair of congenital pseudarthrosis, tibia	80 ⟷ 50
27730	Arrest, epiphyseal (epiphysiodesis), any method; distal tibia	② ⟷ 50
27732	distal fibula	② ⟷ 50
27734	distal tibia and fibula	② ⟷ 50
27740	Arrest, epiphyseal (epiphysiodesis), any method, combined, proximal and distal tibia and fibula;	② 80 ⟷ 50
27742	and distal femur	② 80 ⟷ 50

If epiphyseal arrest of proximal tibia and fibula occurs, consult CPT code 27477.

27745	Prophylactic treatment (nailing, pinning, plating or wiring) with or without methylmethacrylate, tibia	③ 80 ⟷ 50

FRACTURE AND/OR DISLOCATION

27750	Closed treatment of tibial shaft fracture (with or without fibular fracture); without manipulation	① ⟷ 50
27752	with manipulation, with or without skeletal traction	① ⟷ 50
27756	Percutaneous skeletal fixation of tibial shaft fracture (with or without fibular fracture) (eg, pins or screws)	③ 80 ⟷ 50
27758	Open treatment of tibial shaft fracture, (with or without fibular fracture) with plate/screws, with or without cerclage	④ 80 ⟷ 50
27759	Open treatment of tibial shaft fracture (with or without fibular fracture) by intramedullary implant, with or without interlocking screws and/or cerclage	④ 80 ⟷ 50
27760	Closed treatment of medial malleolus fracture; without manipulation	① ⟷ 50
27762	with manipulation, with or without skin or skeletal traction	① ⟷ 50
27766	Open treatment of medial malleolus fracture, with or without internal or external fixation	③ ⟷ 50
27780	Closed treatment of proximal fibula or shaft fracture; without manipulation	① ⟷ 50
27781	with manipulation	① ⟷ 50
27784	Open treatment of proximal fibula or shaft fracture, with or without internal or external fixation	③ ⟷ 50
27786	Closed treatment of distal fibular fracture (lateral malleolus); without manipulation	① ⟷ 50
27788	with manipulation	① ⟷ 50

27792	Open treatment of distal fibular fracture (lateral malleolus), with or without internal or external fixation	③ ⟷ 50
27808	Closed treatment of bimalleolar ankle fracture, (including Potts); without manipulation	① ⟷ 50
27810	with manipulation	① ⟷ 50
27814	Open treatment of bimalleolar ankle fracture, with or without internal or external fixation	③ 80 ⟷ 50
27816	Closed treatment of trimalleolar ankle fracture; without manipulation	① ⟷ 50
27818	with manipulation	① ⟷ 50
27822	Open treatment of trimalleolar ankle fracture, with or without internal or external fixation, medial and/or lateral malleolus; without fixation of posterior lip	③ 80 ⟷ 50
27823	with fixation of posterior lip	③ 80 ⟷ 50
27824	Closed treatment of fracture of weight bearing articular portion of distal tibia (eg, pilon or tibial plafond), with or without anesthesia; without manipulation	① ⟷ 50
27825	with skeletal traction and/or requiring manipulation	② 80 ⟷ 50
27826	Open treatment of fracture of weight bearing articular surface/portion of distal tibia (eg, pilon or tibial plafond), with internal or external fixation; of fibula only	③ 80 ⟷ 50
27827	of tibia only	③ 80 ⟷ 50
27828	of both tibia and fibula	④ 80 ⟷ 50
27829	Open treatment of distal tibiofibular joint (syndesmosis) disruption, with or without internal or external fixation	② 80 ⟷ 50
27830	Closed treatment of proximal tibiofibular joint dislocation; without anesthesia	① 80 ⟷ 50
27831	requiring anesthesia	① 80 ⟷ 50
27832	Open treatment of proximal tibiofibular joint dislocation, with or without internal or external fixation, or with excision of proximal fibula	② 80 ⟷ 50
27840	Closed treatment of ankle dislocation; without anesthesia	① ⟷ 50
27842	requiring anesthesia, with or without percutaneous skeletal fixation	① ⟷ 50
27846	Open treatment of ankle dislocation, with or without percutaneous skeletal fixation; without repair or internal fixation	③ 80 ⟷ 50
27848	with repair or internal or external fixation	③ 80 ⟷ 50

MANIPULATION

27860*	Manipulation of ankle under general anesthesia (includes application of traction or other fixation apparatus)	① 80 ⟷

ARTHRODESIS

27870	Arthrodesis, ankle, any method	④ 80 ⟷ 50
27871	Arthrodesis, tibiofibular joint, proximal or distal	④ 80 ⟷ 50

AMPUTATION

27880	Amputation, leg, through tibia and fibula;	80 ⟷ 50

Burgess amputation

27881	with immediate fitting technique including application of first cast	80 ⟷ 50
27882	open, circular (guillotine)	80 ⟷ 50
27884	secondary closure or scar revision	③ ⟷ 50

27886	re-amputation	

| 27888 | Amputation, ankle, through malleoli of tibia and fibula (eg, Syme, Pirogoff type procedures), with plastic closure and resection of nerves | 80 ⬛ 50 |

| 27889 | Ankle disarticulation | ⬛ 50 |

OTHER PROCEDURES

| 27892 | Decompression fasciotomy, leg; anterior and/or lateral compartments only, with debridement of nonviable muscle and/or nerve | 80 ⬛ 50 |

If decompression fasciotomy is performed on the leg without debridement, consult CPT code 27600.

| 27893 | posterior compartment(s) only, with debridement of nonviable muscle and/or nerve | 80 ⬛ 50 |

If decompression fasciotomy is performed on the leg without debridement, consult CPT code 27601.

| 27894 | anterior and/or lateral, and posterior compartment(s), with debridement of nonviable muscle and/or nerve | 80 ⬛ 50 |

If decompression fasciotomy is performed on the leg without debridement, consult CPT code 27602.

| 27899 | Unlisted procedure, leg or ankle | 80 50 |

FOOT AND TOES

Codes listed in the Musculoskeletal chapter include the application and removal of the first cast or traction device. Replacement of casts and/or traction devices subsequent to the first should be reported separately. CPT codes for other additional procedures, such as obtaining grafts and external fixation, should only be used if the procedure is not already listed as included as part of the basic procedure. Consult the glossary for additional terms and guidelines.

INCISION

| 28001* | Incision and drainage, bursa, foot | ⬛ |

If superficial incision and drainage procedures are performed, consult CPT codes 10040-10160

| 28002* | Incision and drainage below fascia, with or without tendon sheath involvement, foot; single bursal space | ❸ ⬛ |

| 28003 | multiple areas | ❸ ⬛ |

| 28005 | Incision, bone cortex (eg, osteomyelitis or bone abscess), foot | ❸ ⬛ |

| 28008 | Fasciotomy, foot and/or toe | ❸ ⬛ |

Consult also CPT codes 28060, 28062, and 28250.

| 28010 | Tenotomy, percutaneous, toe; single tendon | ⬛ |

| 28011 | multiple tendons | ⬛ |

If an open tenotomy is performed, consult CPT codes 28230-28234.

| 28020 | Arthrotomy, including exploration, drainage, or removal of loose or foreign body; intertarsal or tarsometatarsal joint | ❷ ⬛ |

| 28022 | metatarsophalangeal joint | ⬛ |

| 28024 | interphalangeal joint | ⬛ |

| 28030 | Neurectomy, intrinsic musculature of foot | ❹ 80 ⬛ |

| 28035 | Release, tarsal tunnel (posterior tibial nerve decompression) | ❹ ⬛ |

If other nerves are entrapped, consult CPT codes 64704 and 64722.

EXCISION

| 28043 | Excision, tumor, foot; subcutaneous tissue | ❷ ⬛ 50 |

| 28045 | deep, subfascial, intramuscular | ❸ 80 ⬛ 50 |

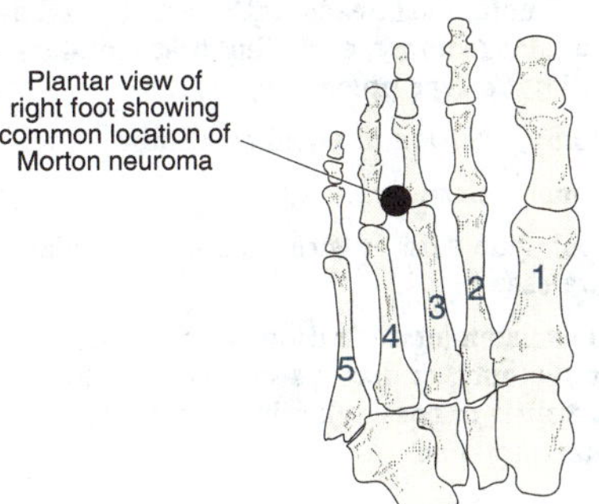

Morton neuroma is a chronic inflammation or irritation of the nerves in the web space between the heads of the metatarsals and phalanges

| 28046 | Radical resection of tumor (eg, malignant neoplasm), soft tissue of foot | ❸ ⬛ 50 |

| 28050 | Arthrotomy with biopsy; intertarsal or tarsometatarsal joint | ❷ ⬛ 50 |

| 28052 | metatarsophalangeal joint | ⬛ 50 |

| 28054 | interphalangeal joint | ❷ 80 ⬛ 50 |

| 28060 | Fasciectomy, plantar fascia; partial (separate procedure) | ❷ ⬛ 50 |

| 28062 | radical (separate procedure) | ❸ ⬛ |

If a plantar fasciotomy is performed, consult CPT codes 28008 and 28250.

| 28070 | Synovectomy; intertarsal or tarsometatarsal joint, each | ❸ ⬛ |

| 28072 | metatarsophalangeal joint, each | ❸ ⬛ |

| 28080 | Excision, interdigital (Morton) neuroma, single, each | ❸ 80 ⬛ 50 |

| 28086 | Synovectomy, tendon sheath, foot; flexor | ❷ 80 ⬛ 50 |

| 28088 | extensor | ❷ 80 ⬛ 50 |

| 28090 | Excision of lesion, tendon, tendon sheath, or capsule (including synovectomy) (eg, cyst or ganglion); foot | ❸ ⬛ 50 |

| 28092 | toe(s), each | ❸ ⬛ |

| 28100 | Excision or curettage of bone cyst or benign tumor, talus or calcaneus; | ❷ 80 ⬛ 50 |

| 28102 | with iliac or other autograft (includes obtaining graft) | ❸ 80 ⬛ 50 |

| 28103 | with allograft | ❸ 80 ⬛ 50 |

| ▲ 28104 | Excision or curettage of bone cyst or benign tumor, tarsal or metatarsal, except talus or calcaneus; | ❷ 80 |

| 28106 | with iliac or other autograft (includes obtaining graft) | ❸ 80 ⬛ |

| 28107 | with allograft | ❸ 80 ⬛ |

| 28108 | Excision or curettage of bone cyst or benign tumor, phalanges of foot | ⬛ |

If a partial ostectomy (eg. hallux valgus, Silver type procedure) is performed, consult CPT code 28290.

| 28110 | Ostectomy, partial excision, fifth metatarsal head (bunionette) (separate procedure) | ❸ ⬛ 50 |

| 28111 | Ostectomy, complete excision; first metatarsal head | ❸ ⬛ 50 |

| 28112 | other metatarsal head (second, third or fourth) | ❸ ⬛ 50 |

| 28113 | fifth metatarsal head | ❸ 80 ⬛ 50 |

Musculoskeletal System

28114 — 28308

28114	all metatarsal heads, with partial proximal phalangectomy, excluding first metatarsal (eg, Clayton type procedure)	③ 80 ⊠ 50
28116	Ostectomy, excision of tarsal coalition	③ ⊠ 50
28118	Ostectomy, calcaneus;	④ 80 ⊠ 50
28119	for spur, with or without plantar fascial release	④ ⊠ 50
28120	Partial excision (craterization, saucerization, sequestrectomy, or diaphysectomy) bone (eg, osteomyelitis or bossing); talus or calcaneus **Barker operation**	⑦ ⊠ 50
28122	tarsal or metatarsal bone, except talus or calcaneus	③ 80 ⊠ 50

If a partial excision of talus or calcaneus is performed, consult CPT code 28120. If a cheilectomy is performed for hallux rigidus, consult CPT code 28289.

28124	phalanx of toe	⊠ 50
28126	Resection, partial or complete, phalangeal base, each toe	⊠
28130	Talectomy (astragalectomy) **Whitman astragalectomy**	③ 80 ⊠ 50
28140	Metatarsectomy	③ ⊠
28150	Phalangectomy, toe, each toe	③ ⊠
28153	Resection, condyle(s), distal end of phalanx, each toe	⊠
28160	Hemiphalangectomy or interphalangeal joint excision, toe, proximal end of phalanx, each	⊠
28171	Radical resection of tumor, bone; tarsal (except talus or calcaneus)	③ 80 ⊠
28173	metatarsal	③ ⊠
28175	phalanx of toe	③ ⊠

If a radical resection of a talus or a calcaneus tumor is performed, consult CPT code 27647.

INTRODUCTION OR REMOVAL

28190*	Removal of foreign body, foot; subcutaneous	⊠ 50
28192	deep	② ⊠ 50
28193	complicated	④ ⊠ 50

REPAIR, REVISION, AND/OR RECONSTRUCTION

28200	Repair, tendon, flexor, foot; primary or secondary, without free graft, each tendon	③ ⊠
28202	secondary with free graft, each tendon (includes obtaining graft)	③ 80 ⊠
28208	Repair, tendon, extensor, foot; primary or secondary, each tendon	③ ⊠
28210	secondary with free graft, each tendon (includes obtaining graft)	③ 80 ⊠
28220	Tenolysis, flexor, foot; single tendon	⊠
28222	multiple tendons	① ⊠
28225	Tenolysis, extensor, foot; single tendon	① ⊠
28226	multiple tendons	① ⊠
28230	Tenotomy, open, tendon flexor; foot, single or multiple tendon(s) (separate procedure)	⊠
28232	toe, single tendon (separate procedure)	⊠
28234	Tenotomy, open, extensor, foot or toe, each tendon	⊠

▲ 28238 Reconstruction (advancement), posterior tibial tendon with excision of accessory tarsal navicular bone (eg, Kidner type procedure) ③ 80 ⊠ 50

If a subcutaneous tenotomy is performed, consult CPT codes 28010 and 28011. If a transfer or transplant of a tendon with muscle redirection or rerouting is performed, consult CPT codes 27690-27692. If an extensor hallucis longus transfer with a great toe IP fusion (Jones procedure) is performed, consult CPT code 28760.

28240	Tenotomy, lengthening, or release, abductor hallucis muscle	② ⊠ 50
28250	Division of plantar fascia and muscle (eg, Steindler stripping) (separate procedure)	③ 80 ⊠ 50
28260	Capsulotomy, midfoot; medial release only (separate procedure)	③ 80 ⊠ 50
28261	with tendon lengthening	③ 80 ⊠ 50
28262	extensive, including posterior talotibial capsulotomy and tendon(s) lengthening (eg, resistant clubfoot deformity)	④ 80 ⊠ 50
28264	Capsulotomy, midtarsal (eg, Heyman type procedure)	① 80 ⊠ 50
28270	Capsulotomy; metatarsophalangeal joint, with or without tenorrhaphy, each joint (separate procedure)	⊠ 50
28272	interphalangeal joint, each joint (separate procedure)	⊠ 50
28280	Syndactylization, toes (eg, webbing or Kelikian type procedure)	② 80 ⊠ 50
28285	Correction, hammertoe (eg, interphalangeal fusion, partial or total phalangectomy)	③ ⊠
28286	Correction, cock-up fifth toe, with plastic skin closure (eg, Ruiz-Mora type procedure)	④ ⊠
28288	Ostectomy, partial, exostectomy or condylectomy, metatarsal head, each metatarsal head	③ ⊠
28289	Hallux rigidus correction with cheilectomy, debridement and capsular release of the first metatarsophalangeal joint	80 ⊠ 50
28290	Correction, hallux valgus (bunion), with or without sesamoidectomy; simple exostectomy (eg, Silver type procedure)	② ⊠ 50
28292	Keller, McBride or Mayo type procedure	② 80 ⊠ 50
28293	resection of joint with implant	③ 80 ⊠ 50
28294	with tendon transplants (eg, Joplin type procedure)	③ 80 ⊠ 50
28296	with metatarsal osteotomy (eg, Mitchell, Chevron, or concentric type procedures)	③ 80 ⊠ 50
28297	Lapidus type procedure	③ 80 ⊠ 50
28298	by phalanx osteotomy	③ 80 ⊠ 50
▲ 28299	by double osteotomy	⑤ 80 ⊠ 50
28300	Osteotomy; calcaneus (eg, Dwyer or Chambers type procedure), with or without internal fixation	② 80 ⊠ 50
28302	talus	② 80 ⊠ 50
28304	Osteotomy, tarsal bones, other than calcaneus or talus;	② 80 ⊠
28305	with autograft (includes obtaining graft) (eg, Fowler type)	③ 80 ⊠
28306	Osteotomy, with or without lengthening, shortening or angular correction, metatarsal; first metatarsal	④ 80 ⊠
28307	first metatarsal with autograft (other than first toe)	④ 80 ⊠
28308	other than first metatarsal, each	② 80 ⊠

28309	multiple (eg, Swanson type cavus foot procedure)	❹ 80 ⊡
28310	Osteotomy, shortening, angular or rotational correction; proximal phalanx, first toe (separate procedure)	❸ ⊡
28312	other phalanges, any toe	❸ ⊡
28313	Reconstruction, angular deformity of toe, soft tissue procedures only (eg, overlapping second toe, fifth toe, curly toes)	❷ ⊡
28315	Sesamoidectomy, first toe (separate procedure)	❹ ⊡ 50
28320	Repair, nonunion or malunion; tarsal bones	❹ 80 ⊡
28322	metatarsal, with or without bone graft (includes obtaining graft)	❹ 80 ⊡
28340	Reconstruction, toe, macrodactyly; soft tissue resection	❹ ⊡
28341	requiring bone resection	❹ ⊡
28344	Reconstruction, toe(s); polydactyly	❹ ⊡
28345	syndactyly, with or without skin graft(s), each web	❹ 80 ⊡
28360	Reconstruction, cleft foot	80 ⊡

FRACTURE AND/OR DISLOCATION

28400	Closed treatment of calcaneal fracture; without manipulation	❶ ⊡ 50
28405	with manipulation	❷ 80 ⊡ 50
	Bohler reduction	
28406	Percutaneous skeletal fixation of calcaneal fracture, with manipulation	❷ 80 ⊡ 50
28415	Open treatment of calcaneal fracture, with or without internal or external fixation;	❸ 80 ⊡ 50
28420	with primary iliac or other autogenous bone graft (includes obtaining graft)	❹ 80 ⊡ 50
28430	Closed treatment of talus fracture; without manipulation	⊡ 50
28435	with manipulation	❷ 80 ⊡ 50
28436	Percutaneous skeletal fixation of talus fracture, with manipulation	❷ ⊡ 50
28445	Open treatment of talus fracture, with or without internal or external fixation	❸ 80 ⊡ 50
28450	Treatment of tarsal bone fracture (except talus and calcaneus); without manipulation, each	⊡
28455	with manipulation, each	80 ⊡
28456	Percutaneous skeletal fixation of tarsal bone fracture (except talus and calcaneus), with manipulation, each	❷ ⊡
28465	Open treatment of tarsal bone fracture (except talus and calcaneus), with or without internal or external fixation, each	❸ ⊡
28470	Closed treatment of metatarsal fracture; without manipulation, each	⊡
28475	with manipulation, each	⊡
28476	Percutaneous skeletal fixation of metatarsal fracture, with manipulation, each	❷ 80 ⊡
28485	Open treatment of metatarsal fracture, with or without internal or external fixation, each	❹ ⊡
28490	Closed treatment of fracture great toe, phalanx or phalanges; without manipulation	⊡
28495	with manipulation	⊡
28496	Percutaneous skeletal fixation of fracture great toe, phalanx or phalanges, with manipulation	❷ ⊡
28505	Open treatment of fracture great toe, phalanx or phalanges, with or without internal or external fixation	❸ ⊡
28510	Closed treatment of fracture, phalanx or phalanges, other than great toe; without manipulation, each	⊡
28515	with manipulation, each	⊡
28525	Open treatment of fracture, phalanx or phalanges, other than great toe, with or without internal or external fixation, each	❸ 80 ⊡
28530	Closed treatment of sesamoid fracture	80 ⊡
28531	Open treatment of sesamoid fracture, with or without internal fixation	⊡
28540	Closed treatment of tarsal bone dislocation, other than talotarsal; without anesthesia	80 ⊡
28545	requiring anesthesia	❶ 80 ⊡
28546	Percutaneous skeletal fixation of tarsal bone dislocation, other than talotarsal, with manipulation	❷ 80 ⊡
28555	Open treatment of tarsal bone dislocation, with or without internal or external fixation	❷ 80 ⊡
28570	Closed treatment of talotarsal joint dislocation; without anesthesia	80 ⊡
28575	requiring anesthesia	❶ 80 ⊡
28576	Percutaneous skeletal fixation of talotarsal joint dislocation, with manipulation	❸ 80 ⊡
28585	Open treatment of talotarsal joint dislocation, with or without internal or external fixation	❸ 80 ⊡
28600	Closed treatment of tarsometatarsal joint dislocation; without anesthesia	80 ⊡
28605	requiring anesthesia	❶ 80 ⊡
28606	Percutaneous skeletal fixation of tarsometatarsal joint dislocation, with manipulation	❷ ⊡
28615	Open treatment of tarsometatarsal joint dislocation, with or without internal or external fixation	❸ 80 ⊡
28630*	Closed treatment of metatarsophalangeal joint dislocation; without anesthesia	80 ⊡
28635*	requiring anesthesia	❶ 80 ⊡
28636	Percutaneous skeletal fixation of metatarsophalangeal joint dislocation, with manipulation	❸ ⊡
28645	Open treatment of metatarsophalangeal joint dislocation, with or without internal or external fixation	❸ ⊡
28660*	Closed treatment of interphalangeal joint dislocation; without anesthesia	⊡
28665*	requiring anesthesia	❶ 80 ⊡
28666	Percutaneous skeletal fixation of interphalangeal joint dislocation, with manipulation	❸ ⊡
28675	Open treatment of interphalangeal joint dislocation, with or without internal or external fixation	❸ ⊡

ARTHRODESIS

28705	Arthrodesis; pantalar	❹ 80 ⊡
28715	triple	❹ 80 ⊡
28725	subtalar	❹ 80 ⊡
	Dunn arthrodesis	
28730	Arthrodesis, midtarsal or tarsometatarsal, multiple or transverse;	❹ 80 ⊡
	Lambrinudi arthrodesis	
28735	with osteotomy (eg, flatfoot correction)	❹ 80 ⊡

▲ 28737 Arthrodesis, with tendon lengthening and advancement, midtarsal, tarsal navicular-cuneiform (eg, Miller type procedure)

28740 Arthrodesis, midtarsal or tarsometatarsal, single joint

28750 Arthrodesis, great toe; metatarsophalangeal joint

28755 interphalangeal joint

28760 Arthrodesis, with extensor hallucis longus transfer to first metatarsal neck, great toe, interphalangeal joint (eg, Jones type procedure)

If a hammertoe operation or interpphalangeal joint fusion is performed, consult CPT code 28285

AMPUTATION

28800 Amputation, foot; midtarsal (eg, Chopart type procedure)

28805 transmetatarsal

28810 Amputation, metatarsal, with toe, single

28820 Amputation, toe; metatarsophalangeal joint

28825 interphalangeal joint

If the tuft of the distal phalanx is amputated, consult CPT code 11752.

OTHER PROCEDURES

To report extracorporeal shock wave therapy involving musculoskeletal system, or plantar fascia, consult CPT Category III codes 0019T, 0020T.

28899 Unlisted procedure, foot or toes

APPLICATION OF CASTS AND STRAPPING

BODY AND UPPER EXTREMITY, CASTS

Codes listed in the Musculoskeletal chapter include the application and removal of the first cast or traction device. Replacement of casts and/or traction devices subsequent to the first should be reported separately. CPT codes for other additional procedures, such as obtaining grafts and external fixation, should only be used if the procedure is not already listed as included as part of the basic procedure. Consult the glossary for additional terms and guidelines.

Use these codes when replacing a cast or strap during or after follow-up care. They also apply when the application is an initial service without treatment or procedure to protect an injury.

Casts are rigid dressings, often made of fiberglass or plaster.

Strapping is the application of tape to bind, correct, or protect an anatomical part.

If orthotics fitting and training are necessary, consult CPT code 97504.

29000 Application of halo type body cast (see 20661-20663 for insertion)

29010 Application of Risser jacket, localizer, body; only

29015 including head

29020 Application of turnbuckle jacket, body; only

29025 including head

29035 Application of body cast, shoulder to hips;

29040 including head, Minerva type

29044 including one thigh

29046 including both thighs

▲ 29049 Application, cast; figure-of-eight

29055 shoulder spica

29058 plaster Velpeau

29065 shoulder to hand (long arm)

29075 elbow to finger (short arm)

29085 hand and lower forearm (gauntlet)

● 29086 finger (eg, contracture)

BODY AND UPPER EXTREMITY, SPLINTS

29105 Application of long arm splint (shoulder to hand)

29125 Application of short arm splint (forearm to hand); static

29126 dynamic

29130 Application of finger splint; static

29131 dynamic

BODY AND UPPER EXTREMITY, STRAPPING - ANY AGE

29200 Strapping; thorax

29220 low back

29240 shoulder (eg, Velpeau)

29260 elbow or wrist

29280 hand or finger

LOWER EXTREMITY, CASTS

29305 Application of hip spica cast; one leg

29325 one and one-half spica or both legs

29345 Application of long leg cast (thigh to toes);

29355 walker or ambulatory type

29358 Application of long leg cast brace

29365 Application of cylinder cast (thigh to ankle)

29405 Application of short leg cast (below knee to toes);

29425 walking or ambulatory type

29435 Application of patellar tendon bearing (PTB) cast

29440 Adding walker to previously applied cast

29445 Application of rigid total contact leg cast

29450 Application of clubfoot cast with molding or manipulation, long or short leg

LOWER EXTREMITY, SPLINTS

29505 Application of long leg splint (thigh to ankle o toes)

29515 Application of short leg splint (calf to foot)

LOWER EXTREMITY, STRAPPING-ANY AGE

29520 Strapping; hip

29530 knee

29540 ankle

29550 toes

29580 Unna boot

29590 Denis-Browne splint strapping

REMOVAL OR REPAIR

These codes are only used for casts applied by another physician.

29700 Removal or bivalving; gauntlet, boot or body cast

29705 full arm or full leg cast

29710 shoulder or hip spica, Minerva, or Risser jacket, etc.

29715 turnbuckle jacket

29720	Repair of spica, body cast or jacket	▣
29730	Windowing of cast	▣
29740	Wedging of cast (except clubfoot casts)	▣
29750	Wedging of clubfoot cast	80 ▣ 50

OTHER PROCEDURES

29799	Unlisted procedure, casting or strapping	80

ENDOSCOPY/ARTHROSCOPY

Codes listed in the Musculoskeletal chapter include the application and removal of the first cast or traction device. Replacement of casts and/or traction devices subsequent to the first should be reported separately. CPT codes for other additional procedures, such as obtaining grafts and external fixation, should only be used if the procedure is not already listed as included as part of the basic procedure. Consult the glossary for additional terms and guidelines.

When arthrotomy is performed in addition to the arthroscopy, append arthrotomy with modifier -51 or 09951.

CIM 35-59 ENDOSCOPY

Although endoscopy is primarily a diagnostic tool, it includes certain therapeutic procedures such as removal of polyps, and endoscopic papillotomy, by which stones are removed from the bile duct. Endoscopic procedures are covered when reasonable and necessary for the individual patient.

MCM 15038 MULTIPLE SURGERIES (CPT MODIFIER 51)

A. General—When more than one surgical service is performed on the same patient, by the same physician, and on the same day:

- The fee schedule amount for a second procedure is 50 percent of the fee schedule amount that would have been otherwise applicable for that procedure; and

- The fee schedule amount for the third through fifth procedures is 50 percent of the fee schedule amount that would have been otherwise applicable for that procedure. Prior to January 1, 1995, the third through fifth procedures were paid at 25 percent of the fee schedule amount. Surgical procedures beyond the fifth are priced "by report" based on documentation of the services furnished.

  Sequence the procedures from the one which has the highest regular fee schedule amount to the one with the lowest.

B. Multiple Endoscopies—For multiple endoscopic procedures, use the full value of the highest valued endoscopy plus the difference between the next highest and the base endoscopy. For example, in the course of performing a fiberoptic colonoscopy (code 45378), a physician performs a biopsy (code 45380) and removes a polyp (code 45385). Both codes 45380 and 45385 contain the values of the base endoscopy, code 45378. Use the actual value of code 45385 plus the difference between codes 45380 and 45378. The endoscopic base codes are listed in the Physician Fee Schedule.

29800	Arthroscopy, temporomandibular joint, diagnostic, with or without synovial biopsy (separate procedure)	80 ▣ 50
29804	Arthroscopy, temporomandibular joint, surgical	③ 80 ▣ 50
	To report an open procedure, consult CPT code 21010.	
● 29805	Arthroscopy, shoulder, diagnostic, with or without synovial biopsy (separate procedure)	③
	To report an open procedure, consult CPT codes 23065-23066, 23100-23101.	
● 29806	Arthroscopy, shoulder, surgical; capsulorrhaphy	③
	If an open procedure is performed, consult CPT codes 23450-23466.	
	If thermal capsulorrhaphy is performed, consult CPT code 29999.	
● 29807	repair of slap lesion	③

29815	~~Arthroscopy, shoulder, diagnostic, with or without synovial biopsy (separate procedure)~~ This code is deleted in 2002. See code 29805.	③ ▣ 50
29819	Arthroscopy, shoulder, surgical; with removal of loose body or foreign body	③ ▣ 50
	To report an open procedure, consult CPT codes 23040-23044, 23107.	
29820	synovectomy, partial	③ 80 ▣ 50
	To report an open procedure, consult CPT code 23105.	
29821	synovectomy, complete	③ 80 ▣ 50
	To report an open procedure, consult CPT code 23105.	
29822	debridement, limited	③ 80 ▣ 50
	For open procedure, see specific open shoulder procedure performed.	
29823	debridement, extensive	③ 80 ▣ 50
	For open procedure, see specific open shoulder procedure performed.	
● 29824	distal claviculectomy including distal articular surface (Mumford procedure)	⑤
	For open procedure, consult CPT code 23120.	
29825	with lysis and resection of adhesions, with or without manipulation	③ 80 ▣ 50
	For open procedure, see specific open shoulder procedure performed.	
29826	decompression of subacromial space with partial acromioplasty, with or without coracoacromial release	③ 80 ▣ 50
	To report an open procedure, consult CPT codes 23130 or 23415.	
29830	Arthroscopy, elbow, diagnostic, with or without synovial biopsy (separate procedure)	③ ▣ 50
29834	Arthroscopy, elbow, surgical; with removal of loose body or foreign body	③ 80 ▣ 50
29835	synovectomy, partial	③ 80 ▣ 50
29836	synovectomy, complete	③ 80 ▣ 50
29837	debridement, limited	③ 80 ▣ 50
29838	debridement, extensive	③ 80 ▣ 50
29840	Arthroscopy, wrist, diagnostic, with or without synovial biopsy (separate procedure)	③ 80 ▣ 50
29843	Arthroscopy, wrist, surgical; for infection, lavage and drainage	③ 80 ▣ 50
29844	synovectomy, partial	③ 80 ▣ 50
29845	synovectomy, complete	③ 80 ▣ 50
29846	excision and/or repair of triangular fibrocartilage and/or joint debridement	③ 80 ▣ 50
29847	internal fixation for fracture or instability	③ 80 ▣ 50
29848	Endoscopy, wrist, surgical, with release of transverse carpal ligament	▣ 50
	If this is an open procedure, consult CPT code 64721.	
29850	Arthroscopically aided treatment of intercondylar spine(s) and/or tuberosity fracture(s) of the knee, with or without manipulation; without internal or external fixation (includes arthroscopy)	④ 80 ▣ 50
	If a bone graft is performed, consult CPT codes 20900 and 20902.	
29851	with internal or external fixation (includes arthroscopy)	④ 80 ▣ 50

▣ CCI Comprehensive Code	50 Bilateral Procedure	✚ CPT Add-on Code	◊ Modifier -51 Exempt Code	● New Code	▲ Revised Code

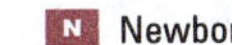 Maternity

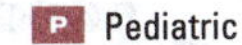 Newborn

P Pediatric

N/P Newborn/Pediatric

Musculoskeletal System

29855 — 29999

29855 **Arthroscopically aided treatment of tibial fracture, proximal (plateau); unicondylar, with or without internal or external fixation (includes arthroscopy)** ④ 80 ↔ 50
    If a bone graft is performed, consult CPT codes 20900 and 20902.

29856 **bicondylar, with or without internal or external fixation (includes arthroscopy)** ④ 80 ↔ 50

29860 **Arthroscopy, hip, diagnostic with or without synovial biopsy (separate procedure)** 80 ↔ 50

29861 **Arthroscopy, hip, surgical; with removal of loose body or foreign body** 80 ↔ 50

29862 **Arthroscopy, hip, surgical; with debridement/shaving of articular cartilage (chondroplasty), abrasion arthroplasty, and/or resection of labrum** 80 ↔ 50

29863 **Arthroscopy, hip, surgical; with synovectomy** 80 ↔ 50

29870 **Arthroscopy, knee, diagnostic, with or without synovial biopsy (separate procedure)** ③ ↔ 50
    To report surgical arthroscopy with implantation of graft for treatment of surface defect, consult CPT Category III codes 0012T, 0013T.

    To report meniscal transplantation, medial or lateral, knee, consult CPT Category III code 0014T.

29871 **Arthroscopy, knee, surgical; for infection, lavage and drainage** ③ ↔ 50

29874 **for removal of loose body or foreign body (eg, osteochondritis dissecans fragmentation, chondral fragmentation)** ③ 80 ↔ 50

29875 **synovectomy, limited (eg, plica or shelf resection) (separate procedure)** ④ 80 ↔ 50

29876 **synovectomy, major, two or more compartments (eg, medial or lateral)** ④ ↔ 50

29877 **debridement/shaving of articular cartilage (chondroplasty)** ④ 80 ↔ 50

29879 **abrasion arthroplasty (includes chondroplasty where necessary) or multiple drilling or microfracture** ③ 80 ↔ 50

29880 **with meniscectomy (medial AND lateral, including any meniscal shaving)** ④ 80 ↔ 50

29881 **with meniscectomy (medial OR lateral, including any meniscal shaving)** ④ 80 ↔ 50

29882 **with meniscus repair (medial OR lateral)** ③ ↔ 50

29883 **with meniscus repair (medial AND lateral)** ③ 80 ↔ 50

29884 **with lysis of adhesions, with or without manipulation (separate procedure)** ③ 80 ↔ 50

29885 **drilling for osteochondritis dissecans with bone grafting, with or without internal fixation (including debridement of base of lesion)** ③ 80 ↔ 50

29886 **drilling for intact osteochondritis dissecans lesion** ③ ↔ 50

29887 **drilling for intact osteochondritis dissecans lesion with internal fixation** ③ 80 ↔ 50

29888 **Arthroscopically aided anterior cruciate ligament repair/augmentation or reconstruction** ③ 80 ↔ 50
    Note that 29888 and 29889 should not be used in conjunction with reconstructive procedures 27427-27429.

29889 **Arthroscopically aided posterior cruciate ligament repair/augmentation or reconstruction** ③ 80 ↔ 50

29891 **Arthroscopy, ankle, surgical; excision of osteochondral defect of talus and/or tibia, including drilling of the defect** 80 ↔ 50

29892 **Arthroscopically aided repair of large osteochondritis dissecans lesion, talar dome fracture, or tibial plafond fracture, with or without internal fixation (includes arthroscopy)** 80 ↔ 50

29893 **Endoscopic plantar fasciotomy** 80 ↔ 50

29894 **Arthroscopy, ankle (tibiotalar and fibulotalar joints), surgical; with removal of loose body or foreign body** ③ 80 ↔ 50

29895 **synovectomy, partial** ③ 80 ↔ 50

29897 **debridement, limited** ③ 80 ↔ 50

29898 **debridement, extensive** ③ 80 ↔ 50

● **29900** **Arthroscopy, metacarpophalangeal joint, diagnostic, includes synovial biopsy** ③
    Code 29900 should not be reported with 29901, 29902.

● **29901** **Arthroscopy, metacarpophalangeal joint, surgical; with debridement** ③

● **29902** **with reduction of displaced ulnar collateral ligament (eg, Stenar lesion)** ③

~~29909~~ ~~Unlisted procedure, arthroscopy~~ This code is deleted in 2002. See code 29999. 50

● **29999** Unlisted procedure, arthroscopy

RESPIRATORY SYSTEM

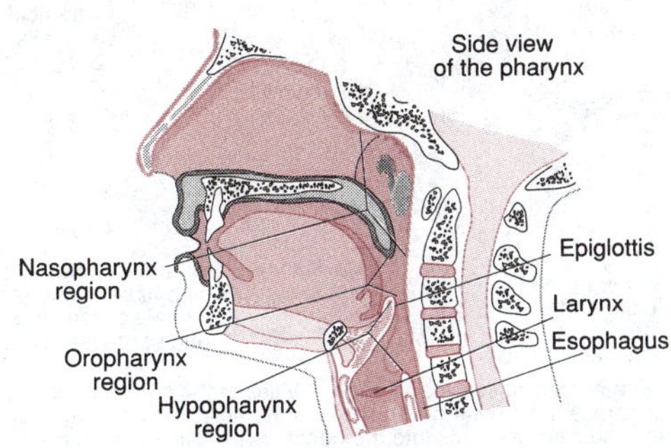

The nasopharynx is the membranous passage above the level of the soft palate; the oropharynx is the region between the soft palate and the upper edge of the epiglottis; the hypopharynx is the region of the epiglottis to the juncture of the larynx and esophagus; the three regions are collectively known as the pharynx

NOSE

INCISION

30000*   **Drainage abscess or hematoma, nasal, internal approach**
If this procedure requires an external approach, consult CPT codes 10060 and 10140.

30020*   **Drainage abscess or hematoma, nasal septum**
If a lateral rhinotomy is performed, consult specific application (eg, 30118, 30320).

EXCISION

30100   **Biopsy, intranasal**
If the skin of the nose is biopsied, consult CPT codes 11100 and 11101.

30110   **Excision, nasal polyp(s), simple**
Note that 30110 is generally completed in an office setting.

30115   **Excision, nasal polyp(s), extensive**
Note that 30115 generally requires the facilities available in a hospital setting.

CIM 35-52 LASER PROCEDURES
Coverage is determined on the basis that the use of lasers to alter, revise, or destroy tissue is a surgical procedure and restricted to practitioners with training in the surgical management of the disease or condition being treated.

▲   **30117**   **Excision or destruction (eg, laser), intranasal lesion; internal approach**

30118   **external approach (lateral rhinotomy)**

30120   **Excision or surgical planing of skin of nose for rhinophyma**

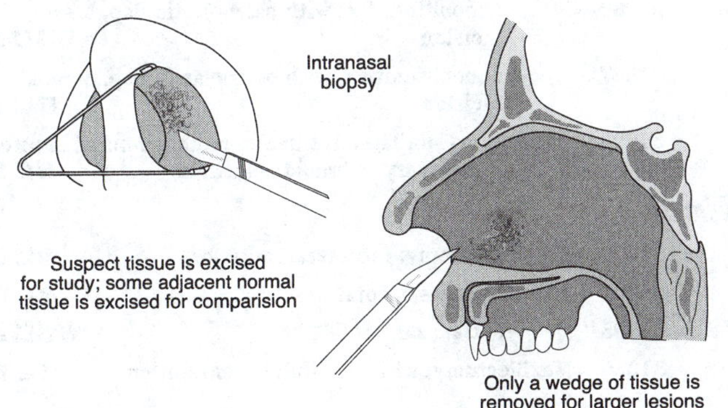

30124   **Excision dermoid cyst, nose; simple, skin, subcutaneous**

30125   **complex, under bone or cartilage**

30130   **Excision turbinate, partial or complete, any method**

30140   **Submucous resection turbinate, partial or complete, any method**
If a submucous resection is performed on the nasal septum, consult CPT code 30520. If a reduction of the turbinates is performed, use 30140 with modifier -52 or 09952.

30150   **Rhinectomy; partial**
If primary or delayed closure and/or reconstruction is needed, consult the Integumentary System (13150-13152, 14060-14300, 15120, 15121, 15260, 15261, 15760, and 20900-20912).

30160   **total**

INTRODUCTION

30200*   **Injection into turbinate(s), therapeutic**

30210*   **Displacement therapy (Proetz type)**

30220   **Insertion, nasal septal prosthesis (button)**

REMOVAL OF FOREIGN BODY

30300*   **Removal foreign body, intranasal; office type procedure**

30310   **requiring general anesthesia**

30320   **by lateral rhinotomy**

REPAIR
If obtaining tissues for a graft, consult CPT codes 20900-20926 and 21210.

30400   **Rhinoplasty, primary; lateral and alar cartilages and/or elevation of nasal tip**
If columellar reconstruction is performed, consult CPT codes 13150-13153.

Carpue's operation

30410   **complete, external parts including bony pyramid, lateral and alar cartilages, and/or elevation of nasal tip**

30420   **including major septal repair**

30430   **Rhinoplasty, secondary; minor revision (small amount of nasal tip work)**

30435   **intermediate revision (bony work with osteotomies)**

30450   **major revision (nasal tip work and osteotomies)**

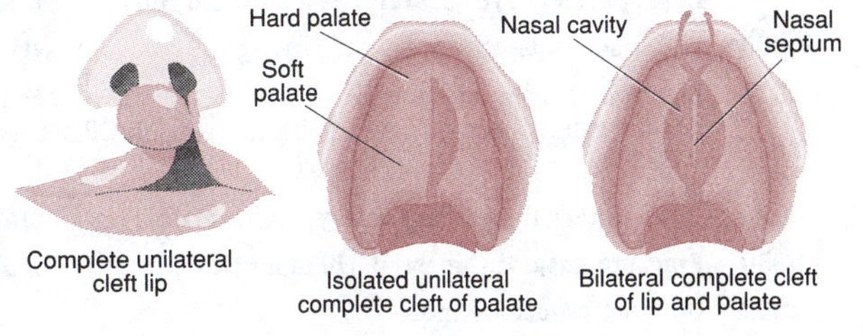

Cleft lip with or without cleft palate is a common birth defect and is seen once or twice per 1000 live births; the condition is twice as common among boys than girls; isolated cleft palate is distinct from cleft lip with or without cleft palate and occurs about once in 2000 births; the condition is more common among girls than boys

---

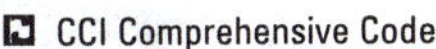 CCI Comprehensive Code   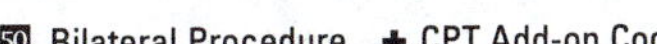 Bilateral Procedure   ✚ CPT Add-on Code   ⊘ Modifier -51 Exempt Code   ● New Code   ▲ Revised Code

M Maternity   **N** Newborn   **P** Pediatric   **N/P** Newborn/Pediatric

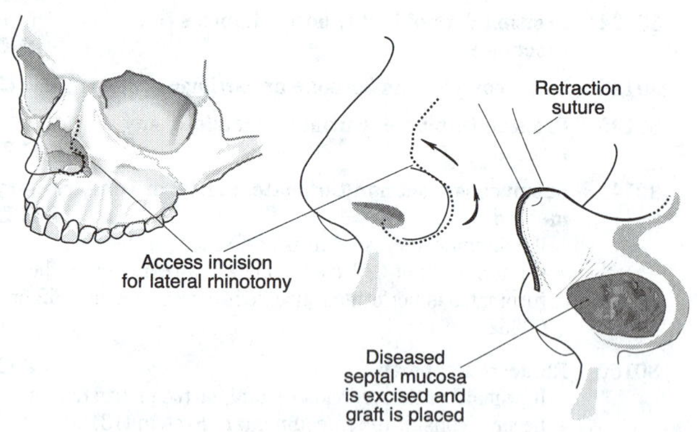

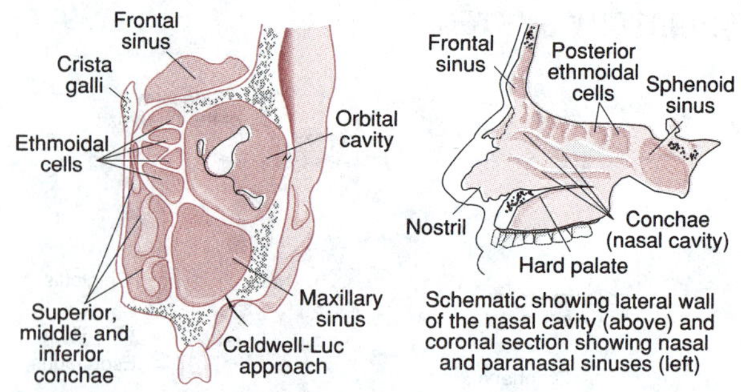

The nasal sinuses are air filled cavities in the cranial bones that bear their names; all are lined with mucous membrane continuous with the nasal cavity and all drain fluids into the nasal cavity. The ethmoid cells vary in size and number and feature very thin septa,or walls. The maxillary sinuses are the largest and are the most frequently infected.

30460 Rhinoplasty for nasal deformity secondary to congenital cleft lip and/or palate, including columellar lengthening; tip only

30462 tip, septum, osteotomies

30465 Repair of nasal vestibular stenosis (eg, spreader grafting, lateral nasal wall reconstruction)
36465 is used to report a bilateral procedure. if procedure is done as a unilateral procedure, append with modifier-52.

30520 Septoplasty or submucous resection, with or without cartilage scoring, contouring or replacement with graft
If submucous resection of the turbinates is performed, consult CPT code 30140.

30540 Repair choanal atresia; intranasal

30545 transpalatine

30560* Lysis intranasal synechia

30580 Repair fistula; oromaxillary (combine with 31030 if antrotomy is included)

30600 oronasal

30620 Septal or other intranasal dermatoplasty (does not include obtaining graft)

30630 Repair nasal septal perforations

DESTRUCTION

▲ **30801*** Cautery and/or ablation, mucosa of turbinates, unilateral or bilateral, any method, (separate procedure); superficial

30802 intramural

OTHER PROCEDURES

30901* Control nasal hemorrhage, anterior, simple (limited cautery and/or packing) any method

30903* Control nasal hemorrhage, anterior, complex (extensive cautery and/or packing) any method

▲ **30905*** Control nasal hemorrhage, posterior, with posterior nasal packs and/or cautery, any method; initial

30906* subsequent

30915 Ligation arteries; ethmoidal
If the external carotid artery is ligated, consult CPT code 37600.

30920 internal maxillary artery, transantral

30930 Fracture nasal turbinate(s), therapeutic

30999 Unlisted procedure, nose

ACCESSORY SINUSES

INCISION

31000* Lavage by cannulation; maxillary sinus (antrum puncture or natural ostium)

31002* sphenoid sinus

31020 Sinusotomy, maxillary (antrotomy); intranasal

31030 radical (Caldwell-Luc) without removal of antrochoanal polyps

31032 radical (Caldwell-Luc) with removal of antrochoanal polyps

31040 Pterygomaxillary fossa surgery, any approach
If a transantral ligation of the internal maxillary artery is performed, consult CPT code 30920.

31050 Sinusotomy, sphenoid, with or without biopsy;

31051 with mucosal stripping or removal of polyp(s)

31070 Sinusotomy frontal; external, simple (trephine operation)
Killian operation

31075 transorbital, unilateral (for mucocele or osteoma, Lynch type)

31080 obliterative without osteoplastic flap, brow incision (includes ablation)
Ridell sinusotomy

31081 obliterative, without osteoplastic flap, coronal incision (includes ablation)

31084 obliterative, with osteoplastic flap, brow incision

31085 obliterative, with osteoplastic flap, coronal incision

31086 nonobliterative, with osteoplastic flap, brow incision

31087 nonobliterative, with osteoplastic flap, coronal incision

31090 Sinusotomy, unilateral, three or more paranasal sinuses (frontal, maxillary, ethmoid, sphenoid)

EXCISION

31200 Ethmoidectomy; intranasal, anterior

31201 intranasal, total

31205 extranasal, total

31225 Maxillectomy; without orbital exenteration

31230	**with orbital exenteration (en bloc)**	80 ☐ 50

If orbital exenteration is performed only, consult CPT codes 65110 and subsequent codes. If skin grafts are necessary, consult CPT code 15120 and subsequent codes.

ENDOSCOPY

Sinus endoscopies include the examination of all parts of the sinuses, including the nasal cavity to the turbinates, and the spheno-ethmoid recess. Any sinusotomy performed during the examination is included in these codes.

Unless otherwise stated, CPT codes 31231-31294 report unilateral procedures. If these procedures are performed bilaterally, append modifier -50 or 09950.

CIM 35-59 ENDOSCOPY

Although endoscopy is primarily a diagnostic tool, it includes certain therapeutic procedures such as removal of polyps, and endoscopic papillotomy, by which stones are removed from the bile duct. Endoscopic procedures are covered when reasonable and necessary for the individual patient.

MCM 15038. MULTIPLE SURGERIES (CPT MODIFIER 51)

A. General—When more than one surgical service is performed on the same patient, by the same physician, and on the same day:

- The fee schedule amount for a second procedure is 50 percent of the fee schedule amount that would have been otherwise applicable for that procedure; and

- The fee schedule amount for the third through fifth procedures is 50 percent of the fee schedule amount that would have been otherwise applicable for that procedure. Prior to January 1, 1995, the third through fifth procedures were paid at 25 percent of the fee schedule amount. Surgical procedures beyond the fifth are priced "by report" based on documentation of the services furnished.

  Sequence the procedures from the one which has the highest regular fee schedule amount to the one with the lowest.

B. Multiple Endoscopies—For multiple endoscopic procedures, use the full value of the highest valued endoscopy plus the difference between the next highest and the base endoscopy. For example, in the course of performing a fiberoptic colonoscopy (code 45378), a physician performs a biopsy (code 45380) and removes a polyp (code 45385). Both codes 45380 and 45385 contain the values of the base endoscopy, code 45378. Use the actual value of code 45385 plus the difference between codes 45380 and 45378. The endoscopic base codes are listed in the Physician Fee Schedule.

31231	**Nasal endoscopy, diagnostic, unilateral or bilateral (separate procedure)**	☐
31233	**Nasal/sinus endoscopy, diagnostic with maxillary sinusoscopy (via inferior meatus or canine fossa puncture)**	❷ ☐ 50
31235	**Nasal/sinus endoscopy, diagnostic with sphenoid sinusoscopy (via puncture of sphenoidal face or cannulation of ostium)**	❶ ☐ 50
31237	**Nasal/sinus endoscopy, surgical; with biopsy, polypectomy or debridement (separate procedure)**	❷ ☐ 50
▲ **31238**	**with control of nasal hemorrhage**	❶ 80 ☐ 50
31239	**with dacryocystorhinostomy**	❹ 80 ☐ 50
31240	**with concha bullosa resection**	❷ 80 ☐ 50
31254	**Nasal/sinus endoscopy, surgical; with ethmoidectomy, partial (anterior)**	❸ ☐ 50
31255	**with ethmoidectomy, total (anterior and posterior)**	❺ ☐ 50
31256	**Nasal/sinus endoscopy, surgical, with maxillary antrostomy;**	❸ ☐ 50

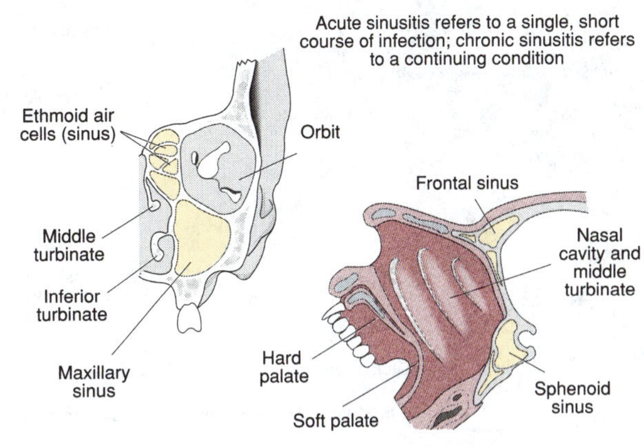

31267	**with removal of tissue from maxillary sinus**	❸ ☐ 50
31276	**Nasal/sinus endoscopy, surgical with frontal sinus exploration, with or without removal of tissue from frontal sinus**	❸ ☐ 50
31287	**Nasal/sinus endoscopy, surgical, with sphenoidotomy;**	❸ 80 ☐ 50
31288	**with removal of tissue from the sphenoid sinus**	❸ 80 ☐ 50
31290	**Nasal/sinus endoscopy, surgical, with repair of cerebrospinal fluid leak; ethmoid region**	80 ☐ 50
31291	**sphenoid region**	80 ☐ 50
31292	**Nasal/sinus endoscopy, surgical; with medial or inferior orbital wall decompression**	80 ☐ 50
31293	**with medial orbital wall and inferior orbital wall decompression**	80 ☐ 50
31294	**with optic nerve decompression**	80 ☐ 50

OTHER PROCEDURES

31299	**Unlisted procedure, accessory sinuses**	80

If a hypophysectomy is performed in a transantral or a transeptal approach, consult CPT code 61548. If a transcranial hypophysectomy is performed, consult CPT code 61546.

LARYNX

EXCISION

31300	**Laryngotomy (thyrotomy, laryngofissure); with removal of tumor or laryngocele, cordectomy**	❺ 80 ☐
31320	**diagnostic**	❷ 80 ☐

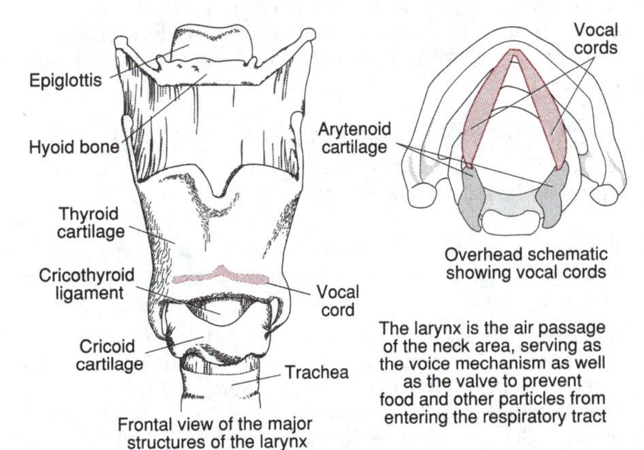

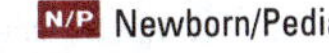

☐ CCI Comprehensive Code	50 Bilateral Procedure ✚ CPT Add-on Code	⊘ Modifier -51 Exempt Code	● New Code	▲ Revised Code
M Maternity	N Newborn	P Pediatric	N/P Newborn/Pediatric

Respiratory System

31360 — 31578

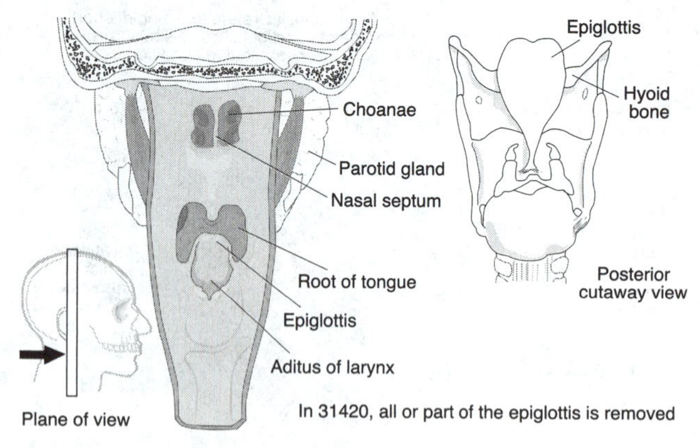

31360	Laryngectomy; total, without radical neck dissection	80
31365	total, with radical neck dissection	80
31367	subtotal supraglottic, without radical neck dissection	80
31368	subtotal supraglottic, with radical neck dissection	80
31370	Partial laryngectomy (hemilaryngectomy); horizontal	80
31375	laterovertical	80
31380	anterovertical	80
31382	antero-latero-vertical	80
31390	Pharyngolaryngectomy, with radical neck dissection; without reconstruction	80
31395	with reconstruction	80
31400	Arytenoidectomy or arytenoidopexy, external approach	80

if performed endoscopically, consult CPT code 31560.

31420	Epiglottidectomy	80

INTRODUCTION

31500 Intubation, endotracheal, emergency procedure

If an injection procedure is used for bronchography, consult CPT codes 31656, 31708, and 31710.

31502 Tracheotomy tube change prior to establishment of fistula tract

ENDOSCOPY

CIM 35-59 ENDOSCOPY

Although endoscopy is primarily a diagnostic tool, it includes certain therapeutic procedures such as removal of polyps, and endoscopic papillotomy, by which stones are removed from the bile duct. Endoscopic procedures are covered when reasonable and necessary for the individual patient.

MCM 15038 MULTIPLE SURGERIES (CPT MODIFIER 51)

A. General—When more than one surgical service is performed on the same patient, by the same physician, and on the same day:

- The fee schedule amount for a second procedure is 50 percent of the fee schedule amount that would have been otherwise applicable for that procedure; and

- The fee schedule amount for the third through fifth procedures is 50 percent of the fee schedule amount that would have been otherwise applicable for that procedure. Prior to January 1, 1995, the third through fifth procedures were paid at 25 percent of the fee schedule amount. Surgical procedures beyond the fifth are priced "by report" based on documentation of the services furnished.

Sequence the procedures from the one which has the highest regular fee schedule amount to the one with the lowest.

B. Multiple Endoscopies—For multiple endoscopic procedures, use the full value of the highest valued endoscopy plus the difference between the next highest and the base endoscopy. For example, in the course of performing a fiberoptic colonoscopy (code 45378), a physician performs a biopsy (code 45380) and removes a polyp (code 45385). Both codes 45380 and 45385 contain the values of the base endoscopy, code 45378. Use the actual value of code 45385 plus the difference between codes 45380 and 45378. The endoscopic base codes are listed in the Physician Fee Schedule.

31505	Laryngoscopy, indirect; diagnostic (separate procedure)	
31510	with biopsy	2 80
31511	with removal of foreign body	2
31512	with removal of lesion	2 80
31513	with vocal cord injection	2 80
31515	Laryngoscopy direct, with or without tracheoscopy; for aspiration	1
31520	diagnostic, newborn	N 80
31525	diagnostic, except newborn	1
31526	diagnostic, with operating microscope	2

Do not report 69990 in addition to 31526 as the operating microscope is considered an inclusive component of the surgery.

31527	with insertion of obturator	1 80
31528	with dilation, initial	2 80
31529	with dilation, subsequent	2 80
31530	Laryngoscopy, direct, operative, with foreign body removal;	2
31531	with operating microscope	3 80

Do not report 69990 in addition to 31531 as the operating microscope is considered an inclusive component of the surgery.

31535	Laryngoscopy, direct, operative, with biopsy;	2
31536	with operating microscope	3

Do not report 69990 in addition to 31536 as the operating microscope is considered an inclusive component of the surgery.

31540	Laryngoscopy, direct, operative, with excision of tumor and/or stripping of vocal cords or epiglottis;	3
31541	with operating microscope	4

Do not report 69990 in addition to 31541 as the operating microscope is considered an inclusive component of the surgery.

31560	Laryngoscopy, direct, operative, with arytenoidectomy;	5 80
31561	with operating microscope	5 80

Do not report 69990 in addition to 31561 as the operating microscope is considered an inclusive component of the surgery.

31570	Laryngoscopy, direct, with injection into vocal cord(s), therapeutic;	2
31571	with operating microscope	2

Do not report 69990 in addition to 31571 as the operating microscope is considered an inclusive component of the surgery.

31575	Laryngoscopy, flexible fiberoptic; diagnostic	
31576	with biopsy	2
31577	with removal of foreign body	2 80
31578	with removal of lesion	2 80

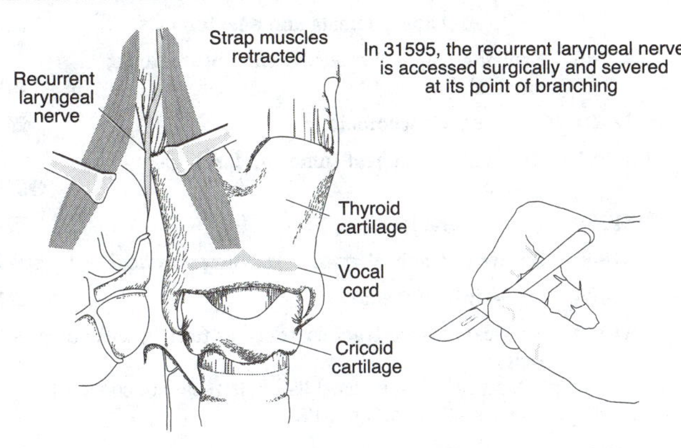

31579	Laryngoscopy, flexible or rigid fiberoptic, with stroboscopy	⌷

REPAIR

31580	Laryngoplasty; for laryngeal web, two stage, with keel insertion and removal	⑤80⌷
31582	for laryngeal stenosis, with graft or core mold, including tracheotomy	⑤⌷
31584	with open reduction of fracture	④80⌷
31585	Treatment of closed laryngeal fracture; without manipulation	①80⌷
31586	with closed manipulative reduction	②80⌷
31587	Laryngoplasty, cricoid split	80⌷
31588	Laryngoplasty, not otherwise specified (eg, for burns, reconstruction after partial laryngectomy)	⑤80⌷
31590	Laryngeal reinnervation by neuromuscular pedicle	⑤80⌷

DESTRUCTION

31595	Section recurrent laryngeal nerve, therapeutic (separate procedure), unilateral	②80⌷

OTHER PROCEDURES

31599	Unlisted procedure, larynx	80

TRACHEA AND BRONCHI

INCISION

31600	Tracheostomy, planned (separate procedure);	②⌷
	If endotracheal intubation is necessary, consult CPT code 31500.	
31601	under two years	N/P 80⌷
31603	Tracheostomy, emergency procedure; transtracheal	⌷
31605	cricothyroid membrane	⌷
31610	Tracheostomy, fenestration procedure with skin flaps	⌷
31611	Construction of tracheoesophageal fistula and subsequent insertion of an alaryngeal speech prosthesis (eg, voice button, Blom-Singer prosthesis)	③80⌷
31612	Tracheal puncture, percutaneous with transtracheal aspiration and/or injection	①80⌷
	If tracheal aspiration under direct vision is performed, consult CPT code 31515.	
31613	Tracheostoma revision; simple, without flap rotation	②⌷
31614	complex, with flap rotation	②⌷

ENDOSCOPY

If a tracheoscopy is performed, consult laryngoscopy codes 31515-31578.

Fluoroscopic guidance, when performed with CPT codes 31622-31646, should not be reported separately.

CIM 35-59 ENDOSCOPY

Although endoscopy is primarily a diagnostic tool, it includes certain therapeutic procedures such as removal of polyps, and endoscopic papillotomy, by which stones are removed from the bile duct. Endoscopic procedures are covered when reasonable and necessary for the individual patient.

MCM 15038. MULTIPLE SURGERIES (CPT MODIFIER 51)

A. General—When more than one surgical service is performed on the same patient, by the same physician, and on the same day:

- The fee schedule amount for a second procedure is 50 percent of the fee schedule amount that would have been otherwise applicable for that procedure; and

- The fee schedule amount for the third through fifth procedures is 50 percent of the fee schedule amount that would have been otherwise applicable for that procedure. Prior to January 1, 1995, the third through fifth procedures were paid at 25 percent of the fee schedule amount. Surgical procedures beyond the fifth are priced "by report" based on documentation of the services furnished.

Sequence the procedures from the one which has the highest regular fee schedule amount to the one with the lowest.

B. Multiple Endoscopies—For multiple endoscopic procedures, use the full value of the highest valued endoscopy plus the difference between the next highest and the base endoscopy. For example, in the course of performing a fiberoptic colonoscopy (code 45378), a physician performs a biopsy (code 45380) and removes a polyp (code 45385). Both codes 45380 and 45385 contain the values of the base endoscopy, code 45378. Use the actual value of code 45385 plus the difference between codes 45380 and 45378. The endoscopic base codes are listed in the Physician Fee Schedule.

31615	Tracheobronchoscopy through established tracheostomy incision	①⌷
31622	Bronchoscopy (rigid or flexible); diagnostic, with or without cell washing (separate procedure)	①⌷
31623	with brushing or protected brushings	⌷
31624	with bronchial alveolar lavage	⌷
31625	with biopsy	②⌷
31628	with transbronchial lung biopsy, with or without fluoroscopic guidance	②⌷
31629	with transbronchial needle aspiration biopsy	②⌷
31630	with tracheal or bronchial dilation or closed reduction of fracture	②⌷
31631	with tracheal dilation and placement of tracheal stent	②⌷
31635	with removal of foreign body	②⌷
31640	with excision of tumor	②⌷
▲ 31641	Bronchoscopy, (rigid or flexible); with destruction of tumor or relief of stenosis by any method other than excision (eg, laser therapy, cryotherapy)	②⌷
	If bronchoscopic photodynamic therapy is performed, report CPT code 31641 in addition to 96570 and 96571 as appropriate.	
31643	with placement of catheter(s) for intracavitary radioelement application	⌷
	If intracavitary radioelement application is performed, consult CPT codes 77761-77763 and 77781-77784.	

⌷ CCI Comprehensive Code	⑤⓪ Bilateral Procedure	✛ CPT Add-on Code	⊘ Modifier -51 Exempt Code	● New Code	▲ Revised Code

M Maternity	N Newborn	P Pediatric	N/P Newborn/Pediatric

31645	with therapeutic aspiration of tracheobronchial tree, initial (eg, drainage of lung abscess)	❶

If catheter aspiration of the tracheobronchial tree at bedside is performed, consult CPT code 31725.

31646	with therapeutic aspiration of tracheobronchial tree, subsequent	❶

If catheter aspiration of the tracheobronchial tree at bedside is performed, consult CPT code 31725.

31656	with injection of contrast material for segmental bronchography (fiberscope only)	❶ 80

For radiological supervision and interpretation, consult CPT codes 71040 and 71060.

If a tracheoscopy is performed, consult laryngoscopy codes 31515-31578.

INTRODUCTION

If endotracheal intubation is performed, consult CPT code 31500. If tracheal aspiration under direct vision is performed, consult CPT code 31515.

31700	**Catheterization, transglottic (separate procedure)**	❶ 80
31708	**Instillation of contrast material for laryngography or bronchography, without catheterization**	80 50

For radiological supervision interpretation, consult CPT codes 70373, 71040, and 71060.

31710	**Catheterization for bronchography, with or without instillation of contrast material**	❶ 80 50

If bronchoscopic catheterization is performed for bronchography, fiberscope only, consult CPT code 31656. If radiological supervision and interpretation is performed, consult CPT codes 71040 and 71060.

31715	**Transtracheal injection for bronchography**	❶ 80 50

For radiological supervision and interpretation, consult CPT codes 71040 and 71060. If prolonged services are necessary, consult CPT codes 99354-99360.

31717	**Catheterization with bronchial brush biopsy**	❶
31720	**Catheter aspiration (separate procedure); nasotracheal**	❶
31725	**tracheobronchial with fiberscope, bedside**	
31730	**Transtracheal (percutaneous) introduction of needle wire dilator/stent or indwelling tube for oxygen therapy**	❶

REPAIR

31750	**Tracheoplasty; cervical**	❺ 80
31755	**tracheopharyngeal fistulization, each stage**	❷ 80
31760	**intrathoracic**	80
31766	**Carinal reconstruction**	80
31770	**Bronchoplasty; graft repair**	80

If a lobectomy and bronchoplasty are performed, consult CPT code 32501.

31775	**excision stenosis and anastomosis**	80
31780	**Excision tracheal stenosis and anastomosis; cervical**	80
31781	**cervicothoracic**	80
31785	**Excision of tracheal tumor or carcinoma; cervical**	❹ 80
31786	**thoracic**	80
31800	**Suture of tracheal wound or injury; cervical**	❷ 80
31805	**intrathoracic**	80
31820	**Surgical closure tracheostomy or fistula; without plastic repair**	❶ 80

If a tracheoesophageal fistula is repaired, consult CPT codes 43305 and 43312.

31825	**with plastic repair**	❷ 80
31830	**Revision of tracheostomy scar**	❷ 80

OTHER PROCEDURES

31899	Unlisted procedure, trachea, bronchi	80

LUNGS AND PLEURA

INCISION

⊘	32000*	**Thoracentesis, puncture of pleural cavity for aspiration, initial or subsequent**	❶

To report imaging guidance, consult CPT codes 76003, 76360, and 76942.

⊘	32002	**Thoracentesis with insertion of tube with or without water seal (eg, for pneumothorax) (separate procedure)**	❷

To report imaging guidance, consult CPT codes 76003, 76360, and 76942.

32005	**Chemical pleurodesis (eg, for recurrent or persistent pneumothorax)**	❷

⊘	32020	**Tube thoracostomy with or without water seal (eg, for abscess, hemothorax, empyema) (separate procedure)**	❷

To report imaging guidance, consult CPT code 75989.

32035	**Thoracostomy; with rib resection for empyema**	80
32036	**with open flap drainage for empyema**	80
32095	**Thoracotomy, limited, for biopsy of lung or pleura**	80

If wound exploration due to penetrating trauma without thoracotomy is performed, consult CPT code 20102.

32100	**Thoracotomy, major; with exploration and biopsy**	80
32110	**with control of traumatic hemorrhage and/or repair of lung tear**	80
32120	**for postoperative complications**	80
32124	**with open intrapleural pneumonolysis**	80

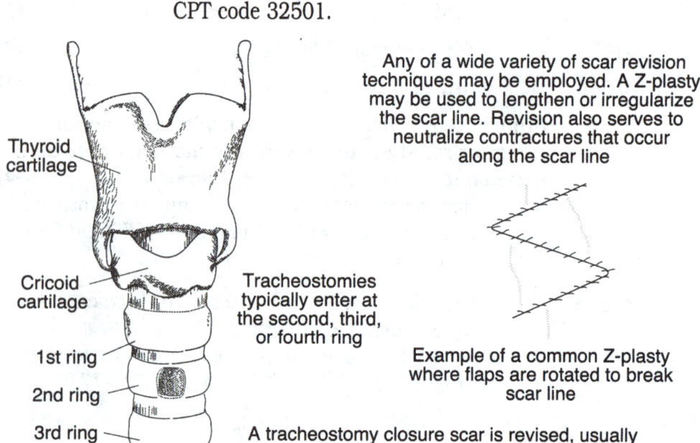

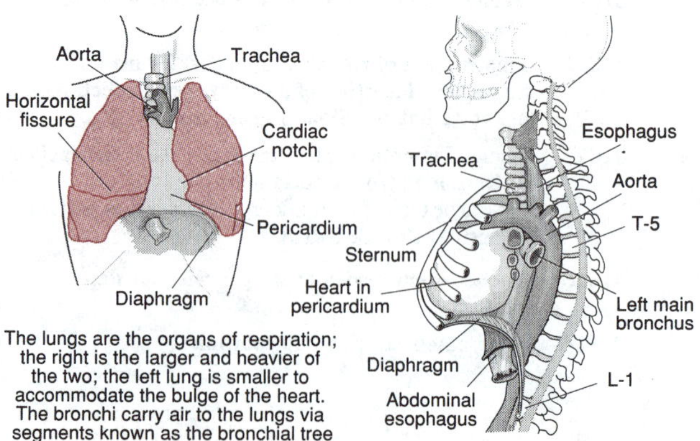

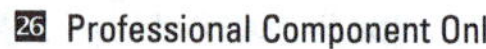
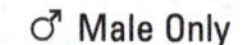

32140	with cyst(s) removal, with or without a pleural procedure	80 ⊡

If segmental or other resections of the lung are performed, consult CPT codes 32480-32525.

32141	with excision-plication of bullae, with or without any pleural procedure	80 ⊡

If lung volume reduction is performed, consult CPT code 32491.

32150	with removal of intrapleural foreign body or fibrin deposit	80 ⊡
32151	with removal of intrapulmonary foreign body	80 ⊡
32160	with cardiac massage	80 ⊡
32200	Pneumonostomy; with open drainage of abscess or cyst	80 ⊡
32201	with percutaneous drainage of abscess or cyst	80 ⊡

For radiological supervision and interpretation, consult CPT code 75989.

32215	Pleural scarification for repeat pneumothorax	80 ⊡
32220	Decortication, pulmonary, (separate procedure); total	80 ⊡
32225	partial	80 ⊡

EXCISION

32310	Pleurectomy, parietal (separate procedure)	80 ⊡
32320	Decortication and parietal pleurectomy	80 ⊡
32400*	Biopsy, pleura; percutaneous needle	❶ ⊡

To report imaging guidance, consult CPT codes 76003, 76360, 76393, and 76942.

To report fine needle aspiration, consult CPT codes 10021 or 10022.

To report evaluation of fine needle aspirate, consult CPT codes 88172, 88173.

32402	open	80 ⊡
32405	Biopsy, lung or mediastinum, percutaneous needle	❶ ⊡

To report radiological supervision and interpretation, consult CPT codes 76003, 76360, 76393, 76942.

To report fine needle aspiration, consult CPT code 10022.

To report evaluation of fine needle aspirate, consult CPT codes 88172, 88173.

▲ 32420*	Pneumocentesis, puncture of lung for aspiration	❶ ⊡
32440	Removal of lung, total pneumonectomy;	80 ⊡
32442	Removal of lung, total pneumonectomy; with resection of segment of trachea followed by broncho-tracheal anastomosis (sleeve pneumonectomy)	80 ⊡

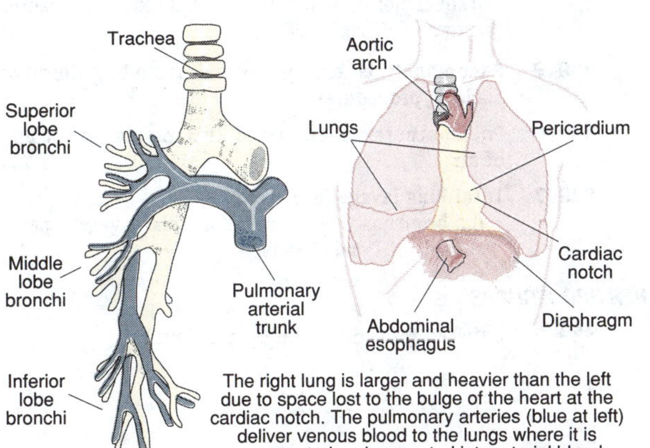

The right lung is larger and heavier than the left due to space lost to the bulge of the heart at the cardiac notch. The pulmonary arteries (blue at left) deliver venous blood to the lungs where it is oxygenated and converted into arterial blood

32445	Removal of lung, total pneumonectomy; extrapleural	80 ⊡
32480	Removal of lung, other than total pneumonectomy; single lobe (lobectomy)	80 ⊡
32482	two lobes (bilobectomy)	80 ⊡
32484	single segment (segmentectomy)	80 ⊡
32486	with circumferential resection of segment of bronchus followed by broncho-bronchial anastomosis (sleeve lobectomy)	80 ⊡
32488	all remaining lung following previous removal of a portion of lung (completion pneumonectomy)	80 ⊡

CIM 35-93 LUNG VOLUME REDUCTION SURGERY (REDUCTION PNEUMOPLASTY, ALSO CALLED LUNG SHAVING OR LUNG CONTOURING) UNILATERAL OR BILATERAL BY OPEN OR THORACOSCOPIC APPROACH FOR TREATMENT OF EMPHYSEMA OR CHRONIC OBSTRUCTIVE PULMONARY DISEASE - NOT GENERALLY COVERED

Unilateral or bilateral LVRS by open or thoracoscopic approach is not generally covered due to the insufficiency of medical evidence available. On April 24, 1996, HCFA and the National Heart, Lung and Blood Institute (NHLBI) of the National Institutes of Health initiated a joint, multi-center, randomized clinical study evaluating the effectiveness of LVRS. Subsequent to the clinical study, Medicare covers beneficiaries' services integral to the study (i.e., tests to determine whether a beneficiary qualifies for randomization, LVRS, and follow-up tests). Medicare does not cover services that are prohibited. For example, Medicare does not cover oral steroids provided as part of a physician's service because they are self-administrable and statutorily excluded from coverage. Part A services are paid according to the DRG system, and Part B physician services are paid according to the physician fee schedule.

MCM 4900 NATIONAL EMPHYSEMA TREATMENT TRIAL (NETT)

On August 1, 1997, The National Heart, Lung, and Blood Institute (NHLBI), part of the National Institutes of Health (NIH), began a 7-year study to examine the role of lung volume reduction surgery (LVRS) and evaluate the long-term outcome of the procedure on function, morbidity, and mortality, as well as to define appropriate patient selection criteria. The Health Care Financing Administration (HCFA) entered into an interagency agreement with NHLBI to cosponsor the study by providing payment for the clinical procedures provided in the trial to Medicare beneficiaries. Johns Hopkins University (JHU) is the coordinating center for this study. In general, HCFA covers payment for patient visits associated with postoperative management and completing forms such as the Interim History (HI), Surgical Summary Report (XS) and the Postoperative Summary Report (XP). Do not pay separately for these visits. The NETT trial includes 32491, 32655, and 32663:

32491 Removal of lung, other than total pneumonectomy; excision-plication of emphysematous lung(s) (bullous or non-bullous) for lung volume reduction, sternal split or transthoracic approach, with or without any pleural procedure Lung volume reduction

32655 Thoracoscopy, surgical; with excision-plication of bullae, including any pleural procedure Thoracoscopy, surgical

32663 Thoracoscopy, surgical; with lobectomy, total or segmental Thoracoscopy, surgical

Claims for NETT services and procedures are to be submitted on Health Insurance Claim Form HCFA-1500 or electronic equivalent.

32491	excision-plication of emphysematous lung(s) (bullous or non-bullous) for lung volume reduction, sternal split or transthoracic approach, with or without any pleural procedure	80 ⊡ 50
32500	wedge resection, single or multiple	80 ⊡

+ **32501** **Resection and repair of portion of bronchus (bronchoplasty) when performed at time of lobectomy or segmentectomy (List separately in addition to code for primary procedure)** `80` `50`

> Note that 32501 is an add-on code and must be used in conjunction with 32480, 32482, and 32484. Note also that 32501 is to be used when a portion of the bronchus is removed in order to preserve the lung and consequently requires plastic closure to preserve function of that preserved lung. This code is not to be used when the proximal end of a resected bronchus is closed.

32520 **Resection of lung; with resection of chest wall** `80` `↱`

32522 **with reconstruction of chest wall, without prosthesis** `80` `↱`

32525 **with major reconstruction of chest wall, with prosthesis** `80` `↱`

32540 **Extrapleural enucleation of empyema (empyemectomy)** `80` `↱`

ENDOSCOPY

CIM 35-59 ENDOSCOPY

Although endoscopy is primarily a diagnostic tool, it includes certain therapeutic procedures such as removal of polyps, and endoscopic papillotomy, by which stones are removed from the bile duct. Endoscopic procedures are covered when reasonable and necessary for the individual patient.

MCM 15038. MULTIPLE SURGERIES (CPT MODIFIER 51)

A. General—When more than one surgical service is performed on the same patient, by the same physician, and on the same day:

- The fee schedule amount for a second procedure is 50 percent of the fee schedule amount that would have been otherwise applicable for that procedure; and

- The fee schedule amount for the third through fifth procedures is 50 percent of the fee schedule amount that would have been otherwise applicable for that procedure. Prior to January 1, 1995, the third through fifth procedures were paid at 25 percent of the fee schedule amount. Surgical procedures beyond the fifth are priced "by report" based on documentation of the services furnished.

Sequence the procedures from the one which has the highest regular fee schedule amount to the one with the lowest.

B. Multiple Endoscopies—For multiple endoscopic procedures, use the full value of the highest valued endoscopy plus the difference between the next highest and the base endoscopy. For example, in the course of performing a fiberoptic colonoscopy (code 45378), a physician performs a biopsy (code 45380) and removes a polyp (code 45385). Both codes 45380 and 45385 contain the values of the base endoscopy, code 45378. Use the actual value of code 45385 plus the difference between codes 45380 and 45378. The endoscopic base codes are listed in the Physician Fee Schedule.

32601 **Thoracoscopy, diagnostic (separate procedure); lungs and pleural space, without biopsy** `80` `↱`

> Surgical thoracoscopy always includes diagnostic thoracoscopy.

32602 **lungs and pleural space, with biopsy** `80` `↱`

32603 **pericardial sac, without biopsy** `80` `↱`

32604 **pericardial sac, with biopsy** `80` `↱`

32605 **mediastinal space, without biopsy** `80` `↱`

32606 **mediastinal space, with biopsy** `80` `↱`

▲ **32650** **Thoracoscopy, surgical; with pleurodesis (eg, mechanical or chemical)** `80` `↱`

32651 **with partial pulmonary decortication** `80` `↱`

32652 **with total pulmonary decortication, including intrapleural pneumonolysis** `80` `↱`

32653 **with removal of intrapleural foreign body or fibrin deposit** `80` `↱`

32654 **with control of traumatic hemorrhage** `80` `↱`

32655 **with excision-plication of bullae, including any pleural procedure** `80` `↱`

32656 **with parietal pleurectomy** `80` `↱`

32657 **with wedge resection of lung, single or multiple** `80` `↱`

32658 **with removal of clot or foreign body from pericardial sac** `80` `↱`

32659 **with creation of pericardial window or partial resection of pericardial sac for drainage** `80` `↱`

32660 **with total pericardiectomy** `80` `↱`

32661 **with excision of pericardial cyst, tumor, or mass** `80` `↱`

32662 **with excision of mediastinal cyst, tumor, or mass** `80` `↱`

32663 **with lobectomy, total or segmental** `80` `↱`

32664 **with thoracic sympathectomy** `80` `↱` `50`

32665 **with esophagomyotomy (Heller type)** `80` `↱`

REPAIR

32800 **Repair lung hernia through chest wall** `80` `↱`

32810 **Closure of chest wall following open flap drainage for empyema (Clagett type procedure)** `80` `↱`

32815 **Open closure of major bronchial fistula** `80` `↱`

32820 **Major reconstruction, chest wall (post-traumatic)** `80` `↱`

LUNG TRANSPLANTATION

32850 **Donor pneumonectomy(ies) with preparation and maintenance of allograft (cadaver)** `↱`

32851 **Lung transplant, single; without cardiopulmonary bypass** `80` `↱`

32852 **with cardiopulmonary bypass** `80` `↱`

32853 **Lung transplant, double (bilateral sequential or en bloc); without cardiopulmonary bypass** `80` `↱`

32854 **with cardiopulmonary bypass** `80` `↱`

SURGICAL COLLAPSE THERAPY; THORACOPLASTY

Consult also CPT codes 32520-32525.

32900 **Resection of ribs, extrapleural, all stages** `80` `↱`

32905 **Thoracoplasty, Schede type or extrapleural (all stages);** `80` `↱`

32906 **with closure of bronchopleural fistula** `80` `↱`

> If the first rib for thoracic outer compression is resected, consult CPT codes 21615 and 21616.
>
> If the major bronchial fistula required open closure, consult CPT code 32815.

32940 **Pneumonolysis, extraperiosteal, including filling or packing procedures** `80` `↱`

32960* **Pneumothorax, therapeutic, intrapleural injection of air** `↱`

32997 **Total lung lavage (unilateral)** `↱`

> If a bronchoscopic bronchial alveolar lavage is performed, consult CPT code 31624.

OTHER PROCEDURES

32999 **Unlisted procedure, lungs and pleura** `80`

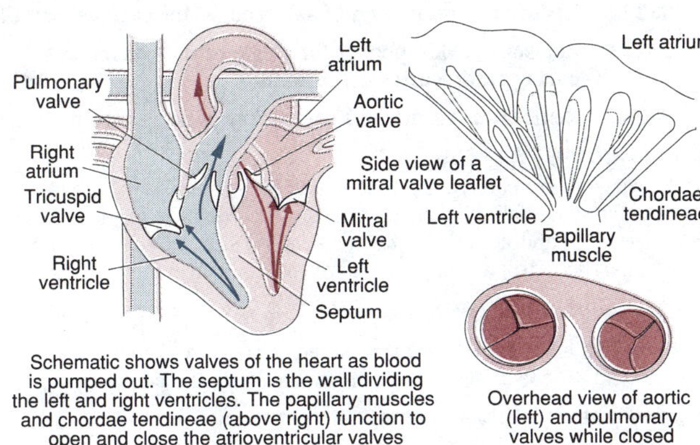

Schematic shows valves of the heart as blood is pumped out. The septum is the wall dividing the left and right ventricles. The papillary muscles and chordae tendineae (above right) function to open and close the atrioventricular valves

CARDIOVASCULAR SYSTEM

Code vascular catheterization to include introduction and all lesser order catheterization used in the approach. Use 36218 and 36248 to report additional second and third order arterial catheterization within the same family of arteries. Code separately catheterization in first order vessels different from the family originally coded.

If monitoring and the operation of pump and other nonsurgical services is performed, consult CPT codes 99190-99192, 99291, 99292, and 99354-99360. If other medical or laboratory related services are performed, consult the appropriate section of CPT. If radiological supervision and interpretation is needed, consult CPT codes 75600-75978.

HEART AND PERICARDIUM

PERICARDIUM

33010* **Pericardiocentesis; initial**
If radiological supervision and interpretation is performed, consult CPT code 76930.

33011* **subsequent**
If radiological supervision and interpretation is performed, consult CPT code 76930.

33015 **Tube pericardiostomy**

33020 **Pericardiotomy for removal of clot or foreign body (primary procedure)**

33025 **Creation of pericardial window or partial resection for drainage**

33030 **Pericardiectomy, subtotal or complete; without cardiopulmonary bypass**
Delorme pericardiectomy

33031 **with cardiopulmonary bypass**

33050 **Excision of pericardial cyst or tumor**

CARDIAC TUMOR

33120 **Excision of intracardiac tumor, resection with cardiopulmonary bypass**

33130 **Resection of external cardiac tumor**

TRANSMYOCARDIAL REVASCULARIZATION

CIM35-94 TRANSMYOCARDIAL REVASCULARIZATION (TMR) FOR TREATMENT OF SEVERE ANGINA

Transmyocardial revascularization (TMR) uses a laser to bore holes through the myocardium of the heart to restore perfusion in areas of the heart inaccessible due to diseased or clogged arteries. This technique is used as a late or last resort for relief of symptoms of severe angina for patients with ischemic heart disease not amenable to direct coronary revascularization interventions, such as angioplasty, stenting or open coronary bypass. Studies indicate that reduction both in pain and hospitalization is significant for most patients treated. Consequently, Medicare covers TMR as a late or last resort

for patients with severe angina (stable or unstable), which has been found refractory to standard medical therapy, including drug therapy at the maximum tolerated or maximum safe dosages. Coverage is further limited to lasers approved by the Food and Drug Administration for TMR.

Patients must meet the following selection guidelines:

- An ejection fraction of 25 percent or greater
- Have areas of viable ischemic myocardium (as demonstrated by diagnostic study) incapable of being revascularized by direct coronary intervention
- Have been stabilized, or have had maximal efforts to stabilize acute conditions such as severe ventricular arrhythmias, decompensated congestive heart failure or acute myocardial infarction

Coverage is limited to physicians properly trained in the procedure. Providers must document that all ancillary personnel are trained in the procedure and the proper use of the equipment. Coverage is further limited to providers dedicated to cardiac care units, including the diagnostic and support services necessary for care of patients undergoing this therapy. In addition, these providers must conform to the standards for laser safety set by the American National Standards Institute.

33140 **Transmyocardial laser revascularization, by thoracotomy (separate procedure)**

+ 33141 **performed at the time of other open cardiac procedure(s) (List separately in addition to code for primary procedure)**
Note that 33141 is an add-on procedure and must be used in conjunction with 33400-33496 and 33510-33536.

PACEMAKER OR PACING CARDIOVERTER-DEFIBRILLATOR

Pacemakers differ from pacing cardioverter-defibrillator pulse generators. In their simplicity. Pacemakers maintain the rhythm of the heart through electrodes placed on the heart or in an artery. The electronics within stimulate one or more chambers in the heart. Pacing cardioverter-defibrillators also include a generator that stimulates the heart but also apply defibrillating shocks to treat ventricular tachycardia or ventricular fibrillation. Most are placed in a "pocket" below the clavicle or below the ribcage.

If an electronic, telephonic analysis of the internal pacemaker system is performed, consult CPT codes 93731-93736.

If radiological supervision and interpretation with insertion of pacemaker is performed, consult CPT code 71090.

CIM 65-6 CARDIAC PACEMAKERS

Cardiac pacemakers are covered as prosthetic devices under the Medicare program, subject to the following conditions, provided that the conditions are chronic or recurrent and not due to transient causes such as acute myocardial infarction, drug toxicity, or electrolyte imbalance:

1. Acquired complete AV heart block.

2. Congenital complete heart block with severe bradycardia or significant physiological deficits or significant symptoms due to the bradycardia.

3. Second degree AV heart block of Type II.

4. Second degree AV heart block of Type I, with significant symptoms due to hemodynamic instability associated with the heart block.

5. Sinus bradycardia associated with major symptoms or substantial sinus bradycardia associated with dizziness or confusion. *

6. Sinus bradycardia of lesser severity, accompanied by dizziness or confusion. *

7. Sinus bradycardia that is the consequence of long-term necessary drug treatment for which there is no acceptable alternative, accompanied by significant symptoms dizziness or confusion. *

8. Sinus node dysfunction with or without tachyarrhythmias or AV conduction block, accompanied by significant symptoms.*

9. Sinus node dysfunction with or without symptoms, accompanied by life-threatening ventricular arrhythmias or tachycardia secondary to the bradycardia.

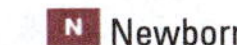

CCI Comprehensive Code   Bilateral Procedure   + CPT Add-on Code   Modifier -51 Exempt Code   ● New Code   ▲ Revised Code

M Maternity   **N** Newborn   **P** Pediatric   **N/P** Newborn/Pediatric

10. Bradycardia associated with supraventricular tachycardia with high degree AV block that is unresponsive to appropriate pharmacological management and when the bradycardia is associated with significant symptoms.

11. The patient with hypersensitive carotid sinus syndrome with syncope due to bradycardia and unresponsive to prophylactic medical measures.

12. Bifascicular or trifascicular block accompanied by syncope that is attributed to transient complete heart block after other plausible causes of syncope have been reasonably excluded.

13. Prophylactic pacemaker use following recovery from acute myocardial infarction during which there was temporary complete and/or Mobitz Type II AV block in association with bundle branch block.

14. Recurrent and refractory ventricular tachycardia, "overdrive pacing," to prevent ventricular tachycardia.

15. Second degree AV heart block of Type I with the QRS complexes prolonged.

* The correlation between symptoms and bradycardia must be documented, or the symptoms must be clearly attributable to the bradycardia rather than to some other cause.

33200 Insertion of permanent pacemaker with epicardial electrode(s); by thoracotomy

33201 by xiphoid approach

CIM 35-79 ANESTHESIA IN CARDIAC PACEMAKER SURGERY

The use of general or monitored anesthesia during transvenous cardiac pacemaker surgery may be covered under Medicare only if adequate documentation of medical necessity is provided on a case-by-case basis. A second type of pacemaker surgery that is sometimes performed involves the use of the thoracic method of implantation, which requires open surgery. Where the thoracic method is employed, general anesthesia is always used and should not require special medical documentation.

Note that 33206–33208 include subcutaneous insertion of the pulse generator and transvenous placement of electrode(s).

33206 Insertion or replacement of permanent pacemaker with transvenous electrode(s); atrial

33207 ventricular

33208 atrial and ventricular

33210 Insertion or replacement of temporary transvenous single chamber cardiac electrode transvenous single chamber cardiac electrode or pacemaker catheter (separate procedure)

33211 Insertion or replacement of temporary transvenous dual chamber pacing electrodes (separate procedure)

33212 Insertion or replacement of pacemaker pulse generator only; single chamber, atrial or ventricular

33213 dual chamber

33214 Upgrade of implanted pacemaker system, conversion of single chamber system to dual chamber system (includes removal of previously placed pulse generator, testing of existing lead, insertion of new lead, insertion of new pulse generator)

33216 Insertion or repositioning of a transvenous electrode (15 days or more after initial insertion); single chamber (one electrode) permanent pacemaker or single chamber pacing cardioverter-defibrillator

33217 dual chamber (two electrodes) permanent pacemaker or dual chamber pacing cardioverter-defibrillator
Codes 33216-33217 should not be reported with 33214.

33218 Repair of single transvenous electrode for a single chamber, permanent pacemaker or single chamber pacing cardioverter-defibrillator

33220 Repair of two transvenous electrodes for a dual chamber permanent pacemaker or dual chamber pacing cardioverter-defibrillator

33222 Revision or relocation of skin pocket for pacemaker

33223 Revision of skin pocket for single or dual chamber pacing cardioverter-defibrillator

33233 Removal of permanent pacemaker pulse generator

CIM 65-6 CARDIAC PACEMAKERS

Cardiac pacemakers are covered as prosthetic devices under the Medicare program, subject to the following conditions, provided that the conditions are chronic or recurrent and not due to transient causes such as acute myocardial infarction, drug toxicity, or electrolyte imbalance:

1. Acquired complete AV heart block.

2. Congenital complete heart block with severe bradycardia or significant physiological deficits or significant symptoms due to the bradycardia.

3. Second degree AV heart block of Type II.

4. Second degree AV heart block of Type I, with significant symptoms due to hemodynamic instability associated with the heart block.

5. Sinus bradycardia associated with major symptoms or substantial sinus bradycardia associated with dizziness or confusion. *

6. Sinus bradycardia of lesser severity, accompanied by dizziness or confusion. *

7. Sinus bradycardia that is the consequence of long-term necessary drug treatment for which there is no acceptable alternative, accompanied by significant symptoms dizziness or confusion. *

8. Sinus node dysfunction with or without tachyarrhythmias or AV conduction block, accompanied by significant symptoms.*

9. Sinus node dysfunction with or without symptoms, accompanied by life-threatening ventricular arrhythmias or tachycardia secondary to the bradycardia.

10. Bradycardia associated with supraventricular tachycardia with high degree AV block that is unresponsive to appropriate pharmacological management and when the bradycardia is associated with significant symptoms.

11. The patient with hypersensitive carotid sinus syndrome with syncope due to bradycardia and unresponsive to prophylactic medical measures.

12. Bifascicular or trifascicular block accompanied by syncope that is attributed to transient complete heart block after other plausible causes of syncope have been reasonably excluded.

13. Prophylactic pacemaker use following recovery from acute myocardial infarction during which there was temporary complete and/or Mobitz Type II AV block in association with bundle branch block.

14. Recurrent and refractory ventricular tachycardia, "overdrive pacing," to prevent ventricular tachycardia.

15. Second degree AV heart block of Type I with the QRS complexes prolonged.

* The correlation between symptoms and bradycardia must be documented, or the symptoms must be clearly attributable to the bradycardia rather than to some other cause.

33234 Removal of transvenous pacemaker electrode(s); single lead system, atrial or ventricular

33235 dual lead system

33236 Removal of permanent epicardial pacemaker and electrodes by thoracotomy; single lead system, atrial or ventricular

33237 dual lead system

33238 Removal of permanent transvenous electrode(s) by thoracotomy

CIM 35-85 IMPLANTATION OF AUTOMATIC DEFIBRILLATORS

Medicare covers the implantation of an automatic defibrillator (ICD-9-CM codes 37.94-37.96 or CPT code 33246) when used as a treatment of last resort for patients who have had a documented episode of life-threatening ventricular tachyarrhythmia or cardiac arrest not associated with myocardial infarction. Patients must also be found, by electrophysiologic testing, to have an inducible tachyarrhythmia that proves unresponsive to medication or surgical therapy (or be considered unsuitable candidates for surgical therapy). It must be emphasized that unless all of the above described conditions and stipulations are met in a particular case, implantation may not be covered.

33240 **Insertion of single or dual chamber pacing cardioverter-defibrillator pulse generator**

33241 **Subcutaneous removal of single or dual chamber pacing cardioverter-defibrillator pulse generator**

If an electrode(s) is removed by thoracotomy, consult CPT code 33243 in conjunction with 33241.

If an electrode(s) is removed transvenously, report 33244 in conjunction with 33241.

If the complete pacing defibrillator system is removed and replaced, report 33241 and 33243 or 33244 and 33249.

33243 **Removal of single or dual chamber pacing cardioverter-defibrillator electrode(s); by thoracotomy**

33244 **by transvenous extraction**

33245 **Insertion of epicardial single or dual chamber pacing cardioverter-defibrillator electrodes by thoracotomy;**

33246 **with insertion of pulse generator**

33249 **Insertion or repositioning of electrode lead(s) for single or dual chamber pacing cardioverter-defibrillator and insertion of pulse generator**

ELECTROPHYSIOLOGIC OPERATIVE PROCEDURES

▲ **33250** **Operative ablation of supraventricular arrhythmogenic focus or pathway (eg, Wolff-Parkinson-White, atrioventricular node re-entry), tract(s) and/or focus (foci); without cardiopulmonary bypass**

33251 **with cardiopulmonary bypass**

33253 **Operative incisions and reconstruction of atria for treatment of atrial fibrillation or atrial flutter (eg, maze procedure)**

33261 **Operative ablation of ventricular arrhythmogenic focus with cardiopulmonary bypass**

PATIENT-ACTIVATED EVENT RECORDER

Note that initial implantation includes programming. If subsequent electronic analysis and/or reprogramming is performed, consult CPT code 93727.

33282 **Implantation of patient-activated cardiac event recorder**

33284 **Removal of an implantable, patient-activated cardiac event recorder**

WOUNDS OF THE HEART AND GREAT VESSELS

33300 **Repair of cardiac wound; without bypass**

33305 **with cardiopulmonary bypass**

33310 **Cardiotomy, exploratory (includes removal of foreign body); without bypass**

33315 **with cardiopulmonary bypass**

33320 **Suture repair of aorta or great vessels; without shunt or cardiopulmonary bypass**

33321 **with shunt bypass**

33322 **with cardiopulmonary bypass**

33330 **Insertion of graft, aorta or great vessels; without shunt, or cardiopulmonary bypass**

33332 **with shunt bypass**

33335 **with cardiopulmonary bypass**

CARDIAC VALVES, AORTIC VALVE

33400 **Valvuloplasty, aortic valve; open, with cardiopulmonary bypass**

Stenosis means the cusps are fused, usually leaving a small central opening. When cusps become thick and inflexible, closure is incomplete (incompetent) and a back-rush or regurgitation results

33401 **open, with inflow occlusion**

33403 **using transventricular dilation, with cardiopulmonary bypass**

33404 **Construction of apical-aortic conduit**

33405 **Replacement, aortic valve, with cardiopulmonary bypass; with prosthetic valve other than homograft or stentless valve**

▲ **33406** **with allograft valve (freehand)**

33410 **with stentless tissue valve**

33411 **Replacement, aortic valve; with aortic annulus enlargement, noncoronary cusp**

33412 **with transventricular aortic annulus enlargement (Konno procedure)**

▲ **33413** **by translocation of autologous pulmonary valve with allograft replacement of pulmonary valve (Ross procedure)**

33414 **Repair of left ventricular outflow tract obstruction by patch enlargement of the outflow tract**

33415 **Resection or incision of subvalvular tissue for discrete subvalvular aortic stenosis**

33416 **Ventriculomyotomy (-myectomy) for idiopathic hypertrophic subaortic stenosis (eg, asymmetric septal hypertrophy)**

33417 **Aortoplasty (gusset) for supravalvular stenosis**

CARDIAC VALVES, MITRAL VALVE

33420 **Valvotomy, mitral valve; closed heart**

33422 **open heart, with cardiopulmonary bypass**

33425 **Valvuloplasty, mitral valve, with cardiopulmonary bypass;**

33426 **with prosthetic ring**

33427 **radical reconstruction, with or without ring**

33430 **Replacement, mitral valve, with cardiopulmonary bypass**

CARDIAC VALVES, TRICUSPID VALVE

33460 **Valvectomy, tricuspid valve, with cardiopulmonary bypass**

33463 **Valvuloplasty, tricuspid valve; without ring insertion**

33464 **with ring insertion**

33465 **Replacement, tricuspid valve, with cardiopulmonary bypass**

33468 **Tricuspid valve repositioning and plication for Ebstein anomaly**

☐ CCI Comprehensive Code   50 Bilateral Procedure   + CPT Add-on Code   ⊘ Modifier -51 Exempt Code   ● New Code   ▲ Revised Code

M Maternity   N Newborn   P Pediatric   N/P Newborn/Pediatric

CARDIAC VALVES, PULMONARY VALVE

33470 Valvotomy, pulmonary valve, closed heart; transventricular   [80] [▸]

Brock's operation

33471 via pulmonary artery   [80] [▸]
If percutaneous valvuloplasty of the pulmonary valve is performed, consult CPT code 92990.

Brock's operation

33472 Valvotomy, pulmonary valve, open heart; with inflow occlusion   [80] [▸]

Brock's operation

33474 with cardiopulmonary bypass   [80] [▸]

Brock's operation

33475 Replacement, pulmonary valve   [80] [▸]

33476 Right ventricular resection for infundibular stenosis, with or without commissurotomy   [80] [▸]

Brock's operation

33478 Outflow tract augmentation (gusset), with or without commissurotomy or infundibular resection   [80] [▸]

OTHER VALVULAR PROCEDURES

33496 Repair of non-structural prosthetic valve dysfunction with cardiopulmonary bypass (separate procedure)   [80] [▸]
If this procedure is a reoperation, use CPT code 33530 in addition to 33496.

CORONARY ARTERY ANOMALIES

33500 Repair of coronary arteriovenous or arteriocardiac chamber fistula; with cardiopulmonary bypass   [80] [▸]

33501 without cardiopulmonary bypass   [80] [▸]

33502 Repair of anomalous coronary artery; by ligation   [80] [▸]

33503 by graft, without cardiopulmonary bypass   [80] [▸]

33504 by graft, with cardiopulmonary bypass   [80] [▸]

33505 with construction of intrapulmonary artery tunnel (Takeuchi procedure)   [80] [▸]

33506 by translocation from pulmonary artery to aorta   [80] [▸]

VENOUS GRAFTING ONLY FOR CORONARY ARTERY BYPASS

CPT codes 33510-33516 include the harvesting of the saphenous vein graft and it should not be reportedly separately. These codes report bypass procedures using venous grafts only.

33510 Coronary artery bypass, vein only; single coronary venous graft   [80] [▸]

33511 two coronary venous grafts   [80] [▸]

33512 three coronary venous grafts   [80] [▸]

33513 four coronary venous grafts   [80] [▸]

33514 five coronary venous grafts   [80] [▸]

33516 six or more coronary venous grafts   [80] [▸]

COMBINED ARTERIAL-VENOUS GRAFTING FOR CORONARY BYPASS

Use these codes to report coronary artery bypass procedures using both venous and arterial grafts during the same procedure, but don't use them alone. They must be reported with a code from range 33533-33536.

CPT codes 33517-33523 include the harvesting of the saphenous vein graft and it should not be reported separately.

⊘ 33517 Coronary artery bypass, using venous graft(s) and arterial graft(s); single vein graft (list separately in addition to code for arterial graft)   [80] [▸]

⊘ 33518 two venous grafts (list separately in addition to code for arterial graft)   [80] [▸]

⊘ 33519 three venous grafts (list separately in addition to code for arterial graft)   [80] [▸]

⊘ 33521 four venous grafts (list separately in addition to code for arterial graft)   [80] [▸]

⊘ 33522 five venous grafts (list separately in addition to code for arterial graft)   [80] [▸]

⊘ 33523 six or more venous grafts (list separately in addition to code for arterial graft)   [80] [▸]

+ 33530 Reoperation, coronary artery bypass procedure or valve procedure, more than one month after original operation (list separately in addition to code for primary procedure)
Note that 33530 is an add-on code and must be used in conjunction with 33400-33496, 33510-33536, and 33863.

ARTERIAL GRAFTING FOR CORONARY ARTERY BYPASS

Use these codes to report coronary artery bypass using either arterial grafts only or a combination of arterial-venous grafts using the internal mammary, gastroepiploic, epigastric, and radial arteries.

CPT codes 33533-33536 include the harvesting of the artery for grafting with the exception of when an upper extremity artery is harvested. Consult CPT code 35600 and use it in addition to the bypass procedure for upper extremity artery harvest.

33533 Coronary artery bypass, using arterial graft(s); single arterial graft   [80] [▸]

33534 two coronary arterial grafts   [80] [▸]

33535 three coronary arterial grafts   [80] [▸]

33536 four or more coronary arterial grafts   [80] [▸]

33542 Myocardial resection (eg, ventricular aneurysmectomy)   [80] [▸]

33545 Repair of postinfarction ventricular septal defect, with or without myocardial resection   [80] [▸]

CORONARY ENDARTERECTOMY

+ 33572 Coronary endarterectomy, open, any method, of left anterior descending, circumflex, or right coronary artery performed in conjunction with coronary artery bypass graft procedure, each vessel (list separately in addition to primary procedure)   [80] [▸]
Note that 33572 is an add-on code and must be used in conjunction with 33510-33516 and 33533-33536.

SINGLE VENTRICLE AND OTHER COMPLEX CARDIAC ANOMALIES

33600 Closure of atrioventricular valve (mitral or tricuspid) by suture or patch   [80] [▸]

33602 Closure of semilunar valve (aortic or pulmonary) by suture or patch   [80] [▸]

33606 Anastomosis of pulmonary artery to aorta (Damus-Kaye-Stansel procedure)   [80] [▸]

33608 Repair of complex cardiac anomaly other than pulmonary atresia with ventricular septal defect by construction or replacement of conduit from right or left ventricle to pulmonary artery   [80] [▸]
If repair of the pulmonary atresia with a ventricular septal defect is performed, consult CPT codes 33918, 33919, and 33920.

▲ 33610 Repair of complex cardiac anomalies (eg, single ventricle with subaortic obstruction) by surgical enlargement of ventricular septal defect   [80] [▸]

33611 Repair of double outlet right ventricle with intraventricular tunnel repair;   [80] [▸]

| 33612 | with repair of right ventricular outflow tract obstruction | 80 |

33615 Repair of complex cardiac anomalies (eg, tricuspid atresia) by closure of atrial septal defect and anastomosis of atria or vena cava to pulmonary artery (simple Fontan procedure) 80

33617 Repair of complex cardiac anomalies (eg, single ventricle) by modified Fontan procedure 80

33619 Repair of single ventricle with aortic outflow obstruction and aortic arch hypoplasia (hypoplastic left heart syndrome) (eg, Norwood procedure) 80

SEPTAL DEFECT

33641 Repair atrial septal defect, secundum, with cardiopulmonary bypass, with or without patch 80

33645 Direct or patch closure, sinus venosus, with or without anomalous pulmonary venous drainage 80

33647 Repair of atrial septal defect and ventricular septal defect, with direct or patch closure 80

33660 Repair of incomplete or partial atrioventricular canal (ostium primum atrial septal defect), with or without atrioventricular valve repair 80

33665 Repair of intermediate or transitional atrioventricular canal, with or without atrioventricular valve repair 80

33670 Repair of complete atrioventricular canal, with or without prosthetic valve 80

33681 Closure of ventricular septal defect, with or without patch 80

33684 with pulmonary valvotomy or infundibular resection (acyanotic) 80

33688 with removal of pulmonary artery band, with or without gusset 80

33690 Banding of pulmonary artery 80

33692 Complete repair tetralogy of Fallot without pulmonary atresia; 80

33694 with transannular patch 80

33697 Complete repair tetralogy of Fallot with pulmonary atresia including construction of conduit from right ventricle to pulmonary artery and closure of ventricular septal defect 80

SINUS OF VALSALVA

33702 Repair sinus of Valsalva fistula, with cardiopulmonary bypass; 80

33710 with repair of ventricular septal defect 80

33720 Repair sinus of Valsalva aneurysm, with cardiopulmonary bypass 80

33722 Closure of aortico-left ventricular tunnel 80

TOTAL ANOMALOUS PULMONARY VENOUS DRAINAGE

33730 Complete repair of anomalous venous return (supracardiac, intracardiac, or infracardiac types) 80

To code a partial anomalous return, see atrial septal defect.

33732 Repair of cor triatriatum or supravalvular mitral ring by resection of left atrial membrane 80

SHUNTING PROCEDURES

33735 Atrial septectomy or septostomy; closed heart (Blalock-Hanlon type operation) 80

33736 open heart with cardiopulmonary bypass 80

33737 open heart, with inflow occlusion 80

33750 Shunt; subclavian to pulmonary artery (Blalock-Taussig type operation) 80

33755 ascending aorta to pulmonary artery (Waterston type operation) 80

33762 descending aorta to pulmonary artery (Potts-Smith type operation) 80

33764 central, with prosthetic graft 80

33766 superior vena cava to pulmonary artery for flow to one lung (classical Glenn procedure) 80

33767 superior vena cava to pulmonary artery for flow to both lungs (bidirectional Glenn procedure) 80

TRANSPOSITION OF THE GREAT VESSELS

33770 Repair of transposition of the great arteries with ventricular septal defect and subpulmonary stenosis; without surgical enlargement of ventricular septal defect 80

33771 with surgical enlargement of ventricular septal defect 80

33774 Repair of transposition of the great arteries, atrial baffle procedure (eg, Mustard or Senning type) with cardiopulmonary bypass; 80

33775 with removal of pulmonary band 80

33776 with closure of ventricular septal defect 80

33777 with repair of subpulmonic obstruction 80

33778 Repair of transposition of the great arteries, aortic pulmonary artery reconstruction (eg, Jatene type); 80

33779 with removal of pulmonary band 80

33780 with closure of ventricular septal defect 80

33781 with repair of subpulmonic obstruction 80

TRUNCUS ARTERIOSUS

33786 Total repair, truncus arteriosus (Rastelli type operation) 80

33788 Reimplantation of an anomalous pulmonary artery 80

If banding of the pulmonary artery is performed, consult CPT code 33690.

AORTIC ANOMALIES

33800 Aortic suspension (aortopexy) for tracheal decompression (eg, for tracheomalacia) (separate procedure) 80

33802 Division of aberrant vessel (vascular ring); 80

33803 with reanastomosis 80

33813 Obliteration of aortopulmonary septal defect; without cardiopulmonary bypass 80

33814 with cardiopulmonary bypass 80

33820 Repair of patent ductus arteriosus; by ligation 80

33822 by division, under 18 years P 80

33824 by division, 18 years and older 80

33840 Excision of coarctation of aorta, with or without associated patent ductus arteriosus; with direct anastomosis 80

33845 with graft 80

33851 repair using either left subclavian artery or prosthetic material as gusset for enlargement 80

33852 Repair of hypoplastic or interrupted aortic arch using autogenous or prosthetic material; without cardiopulmonary bypass 80

33853 with cardiopulmonary bypass 80

□ CCI Comprehensive Code   50 Bilateral Procedure   + CPT Add-on Code   ⊘ Modifier -51 Exempt Code   ● New Code   ▲ Revised Code

M Maternity   N Newborn   P Pediatric   N/P Newborn/Pediatric

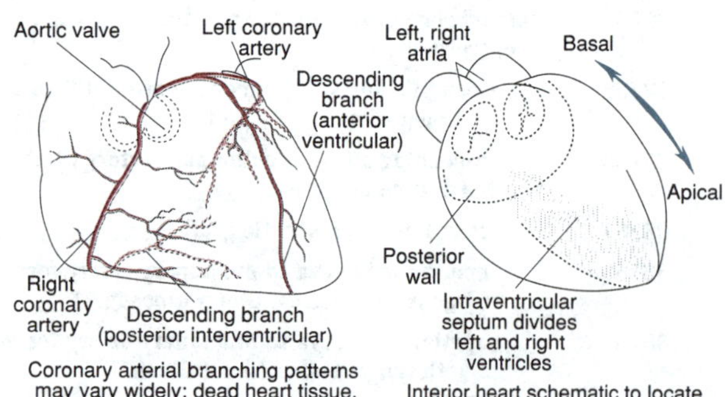

Coronary arterial branching patterns may vary widely; dead heart tissue, usually caused by arterial occlusion, is called a myocardial infarct and about 1.5 million cases are reported annually. Inadequate blood supply can lead to "angina pectoris," or chest pain

Interior heart schematic to locate a myocardial infarction; walls of the left ventrical are much thicker and more than half of MI occurrences will see some degree of transient impairment to the left ventricle

THORACIC AORTIC ANEURYSM

33860   Ascending aorta graft, with cardiopulmonary bypass, with or without valve suspension;   80

33861   with coronary reconstruction   80

33863   with aortic root replacement using composite prosthesis and coronary reconstruction   80

33870   Transverse arch graft, with cardiopulmonary bypass   80

33875   Descending thoracic aorta graft, with or without bypass   80

33877   Repair of thoracoabdominal aortic aneurysm with graft, with or without cardiopulmonary bypass   80

PULMONARY ARTERY

CIM 35-55 TRANSVENOUS (CATHETER) PULMONARY EMBOLECTOMY - NOT COVERED

Transvenous (catheter) pulmonary embolectomy is an experimental procedure for removing pulmonary emboli by passing a catheter through the femoral vein. It is not covered under Medicare.

33910   Pulmonary artery embolectomy; with cardiopulmonary bypass   80

33915   without cardiopulmonary bypass   80

33916   Pulmonary endarterectomy, with or without embolectomy, with cardiopulmonary bypass   80

33917   Repair of pulmonary artery stenosis by reconstruction with patch or graft   80

33918   Repair of pulmonary atresia with ventricular septal defect, by unifocalization of pulmonary arteries; without cardiopulmonary bypass   80

33919   with cardiopulmonary bypass   80

33920   Repair of pulmonary atresia with ventricular septal defect, by construction or replacement of conduit from right or left ventricle to pulmonary artery   80

If other complex cardiac anomalies are repaired by construction of right or left ventricle to pulmonary artery conduit, consult CPT code 33608.

33922   Transection of pulmonary artery with cardiopulmonary bypass   80

+ 33924   Ligation and takedown of a systemic-to-pulmonary artery shunt, performed in conjunction with a congenital heart procedure (List separately in addition to code for primary procedure)   80

Note that 33924 is an add-on code and must be used in conjunction with 33470-33475, 33600-33619, 33684-33688, 33692-33697, 33735-33767, 33770-33781, 33786, and 33918-33922.

HEART/LUNG TRANSPLANTATION

33930   Donor cardiectomy-pneumonectomy, with preparation and maintenance of allograft

CIM 35-87 HEART TRANSPLANTS

(See Intermediary Manual §3101.l4 and Carriers Manual §2300.1.)

(See Intermediary Manual §3660.8 and Carriers Manual §§2050.3, 4471 and 5249.)

Cardiac transplantation is covered under Medicare when performed in a facility approved by Medicare as meeting institutional coverage criteria. Under no circumstances will exceptions be made for facilities with transplant programs in existence for less than two years. Applications from consortia will not be approved. Consideration is given to heart transplant facilities that consist of more than one hospital where all of the following conditions exist:

- Under the common control or have a formal affiliation under the auspices of an organization such as a university or medical research institute

- Share resources by routinely using the same personnel or services in their transplant programs

- Submit, in the Kaplan-Meier method, the individual and pooled experience and survival data

- Meet the remaining Medicare criteria for heart transplant facilities (i.e., criteria regarding patient selection, patient management, and program commitment)

Pediatric cardiac transplantation is covered for Medicare beneficiaries when performed in a pediatric hospital if the hospital submits an application to HCFA that documents:

- The hospital's pediatric heart transplant program is operated jointly by the hospital and another facility that has been found by HCFA to meet the institutional coverage criteria

- The unified program shares the same transplant surgeons and quality assurance program (including oversight committee, patient protocol, and patient selection criteria)

- The hospital is able to provide the specialized facilities, services, and personnel that are required by pediatric heart transplant patients

Medicare covers follow-up care as a result of a covered and noncovered heart transplants.

Medicare does not cover the use of artificial hearts or ventricular assist devices, either as a permanent replacement for a human heart or as a temporary/life-support system until a human heart becomes available for transplant (often referred to as a "bridge to transplant").

MCM 2300.1 SERVICES RELATED TO AND REQUIRED AS A RESULT OF SERVICES WHICH ARE NOT COVERED UNDER MEDICARE

Medical and hospital services may be required to treat a condition that arises as a result of services not covered because they are not reasonable and necessary or excluded for other reasons. Services "related to" noncovered services (e.g., cosmetic surgery, noncovered organ transplants, noncovered artificial organ implants), including services related to follow-up care and complications of noncovered services that require treatment during a hospital stay when noncovered service were performed, are not covered services under Medicare. Services "not related to" noncovered services are covered under Medicare.

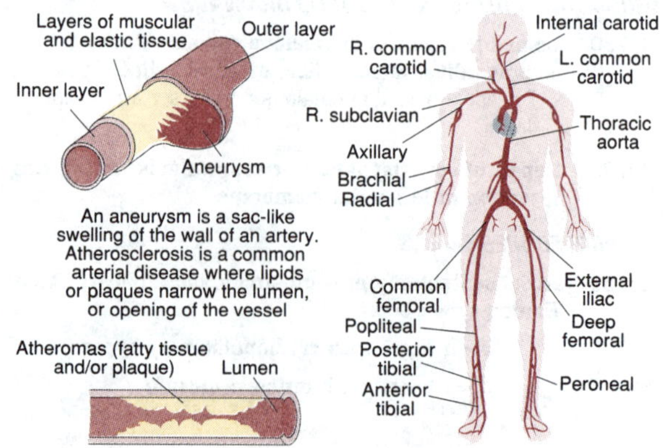

MCM 2050.3 INCIDENT TO PHYSICIAN'S SERVICE IN CLINIC

A physician directed clinic is one where:

10. A physician (or a number of physicians) is present to perform medical (rather than administrative) services at all times the clinic is open

11. Each patient is under the care of a clinic physician

12. The nonphysician services are under medical supervision

In highly organized clinics, particularly those that are departmentalized, direct personal physician supervision may be the responsibility of several physicians as opposed to an individual attending physician. In this situation, medical management of all services provided in the clinic is assured. The physician ordering a particular service need not be the physician who is supervising the service. Supplies provided by the clinic during the course of treatment are also covered. When the auxiliary personnel perform services outside the clinic premises, the services are covered only if performed under the direct personal supervision of a clinic physician. If the clinic refers a patient for auxiliary services performed by personnel who are not employed by the clinic, such services are not incident to a physician's service.

MCM 4471.2 DETERMINATION OF ELIGIBILITY

Benefit eligibility is limited to the one-year period following the date of the beneficiary's discharge from a hospital or transplant center after a Medicare covered kidney, heart or liver transplant. The specialty carrier consults one of three alternative sources of information to determine the date of kidney transplant:

4. HCFA compiles and furnishes in hardcopy or tape format to specialty carriers a monthly listing of beneficiaries who have received kidney transplants. HCFA's system is not yet equipped to handle heart and liver transplant data. The initial listing included all beneficiaries who had received a kidney transplant since January 1, 1986. It is updated monthly.

5. Intermediaries send copies of the Part A Medicare Benefit Notice that contains the date of transplant to the specialty carriers. The specialty carriers maintain the data and release it to area carriers upon request.

6. If you are unable to locate the beneficiary's transplant information above, refer to the discharge date listed on the prescription form. The prescription form should accompany the initial claim and indicate the date of discharge. You may contact the prescribing physician for substantiation of the discharge date. If there is no other eligibility information other than the prescription regarding the discharge date, the beneficiary may pay for a one month's supply of immunosuppressive drugs based upon the discharge date listed. If the information obtained indicates transplant failure, do not approve payment for drugs in subsequent periods.

MCM 5249. PAYMENT FOR IMMUNOSUPPRESSIVE DRUGS FURNISHED TO TRANSPLANT PATIENTS

Medicare pays for FDA approved immunosuppressive drugs. This benefit is subject to the Part B deductible and coinsurance provision and is limited to the one-year period after the date of the transplant procedure. Medicare pays for immunosuppressive drugs provided outside the one-year period if the drugs are covered under some other provision of the law (e.g., when the drugs are covered as inpatient hospital services or are furnished incident to a physician's service). We interpret "1-year period after the date of the transplant procedure" to mean 365 days from the day an inpatient is discharged from the hospital; from surgery until hospital discharge, payment for these drugs is included in Medicare's Part A payment to the hospital. If the same patient receives a subsequent transplant operation within 365 days, the period for this benefit begins anew.

The physician should supply the patient with a non-refillable 30-day prescription for the immunosuppressive drugs and to the carrier the date of that patient's discharge from the hospital on the first immunosuppressive drug prescription for subsequent transplant patients. The date is used for limitation purposes because the dosage of these drugs frequently diminishes over a period of time and prescription changes.

33935	**Heart-lung transplant with recipient cardiectomy-pneumonectomy**	80 ↻
33940	**Donor cardiectomy, with preparation and maintenance of allograft**	↻

33945	**Heart transplant, with or without recipient cardiectomy**	80 ↻

CARDIAC ASSIST

33960   **Prolonged extracorporeal circulation for cardiopulmonary insufficiency; initial 24 hours**   80 ↻

If an insertion of a cannula is performed for prolonged extracorporeal circulation, consult CPT code 36822.

+ **33961**   **each additional 24 hours (List separately in addition to code for primary procedure)**   80 ↻

If an insertion of a cannula is performed for prolonged extracorporeal circulation, consult CPT code 36822.

Note that 33961 is an add-on code and must be used in conjunction with 33960.

● **33967**   **Insertion of intra-aortic balloon assist device, percutaneous**

33968   **Removal of intra-aortic balloon assist device, percutaneous**   ↻

33970   **Insertion of intra-aortic balloon assist device through the femoral artery, open approach**   80 ↻

If the insertion is performed percutaneously, consult CPT code 33967.

33971   **Removal of intra-aortic balloon assist device including repair of femoral artery, with or without graft**   ↻

33973   **Insertion of intra-aortic balloon assist device through the ascending aorta**   80 ↻

33974   **Removal of intra-aortic balloon assist device from the ascending aorta, including repair of the ascending aorta, with or without graft**   ↻

CIM 65-15 ARTIFICIAL HEARTS AND RELATED DEVICES

All of the following criteria must be fulfilled in order for Medicare coverage to be provided for a ventricular assist device (VAD) used as a bridge to transplant:

- The VAD must be used in accordance with the FDA approved labeling instructions. This means that the VAD is used as a temporary mechanical circulatory support for approved transplant candidates as a bridge to cardiac transplantation

- The patient is approved and listed as a candidate for heart transplantion by a Medicare approved heart transplant center

- The VAD is implanted in a Medicare approved heart transplant center on a patient who is listed by that center. If the patient is listed by another Medicare approved transplant center, the implanting center must receive written permission from the center under which the patient is listed

Centers implanting VADs should make every reasonable effort to transplant patients on such devices as soon as medically reasonable.

▲ **33975**   **Insertion of ventricular assist device; extracorporeal, single ventricle**   80 ↻

▲ **33976**   **extracorporeal, biventricular**   80 ↻

▲ **33977**   **Removal of ventricular assist device; extracorporeal, single ventricle**   80 ↻

▲ **33978**   **extracorporeal, biventricular**   80 ↻

● **33979**   **Insertion of ventricular assist device, implantable intracorporeal, single ventricle**

● **33980**   **Removal of ventricular assist device, implantable intracorporeal, single ventricle**

OTHER PROCEDURES

33999   **Unlisted procedure, cardiac surgery**   80

Cardiovascular System

34001 — 35001

ARTERIES AND VEINS

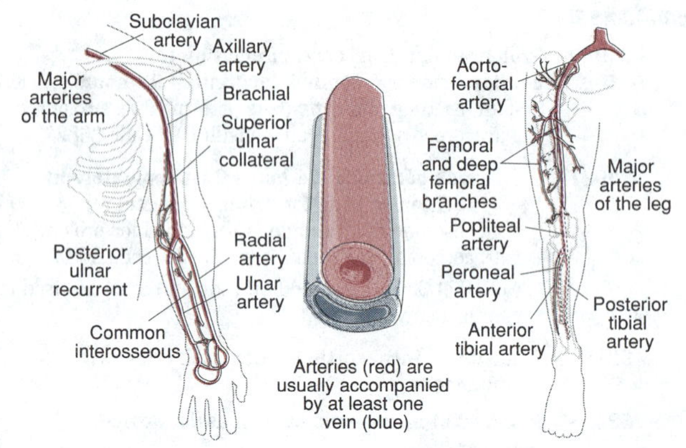

EMBOLECTOMY/THROMBECTOMY, ARTERIAL, WITH OR WITHOUT CATHETER

34001   Embolectomy or thrombectomy, with or without catheter; carotid, subclavian or innominate artery, by neck incision   80 ⬈ 50

34051   innominate, subclavian artery, by thoracic incision   80 ⬈ 50

34101   axillary, brachial, innominate, subclavian artery, by arm incision   ③ 80 ⬈ 50

34111   radial or ulnar artery, by arm incision   80 ⬈ 50

34151   renal, celiac, mesentery, aortoiliac artery, by abdominal incision   80 ⬈ 50

34201   femoropopliteal, aortoiliac artery, by leg incision   80 ⬈ 50

34203   popliteal-tibio-peroneal artery, by leg incision   80 ⬈ 50

EMBOLECTOMY/THROMBECTOMY, VENOUS, DIRECT OR WITH CATHETER

34401   Thrombectomy, direct or with catheter; vena cava, iliac vein, by abdominal incision   80 ⬈ 50

34421   vena cava, iliac, femoropopliteal vein, by leg incision   80 ⬈ 50

34451   vena cava, iliac, femoropopliteal vein, by abdominal and leg incision   80 ⬈ 50

34471   subclavian vein, by neck incision   ⬈ 50

34490   axillary and subclavian vein, by arm incision   ⬈ 50

VENOUS RECONSTRUCTION

34501   Valvuloplasty, femoral vein   80 ⬈ 50

34502   Reconstruction of vena cava, any method   80 ⬈

34510   Venous valve transposition, any vein donor   80 ⬈ 50

34520   Cross-over vein graft to venous system   80 ⬈ 50

34530   Saphenopopliteal vein anastomosis   80 ⬈ 50

ENDOVASCULAR REPAIR OF ABDOMINAL AORTIC ANEURYSM

CPT codes 38000-34832 address the repair of a weakness of the aorta with codes describing an endovascular graft under fluoroscopic guidance. These codes include balloon angioplasty with the prosthesis, catheter manipulations, vascular access, and closure.

If extensive repair or replacement of an artery is required, report as an additional procedure.

For endovascular repair of infrarenal abdominal aortic aneurysm or dissection using a modular bifurcated prostheseis (two docking limbs), use Category III code 0001T.

Report 34825 and 34826 in addition to codes 34800-34808 as appropriate. If procedure is done as a staged procedure append modifier-58 or 09958.

For open approach use 34812-34820 in conjunction with 34800, 34802, 34804, and 34808 as appropriate.

Note that 34808 is an add-on code and must be used in conjunction with codes 34800, 34813, 34825 and 34826.

34800   Endovascular repair of infrarenal abdominal aortic aneurysm or dissection; using aorto-aortic tube prosthesis   80

34802   using modular bifurcated prosthesis (one docking limb)   80
When repaired using a modular bifurcated prosthesis with two docking limbs, consult CPT Category III code 0001T.

34804   using unibody bifurcated prosthesis   80
When repaired using an aorto-uniiliac or aorto-unifemoral prosthesis, consult CPT Category III code 0002T.

+ 34808   Endovascular placement of iliac artery occlusion device (List separately in addition to code for primary procedure)   80

34812   Open femoral artery exposure for delivery of aortic endovascular prosthesis, by groin incision, unilateral   80

34813   Placement of femoral-femoral prosthetic graft during endovascular aortic aneurysm repair (List separately in addition to code for primary procedure)   80
If femoral artery grafting is performed, consult CPT codes 35521, 35533, 35546, 35551-35558, 35566, 25646, 35651-35661, 35666 and 35700.

34820   Open iliac artery exposure for delivery of endovascular prosthesis or iliac occlusion during endovascular therapy, by abdominal or retroperitoneal incision, unilateral   80 ⬈

34825   Placement of proximal or distal extension prosthesis for endovascular repair of infrarenal abdominal aortic aneurysm; initial vessel   80
For radiological supervision and interpretation, consult code 75953.

+ 34826   each additional vessel (List separately in addition to code for primary procedure)   80

34830   Open repair of infrarenal aortic aneurysm or dissection, plus repair of associated arterial trauma, following unsuccessful endovascular repair; tube prosthesis   80 ⬈

34831   aorto-bi-iliac prosthesis   80 ⬈

34832   aorto-bifemoral prosthesis   80 ⬈

DIRECT REPAIR OF ANEURYSM OR EXCISION (PARTIAL OR TOTAL) AND GRAFT INSERTION FOR ANEURYSM, FALSE ANEURYSM, RUPTURED ANEURYSM, AND ASSOCIATED OCCLUSIVE DISEASE

Preparation of the artery for anastomosis, including endarterectomy is included in CPT codes 35001-35162.

If direct repairs associated with occlusive disease only are performed, consult CPT codes 35201-35286.

If a thoracic aortic aneurysm is repaired, consult CPT codes 33860-33875.

If an intracranial aneurysim is repaired, consult CPT code 61700 and subsequent codes.

▲ **35001**   Direct repair of aneurysm, pseudoaneurysm, or excision (partial or total) and graft insertion, with or without patch graft; for aneurysm and associated occlusive disease, carotid, subclavian artery, by neck incision   80 ⬈ 50

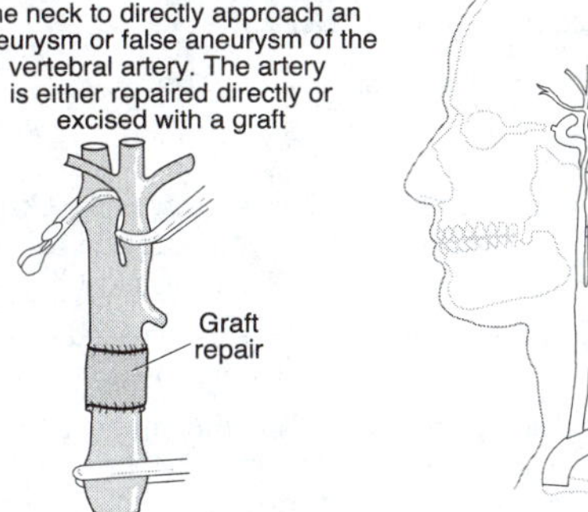

	35002	for ruptured aneurysm, carotid, subclavian artery, by neck incision	80 ⬑ 50
▲	35005	for aneurysm, pseudoaneurysm, and associated occlusive disease, vertebral artery	80 ⬑ 50
	35011	for aneurysm and associated occlusive disease, axillary-brachial artery, by arm incision	80 ⬑ 50
	35013	for ruptured aneurysm, axillary-brachial artery, by arm incision	80 ⬑ 50
▲	35021	for aneurysm, pseudoaneurysm, and associated occlusive disease, innominate, subclavian artery, by thoracic incision	80 ⬑ 50
	35022	for ruptured aneurysm, innominate, subclavian artery, by thoracic incision	80 ⬑ 50
▲	35045	for aneurysm, pseudoaneurysm, and associated occlusive disease, radial or ulnar artery	80 ⬑ 50
▲	35081	for aneurysm, pseudoaneurysm, and associated occlusive disease, abdominal aorta	80 ⬑
	35082	for ruptured aneurysm, abdominal aorta	80 ⬑
▲	35091	for aneurysm, pseudoaneurysm, and associated occlusive disease, abdominal aorta involving visceral vessels (mesenteric, celiac, renal)	80 ⬑ 50
	35092	for ruptured aneurysm, abdominal aorta involving visceral vessels (mesenteric, celiac, renal)	80 ⬑ 50
▲	35102	for aneurysm, pseudoaneurysm, and associated occlusive disease, abdominal aorta involving iliac vessels (common, hypogastric, external)	80 ⬑ 50
	35103	for ruptured aneurysm, abdominal aorta involving iliac vessels (common, hypogastric, external)	80 ⬑ 50
▲	35111	for aneurysm, pseudoaneurysm, and associated occlusive disease, splenic artery	80 ⬑ 50
	35112	for ruptured aneurysm, splenic artery	80 ⬑ 50
▲	35121	for aneurysm, pseudoaneurysm, and associated occlusive disease, hepatic, celiac, renal, or mesenteric artery	80 ⬑ 50
	35122	for ruptured aneurysm, hepatic, celiac, renal, or mesenteric artery	80 ⬑ 50
▲	35131	for aneurysm, pseudoaneurysm, and associated occlusive disease, iliac artery (common, hypogastric, external)	80 ⬑ 50
	35132	for ruptured aneurysm, iliac artery (common, hypogastric, external)	80 ⬑ 50
▲	35141	for aneurysm, pseudoaneurysm, and associated occlusive disease, common femoral artery (profunda femoris, superficial femoral)	80 ⬑ 50
	35142	for ruptured aneurysm, common femoral artery (profunda femoris, superficial femoral)	80 ⬑ 50
▲	35151	for aneurysm, pseudoaneurysm, and associated occlusive disease, popliteal artery	80 ⬑ 50
	35152	for ruptured aneurysm, popliteal artery	80 ⬑ 50
▲	35161	for aneurysm, pseudoaneurysm, and associated occlusive disease, other arteries	80 ⬑ 50
	35162	for ruptured aneurysm, other arteries	80 ⬑ 50

REPAIR ARTERIOVENOUS FISTULA

35180	Repair, congenital arteriovenous fistula; head and neck	80 ⬑
35182	thorax and abdomen	80 ⬑
35184	extremities	80 ⬑
35188	Repair, acquired or traumatic arteriovenous fistula; head and neck	80 ⬑
35189	thorax and abdomen	80 ⬑
35190	extremities	80 ⬑

REPAIR BLOOD VESSEL OTHER THAN FOR FISTULA, WITH OR WITHOUT PATCH ANGIOPLASTY

If an AV fistula is repaired, consult CPT codes 35180-35190.

35201	Repair blood vessel, direct; neck	80 ⬑ 50
35206	upper extremity	80 ⬑ 50
35207	hand, finger	⬑ 50
35211	intrathoracic, with bypass	80 ⬑ 50
35216	intrathoracic, without bypass	80 ⬑ 50
35221	intra-abdominal	80 ⬑ 50
35226	lower extremity	80 ⬑ 50
35231	Repair blood vessel with vein graft; neck	80 ⬑ 50
35236	upper extremity	80 ⬑ 50
35241	intrathoracic, with bypass	80 ⬑ 50
35246	intrathoracic, without bypass	80 ⬑ 50
35251	intra-abdominal	80 ⬑ 50
35256	lower extremity	80 ⬑ 50
35261	Repair blood vessel with graft other than vein; neck	80 ⬑ 50
35266	upper extremity	80 ⬑ 50
35271	intrathoracic, with bypass	80 ⬑ 50
35276	intrathoracic, without bypass	80 ⬑ 50
35281	intra-abdominal	80 ⬑ 50
35286	lower extremity	80 ⬑ 50

THROMBOENDARTERECTOMY

CIM 35-32 VERTEBRAL ARTERY SURGERY

Five types of surgical procedures performed to relieve obstructions blocking the flow of blood through the vertebral artery are:

- Vertebral artery endarterectomy, a procedure which cleans out arteriosclerotic plaques which are inside the vertebral artery
- Vertebral artery by-pass or resection with anastomosis or graft
- Subclavian artery resection with or without endarterectomy
- Removal of laterally located osteophytes anywhere in the C6(C7)-C2 course of the vertebral artery
- Arteriolysis which frees the artery from surrounding tissue, with or without arteriopexy (fixation of the vessel)

These procedures are covered if each of the following conditions is met:

- Symptoms of vertebral artery obstruction exist
- Other causes have been considered and ruled out
- There is radiographic evidence of a valid vertebral artery obstruction

Cardiovascular System

35301 — 35481

- Contraindications to the procedure do not exist, such as coexistent obstructions of multiple cerebral vessels

Angiograms should show the aortic arch with the vessels off the arch and the vessels in the neck and head (providing biplane views of the carotid and vertebral vascular system). In addition, serial views are needed to diagnose "subclavian steal," the subclavian artery obstruction that causes the symptoms of vertebral artery obstruction. In addition to vertebral artery obstruction, the differential diagnosis should include various degenerative disorders of the brain, orthostatic hypotension, acoustic neuroma, labyrinthitis, diabetes mellitus and hypoglycemia related disorders. Obstructions which can cause symptoms of blocked vertebral artery blood flow and which can be documented by an angiogram include:

- Intravascular obstructions—arteriosclerotic lesions within the vertebral artery or in other arteries

- Extravascular obstructions

- Bony tissue or osteophytes, located laterally in the C6 (C7)-C2 cervical vertebral area course of the vertebral artery, most commonly at C5 - C6

- Anatomical variations—Anomalous location of the origin of the vertebral artery, a congenital aberration, and tortuosity and kinks of the vertebral artery

- Fibrous tissue—Tissue changed as a result of manipulation of the neck for neck pain or injury associated with hematoma

Claims for this type of procedure require identification of the obstruction and the surgical procedure performed.

If a coronary artery bypass is performed, consult CPT codes 33510-33536 and 33572.

Code	Description		
35301	**Thromboendarterectomy, with or without patch graft; carotid, vertebral, subclavian, by neck incision**	80 ↻	50
35311	subclavian, innominate, by thoracic incision	80 ↻	50
35321	axillary-brachial	80 ↻	50
35331	abdominal aorta	80 ↻	50
35341	mesenteric, celiac, or renal	80 ↻	50
35351	iliac	80 ↻	50
35355	iliofemoral	80 ↻	50
35361	combined aortoiliac	80 ↻	50
35363	combined aortoiliofemoral	80 ↻	50
35371	common femoral	80 ↻	50
35372	deep (profunda) femoral	80 ↻	50
35381	femoral and/or popliteal, and/or tibioperoneal	80 ↻	50
+ 35390	**Reoperation, carotid, thromboendarterectomy, more than one month after original operation (List separately in addition to code for primary procedure)**	80 ↻	50

Note that 35390 is an add-on code and must be used in conjunction with 35301.

ANGIOSCOPY

Code	Description	
+ 35400	**Angioscopy (non-coronary vessels or grafts) during therapeutic intervention (List separately in addition to code for primary procedure)**	80 ↻

Note that 35400 is an add-on code and must be used in conjunction with a code for the therapeutic intervention.

TRANSLUMINAL ANGIOPLASTY, OPEN

CIM 50-32 PERCUTANEOUS TRANSLUMINAL ANGIOPLASTY (PTA)

Percutaneous transluminal angioplasty (PTA) PTA is covered to treat the following indications:

- Atherosclerotic obstructive lesions

- In the lower extremities (upper extremities do not include head or neck vessels)

- Of a single coronary artery for patients who exhibit the following characteristics:

Angina refractory to optimal medical management

Objective evidence of myocardial ischemia

Lesions amenable to angioplasty

- Of the renal arteries for patients for whom surgery is the likely alternative (i.e., PTA for this group of patients is an alternative to surgery, not simply an addition to medical management.)

- Obstructive lesions of arteriovenous dialysis fistulas and grafts when performed through either a venous or arterial approach

Effective July 1, 2001, Medicare will cover PTA of the carotid artery concurrent with carotid stent placement when furnished in accordance with the Food and Drug Administration (FDA) approved protocols governing Category B Investigational Device Exemption (IDE) clinical trials.

For radiological supervision and interpretation, consult CPT codes 75962-75968 and 75978.

Code	Description		
35450	**Transluminal balloon angioplasty, open; renal or other visceral artery**	80 ↻	50
35452	aortic	80 ↻	50
35454	iliac	80 ↻	50
35456	femoral-popliteal	80 ↻	50
35458	brachiocephalic trunk or branches, each vessel	80 ↻	50
35459	tibioperoneal trunk and branches	80 ↻	50
35460	venous	↻	50

TRANSLUMINAL ANGIOPLASTY, PERCUTANEOUS

For radiological supervision and interpretation, consult CPT codes 75962-75968 and 75978.

Code	Description		
35470	**Transluminal balloon angioplasty, percutaneous; tibioperoneal trunk or branches, each vessel**	↻	50
35471	renal or visceral artery	↻	50
35472	aortic	80 ↻	50
35473	iliac	↻	50
35474	femoral-popliteal	↻	50
35475	brachiocephalic trunk or branches, each vessel	↻	50
35476	venous	↻	50

TRANSLUMINAL ATHERECTOMY, OPEN

If radiological supervision and interpretation is needed, consult CPT codes 75992-75996.

Code	Description	
35480	**Transluminal peripheral atherectomy, open; renal or other visceral artery**	80 ↻
35481	aortic	80 ↻

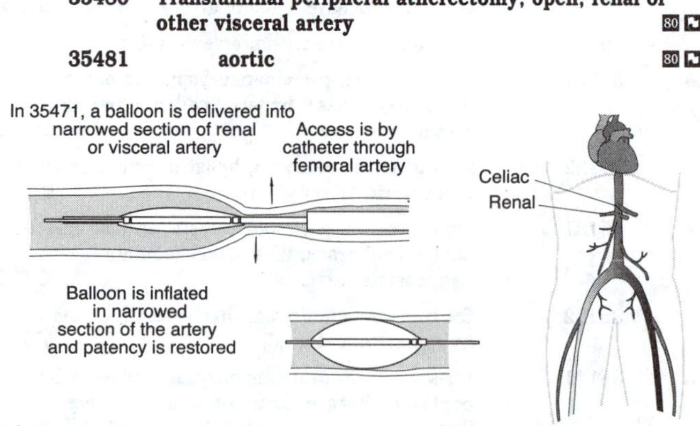

A balloon angioplasty is performed on the renal or visceral artery in a percutaneous procedure

35482	iliac	80 CCI
35483	femoral-popliteal	80 CCI
35484	brachiocephalic trunk or branches, each vessel	80 CCI
35485	tibioperoneal trunk and branches	80 CCI

TRANSLUMINAL ATHERECTOMY, PERCUTANEOUS

For radiological supervision and interpretation, consult CPT codes 75992-75996.

35490	Transluminal peripheral atherectomy, percutaneous; renal or other visceral artery	80 CCI
35491	aortic	80 CCI
35492	iliac	80 CCI
35493	femoral-popliteal	CCI
35494	brachiocephalic trunk or branches, each vessel	CCI
35495	tibioperoneal trunk and branches	80 CCI

BYPASS GRAFT, VEIN

+ **35500** Harvest of upper extremity vein, one segment, for lower extremity or coronary artery bypass procedure (List separately in addition to code for primary procedure)   80 50

> Note that 35500 is an add-on code and must be used in conjunction with codes 33510-33536, 35556, 35566, 35571, 35583-35587.
>
> If more than one vein segment is harvested, consult CPT codes 35682 and 35683.

35501	Bypass graft, with vein; carotid	80 CCI 50
35506	carotid-subclavian	80 CCI 50
35507	subclavian-carotid	80 CCI 50
35508	carotid-vertebral	80 CCI 50
35509	carotid-carotid	80 CCI 50
35511	subclavian-subclavian	80 CCI 50
35515	subclavian-vertebral	80 CCI 50
35516	subclavian-axillary	80 CCI 50
35518	axillary-axillary	80 CCI 50
35521	axillary-femoral	80 CCI 50

If a bypass graft is performed with a synthetic graft, consult CPT code 35621.

35526	aortosubclavian or carotid	80 CCI 50

If a bypass graft is performed with a synthetic graft, consult CPT code 35626.

35531	aortoceliac or aortomesenteric	80 CCI 50
35533	axillary-femoral-femoral	80 CCI 50

If a bypass graft is performed with a synthetic graft, consult CPT code 35654.

35536	splenorenal	80 CCI 50
35541	aortoiliac or bi-iliac	80 CCI

If a bypass graft is performed with a synthetic graft, consult CPT code 35641.

35546	aortofemoral or bifemoral	80 CCI 50

If a bypass graft is performed with a synthetic graft, consult CPT code 35646.

35548	aortoiliofemoral, unilateral	80 CCI

If a bypass graft is performed with a synthetic graft, consult CPT code 37799.

35549	aortoiliofemoral, bilateral	80 CCI

If a bypass graft is performed with a synthetic graft, consult CPT code 37799.

35551	aortofemoral-popliteal	80 CCI 50
35556	femoral-popliteal	80 CCI 50
35558	femoral-femoral	80 CCI 50
35560	aortorenal	80 CCI 50
35563	ilioiliac	80 CCI 50
35565	iliofemoral	80 CCI 50
35566	femoral-anterior tibial, posterior tibial, peroneal artery or other distal vessels	80 CCI 50
35571	popliteal-tibial, -peroneal artery or other distal vessels	80 CCI 50

BYPASS GRAFT, IN-SITU VEIN

35582	In-situ vein bypass; aortofemoral-popliteal (only femoral-popliteal portion in-situ)	80 CCI 50
35583	femoral-popliteal	80 CCI 50
35585	femoral-anterior tibial, posterior tibial, or peroneal artery	80 CCI 50
35587	popliteal-tibial, peroneal	80 CCI 50

BYPASS GRAFT, OTHER THAN VEIN

⊘	35600	Harvest of upper extremity artery, one segment, for coronary artery bypass procedure	80 50
	35601	Bypass graft, with other than vein; carotid	80 CCI 50
	35606	carotid-subclavian	80 CCI 50
	35612	subclavian-subclavian	80 CCI 50
	35616	subclavian-axillary	80 CCI 50
	35621	axillary-femoral	80 CCI 50
	35623	axillary-popliteal or -tibial	80 CCI 50
	35626	aortosubclavian or carotid	80 CCI 50
	35631	aortoceliac, aortomesenteric, aortorenal	80 CCI 50
	35636	splenorenal (splenic to renal arterial anastomosis)	80 CCI 50
	35641	aortoiliac or bi-iliac	80 CCI
	35642	carotid-vertebral	80 CCI 50
	35645	subclavian-vertebral	80 CCI 50
▲	35646	aortobifemoral	80 CCI 50
●	35647	aortofemoral	
	35650	axillary-axillary	80 CCI 50
	35651	aortofemoral-popliteal	80 CCI 50
	35654	axillary-femoral-femoral	80 CCI 50
	35656	femoral-popliteal	80 CCI 50
	35661	femoral-femoral	80 CCI 50
	35663	ilioiliac	80 CCI 50
	35665	iliofemoral	80 CCI 50

Vena cava and renal veins
Celiac trunk
Superior mesenteric
Renal
Abdominal aorta as it exits diaphragm
Abdominal aorta
Synthetic graft
Blockage

In 35631, a bypass graft of material other than vein is surgically installed from the aorta to the celiac, mesenteric, or renal arteries. The graft is typically placed in an end-to-side fashion on both the aorta and the recipient vessel downstream from the blockage

---

☐ CCI Comprehensive Code   50 Bilateral Procedure   + CPT Add-on Code   ⊘ Modifier -51 Exempt Code   ● New Code   ▲ Revised Code

M Maternity   N Newborn   P Pediatric   N/P Newborn/Pediatric

| 35666 | femoral-anterior tibial, posterior tibial, or peroneal artery | 80 ⤵ 50 |
| 35671 | popliteal-tibial or -peroneal artery | 80 ⤵ 50 |

COMPOSITE GRAFTS

Use the following codes to report harvest and anastomosis of two or more vein segments from sites distant to that where the bypass is being performed.

+ 35681   Bypass graft; composite, prosthetic and vein (List separately in addition to code for primary procedure)   80 ⤵ 50

> Note that 35681 is not to be reported in addition to 35682 and 35683.

+ 35682   autogenous composite, two segments of veins from two locations (List separately in addition to code for primary procedure)   80 ⤵

> Note that 35682 is not to be reported in addition to 35681 and 35683.

+ 35683   autogenous composite, three or more segments of vein from two or more locations (List separately in addition to code for primary procedure)   80 ⤵

> Note that 35683 is not to be reported in addition to 35681 and 35682.

ADJUVANT TECHNIQUES

● **+ 35685**   Placement of vein patch or cuff at distal anastomosis of bypass graft, synthetic conduit (List separately in addition to code for primary procedure)

> Note that 35685 is an add-on code and must be used in conjunction with codes 35656, 35666 or 35671.

● **+ 35686**   Creation of distal arteriovenous fistula during lower extremity bypass surgery (non-hemodialysis) (List separately in addition to code for primary procedure)

> Note that 35686 is an add-on code and must be used in conjunction with codes 35556, 35566, 35571, 35583-35587, 35656, 35666, or 35671.

ARTERIES AND VEINS

ARTERIAL TRANSPOSITION

35691	Transposition and/or reimplantation; vertebral to carotid artery	80 ⤵ 50
35693	vertebral to subclavian artery	80 ⤵ 50
35694	subclavian to carotid artery	80 ⤵ 50
35695	carotid to subclavian artery	80 ⤵ 50

EXPLORATION/REVISION

+ 35700   Reoperation, femoral-popliteal or femoral (popliteal) - anterior tibial, posterior tibial, peroneal artery or other distal vessels, more than one month after original operation (List separately in addition to code for primary procedure)   80 50

> Note that 35700 is an add-on code and must be used in conjunction with 35556, 35566, 35571, 35583, 35585, 35587, 35656, 35666, and 35671.

35701	Exploration (not followed by surgical repair), with or without lysis of artery; carotid artery	80 ⤵ 50
35721	femoral artery	80 ⤵ 50
35741	popliteal artery	80 ⤵ 50
35761	other vessels	80 ⤵ 50
35800	Exploration for postoperative hemorrhage, thrombosis or infection; neck	80 ⤵
35820	chest	80 ⤵
35840	abdomen	80 ⤵
35860	extremity	80 ⤵
35870	Repair of graft-enteric fistula	80 ⤵

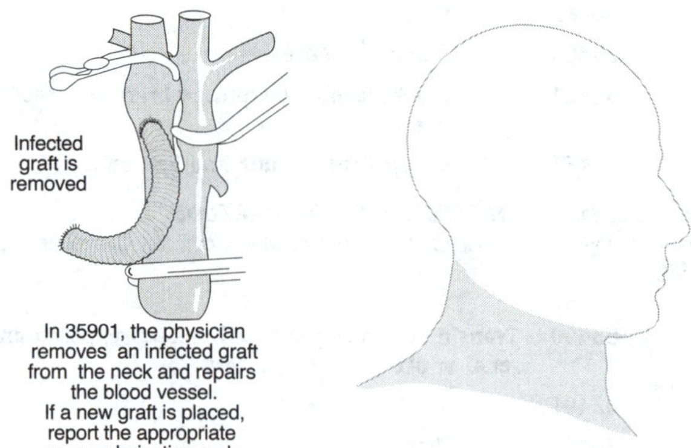

| 35875 | Thrombectomy of arterial or venous graft (other than hemodialysis graft or fistula); | ⤵ |
| 35876 | with revision of arterial or venous graft | 80 ⤵ |

> If thrombectomy of hemodialysis graft or fistula is performed, consult CPT codes 36831 and 36833.

35879	Revision, lower extremity arterial bypass, without thrombectomy, open; with vein patch angioplasty	80 ⤵ 50
35881	with segmental vein interposition	80 ⤵ 50
35901	Excision of infected graft; neck	80 ⤵
35903	extremity	80 ⤵
35905	thorax	80 ⤵
35907	abdomen	80 ⤵

INTRAVENOUS

Use these codes for cardiovascular procedures requiring local anesthesia, injection of contrast media, introduction of needles, and introduction of catheters. They also include care associated before and after the injection procedures themselves. The cost of catheters, contrast media, and drugs are not included.

If introduction of needle or intracatheter, vein is performed as part of critical care services (99291-99292) do not report separately.

| 36000* | Introduction of needle or intracatheter, vein | ⤵ 50 |
| ● 36002 | Injection procedures (eg, thrombin) for percutaneous treatment of extremity pseudoaneurysm | |

> To report imaging guidance, consult CPT codes 76003, 76360, 76393, or 76942.
>
> To report ultrasound guided compression repair of pseudoaneurysms, consult CPT code 76936.
>
> Code 36002 should not be used to report vascular sealant of an arteriotomy site.

| ▲ 36005 | Injection procedure for extremity venography (including introduction of needle or intracatheter) | 80 ⤵ |

> To report radiological supervision and interpretation, consult CPT codes 75820 and 75822.

36010	Introduction of catheter, superior or inferior vena cava	⤵ 50
36011	Selective catheter placement, venous system; first order branch (eg, renal vein, jugular vein)	⤵ 50
36012	second order, or more selective, branch (eg, left adrenal vein, petrosal sinus)	⤵ 50
36013	Introduction of catheter, right heart or main pulmonary artery	⤵
36014	Selective catheter placement, left or right pulmonary artery	⤵ 50
36015	Selective catheter placement, segmental or subsegmental pulmonary artery	⤵ 50

If a flow directed catheter is inserted (eg. Swan-Ganz), consult CPT code 93503. If venous catheterization is performed for selective organ blood sampling, consult CPT code 36500.

INTRA-ARTERIAL - INTRA-AORTIC

If angioplasty is performed, consult CPT codes 35470-35475. If transcatheter therapies are performed, consult CPT codes 37200-37208, 61624, and 61626.

If radiological supervision and interpretation is needed, see the Radiology section of CPT. If an angiography is performed, consult CPT codes 75600-75790.

36100   **Introduction of needle or intracatheter, carotid or vertebral artery**

36120   **Introduction of needle or intracatheter; retrograde brachial artery**

36140   **extremity artery**

36145   **arteriovenous shunt created for dialysis (cannula, fistula, or graft)**

> To report insertion of arteriovenous cannula, consult CPT codes 36810-36821.

36160   **Introduction of needle or intracatheter, aortic, translumbar**

36200   **Introduction of catheter, aorta**

36215   **Selective catheter placement, arterial system; each first order thoracic or brachiocephalic branch, within a vascular family**

> If catheter placement is performed for cornary angiography, consult CPT code 93508.

36216   **initial second order thoracic or brachiocephalic branch, within a vascular family**

36217   **initial third order or more selective thoracic or brachiocephalic branch, within a vascular family**

+ 36218   **additional second order, third order, and beyond, thoracic or brachiocephalic branch, within a vascular family (List in addition to code for initial second or third order vessel as appropriate)**

36245   **Selective catheter placement, arterial system; each first order abdominal, pelvic, or lower extremity artery branch, within a vascular family**

36246   **initial second order abdominal, pelvic, or lower extremity artery branch, within a vascular family**

36247   **initial third order or more selective abdominal, pelvic, or lower extremity artery branch, within a vascular family**

+ 36248   **additional second order, third order, and beyond, abdominal, pelvic, or lower extremity artery branch, within a vascular family (List in addition to code for initial second or third order vessel as appropriate)**

> Note that 36248 is an add-on code and must be used in conjunction with 36246 and 36247.

36260   **Insertion of implantable intra-arterial infusion pump (eg, for chemotherapy of liver)**

36261   **Revision of implanted intra-arterial infusion pump**

36262   **Removal of implanted intra-arterial infusion pump**

36299   **Unlisted procedure, vascular injection**

VENOUS

▲ **36400**   **Venipuncture, under age 3 years; femoral or jugular**

36405*   **scalp vein**

36406   **other vein**

36410*   **Venipuncture, child over age 3 years or adult, necessitating physician's skill (separate procedure), for diagnostic or therapeutic purposes. Not to be used for routine venipuncture.**

> If venipuncture is performed as part of critical care services (99291-99292) do not report separately.

36415*   **Routine venipuncture or finger/heel/ear stick for collection of specimen(s)**

36420   **Venipuncture, cutdown; under age 1 year**

36425   **age 1 or over**

CIM 35-71 NONSELECTIVE (RANDOM) TRANSFUSIONS AND LIVING - RELATED DONOR SPECIFIC TRANSFUSIONS (DST) IN KIDNEY TRANSPLANTATION

Pretransplant transfusions are covered under Medicare without a specific limit on the number of transfusions, subject to the normal Medicare blood deductible provisions. Where blood is given directly to the transplant patient, (e.g., donor specific transfusions) the blood is considered replaced for purposes of blood deductible provisions.

CIM 45-18 GRANULOCYTE TRANSFUSIONS

Medicare covers granulocyte transfusions to patients suffering from severe infection and granulocytopenia. Granulocytopenia is usually identified as less than 500 granulocytes/mm2 whole blood. Accepted indications for transfusions include:

- Granulocytopenia with evidence of gram negative sepsis
- Granulocytopenia in febrile patients with local progressive infections unresponsive to appropriate antibiotic therapy, thought to be due to gram negative organisms

CIM 45-27 BLOOD TRANSFUSIONS

Blood transfusions are used to restore blood volume after hemorrhage, to improve the oxygen carrying capacity of blood in severe anemia, and to combat shock in acute hemolytic anemia.

Definitions

1. Homologous blood transfusion is the infusion of blood or blood components collected from the general public.

2. An autologous blood transfusion is the collection and infusion of a patient's own blood.

3. A donor directed blood transfusion is the infusion of blood or blood components collected from a specific individual(s) other than the patient and infused into the specific patient for whom the blood is designated.

4. Perioperative blood salvage is the collection and reinfusion of blood lost during and immediately after surgery.

Medicare (Part A and Part B) generally covers medically necessary transfusion of blood, regardless of the type. The following polices apply to the preoperative collection, processing, and storage of autologous and donor-directed blood:

- Non-physician services furnished to hospital patients are covered and paid for as hospital services
- Inclusion of services provided to hospital patients by an outside supplier as part of hospital services is referred to as "bundling"
- The hospital pays the supplier when the facility obtains either autologous or donor-directed blood from an independent supplier, the supplier collects, processes, and stores the blood and, delivers it to the hospital

Under Part A payment, Medicare recognizes only a processing fee charged to the hospital by the independent blood bank. Under the prospective payment system (PPS), the diagnosis related group (DRG) payment to the hospital includes all covered blood and blood processing expenses, whether or not the blood is eventually used.

All patients share the cost of blood provided by a hospital operating its own blood collection.

Under Part B, the collection, processing, and storage of blood for later transfusion into the beneficiary is not recognized as a separate service and no

---

blood supplier can receive direct payment under Part B for blood donation services.

When perioperative blood salvage is used in surgery on a hospital patient, payment to the hospital (under PPS or through cost reimbursement) includes payment for all related costs.

36430	**Transfusion, blood or blood components**	
36440*	**Push transfusion, blood, 2 years or under**	
36450	**Exchange transfusion, blood; newborn**	
36455	**other than newborn**	
36460	**Transfusion, intrauterine, fetal**	

> If radiological supervision and interpretation is performed, consult CPT code 76941.

36468	**Single or multiple injections of sclerosing solutions, spider veins (telangiectasia); limb or trunk**	
36469	**face**	

CIM 35-13 PROLOTHERAPY, JOINT SCLEROTHERAPY, AND LIGAMENTOUS INJECTIONS WITH SCLEROSING AGENTS - NOT COVERED

The medical effectiveness of the above therapies has not been verified by scientifically controlled studies and coverage is denied on the ground that they are not reasonable and necessary.

36470*	**Injection of sclerosing solution; single vein**	
36471*	**multiple veins, same leg**	
36481	**Percutaneous portal vein catheterization by any method**	

> To report radiological supervision and interpretation, consult CPT codes 75885 and 75887.

36488* **Placement of central venous catheter (subclavian, jugular, or other vein) (eg, for central venous pressure, hyperalimentation, hemodialysis, or chemotherapy); percutaneous, age 2 years or under**

36489* **percutaneous, over age 2**
> To report imaging guidance, consult CPT codes 76000, 76003, 76942.

36490* **cutdown, age 2 years or under**

36491* **cutdown, over age 2**
> If examining and instructing a patient for a review of prescription fluids for long-term or permanent hyperalimentation, consult Evaluation and Management codes for office or hospital inpatient category or follow-up inpatient consultation codes as appropriate.

36493 **Repositioning of previously placed central venous catheter under fluoroscopic guidance**
> To report fluoroscopic guidance, consult CPT code 76000.

36500 **Venous catheterization for selective organ blood sampling**
> If the superior or inferior vena cava is catheterized, consult CPT code 36010. If radiological supervision and interpretation is performed, consult CPT code 75893.

36510* **Catheterization of umbilical vein for diagnosis or therapy, newborn**

CIM 35-60 APHERSIS (THERAPEUTIC PHERESIS)

Apheresis is as an autologous procedure (i.e., blood is taken from the patient, processed, and returned to the patient as part of a continuous procedure). Apheresis is covered for the following indications:

- Plasma exchange for acquired myasthenia gravis
- Leukapheresis in the treatment of leukemia

Plasmapheresis in the treatment of primary macroglobulinemia (Waldenstrom).

- Treatment of hyperglobulinemias, including (but not limited to) multiple myelomas, cryoglobulinemia and hyperviscosity syndromes

- Plasmapheresis or plasma exchange as a last resort treatment of thromobotic thrombocytopenic purpura (TTP)
- Plasmapheresis or plasma exchange in the last resort treatment of life threatening rheumatoid vasculitis
- Plasma perfusion of charcoal filters for treatment of pruritus of cholestatic liver disease
- Plasma exchange in the treatment of Goodpasture's Syndrome
- Plasma exchange in the treatment of glomerulonephritis associated with antiglomerular basement membrane antibodies and advancing renal failure or pulmonary hemorrhage
- Treatment of chronic relapsing polyneuropathy for patients with severe or life threatening symptoms who have failed to respond to conventional therapy
- Treatment of life threatening scleroderma and polymyositis when the patient is unresponsive to conventional therapy
- Treatment of Guillain-Barre Syndrome
- Treatment of last resort for life threatening systemic lupus erythematosus (SLE) when conventional therapy has failed to prevent clinical deterioration

Apheresis is covered only when performed in the following settings:

- In a hospital setting (either inpatient or outpatient). Nonphysician services furnished to hospital patients are covered and paid for as hospital services. When covered services are provided to hospital patients by an outside provider/supplier, the hospital is responsible for paying the provider/supplier for the services
- In a nonhospital setting when a physician is present to perform medical services and to respond to medical emergencies at all times during patient care hours and all nonphysician services are furnished under the direct supervision of a physician

36520 **Therapeutic apheresis; plasma and/or cell exchange**

36521 **with extracorporeal affinity column adsorption and plasma reinfusion**

CIM 35-88 EXTRACORPOREAL PHOTOPHERESIS

Medicare covers extracorporeal photopheresis, a treatment for cutaneous T-cell lymphoma (CTCL), when used in the palliative treatment of the skin manifestations of CTCL that has not responded to other therapy.

36522 **Photopheresis, extracorporeal**

36530 **Insertion of implantable intravenous infusion pump**
> To report imaging guidance, consult CPT codes 76000, 76003, 76942.

36531 **Revision of implantable intravenous infusion pump**

36532 **Removal of implantable intravenous infusion pump**
> To report imaging guidance, consult CPT code 76000.

36533 **Insertion of implantable venous access device, with or without subcutaneous reservoir**
> To report refilling and maintenance of an implantable venous access device, and/or subcutaneous reservoir, consult CPT code 96530.
>
> To report imaging guidance, consult CPT codes 76000, 760003, 76942.

36534 **Revision of implantable venous access device, and/or subcutaneous reservoir**
> If the implantable venous access device and/or subcutaneous reservoir is removed, consult CPT code 36535.

36535 **Removal of implantable venous access device, and/or subcutaneous reservoir**
> Note that 36535 can be used in conjunction with 36533 and 36534, as appropriate. Note that 36535 cannot be used in conjunction with 36488-36491.

To report imaging guidance, consult CPT code 76000.

36540   **Collection of blood specimen from a partially or completely implantable venous access device**

36550   **Declotting by thrombolytic agent of implanted vascular access device or catheter** 〔80〕

ARTERIAL

36600*   **Arterial puncture, withdrawal of blood for diagnosis** 〔↑〕
If arterial puncture is performed as part of critical care services (99291-99292) do not report separately.

⊘   **36620**   **Arterial catheterization or cannulation for sampling, monitoring or transfusion (separate procedure); percutaneous** 〔↑〕

36625   **cutdown** 〔↑〕

36640   **Arterial catheterization for prolonged infusion therapy (chemotherapy), cutdown** ❶〔↑〕
Consult also 96420-96425. If arterial catheterization is performed for occlusion therapy, consult CPT code 75894.

⊘   **36660***   **Catheterization, umbilical artery, newborn, for diagnosis or therapy** 〔N〕〔80〕〔↑〕

INTRAOSSEOUS

36680   **Placement of needle for intraosseous infusion** 〔80〕〔↑〕

HEMODIALYSIS ACCESS, INTERVASCULAR CANNULATION FOR EXTRACORPOREAL CIRCULATION, OR SHUNT INSERTION

36800   **Insertion of cannula for hemodialysis, other purpose (separate procedure); vein to vein** ❸〔↑〕

36810   **arteriovenous, external (Scribner type)** ❸〔↑〕

36815   **arteriovenous, external revision, or closure** ❸〔↑〕

▲   **36819**   **Arteriovenous anastomosis, open; by upper arm basilic vein transposition** ❸〔80〕〔↑〕

●   **36820**   **by forearm vein transposition** ❸

36821   **direct, any site (eg, Cimino type) (separate procedure)** ❸〔80〕〔↑〕

36822   **Insertion of cannula(s) for prolonged extracorporeal circulation for cardiopulmonary insufficiency (ECMO) (separate procedure)** 〔↑〕
If maintenance is performed for prolonged extracorporal circulation, consult CPT code 33960.

▲   **36823**   **Insertion of arterial and venous cannula(s) for isolated extracorporeal circulation including regional chemotherapy perfusion to an extremity, with or without hyperthermia, with removal of cannula(s) and repair of arteriotomy and venotomy sites** 〔↑〕
Code 36823 includes chemotherapy perfusion by a membrane oxygenator/perfusion pump, Do not code 96408-96425 with 36823.

36825   **Creation of arteriovenous fistula by other than direct arteriovenous anastomosis (separate procedure); autogenous graft** ❹〔80〕〔↑〕
If direct arteriovenous anastomosis is performed, consult CPT code 36821.

36830   **nonautogenous graft** ❹〔80〕〔↑〕
If direct arteriovenous anastomosis is performed, consult CPT code 36821.

36831   **Thrombectomy, open, arteriovenous fistula without revision, autogenous or nonautogenous dialysis graft (separate procedure)** 〔80〕〔↑〕

36832   **Revision, open, arteriovenous fistula; without thrombectomy, autogenous or nonautogenous dialysis graft (separate procedure)** ❹〔80〕〔↑〕

36833   **with thrombectomy, autogenous or nonautogenous dialysis graft (separate procedure)** ❹〔80〕〔↑〕

36834   **Plastic repair of arteriovenous aneurysm (separate procedure)** 〔80〕〔↑〕

36835   **Insertion of Thomas shunt (separate procedure)** ❹〔↑〕

36860   **External cannula declotting (separate procedure); without balloon catheter** ❷〔↑〕

36861   **with balloon catheter** ❸〔↑〕
To report imaging guidance, consult CPT code 76000.

●   **36870**   **Thrombectomy, percutaneous, arteriovenous fistula, autogenous or nonautogenous graft (includes mechanical thrombus extraction and intra-graft thrombolysis)** 〔↑〕〔50〕
Do not report 36550 with 36870. For catheterization, report code 46145.

If radiological supervision and interpretation is used, consult CPT code 75790.

PORTAL DECOMPRESSION PROCEDURES

37140   **Venous anastomosis; portocaval** 〔↑〕
If peritoneal-venous shunt is inserted, consult CPT code 49425.

37145   **renoportal** 〔80〕〔↑〕

37160   **caval-mesenteric** 〔80〕〔↑〕

37180   **splenorenal, proximal** 〔80〕〔↑〕

37181   **splenorenal, distal (selective decompression of esophagogastric varices, any technique)** 〔80〕〔↑〕

TRANSCATHETER PROCEDURES

The appropriate CPT codes for placement of catheters and radiological supervision and interpretation should be reported in addition to the following therapeutic procedures.

37195   **Thrombolysis, cerebral, by intravenous infusion** 〔80〕〔↑〕

37200   **Transcatheter biopsy** 〔↑〕
For radiological supervision and interpretation, consult CPT code 75970.

37201   **Transcatheter therapy, infusion for thrombolysis other than coronary** 〔↑〕
For radiological supervision and interpretation, consult CPT code 75896.

If thrombolysis of the coronary vessels is performed, consult CPT codes 92975 and 92977.

37202   **Transcatheter therapy, infusion other than for thrombolysis, any type (eg, spasmolytic, vasoconstrictive)** 〔↑〕
For radiological supervision and interpretation, consult CPT code 75896.

37203   **Transcatheter retrieval, percutaneous, of intravascular foreign body (eg, fractured venous or arterial catheter)** 〔↑〕
For radiological supervision and interpretation, consult CPT code 75961.

CIM 35-35 THERAPEUTIC EMBOLIZATION

Therapeutic embolization is covered when done for hemorrhage and for other conditions amenable to treatment by the procedure. Renal embolization for the treatment of renal adenocarcinoma is covered as a type of therapeutic embolization to:

- Reduce tumor vascularity preoperatively
- Reduce tumor bulk in inoperable cases
- Palliate specific symptoms

37204   **Transcatheter occlusion or embolization (eg, for tumor destruction, to achieve hemostasis, to occlude a vascular malformation), percutaneous, any method, non-central nervous system, non-head or neck** 〔↑〕

〔↑〕 CCI Comprehensive Code   〔50〕 Bilateral Procedure   ✚ CPT Add-on Code   ⊘ Modifier -51 Exempt Code   ● New Code   ▲ Revised Code

〔M〕 Maternity   〔N〕 Newborn   〔P〕 Pediatric   〔N/P〕 Newborn/Pediatric

For radiological supervision and interpretation, consult CPT code 75894.

Consult also CPT codes 61624 and 61626.

37205 Transcatheter placement of an intravascular stent(s), (non-coronary vessel), percutaneous; initial vessel [80] [▶]

For radiological supervision and interpretation, consult CPT code 75960.

+ 37206 each additional vessel (List separately in addition to code for primary procedure) [80]

Note that 37206 is an add-on code and must be used in conjunction with 37205.

To reporty transcatheter placement of extracranial cerebrovascular artery stent(s), consult CPT Category III codes 0005T, 0006T.

For radiological supervision and interpretation, consult CPT code 75960.

37207 Transcatheter placement of an intravascular stent(s), (non-coronary vessel), open; initial vessel [80] [▶] [50]

For radiological supervision and interpretation, consult CPT code 75960.

For catheterization, consult CPT codes 36215-36248.

For transcatheter placement of intracoronary stent(s), consult CPT codes 92980, 92981.

+ 37208 each additional vessel (List separately in addition to code for primary procedure) [80]

For radiological supervision and interpretation, consult CPT code 75960.

For catheterization, consult CPT codes 36215-36248.

For transcatheter placement of intracoronary stent(s), consult CPT codes 92980, 92981.

Note that 37208 is an add-on code and must be used in conjunction with 37207.

37209 Exchange of a previously placed arterial catheter during thrombolytic therapy [▶]

For radiological supervision and interpretation, consult CPT code 75900.

INTRAVASCULAR ULTRASOUND SERVICES

Includes all manipulations and repositioning of the transducer within the specific vessel being examined, before and after treatment.

CIM 50-7 ULTRASOUND DIAGNOSTIC PROCEDURES

Medicare coverage is extended to the procedures listed in Category I. Techniques in Category II are considered experimental and should not be covered at this time.

Category I (covered, may be adjunct to radiologic and nuclear medicine diagnostic technique)

1. Echoencephalography, (Diencephalic Midline) (A-Mode)
2. Echoencephalography, Complete (Diencephalic Midline and Ventricular Size)
3. Ocular and Orbital Echography (A-Mode) (includes determining the suitability of aphakic patients for an artificial lens implant following cataract surgery)
4. Ocular and Orbital Sonography (B-Mode)
5. Echocardiography, Pericardial Effusion (M-Mode)
6. Pericardiocentesis, by Ultrasonic Guidance
7. Echocardiography, Cardiac Valve(s) (M-Mode)
8. Echocardiography, Complete (M-Mode)
9. Echocardiography, limited (e.g., follow-up or limited study) (M-Mode)
10. Pleural Effusion Echography
11. Thoracentesis, by Ultrasonic Guidance
12. Abdominal Sonography, complete survey study (B-Scan)
13. Abdominal Sonography, limited (e.g., follow-up or limited study) (B-Scan)
14. Renal Cyst Aspiration, by Ultrasonic Guidance
15. Renal Biopsy, by Ultrasonic Guidance
16. Pancreas Sonography (B-Scan)
17. Spleen Sonography (B-Scan)
18. Abdominal Aorta Echography (A-Mode)
19. Abdominal Aorta Sonography (B-Scan)
20. Retroperitoneal Sonography (B-Scan)
21. Retroperitoneal sonography does not include planning of fields for radiation therapy.
22. Urinary Bladder Sonography (B-Scan)
23. Urinary bladder sonography does not include staging of bladder tumors.
24. Pregnancy Diagnosis sonography (B-Scan)
25. Fetal Age Determination (Biparietal Diameter) Sonography (B-Scan)
26. Fetal Growth Rate Sonography (B-Scan)
27. Placenta Localization Sonography (B-Scan)
28. Pregnancy Sonography, Complete (B-Scan)
29. Molar Pregnancy Diagnosis Sonography (B-Scan)
30. Ectopic Pregnancy Diagnosis sonography (B-Scan)
31. Passive Testing (Antepartum Monitoring of Fetal Heart Rate In the Resting Fetus)
32. Intrauterine Contraceptive Device Sonography (B-Scan)
33. Pelvic Mass Diagnosis Sonography (B-Scan)
34. Amniocentesis, by Ultrasonic Guidance
35. Arterial Flow Study, Peripheral (Doppler)
36. Venous Flow Study, Peripheral (Doppler)
37. Arterial Aneurysm, Peripheral (B-Scan)
38. Radiation Therapy Planning Sonography (B-Scan)
39. Thyroid Echography (A-Mode)
40. Thyroid Sonography (B-Scan)
41. Breast Echography (A-Mode)
42. Breast Sonography (B-Scan)
43. Hepatic Sonography (B-Scan)
44. Gallbladder Sonography
45. Renal Sonography
46. Two-Dimensional Echocardiography (B-Mode)

Category II (clinical reliability and efficacy not proven)

1. B-Scan for atherosclerotic narrowing of peripheral arteries
2. Monitoring of cardiac output (Doppler)

When appropriate, new uses for ultrasound diagnostic procedures should be forwarded to the Bureau of Eligibility, Reimbursement and Coverage, HCFA, so that revisions may be made in the coverage policy when appropriate.

+ 37250 Intravascular ultrasound (non-coronary vessel) during diagnostic evaluation and/or therapeutic intervention; initial vessel (List separately in addition to code for primary procedure) [80] [▶]

If catheterization is performed, consult CPT codes 36215-36248. If transcatheter therapies are performed, consult CPT codes 37200-37208, 61624, and 61626. For radiological supervision and interpretation, consult CPT codes 75945 and 75946.

Note that 37250 is an add-on code and must be used in conjunction with the appropriate CPT code for the diagnostic or therapeutic procedure performed.

+ 37251 each additional vessel (List separately in addition to code for primary procedure) [80]

Note that 37251 is an add-on code and must be used in conjunction with 37250.

LIGATION AND OTHER PROCEDURES

37565   Ligation, internal jugular vein   80 ⊡

CIM 35-57 ELECTROENCEPHALOGRAPHIC MONITORING DURING SURGICAL PROCEDURES INVOLVING THE CEREBRAL VASCULATURE

EEG monitoring as an indirect measure of cerebral perfusion requires the expertise of an electroencephalographer, a neurologist trained in EEG, or an advanced EEG technician for its proper interpretation. The procedure may be covered routinely in carotid endarterectomies and in other neurological procedures where cerebral perfusion could be reduced. Such other procedures might include aneurysm surgery where hypotensive anesthesia is used or other cerebral vascular procedures where cerebral blood flow may be interrupted.

37600   Ligation; external carotid artery   80 ⊡
     If ligation is used to treat an intracranial aneurysm, consult CPT code 61703.

37605   internal or common carotid artery   80 ⊡

37606   internal or common carotid artery, with gradual occlusion, as with Selverstone or Crutchfield clamp   80 ⊡

37607   Ligation or banding of angioaccess arteriovenous fistula   ⊡

37609   Ligation or biopsy, temporal artery   ❷ ⊡

37615   Ligation, major artery (eg, post-traumatic, rupture); neck   80 ⊡
     Touroff ligation

37616   chest   80 ⊡
     Bardenheuer operation

37617   abdomen   80 ⊡

37618   extremity   80 ⊡

37620   Interruption, partial or complete, of inferior vena cava by suture, ligation, plication, clip, extravascular, intravascular (umbrella device)   ⊡
     For radiological supervision and interpretation, consult CPT code 75940.

37650   Ligation of femoral vein   ⊡ 50

37660   Ligation of common iliac vein   80 ⊡

37700   Ligation and division of long saphenous vein at saphenofemoral junction, or distal interruptions   ❷ ⊡ 50

37720   Ligation and division and complete stripping of long or short saphenous veins   ❸ ⊡ 50

37730   Ligation and division and complete stripping of long and short saphenous veins   ❸ ⊡ 50
     Babcock operation

37735   Ligation and division and complete stripping of long or short saphenous veins with radical excision of ulcer and skin graft and/or interruption of communicating veins of lower leg, with excision of deep fascia   ❸ 80 ⊡ 50

37760   Ligation of perforators, subfascial, radical (Linton type), with or without skin graft   ❸ 80 ⊡

37780   Ligation and division of short saphenous vein at saphenopopliteal junction (separate procedure)   ❸ ⊡ 50

37785   Ligation, division, and/or excision of recurrent or secondary varicose veins (clusters), one leg   ❸ ⊡ 50

37788   Penile revascularization, artery, with or without vein graft   ♂ 80 ⊡

37790   Penile venous occlusive procedure   ♂ 80 ⊡

37799   Unlisted procedure, vascular surgery   80

HEMIC AND LYMPHATIC SYSTEMS

SPLEEN

EXCISION

38100   Splenectomy; total (separate procedure)   80 ⊡

38101   partial (separate procedure)   80 ⊡

+ 38102   total, en bloc for extensive disease, in conjunction with other procedure (List in addition to code for primary procedure)   80 ⊡

REPAIR

38115   Repair of ruptured spleen (splenorrhaphy) with or without partial splenectomy   80 ⊡

LAPAROSCOPY

Surgical laparoscopy always includes diagnostic laparoscopy.

38120   Laparoscopy, surgical, splenectomy   80 ⊡

38129   Unlisted laparoscopy procedure, spleen   80

INTRODUCTION

38200   Injection procedure for splenoportography   80 ⊡
     For radiological supervision and interpretation, consult CPT code 75810.

GENERAL

BONE MARROW OR STEM CELL SERVICES/PROCEDURES

● **38220**   Bone marrow aspiration

● **38221**   Bone marrow biopsy, needle or trocar
     For bone marrow biopsy interpretation, use 88305.

MCM 2070 DIAGNOSTIC X-RAY, DIAGNOSTIC LABORATORY, AND OTHER DIAGNOSTIC TESTS

Medicare covers diagnostic x-ray, diagnostic laboratory, and other diagnostic tests, including materials and the services of technicians. Medicare covers diagnostic X-ray services performed in a facility directed by a physician or group of physicians if they are performed under the direct supervision of a physician. Certain diagnostic X-ray procedures are also covered when performed by technicians without direct personal physician supervision if the technicians' general supervision and training, as well as the maintenance of the necessary equipment and supplies, are the continuing responsibility of a physician. Covered diagnostic tests include:

Histopathology

Tissue Decalcification

Bone Marrow Biopsy

Tissue Pathology

Surgical pathology

Frozen sections

Autopsy and sections

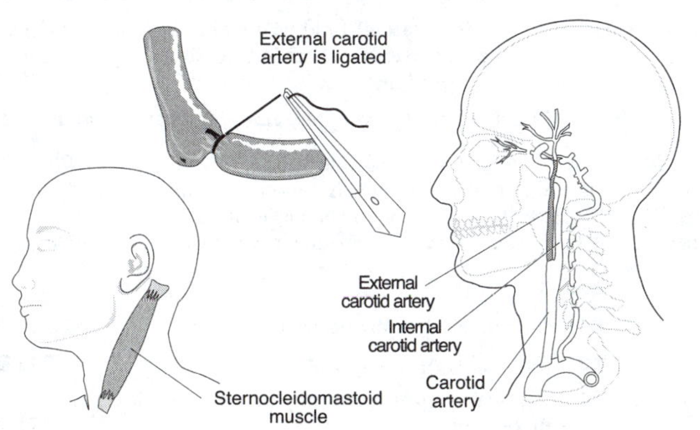

CIM 50-23 HISTOCOMPATIBILITY TESTING

Histocompatibility testing is covered when it is performed on patients:

- In preparation for a kidney transplant
- In preparation for bone marrow transplantation
- In preparation for blood platelet transfusions (particularly where multiple infusions are involved)
- Who are suspected of having ankylosing spondylitis

It is covered for ankylosing spondylitis when other methods of diagnosis would not be appropriate or have yielded inconclusive results. Documentation is required.

38230 **Bone marrow harvesting for transplantation** 80 ▣

38231 **Blood-derived peripheral stem cell harvesting for transplantation, per collection** 80 ▣

If cryopreservation, freezing, and storage of blood-derived stem cells is performed for transplantation, consult CPT code 88240. If thawing and expansion of blood-derived stem cells is performed for transplantation, consult CPT code 88241.

If modification, treatment, and processing of bone marrow or blood-derived stem cell specimens is performed for transplantation, consult CPT ode 86915.

38240 **Bone marrow or blood-derived peripheral stem cell transplantation; allogenic** 80 ▣

If bone marrow aspiration is performed, consult CPT code 85095.

If modification, treatment, and processing of bone marrow or blood-derived stem cell specimens is performed for transplantation, consult CPT ode 86915.

38241 **autologous** 80 ▣

If bone marrow aspiration is performed, consult CPT code 38220.

If compatibility studies are performed, consult CPT codes 86812-86822.

If modification, treatment, and processing of bone marrow or blood-derived stem cell specimens is performed for transplantation, consult CPT ode 86915.

LYMPH NODES AND LYMPHATIC CHANNELS

INCISION

38300* **Drainage of lymph node abscess or lymphadenitis; simple** ❶ ▣

38305 **extensive** ❷ ▣

38308 **Lymphangiotomy or other operations on lymphatic channels** ❷ 80 ▣

38380 **Suture and/or ligation of thoracic duct; cervical approach** 80 ▣

38381 **thoracic approach** 80 ▣

38382 **abdominal approach** 80 ▣

Cancers of the lymphatic system are called lymphomas; they are more common after age 50 and occur most frequently in the groin (inguinal), neck (cervical), and armpit (axillary) nodes

About 14 percent of malignant lymphomas are Hodgkin's disease, a form of cancer distinguished by the presence of unique, large, R-S cells; incidence peaks in the late 20s. Because the malignant lymphomas occur early in life, they account for more years of potential life lost than many of the more common cancers

EXCISION

If injection is performed for sentinel node identification, consult CPT code 38792.

38500 **Biopsy or excision of lymph node(s); open, superficial** ❷ ▣ 50

Do not report code 38500 in conjunction with 38700-38780.

38505 **by needle, superficial (eg, cervical, inguinal, axillary)** ❶ ▣ 50

To report imaging guidance, consult CPT codes 76360, 76393, 76942.

If fine needle aspiration is performed, consult CPT code 10021 or 10022.

To report evaluation of fine needle aspirate, consult CPT codes 88172, 88173.

38510 **open, deep cervical node(s)** ❷ ▣ 50

38520 **open, deep cervical node(s) with excision scalene fat pad** ❷ ▣ 50

38525 **open, deep axillary node(s)** ❷ ▣ 50

38530 **open, internal mammary node(s)** ❷ 80 ▣ 50

If percutaneous needle biopsy is performed on a retroperitoneal lymph node or mass, consult CPT code 49180; if fine needle aspiration is performed, consult CPT code 10022.

Do not report CPT code 38530 in conjuction with 38720-38746.

38542 **Dissection, deep jugular node(s)** ❷ 80 ▣ 50

If radical cervical neck dissection is performed, consult CPT code 38720.

38550 **Excision of cystic hygroma, axillary or cervical; without deep neurovascular dissection** ❸ 80 ▣

38555 **with deep neurovascular dissection** ❹ 80 ▣

LIMITED LYMPHADENECTOMY FOR STAGING

38562 **Limited lymphadenectomy for staging (separate procedure); pelvic and para-aortic** 80 ▣

If this procedure is combined with prostatectomy, consult CPT code 55812 or 55842. If this procedure is combined with the insertion of a radioactive substance into the prostate, consult CPT code 55862.

38564 **retroperitoneal (aortic and/or splenic)** 80 ▣

LAPAROSCOPY

38570 **Laparoscopy, surgical; with retroperitoneal lymph node sampling (biopsy), single or multiple** 80 ▣

If drainage of a lymphocele to the peritoneal cavity is performed, consult CPT code 49323.

38571 **with bilateral total pelvic lymphadenectomy** 80 ▣

38572 **with bilateral total pelvic lymphadenectomy and peri-aortic lymph node sampling (biopsy), single or multiple** 80 ▣

38589 **Unlisted laparoscopy procedure, lymphatic system** 80 50

RADICAL LYMPHADENECTOMY (RADICAL RESECTION OF LYMPH NODES)

If limited pelvic and retroperitoneal lymphadenectomies are performed, consult CPT codes 38562 and 38564. If lymphedematous skin and subcutaneous tissue are excised and repaired, consult CPT codes 15000 and 15570-15650.

38700 **Suprahyoid lymphadenectomy** ❷ 80 ▣ 50

38720 **Cervical lymphadenectomy (complete)** 80 ▣ 50

38724 **Cervical lymphadenectomy (modified radical neck dissection)** 80 ▣ 50

38740 **Axillary lymphadenectomy; superficial** ❷ 80 ▣

    CPT only © 2001 American Medical Association. All Rights Reserved. (Black Ink)   ©2001 Ingenix, Inc. (Blue Ink)

	38745	complete	④ 80 ⬚
+	38746	Thoracic lymphadenectomy, regional, including mediastinal and peritracheal nodes (List in addition to code for primary procedure)	80
+	38747	Abdominal lymphadenectomy, regional, including celiac, gastric, portal, peripancreatic, with or without para-aortic and vena caval nodes (List separately in addition to code for primary procedure)	80 ⬚
	38760	Inguinofemoral lymphadenectomy, superficial, including Cloquet's node (separate procedure)	❷ 80 ⬚ 50
	38765	Inguinofemoral lymphadenectomy, superficial, in continuity with pelvic lymphadenectomy, including external iliac, hypogastric, and obturator nodes (separate procedure)	80 ⬚ 50
	38770	Pelvic lymphadenectomy, including external iliac, hypogastric, and obturator nodes (separate procedure)	80 ⬚ 50
	38780	Retroperitoneal transabdominal lymphadenectomy, extensive, including pelvic, aortic, and renal nodes (separate procedure)	80 ⬚

INTRODUCTION

| | 38790 | Injection procedure; lymphangiography | ❶ ⬚ 50 |

If radiological supervision and interpretation is performed, consult CPT codes 75801-75807.

| ⊘ | 38792 | for identification of sentinel node | ⬚ 50 |

If the sentinel node is excised, consult CPT codes 38500-38542. If nuclear medicine lymphatics and lymph gland imaging is performed, consult CPT code 78195.

| | 38794 | Cannulation, thoracic duct | 80 ⬚ |

OTHER PROCEDURES

| | 38999 | Unlisted procedure, hemic or lymphatic system | 80 |

MEDIASTINUM AND DIAPHRAGM

MEDIASTINUM

INCISION

| | 39000 | Mediastinotomy with exploration, drainage, removal of foreign body, or biopsy; cervical approach | 80 ⬚ |
| | 39010 | transthoracic approach, including either transthoracic or median sternotomy | 80 ⬚ |

EXCISION

| | 39200 | Excision of mediastinal cyst | 80 ⬚ |
| | 39220 | Excision of mediastinal tumor | 80 ⬚ |

If a substernal thyroidectomy is performed, consult CPT code 60270. If a thymectomy is performed, consult CPT code 60520.

ENDOSCOPY

| | 39400 | Mediastinoscopy, with or without biopsy | ⬚ |

OTHER PROCEDURES

| | 39499 | Unlisted procedure, mediastinum | 80 |

DIAPHRAGM

REPAIR

	39501	Repair, laceration of diaphragm, any approach	80 ⬚
	39502	Repair, paraesophageal hiatus hernia, transabdominal, with or without fundoplasty, vagotomy, and/or pyloroplasty, except neonatal	80 ⬚
	39503	Repair, neonatal diaphragmatic hernia, with or without chest tube insertion and with or without creation of ventral hernia	N 80 ⬚
	39520	Repair, diaphragmatic hernia (esophageal hiatal); transthoracic	80 ⬚
	39530	combined, thoracoabdominal	80 ⬚
	39531	combined, thoracoabdominal, with dilation of stricture (with or without gastroplasty)	80 ⬚
	39540	Repair, diaphragmatic hernia (other than neonatal), traumatic; acute	80 ⬚
	39541	chronic	80 ⬚
	39545	Imbrication of diaphragm for eventration, transthoracic or transabdominal, paralytic or nonparalytic	80 ⬚
	39560	Resection, diaphragm; with simple repair (eg, primary suture)	80 ⬚
	39561	with complex repair (eg, prosthetic material, local muscle flap)	80 ⬚

OTHER PROCEDURES

| | 39599 | Unlisted procedure, diaphragm | 80 |

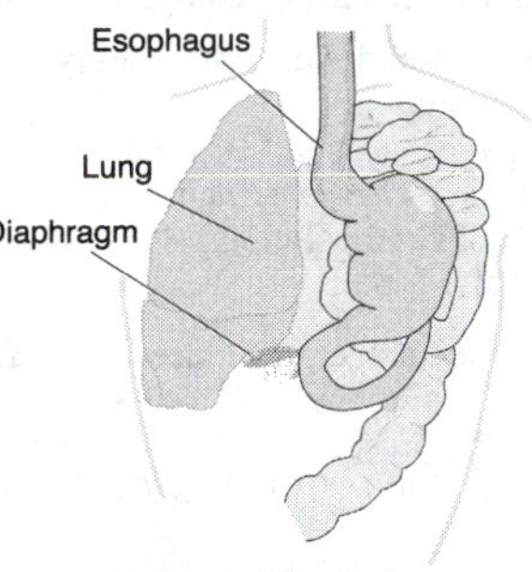

A defect of the diaphragm can allow abdominal contents to herniate into the thoracic cavity

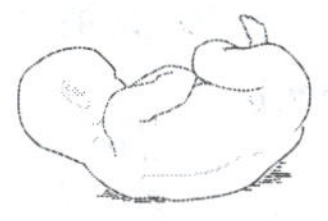

Code 39503 reports the repair of a diaphragmatic hernia in a neonate. The nature of the repair may necessitate the creation of a ventral hernia (an opening in the anterior abdomen to accommodate the viscera). A chest tube may or may not be required

The code is reserved for procedures on neonates

DIGESTIVE SYSTEM

LIPS

To report procedures performed on the skin of the lips, consult CPT code 10040 and subsequent codes.

EXCISION

40490	Biopsy of lip	TC
40500	Vermilionectomy (lip shave), with mucosal advancement	❷ TC
40510	Excision of lip; transverse wedge excision with primary closure	❷ TC

If mucous lesions are excised, consult CPT codes 40810-40816.

40520	V-excision with primary direct linear closure	❷ TC

If mucous lesions are excised, consult CPT codes 40810-40816.

40525	full thickness, reconstruction with local flap (eg, Estlander or fan)	❷ TC
40527	full thickness, reconstruction with cross lip flap (Abbe-Estlander)	❷ 80 TC
40530	Resection of lip, more than one-fourth, without reconstruction	❷ TC

If reconstruction is performed, consult CPT code 13131 and subsequent codes.

REPAIR (CHEILOPLASTY)

40650	Repair lip, full thickness; vermilion only	❸ 80 TC
40652	up to half vertical height	❸ 80 TC
40654	over one-half vertical height, or complex	❸ TC
40700	Plastic repair of cleft lip/nasal deformity; primary, partial or complete, unilateral	80 TC

If the cleft palate is repaired, consult CPT codes 42200 and subsequent codes. If other reconstructive procedures are performed, consult CPT codes 14060, 14061, 15120-15261, 15574, 15576, and 15630.

40701	primary bilateral, one stage procedure	80 TC

If the cleft palate is repaired, consult CPT codes 42200 et seq. If other reconstructive procedures are performed, consult CPT codes 14060, 14061, 15120-15261, 15574, 15576, and 15630.

40702	primary bilateral, one of two stages	80 TC
40720	secondary, by recreation of defect and reclosure	80 TC 50

If rhinoplasty only is performed for nasal deformity secondary to a congenital cleft lip, consult CPT codes 30460 and 30462.

40761	with cross lip pedicle flap (Abbe-Estlander type), including sectioning and inserting of pedicle	TC

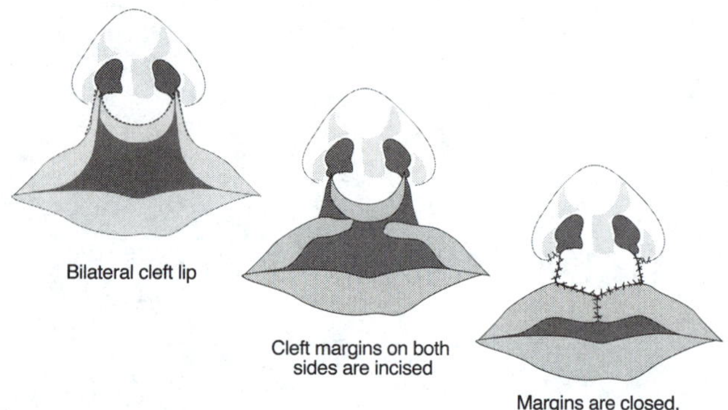

OTHER PROCEDURES

40799	Unlisted procedure, lips	80

VESTIBULE OF MOUTH

INCISION

40800*	Drainage of abscess, cyst, hematoma, vestibule of mouth; simple	TC
40801	complicated	❷ TC
40804*	Removal of embedded foreign body, vestibule of mouth; simple	80 TC
40805	complicated	❷ 80 TC
40806	Incision of labial frenum (frenotomy)	❶ 80 TC

EXCISION, DESTRUCTION

40808	Biopsy, vestibule of mouth	TC
40810	Excision of lesion of mucosa and submucosa, vestibule of mouth; without repair	TC
40812	with simple repair	TC
40814	with complex repair	❷ TC
40816	complex, with excision of underlying muscle	❷ TC
40818	Excision of mucosa of vestibule of mouth as donor graft	❶ 80 TC
40819	Excision of frenum, labial or buccal (frenumectomy, frenulectomy, frenectomy)	❶ 80 TC

<u>CIM 35-52 LASER PROCEDURES</u>

Coverage is determined on the basis that the use of lasers to alter, revise, or destroy tissue is a surgical procedure and restricted to practitioners with training in the surgical management of the disease or condition being treated.

40820	Destruction of lesion or scar of vestibule of mouth by physical methods (eg, laser, thermal, cryo, chemical)	❶ TC

REPAIR

40830	Closure of laceration, vestibule of mouth; 2.5 cm or less	80 TC
40831	over 2.5 cm or complex	❶ 80 TC
40840	Vestibuloplasty; anterior	❷ 80 TC
40842	posterior, unilateral	❸ 80 TC
40843	posterior, bilateral	❸ 80 TC
40844	entire arch	❺ 80 TC
40845	complex (including ridge extension, muscle repositioning)	❺ 80 TC

If skin grafts are performed, consult CPT code 15000 and subsequent codes.

OTHER PROCEDURES

40899	Unlisted procedure, vestibule of mouth	80

TONGUE AND FLOOR OF MOUTH

INCISION

41000*	Intraoral incision and drainage of abscess, cyst, or hematoma of tongue or floor of mouth; lingual	❶ TC
41005*	sublingual, superficial	❶ 80 TC
41006	sublingual, deep, supramylohyoid	❶ 80 TC
41007	submental space	❶ 80 TC
41008	submandibular space	❶ 80 TC
41009	masticator space	❶ 80 TC
41010	Incision of lingual frenum (frenotomy)	❶ 80 TC
41015	Extraoral incision and drainage of abscess, cyst, or hematoma of floor of mouth; sublingual	❶ 80 TC

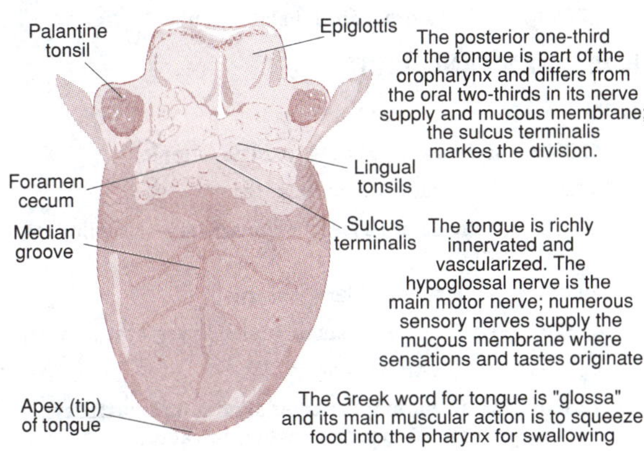

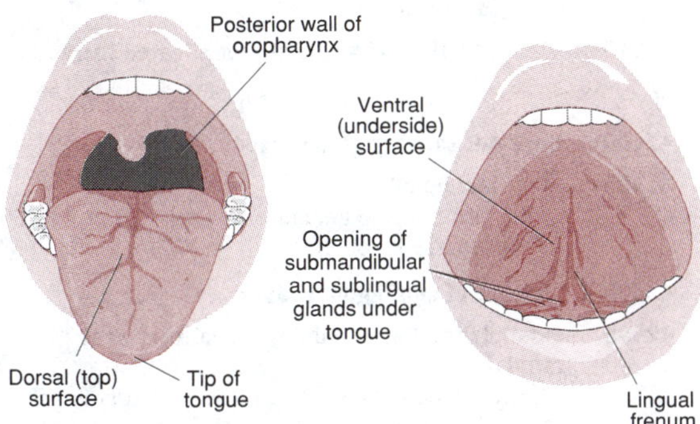

Anterior (front) two-thirds of tongue comprises most of easily visible portions; the base, or root, comprises the remainder of tongue

41016	submental	❶ 80 ▣
41017	submandibular	❶ 80 ▣
41018	masticator space	❶ 80 ▣

If a frenoplasty is performed, consult CPT code 41520.

EXCISION

41100	Biopsy of tongue; anterior two-thirds	▣
41105	posterior one-third	❷ ▣
41108	Biopsy of floor of mouth	▣
41110	Excision of lesion of tongue without closure	❶ ▣
41112	Excision of lesion of tongue with closure; anterior two-thirds	❷ ▣
41113	posterior one-third	❷ ▣
41114	with local tongue flap	❷ 80 ▣

Note that 41114 must be listed in addition to 41112 or 41113.

41115	Excision of lingual frenum (frenectomy)	❶ 80 ▣
41116	Excision, lesion of floor of mouth	❶ ▣
41120	Glossectomy; less than one-half tongue	❺ 80 ▣
41130	hemiglossectomy	80 ▣
41135	partial, with unilateral radical neck dissection	80 ▣
41140	complete or total, with or without tracheostomy, without radical neck dissection	80 ▣

Regnolli's excision

41145	complete or total, with or without tracheostomy, with unilateral radical neck dissection	80 ▣

41150	composite procedure with resection floor of mouth and mandibular resection, without radical neck dissection	80 ▣
41153	composite procedure with resection floor of mouth, with suprahyoid neck dissection	80 ▣
41155	composite procedure with resection floor of mouth, mandibular resection, and radical neck dissection (Commando type)	80 ▣

REPAIR

41250*	Repair of laceration 2.5 cm or less; floor of mouth and/or anterior two-thirds of tongue	❷ 80 ▣
41251*	posterior one-third of tongue	❷ 80 ▣
41252*	Repair of laceration of tongue, floor of mouth, over 2.6 cm or complex	❷ 80 ▣

OTHER PROCEDURES

41500	Fixation of tongue, mechanical, other than suture (eg, K-wire)	❶ 80 ▣
41510	Suture of tongue to lip for micrognathia (Douglas type procedure)	❶ 80 ▣
41520	Frenoplasty (surgical revision of frenum, eg, with Z-plasty)	❷ 80 ▣

If a frenotomy is performed, consult CPT codes 40806 and 41010.

41599	Unlisted procedure, tongue, floor of mouth	80

DENTOALVEOLAR STRUCTURES

INCISION

41800*	Drainage of abscess, cyst, hematoma from dentoalveolar structures	❶ ▣
41805	Removal of embedded foreign body from dentoalveolar structures; soft tissues	❶ 80 ▣
41806	bone	❶ 80 ▣

EXCISION, DESTRUCTION

41820	Gingivectomy, excision gingiva, each quadrant	80 ▣
41821	Operculectomy, excision pericoronal tissues	80 ▣
41822	Excision of fibrous tuberosities, dentoalveolar structures	80 ▣
41823	Excision of osseous tuberosities, dentoalveolar structures	80 ▣
41825	Excision of lesion or tumor (except listed above), dentoalveolar structures; without repair	▣
41826	with simple repair	▣
41827	with complex repair	❷ ▣

If the destruction of lesion is nonexcisional, consult CPT code 41850.

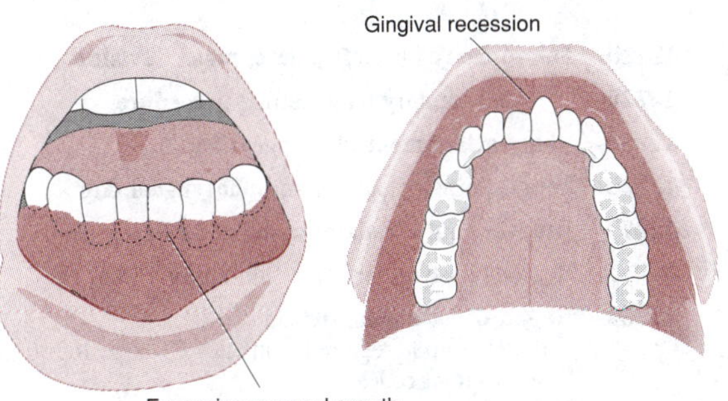

Gingivitis is an inflammatory response to bacteria on the teeth; it is characterized by tender, red, swollen gums and can lead to gingival recession

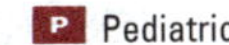

Digestive System

41828 — 42505

41828	Excision of hyperplastic alveolar mucosa, each quadrant (specify)	80 ▣
41830	Alveolectomy, including curettage of osteitis or sequestrectomy	80 ▣
41850	Destruction of lesion (except excision), dentoalveolar structures	80 ▣

OTHER PROCEDURES

41870	Periodontal mucosal grafting	80 ▣
41872	Gingivoplasty, each quadrant (specify)	80 ▣
41874	Alveoloplasty, each quadrant (specify)	80 ▣

If laceration closure is performed, consult CPT codes 40830 and 40831. If a segmental osteotomy is performed, consult CPT code 21206. If fractures are reduced, consult CPT codes 21421-21490.

41899	Unlisted procedure, dentoalveolar structures	80

PALATE AND UVULA

INCISION

42000*	Drainage of abscess of palate, uvula	❷ 80 ▣

EXCISION, DESTRUCTION

42100	Biopsy of palate, uvula	▣
42104	Excision, lesion of palate, uvula; without closure	❷ ▣
42106	with simple primary closure	❷ ▣
42107	with local flap closure	❷ ▣

If a skin graft is performed, consult CPT codes 14040-14300. If a mucosal graft is performed, consult CPT code 40818.

42120	Resection of palate or extensive resection of lesion	❹ 80 ▣

If reconstruction of palate with extraoral tissue is performed, consult CPT codes 14040-14300, 15050, 15120, 15240, and 15576.

42140	Uvulectomy, excision of uvula	❷ ▣
42145	Palatopharyngoplasty (eg, uvulopalatopharyngoplasty, uvulopharyngoplasty)	❺ ▣
42160	Destruction of lesion, palate or uvula (thermal, cryo or chemical)	❶ 80 ▣

REPAIR

42180	Repair, laceration of palate; up to 2 cm	❶ 80 ▣
42182	over 2 cm or complex	❷ 80 ▣
42200	Palatoplasty for cleft palate, soft and/or hard palate only	❺ 80 ▣
42205	Palatoplasty for cleft palate, with closure of alveolar ridge; soft tissue only	❻ 80 ▣
42210	with bone graft to alveolar ridge (includes obtaining graft)	❻ 80 ▣
42215	Palatoplasty for cleft palate; major revision	❼ 80 ▣
42220	secondary lengthening procedure	❺ 80 ▣
42225	attachment pharyngeal flap	❻ 80 ▣
42226	Lengthening of palate, and pharyngeal flap	80 ▣
42227	Lengthening of palate, with island flap	80 ▣
42235	Repair of anterior palate, including vomer flap	❻ 80 ▣
42260	Repair of nasolabial fistula	❹ 80 ▣

If a cleft lip is repaired, consult CPT code 40700 and subsequent codes.

42280	Maxillary impression for palatal prosthesis	80 ▣
42281	Insertion of pin-retained palatal prosthesis	❸ 80 ▣

OTHER PROCEDURES

42299	Unlisted procedure, palate, uvula	80

SALIVARY GLAND AND DUCTS

INCISION

42300*	Drainage of abscess; parotid, simple	❶ ▣
42305	parotid, complicated	❷ 80 ▣
42310*	Drainage of abscess; submaxillary or sublingual, intraoral	❶ 80 ▣
42320*	submaxillary, external	❶ 80 ▣
42325	Fistulization of sublingual salivary cyst (ranula);	❷ 80 ▣
42326	with prosthesis	80 ▣
42330	Sialolithotomy; submandibular (submaxillary), sublingual or parotid, uncomplicated, intraoral	▣
42335	submandibular (submaxillary), complicated, intraoral	❸ ▣
42340	parotid, extraoral or complicated intraoral	❷ 80 ▣

EXCISION

42400*	Biopsy of salivary gland; needle	▣
42405	incisional	❷ ▣

To report imaging guidance, consult CPT codes 76003, 76360, 76393, 76942.

42408	Excision of sublingual salivary cyst (ranula)	❸ 80 ▣
42409	Marsupialization of sublingual salivary cyst (ranula)	❸ 80 ▣

If fistulization of a sublingual salivary cyst is performed, consult CPT code 42325.

42410	Excision of parotid tumor or parotid gland; lateral lobe, without nerve dissection	❸ 80 ▣
42415	lateral lobe, with dissection and preservation of facial nerve	80 ▣
42420	total, with dissection and preservation of facial nerve	❼ 80 ▣
42425	total, en bloc removal with sacrifice of facial nerve	❼ 80 ▣
42426	total, with unilateral radical neck dissection	80 ▣

If suture or grafting of a facial nerve is performed, consult CPT codes 64864, 64865, 69740, and 69745.

42440	Excision of submandibular (submaxillary) gland	❸ 80 ▣
42450	Excision of sublingual gland	❷ 80 ▣

REPAIR

42500	Plastic repair of salivary duct, sialodochoplasty; primary or simple	❸ 80 ▣
42505	secondary or complicated	❹ ▣

After the larynx, the oral cavity and oropharynx are the most common sites for squamous cell carcinoma of the head and neck

The parotid gland is a common site for malignant lesions, occurring there several times more frequently than cancers of the other major salivary glands

DIGESTIVE SYSTEM

42507	Parotid duct diversion, bilateral (Wilke type procedure);	❸ 80 ◪
42508	with excision of one submandibular gland	❹ 80 ◪
42509	with excision of both submandibular glands	❹ 80 ◪
42510	with ligation of both submandibular (Wharton's) ducts	❹ 80 ◪

OTHER PROCEDURES

42550	Injection procedure for sialography	◪
	If radiological supervision and interpretation is performed, consult CPT code 70390.	
42600	Closure salivary fistula	❶ 80 ◪
42650*	Dilation salivary duct	◪
42660*	Dilation and catheterization of salivary duct, with or without injection	80 ◪
42665	Ligation salivary duct, intraoral	80 ◪
42699	Unlisted procedure, salivary glands or ducts	80

PHARYNX, ADENOIDS, AND TONSILS

INCISION

42700*	Incision and drainage abscess; peritonsillar	❶ ◪
42720	retropharyngeal or parapharyngeal, intraoral approach	❶ 80 ◪
42725	retropharyngeal or parapharyngeal, external approach	❷ 80 ◪

EXCISION, DESTRUCTION

42800	Biopsy; oropharynx	◪
42802	hypopharynx	❶ ◪
42804	nasopharynx, visible lesion, simple	❶ ◪
42806	nasopharynx, survey for unknown primary lesion	❷ ◪
	If a laryngoscopic biopsy is performed, consult CPT codes 31510, 31535, and 31536.	
42808	Excision or destruction of lesion of pharynx, any method	❷ ◪
42809	Removal of foreign body from pharynx	◪
42810	Excision branchial cleft cyst or vestige, confined to skin and subcutaneous tissues	❸ 80 ◪
42815	Excision branchial cleft cyst, vestige, or fistula, extending beneath subcutaneous tissues and/or into pharynx	❺ 80 ◪
42820	Tonsillectomy and adenoidectomy; under age 12	P 80 ◪
42821	age 12 or over	❺ 80 ◪

The nasal cavities and paranasal sinuses are lined with a continuous mucous membrane

Nasal cavity

Auditory tube

Epiglottis

Orbit

Nasopharynx region

Oropharynx region

Ethmoidal cells

Hypopharynx region

Maxillary sinus

Vocal cord and larynx

Trachea

Middle and inferior meatus

Frontal coronal section of left side of skull showing sinuses

The pharynx is a transitional zone between the oral cavity and the rest of the digestive canal. It is the common route for both air and food

Tonsillar tags or polyps are removed

Snare

Electrocautery tool

In 42860, tags or polyps on the tonsil are removed, usually by simple cauterization or snare

42825	Tonsillectomy, primary or secondary; under age 12	P 80 ◪
42826	age 12 or over	❹ ◪
42830	Adenoidectomy, primary; under age 12	P 80 ◪
42831	age 12 or over	❹ 80 ◪
42835	Adenoidectomy, secondary; under age 12	P 80 ◪
42836	age 12 or over	❹ 80 ◪
42842	Radical resection of tonsil, tonsillar pillars, and/or retromolar trigone; without closure	80 ◪
42844	closure with local flap (eg, tongue, buccal)	80 ◪
42845	closure with other flap	80 ◪
	If closure is performed with another flap(s), consult the appropriate CPT code for the flap(s). If this procedure is combined with a radical neck dissection, consult also CPT code 38720.	
42860	Excision of tonsil tags	❸ 80 ◪
42870	Excision or destruction lingual tonsil, any method (separate procedure)	❸ 80 ◪
	If the nasopharynx is resected by bicoronal and/or transzygomatic approach, consult CPT codes 61586 and 61600.	
42890	Limited pharyngectomy	80 ◪
42892	Resection of lateral pharyngeal wall or pyriform sinus, direct closure by advancement of lateral and posterior pharyngeal walls	80 ◪
	If this procedure is combined with a radical neck dissection, consult also CPT code 38720.	
42894	Resection of pharyngeal wall requiring closure with myocutaneous flap	80 ◪
	If this procedure is combined with a radical neck dissection, consult also CPT code 38720.	

REPAIR

42900	Suture pharynx for wound or injury	❶ 80 ◪
42950	Pharyngoplasty (plastic or reconstructive operation on pharynx)	❷ 80 ◪
	If this procedure involves the pharyngeal flap, consult CPT code 42225.	
42953	Pharyngoesophageal repair	80 ◪
	If closure with myocutaneous or other flap is performed, use the appropriate CPT code in addition to 42953.	

OTHER PROCEDURES

42955	Pharyngostomy (fistulization of pharynx, external for feeding)	❷ 80 ◪
42960	Control oropharyngeal hemorrhage, primary or secondary (eg, post-tonsillectomy); simple	❶ 80 ◪
42961	complicated, requiring hospitalization	80 ◪

◪ CCI Comprehensive Code	🔟 Bilateral Procedure	✚ CPT Add-on Code
⃠ Modifier -51 Exempt Code	● New Code	▲ Revised Code
M Maternity	N Newborn	P Pediatric
N/P Newborn/Pediatric		

42962	with secondary surgical intervention	❷ 80 ↻
▲ 42970	Control of nasopharyngeal hemorrhage, primary or secondary (eg, postadenoidectomy); simple, with posterior nasal packs, with or without anterior packs and/or cautery	↻
42971	complicated, requiring hospitalization	80 ↻
42972	with secondary surgical intervention	80 ↻
42999	Unlisted procedure, pharynx, adenoids, or tonsils	80

ESOPHAGUS

INCISION

If esophageal intubation is performed with a laparotomy, consult CPT code 43510.

43020	Esophagotomy, cervical approach, with removal of foreign body	80 ↻
43030	Cricopharyngeal myotomy	80 ↻
43045	Esophagotomy, thoracic approach, with removal of foreign body	80 ↻

EXCISION

43100	Excision of lesion, esophagus, with primary repair; cervical approach	80 ↻
43101	thoracic or abdominal approach	80 ↻
43107	Total or near total esophagectomy, without thoracotomy; with pharyngogastrostomy or cervical esophagogastrostomy, with or without pyloroplasty (transhiatal)	80 ↻
▲ 43108	with colon interposition or small intestine reconstruction, including intestine mobilization, preparation and anastomosis(es)	80 ↻
43112	Total or near total esophagectomy, with thoracotomy; with pharyngogastrostomy or cervical esophagogastrostomy, with or without pyloroplasty	80 ↻
▲ 43113	with colon interposition or small intestine reconstruction, including intestine mobilization, preparation, and anastomosis(es)	80 ↻
43116	Partial esophagectomy, cervical, with free intestinal graft, including microvascular anastomosis, obtaining the graft and intestinal reconstruction	80 ↻

Do not report 69990 in addition to 43116 as the operating microscope is considered an inclusive component of the surgery. If another physician performs an intestinal or a free jejunal graft with microvascular anastomosis, append modifier -52 to this code. If a free jejunal graft with microvascular anastomosis is performed alone, consult CPT code 43496.

43117	Partial esophagectomy, distal two-thirds, with thoracotomy and separate abdominal incision, with or without proximal gastrectomy; with thoracic esophagogastrostomy, with or without pyloroplasty (Ivor Lewis)	80 ↻
▲ 43118	with colon interposition or small intestine reconstruction, including intestine mobilization, preparation, and anastomosis(es)	80 ↻
43121	Partial esophagectomy, distal two-thirds, with thoracotomy only, with or without proximal gastrectomy, with thoracic esophagogastrostomy, with or without pyloroplasty	80 ↻
43122	Partial esophagectomy, thoracoabdominal or abdominal approach, with or without proximal gastrectomy; with esophagogastrostomy, with or without pyloroplasty	80 ↻
▲ 43123	with colon interposition or small intestine reconstruction, including intestine mobilization, preparation, and anastomosis(es)	80 ↻
43124	Total or partial esophagectomy, without reconstruction (any approach), with cervical esophagostomy	80 ↻
43130	Diverticulectomy of hypopharynx or esophagus, with or without myotomy; cervical approach	80 ↻
43135	thoracic approach	80 ↻

ENDOSCOPY

CIM 35-59 ENDOSCOPY

Although endoscopy is primarily a diagnostic tool, it includes certain therapeutic procedures such as removal of polyps, and endoscopic papillotomy, by which stones are removed from the bile duct. Endoscopic procedures are covered when reasonable and necessary for the individual patient.

43200	Esophagoscopy, rigid or flexible; diagnostic, with or without collection of specimen(s) by brushing or washing (separate procedure)	❶ ↻
43202	with biopsy, single or multiple	❶ ↻

CIM 35-73 INJECTION SCLEROTHERAPY FOR ESOPHAGEAL VARICEAL BLEEDING

Injection sclerotherapy involves the insertion of a flexible fiberoptic endoscope into the esophagus, and the injection of a sclerosing agent or solution into the varicosities to control bleeding. This procedure is covered under Medicare.

43204	with injection sclerosis of esophageal varices	❶ ↻
43205	with band ligation of esophageal varices	80 ↻
43215	with removal of foreign body	❶ ↻

For radiological supervision and interpretation, consult CPT code 74235.

43216	with removal of tumor(s), polyp(s), or other lesion(s) by hot biopsy forceps or bipolar cautery	❶ 80 ↻
43217	with removal of tumor(s), polyp(s), or other lesion(s) by snare technique	❶ ↻
43219	with insertion of plastic tube or stent	❶ ↻
43220	with balloon dilation (less than 30 mm diameter)	❶ ↻

If an endoscopic dilation is performed with a balloon 30 mm in diameter or larger, consult CPT code 43458. If dilation is performed without visualization, consult CPT codes 43450-43453.

If procedure is performed with imaging guidance, consult CPT code 74360.

43226	with insertion of guide wire followed by dilation over guide wire	❶ ↻

For radiological supervision and interpretation of procedure, consult CPT code 74360.

▲ 43227	with control of bleeding (eg, injection, bipolar cautery, unipolar cautery, laser, heater probe, stapler, plasma coagulator)	❷ ↻
43228	with ablation of tumor(s), polyp(s), or other lesion(s), not amenable to removal by hot biopsy forceps, bipolar cautery or snare technique	❷ ↻

If esophagoscopic photodynamic therapy is performed, report 43228 in addition to CPT codes 96570 and 96571 as appropriate.

43231	with endoscopic ultrasound examination	80 ↻

Do not report CPT code 76975 when reporting 43231 and 43232.

43232	with transendoscopic ultrasound-guided intramural or transmural fine needle aspiration/biopsy(s)	80 ↻

To report interpretation of specimen, consult CPT codes 88172 and 88173.

CIM 35-59 ENDOSCOPY
Although endoscopy is primarily a diagnostic tool, it includes certain therapeutic procedures such as removal of polyps, and endoscopic papillotomy, by which stones are removed from the bile duct. Endoscopic procedures are covered when reasonable and necessary for the individual patient.

43234   **Upper gastrointestinal endoscopy, simple primary examination (eg, with small diameter flexible endoscope) (separate procedure)**

43235   **Upper gastrointestinal endoscopy including esophagus, stomach, and either the duodenum and/or jejunum as appropriate; diagnostic, with or without collection of specimen(s) by brushing or washing (separate procedure)**

43239   **with biopsy, single or multiple**
To report upper gastrointestinal endoscopy with suturing of the esophagogastric junction, consult CPT Category III code 0008T.

43240   **with transmural drainage of pseudocyst**

43241   **with transendoscopic intraluminal tube or catheter placement**

43242   **with transendoscopic ultrasound-guided intramural or transmural fine needle aspiration/biopsy(s)**
Do not report CPT code 76975 when reporting 43242.

43243   **with injection sclerosis of esophageal and/or gastric varices**

43244   **with band ligation of esophageal and/or gastric varices**

▲ **43245**   **with dilation of gastric outlet for obstruction (eg, balloon, guide wire, bougie)**

43246   **with directed placement of percutaneous gastrostomy tube**
For radiological supervision and interpretation, consult CPT code 74350.

43247   **with removal of foreign body**
For radiological supervision and interpretation, consult CPT code 74235.

43248   **with insertion of guide wire followed by dilation of esophagus over guide wire**

43249   **with balloon dilation of esophagus (less than 30 mm diameter)**

43250   **with removal of tumor(s), polyp(s), or other lesion(s) by hot biopsy forceps or bipolar cautery**

43251   **with removal of tumor(s), polyp(s), or other lesion(s) by snare technique**

43255   **with control of bleeding, any method**

43256   **with transendoscopic stent placement (includes predilation)**

43258   **with ablation of tumor(s), polyp(s), or other lesion(s) not amenable to removal by hot biopsy forceps, bipolar cautery or snare technique**
If injection sclerosis of esophageal varices is performed, consult CPT code 43204 or 43243.

43259   **with endoscopic ultrasound examination**
For radiological supervision and interpretation, consult CPT code 76975.

43260   **Endoscopic retrograde cholangiopancreatography (ERCP); diagnostic, with or without collection of specimen(s) by brushing or washing (separate procedure)**
For radiological supervision and interpretation, consult CPT codes 74328, 74329, and 74330.

43261   **with biopsy, single or multiple**

43262   **with sphincterotomy/papillotomy**
For radiological supervision and interpretation, consult CPT codes 74328, 74329, and 74330.

43263   **with pressure measurement of sphincter of Oddi (pancreatic duct or common bile duct)**
For radiological supervision and interpretation, consult CPT codes 74328, 74329, and 74330.

▲ **43264**   **with endoscopic retrograde removal of calculus/calculi from biliary and/or pancreatic ducts**
If these procedures (43264-43271) are performed with a sphincterotomy, consult also CPT code 43262. If radiological supervision and interpretation is performed, consult CPT codes 74328, 74329, and 74330.

▲ **43265**   **with endoscopic retrograde destruction, lithotripsy of calculus/calculi, any method**

43267   **with endoscopic retrograde insertion of nasobiliary or nasopancreatic drainage tube**

43268   **with endoscopic retrograde insertion of tube or stent into bile or pancreatic duct**

43269   **with endoscopic retrograde removal of foreign body and/or change of tube or stent**

43271   **with endoscopic retrograde balloon dilation of ampulla, biliary and/or pancreatic duct(s)**

43272   **with ablation of tumor(s), polyp(s), or other lesion(s) not amenable to removal by hot biopsy forceps, bipolar cautery or snare technique**

LAPAROSCOPY

43280   **Laparoscopy, surgical, esophagogastric fundoplasty (eg, Nissen, Toupet procedures)**
If an open approach is used, consult CPT code 43324.

43289   **Unlisted laparoscopy procedure, esophagus**

REPAIR

43300   **Esophagoplasty, (plastic repair or reconstruction), cervical approach; without repair of tracheoesophageal fistula**

43305   **with repair of tracheoesophageal fistula**

43310   **Esophagoplasty, (plastic repair or reconstruction), thoracic approach; without repair of tracheoesophageal fistula**

43312   **with repair of tracheoesophageal fistula**

● **43313**   **Esophagoplasty for congenital defect, (plastic repair or reconstruction), thoracic approach; without repair of congenital tracheoesophageal fistula**

● **43314**   **with repair of congenital tracheoesophageal fistula**

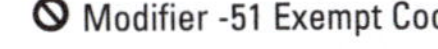

Sections of stomach or bowel are commonly used to repair a resected portion of the esophagus

The esophagus is a muscular tube that delivers food from the oral cavity to the stomach. It spans the cervical, thoracic, and abdominal regions and numerous surgical approaches may be used

---

Digestive System

43320 — 43635

43320 Esophagogastrostomy (cardioplasty), with or without vagotomy and pyloroplasty, transabdominal or transthoracic approach 80

43324 Esophagogastric fundoplasty (eg, Nissen, Belsey IV, Hill procedures) 80

    If a laparoscopic approach is used, consult CPT code 43280.

43325 Esophagogastric fundoplasty; with fundic patch (Thal-Nissen procedure) 80

    If a cricopharyngeal myotomy is performed, consult CPT code 43030.

43326   with gastroplasty (eg, Collis) 80

43330 Esophagomyotomy (Heller type); abdominal approach 80

43331   thoracic approach 80

    If a thoracoscopic esophagomyotomy is performed, consult CPT code 32665.

43340 Esophagojejunostomy (without total gastrectomy); abdominal approach 80

43341   thoracic approach 80

43350 Esophagostomy, fistulization of esophagus, external; abdominal approach 80

43351   thoracic approach 80

43352   cervical approach 80

43360 Gastrointestinal reconstruction for previous esophagectomy, for obstructing esophageal lesion or fistula, or for previous esophageal exclusion; with stomach, with or without pyloroplasty 80

▲ **43361**   with colon interposition or small intestine reconstruction, including intestine mobilization, preparation, and anastomosis(es) 80

43400 Ligation, direct, esophageal varices 80

43401 Transection of esophagus with repair, for esophageal varices 80

43405 Ligation or stapling at gastroesophageal junction for pre-existing esophageal perforation 80

43410 Suture of esophageal wound or injury; cervical approach 80

43415   transthoracic or transabdominal approach 80

43420 Closure of esophagostomy or fistula; cervical approach 80

43425   transthoracic or transabdominal approach 80

    If an esophageal hiatal hernia is repaired, consult CPT code 39520 and subsequent codes.

MANIPULATION

If an associated esophagogram is performed, consult CPT code 74220.

43450* Dilation of esophagus, by unguided sound or bougie, single or multiple passes ❶

43453 Dilation of esophagus, over guide wire ❶

    If dilation is performed with direct visualization, consult CPT code 43220.

43456 Dilation of esophagus, by balloon or dilator, retrograde ❷

43458 Dilation of esophagus with balloon (30 mm diameter or larger) for achalasia ❷

    If dilation is performed with a balloon less than 30 mm in diameter, consult CPT code 43220. If radiological supervision and interpretation is performed, consult CPT code 74360.

43460 Esophagogastric tamponade, with balloon (Sengstaaken type)

    If an esophageal foreign body is removed by balloon catheter, consult CPT codes 43215, 43247, and 74235.

OTHER PROCEDURES

43496 Free jejunum transfer with microvascular anastomosis 80

    Do not report 69990 in addition to 43496 as the operating microscope is considered an inclusive component of the surgery.

43499 Unlisted procedure, esophagus 80

STOMACH

INCISION

43500 Gastrotomy; with exploration or foreign body removal 80

43501   with suture repair of bleeding ulcer 80

43502   with suture repair of pre-existing esophagogastric laceration (eg, Mallory-Weiss) 80

43510   with esophageal dilation and insertion of permanent intraluminal tube (eg, Celestin or Mousseaux-Barbin) 80

43520 Pyloromyotomy, cutting of pyloric muscle (Fredet-Ramstedt type operation) 80

EXCISION

43600 Biopsy of stomach; by capsule, tube, peroral (one or more specimens) ❶

43605   by laparotomy 80

43610 Excision, local; ulcer or benign tumor of stomach 80

43611   malignant tumor of stomach 80

43620 Gastrectomy, total; with esophagoenterostomy 80

43621   with Roux-en-Y reconstruction 80

43622   with formation of intestinal pouch, any type 80

43631 Gastrectomy, partial, distal; with gastroduodenostomy 80
    Billroth operation

43632   with gastrojejunostomy 80
    Polya anastomosis

43633   with Roux-en-Y reconstruction 80

43634   with formation of intestinal pouch 80

+ **43635** Vagotomy when performed with partial distal gastrectomy (List separately in addition to code(s) for primary procedure) 80

    Note that 43635 is an add-on code and must be used in conjunction with 43631, 43632, 43633, and 43634.

---

26 Professional Component Only   80/80 Assist-at-Surgery Allowed/With Documentation   Unlisted   Commonly Miscoded   Not Covered

TC Technical Component Only   **MCM & CIM** Medicare References   ❶❷❸❹❺❻❼❽ ASC Group   ♂ Male Only   ♀ Female Only

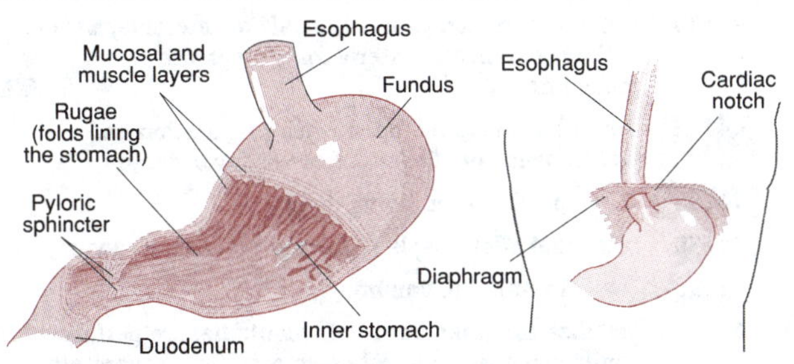

The stomach is a highly distensible organ that serves as a reservoir to mix food and break it down with digestive juices. The esophagus pierces the diaphragm at the cardiac notch, where the stomach begins. The pyloric sphincter marks the inferior border of the stomach. The vagal nerve trunks run down the front and back of the esophagus and serve the stomach by controlling secretion of digestive acids

43638   **Gastrectomy, partial, proximal, thoracic or abdominal approach including esophagogastrostomy, with vagotomy;**   80

43639   **with pyloroplasty or pyloromyotomy**   80
If a regional thoracic lymphadenectomy is performed, consult CPT code 38746. If a regional abdominal lymphadenectomy is performed, consult CPT code 38747.

43640   **Vagotomy including pyloroplasty, with or without gastrostomy; truncal or selective**   80
If pyloroplasty is performed, consult CPT code 43800. If a vagotomy is performed, consult CPT codes 64752-64760.

43641   **parietal cell (highly selective)**   80
If an upper gastrointestinal endoscopy is performed, consult CPT codes 43234-43259.

LAPAROSCOPY

43651   **Laparoscopy, surgical; transection of vagus nerves, truncal**   80

43652   **transection of vagus nerves, selective or highly selective**   80

43653   **gastrostomy, without construction of gastric tube (eg, Stamm procedure) (separate procedure)**   80

43659   **Unlisted laparoscopy procedure, stomach**   80 50

INTRODUCTION

43750   **Percutaneous placement of gastrostomy tube**   2
For radiological supervision and interpretation, consult CPT code 74350.

43752   **Naso- or oro-gastric tube placement, necessitating physician's skill**
Do not report CPT code 43752 when reporting critical care codes 99291-99292 or neonatal intensive care codes, 99295-99298.

If imaging guidance is performed, consult CPT code 76000. For enteric tube placement, consult CPT codes 44500, 74340.

43760*   **Change of gastrostomy tube**   1
If an endoscopic placement of a gastrostomy tube is performed, consult CPT code 43246. For radiological supervision and interpretation, consult CPT code 75984.

43761   **Repositioning of the gastric feeding tube, any method, through the duodenum for enteric nutrition**
If imaging guidance is performed, consult CPT code 75984.

OTHER PROCEDURES

43800   **Pyloroplasty**   80
If pyloroplasty and vagotomy are performed, consult CPT code 43640.

43810   **Gastroduodenostomy**   80

43820   **Gastrojejunostomy; without vagotomy**   80

43825   **with vagotomy, any type**   80

43830   **Gastrostomy, open; without construction of gastric tube (eg, Stamm procedure) (separate procedure)**   80

43831   **neonatal, for feeding**   P 80
If a gastrostomy tube is changed, consult CPT code 43760.

43832   **with construction of gastric tube (eg, Janeway procedure)**   80

CIM 50-9 GASTROPHOTOGRAPHY

Medicare reimburses gastrophotography when required for documenting and evaluating (healing or worsening) of lesions such as the gastric ulcer, facilitates consult between physicians concerning difficult-to-interpret lesions, providing preoperative characterization for the surgeon, and permitting better diagnosis of postoperative gastric bleeding to determine the need for reoperation.

43840   **Gastrorrhaphy, suture of perforated duodenal or gastric ulcer, wound, or injury**   80

CIM 35-26 TREATMENT OF OBESITY

Medicare covers services for obesity when the condition is caused by illnesses such as hypothyroidism, Cushing's disease, and hypothalamic lesions, or when obesity aggravates a number of cardiac and respiratory diseases as well as diabetes and hypertension.

43842   **Gastric restrictive procedure, without gastric bypass, for morbid obesity; vertical-banded gastroplasty**   80

43843   **other than vertical-banded gastroplasty**   80

CIM 35-33 INTESTINAL BY-PASS SURGERY—NOT COVERED

Severe adverse reactions such as steatorrhea, electrolyte depletion, liver failure, arthralgia, hypoplasia of bone marrow, and avitaminosis have sometimes occurred as a result of an intestinal bypass surgery for treatment of obesity and, thus, it is not a covered Medicare procedure.

CIM 35-40 GASTRIC BYPASS SURGERY FOR OBESITY

Gastric bypass surgery, a variation of the gastrojejunostomy, for extreme obesity is covered under the program if (1) it is medically appropriate for the individual to have such surgery; and (2) the surgery is to correct an illness that caused the obesity or was aggravated by the obesity.

43846   **Gastric restrictive procedure, with gastric bypass for morbid obesity; with short limb (less than 100 cm) Roux-en-Y gastroenterostomy**   80

▲ **43847**   **with small intestine reconstruction to limit absorption**   80

43848   **Revision of gastric restrictive procedure for morbid obesity (separate procedure)**   80

43850   **Revision of gastroduodenal anastomosis (gastroduodenostomy) with reconstruction; without vagotomy**   80

43855   **with vagotomy**   80

▲ **43860**   **Revision of gastrojejunal anastomosis (gastrojejunostomy) with reconstruction, with or without partial gastrectomy or intestine resection; without vagotomy**   80

43865   **with vagotomy**   80

43870   **Closure of gastrostomy, surgical**   1 80

43880   **Closure of gastrocolic fistula**   80

43999   **Unlisted procedure, stomach**   80

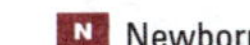 CCI Comprehensive Code   50 Bilateral Procedure   ✛ CPT Add-on Code   ⊘ Modifier -51 Exempt Code   ● New Code   ▲ Revised Code

M Maternity   N Newborn   P Pediatric   N/P Newborn/Pediatric

Digestive System

44005 — 44204

INTESTINES (EXCEPT RECTUM)

INCISION

44005 Enterolysis (freeing of intestinal adhesion) (separate procedure) 80
> Code 44005 is not to be used with 45136.
>
> If a laparoscopic approach is used, consult CPT code 44200.

44010 Duodenotomy, for exploration, biopsy(s), or foreign body removal 80

+ 44015 Tube or needle catheter jejunostomy for enteral alimentation, intraoperative, any method (List separately in addition to primary procedure) 80

▲ **44020** Enterotomy, small intestine, other than duodenum; for exploration, biopsy(s), or foreign body removal 80

44021 for decompression (eg, Baker tube) 80

44025 Colotomy, for exploration, biopsy(s), or foreign body removal 80
> Amussat's operation

44050 Reduction of volvulus, intussusception, internal hernia, by laparotomy 80

44055 Correction of malrotation by lysis of duodenal bands and/or reduction of midgut volvulus (eg, Ladd procedure) 80

EXCISION

44100 Biopsy of intestine by capsule, tube, peroral (one or more specimens) 1

▲ **44110** Excision of one or more lesions of small or large intestine not requiring anastomosis, exteriorization, or fistulization; single enterotomy 80

44111 multiple enterotomies 80

44120 Enterectomy, resection of small intestine; single resection and anastomosis 80
> Code 44120 is not to be used with 45136.

+ 44121 each additional resection and anastomosis (List separately in addition to code for primary procedure) 80
> Note that 44121 is an add-on code and must be used in conjunction with 44120.

44125 with enterostomy 80

● **44126** Enterectomy, resection of small intestine for congenital atresia, single resection and anastomosis of proximal segment of intestine; without tapering

● **44127** with tapering

● **+ 44128** each additional resection and anastomosis (List separately in addition to code for primary procedure)
> Note that 44128 is an add-on code and must be used in conjunction with codes 44126 and 44127.

In 44021, a select portion of intestine is surgically approached and incised. A tube is inserted into the bowel lumen and threaded distally, often to a point of obstruction. The tube is used to decompress the bowel segment it passes through, often during or immediately following surgery for bowel obstruction

---

44130 Enteroenterostomy, anastomosis of intestine, with or without cutaneous enterostomy (separate procedure) 80

44132 Donor enterectomy, open, with preparation and maintenance of allograft; from cadaver donor

44133 partial, from living donor

44135 Intestinal allotransplantation; from cadaver donor

44136 from living donor

+ 44139 Mobilization (take-down) of splenic flexure performed in conjunction with partial colectomy (List separately in addition to primary procedure) 80
> Note that 44139 is an add-on code and must be used in conjunction with 44140-44147.

44140 Colectomy, partial; with anastomosis 80
> if procedure is performed laparoscopically, consult CPT code 44204.

44141 with skin level cecostomy or colostomy 80

44143 with end colostomy and closure of distal segment (Hartmann type procedure) 80

44144 with resection, with colostomy or ileostomy and creation of mucofistula 80

44145 with coloproctostomy (low pelvic anastomosis) 80

44146 with coloproctostomy (low pelvic anastomosis), with colostomy 80

44147 abdominal and transanal approach 80

44150 Colectomy, total, abdominal, without proctectomy; with ileostomy or ileoproctostomy 80
> Lane's operation

44151 with continent ileostomy 80

44152 with rectal mucosectomy, ileoanal anastomosis, with or without loop ileostomy 80

44153 with rectal mucosectomy, ileoanal anastomosis, creation of ileal reservoir (S or J), with or without loop ileostomy 80

44155 Colectomy, total, abdominal, with proctectomy; with ileostomy 80
> Miles' colectomy

44156 with continent ileostomy 80

▲ **44160** Colectomy, partial, with removal of terminal ileum with ileocolostomy 80
> if procedure is performed laparoscopically, consult CPT code 44205.

LAPAROSCOPY

44200 Laparoscopy, surgical; enterolysis (freeing of intestinal adhesion) (separate procedure) 80
> If laparoscopy with salpingolysis or ovariolysis is performed, consult CPT code 58660.

44201 jejunostomy (eg, for decompression or feeding) 80

▲ **44202** enterectomy, resection of small intestine, single resection and anastomosis 80

● **+ 44203** each additional small intestine resection and anastomosis (List separately in addition to code for primary procedure)
> Note that 44203 is an add-on code and must be used in conjunction with code 44202.
>
> To report open procedure, consult CPT codes 44120, 44121.

● **44204** colectomy, partial, with anastomosis
> To report open procedure, consult CPT code 44140.

● 44205   colectomy, partial, with removal of terminal ileum with ileocolostomy
To report open procedure, consult CPT code 44160.

44209   Unlisted laparoscopy procedure, intestine (except rectum)   80 50

ENTEROSTOMY - EXTERNAL FISTULIZATION OF INTESTINES

44300   Enterostomy or cecostomy, tube (eg, for decompression or feeding) (separate procedure)   80

44310   Ileostomy or jejunostomy, non-tube (separate procedure)   80
Code 44310 is not to be used with code 45136.

44312   Revision of ileostomy; simple (release of superficial scar) (separate procedure)   0 80

44314   complicated (reconstruction in-depth) (separate procedure)   80

44316   Continent ileostomy (Kock procedure) (separate procedure)   80
If a fiberoptic evaluation is performed, consult CPT code 44385.

44320   Colostomy or skin level cecostomy; (separate procedure)   80
Mikulicz resection

▲ 44322   with multiple biopsies (eg, for congenital megacolon) (separate procedure)   80
Mikulicz resection

44340   Revision of colostomy; simple (release of superficial scar) (separate procedure)   3

44345   complicated (reconstruction in-depth) (separate procedure)   4 80

44346   with repair of paracolostomy hernia (separate procedure)   4 80

ENDOSCOPY, SMALL INTESTINE AND STOMAL

CIM 35-59 ENDOSCOPY
Although endoscopy is primarily a diagnostic tool, it includes certain therapeutic procedures such as removal of polyps, and endoscopic papillotomy, by which stones are removed from the bile duct. Endoscopic procedures are covered when reasonable and necessary for the individual patient.

Diagnostic endoscopy is included in surgical endoscopy.

44360   Small intestinal endoscopy, enteroscopy beyond second portion of duodenum, not including ileum; diagnostic, with or without collection of specimen(s) by brushing or washing (separate procedure)   2

44361   with biopsy, single or multiple   2

44363   with removal of foreign body   2 80

44364   with removal of tumor(s), polyp(s), or other lesion(s) by snare technique   2 80

44365   with removal of tumor(s), polyp(s), or other lesion(s) by hot biopsy forceps or bipolar cautery   2 80

▲ 44366   with control of bleeding (eg, injection, bipolar cautery, unipolar cautery, laser, heater probe, stapler, plasma coagulator)   2

44369   with ablation of tumor(s), polyp(s), or other lesion(s) not amenable to removal by hot biopsy forceps, bipolar cautery or snare technique   2 80

44370   with transendoscopic stent placement (includes predilation)   80

44372   with placement of percutaneous jejunostomy tube   2

Skin

In 44346, the site of the colostomy may be moved. The bowel is mobilized and trimmed of any herniations. The former site is closed

Herniations that have formed around the site of a colostomy are repaired

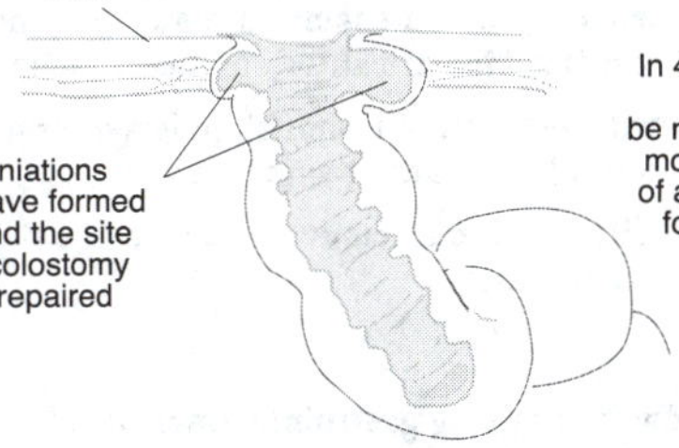

The colon is mobilized, trimmed if necessary, and a new stoma is often created

44373   with conversion of percutaneous gastrostomy tube to percutaneous jejunostomy tube   2

44376   Small intestinal endoscopy, enteroscopy beyond second portion of duodenum, including ileum; diagnostic, with or without collection of specimen(s) by brushing or washing (separate procedure)   80

44377   with biopsy, single or multiple   80

▲ 44378   with control of bleeding (eg, injection, bipolar cautery, unipolar cautery, laser, heater probe, stapler, plasma coagulator)   80

● 44379   with transendoscopic stent placement (includes predilation)   80

44380   Ileoscopy, through stoma; diagnostic, with or without collection of specimen(s) by brushing or washing (separate procedure)   0

44382   with biopsy, single or multiple   0

● 44383   with transendoscopic stent placement (includes predilation)

44385   Endoscopic evaluation of small intestinal (abdominal or pelvic) pouch; diagnostic, with or without collection of specimen(s) by brushing or washing (separate procedure)   0

44386   with biopsy, single or multiple   0 80

44388   Colonoscopy through stoma; diagnostic, with or without collection of specimen(s) by brushing or washing (separate procedure)   0
If colonoscopy is performed via rectum, consult CPT codes 45330-45385.

44389   with biopsy, single or multiple   0

44390   with removal of foreign body   0 80

▲ 44391   with control of bleeding (eg, injection, bipolar cautery, unipolar cautery, laser, heater probe, stapler, plasma coagulator)   0 80

44392   with removal of tumor(s), polyp(s), or other lesion(s) by hot biopsy forceps or bipolar cautery   0

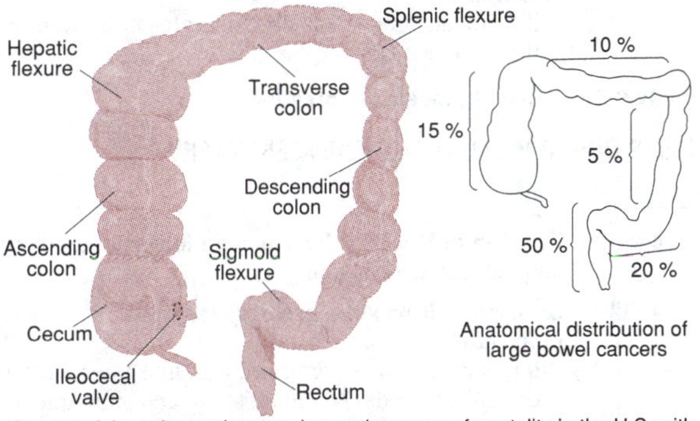

Cancer of the colon and rectum is a major cause of mortality in the U.S. with about 140,000 new cases identified annually; peak incidence is about 70 years of age; rectal cancer is more common among men, colon cancer among women

---

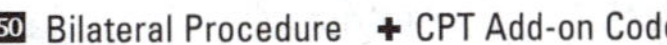 CCI Comprehensive Code   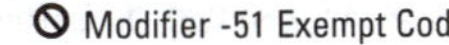 Bilateral Procedure   ✚ CPT Add-on Code   ⊘ Modifier -51 Exempt Code   ● New Code   ▲ Revised Code

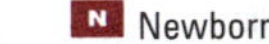 Maternity   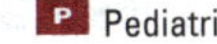 Newborn   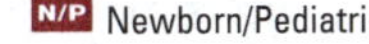 Pediatric   N/P Newborn/Pediatric

Digestive System

44393 — 45100

	44393	with ablation of tumor(s), polyp(s), or other lesion(s) not amenable to removal by hot biopsy forceps, bipolar cautery or snare technique
	44394	with removal of tumor(s), polyp(s), or other lesion(s) by snare technique
	44397	with transendoscopic stent placement (includes predilation)

INTRODUCTION

| ⊘ | 44500 | Introduction of long gastrointestinal tube (eg, Miller-Abbott) (separate procedure) |

For radiological supervision and interpretation, consult CPT code 74340.

For placement of naso- or oro-gastric tube, consult CPT code 43752.

REPAIR

	44602	Suture of small intestine (enterorrhaphy) for perforated ulcer, diverticulum, wound, injury or rupture; single perforation
	44603	multiple perforations
	44604	Suture of large intestine (colorrhaphy) for perforated ulcer, diverticulum, wound, injury or rupture (single or multiple perforations); without colostomy
	44605	with colostomy
	44615	Intestinal strictureplasty (enterotomy and enterorrhaphy) with or without dilation, for intestinal obstruction
	44620	Closure of enterostomy, large or small intestine;
	44625	with resection and anastomosis other than colorectal
	44626	with resection and colorectal anastomosis (eg, closure of Hartmann type procedure)
	44640	Closure of intestinal cutaneous fistula
	44650	Closure of enteroenteric or enterocolic fistula
	44660	Closure of enterovesical fistula; without intestinal or bladder resection
▲	44661	with intestine and/or bladder resection

If closure of a renocolic fistula is performed, consult CPT codes 50525 and 50526. If closure of a gastrocolic fistula is performed, consult CPT code 43880. If closure of a rectovesical fistula is performed, consult CPT codes 45800 and 45805.

| | 44680 | Intestinal plication (separate procedure) |

Noble intestinal plication

OTHER PROCEDURES

| ▲ | 44700 | Exclusion of small intestine from pelvis by mesh or other prosthesis, or native tissue (eg, bladder or omentum) |

If therapeutic radiation clinical treatment is given, consult the Radiation Oncology section.

| | 44799 | Unlisted procedure, intestine |

MECKEL'S DIVERTICULUM AND THE MESENTERY

EXCISION

| | 44800 | Excision of Meckel's diverticulum (diverticulectomy) or omphalomesenteric duct |
| | 44820 | Excision of lesion of mesentery (separate procedure) |

If this procedure is performed with intestine resection, consult CPT codes 44120 or 44140 and subsequent codes.

SUTURE

| | 44850 | Suture of mesentery (separate procedure) |

If an internal hernia is reduced and repaired, consult CPT code 44050.

OTHER PROCEDURES

| | 44899 | Unlisted procedure, Meckels diverticulum and the mesentery |

APPENDIX

INCISION

| | 44900 | Incision and drainage of appendiceal abscess; open |
| | 44901 | percutaneous |

For radiological supervision and interpretation, consult CPT code 75989.

EXCISION

| | 44950 | Appendectomy; |

An incidental appendectomy during other intra-abdominal surgery does not usually warrant a separate identification. However, if it is necessary to report, append modifier -52 or 09952 to 44950.

Battle's operation

| + | 44955 | when done for indicated purpose at time of other major procedure (not as separate procedure) (List separately in addition to code for primary procedure) |
| | 44960 | for ruptured appendix with abscess or generalized peritonitis |

Battle's operation

LAPAROSCOPY

| | 44970 | Laparoscopy, surgical, appendectomy |
| | 44979 | Unlisted laparoscopy procedure, appendix |

RECTUM

INCISION

	45000	Transrectal drainage of pelvic abscess
	45005	Incision and drainage of submucosal abscess, rectum
	45020	Incision and drainage of deep supralevator, pelvirectal, or retrorectal abscess

Consult also CPT codes 46050 and 46060.

EXCISION

| | 45100 | Biopsy of anorectal wall, anal approach (eg, congenital megacolon) |

If an endoscopic biopsy is performed, consult CPT code 45305.

45108	Anorectal myomectomy	②
45110	Proctectomy; complete, combined abdominoperineal, with colostomy	80
45111	partial resection of rectum, transabdominal approach **Luschka proctectomy**	80
45112	Proctectomy, combined abdominoperineal, pull-through procedure (eg, colo-anal anastomosis)	80
	If a colo-anal anastomosis is performed with the creation of a colonic reservoir or pouch, consult CPT code 45119.	
45113	Proctectomy, partial, with rectal mucosectomy, ileoanal anastomosis, creation of ileal reservoir (S or J), with or without loop ileostomy	80
45114	Proctectomy, partial, with anastomosis; abdominal and transsacral approach	80
45116	transsacral approach only (Kraske type)	80
45119	Proctectomy, combined abdominoperineal pull-through procedure (eg, colo-anal anastomosis), with creation of colonic reservoir (eg, J-pouch), with or without proximal diverting ostomy	80
45120	Proctectomy, complete (for congenital megacolon), abdominal and perineal approach; with pull-through procedure and anastomosis (eg, Swenson, Duhamel, or Soave type operation)	80
45121	with subtotal or total colectomy, with multiple biopsies	80
45123	Proctectomy, partial, without anastomosis, perineal approach	80

CIM 45-22 LYMPHOCYTE IMMUNE GLOBULIN, ANTI-THYMOCYTE GLOBULIN (EQUINE)

The Food and Drug Administration (FDA) has approved one lymphocyte immune globulin preparation, anti-thymocyte globulin (equine). Medicare covers equine when used for managing allograft rejection episodes in renal transplantation.

CIM 50-23 HISTOCOMPATIBILITY TESTING

Histocompatibility testing is covered when it is performed on patients:

- In preparation for a kidney transplant
- In preparation for bone marrow transplantation
- In preparation for blood platelet transfusions (particularly where multiple infusions are involved)
- Who are suspected of having ankylosing spondylitis

It is covered for ankylosing spondylitis when other methods of diagnosis would not be appropriate or have yielded inconclusive results. Documentation is required.

45126	Pelvic exenteration for colorectal malignancy, with proctectomy (with or without colostomy), with removal of bladder and ureteral transplantations, and/or hysterectomy, or cervicectomy, with or without removal of tube(s), with or without removal of ovary(s), or any combination thereof	80
45130	Excision of rectal procidentia, with anastomosis; perineal approach **Altemeier procedure**	80
45135	abdominal and perineal approach	80
● 45136	Excision of ileoanal reservoir with ileostomy Code 45136 is not to be used with 44005, 44120, 44310.	
45150	Division of stricture of rectum	② 80
45160	Excision of rectal tumor by proctotomy, transacral or transcoccygeal approach	80
45170	Excision of rectal tumor, transanal approach	② 80

DESTRUCTION

| ▲ | 45190 | Destruction of rectal tumor (eg, electrodessication, electrosurgery, laser ablation, laser resection, cryosurgery) transanal approach | 80 |

ENDOSCOPY

See glossary for additional terms and guidelines.

Diagnostic endoscopy is included in surgical endoscopy.

CIM 35-59 ENDOSCOPY

Although endoscopy is primarily a diagnostic tool, it includes certain therapeutic procedures such as removal of polyps, and endoscopic papillotomy, by which stones are removed from the bile duct. Endoscopic procedures are covered when reasonable and necessary for the individual patient.

	45300	Proctosigmoidoscopy, rigid; diagnostic, with or without collection of specimen(s) by brushing or washing (separate procedure)	
▲	45303	with dilation (eg, balloon, guide wire, bougie)	
		If radiological supervision and interpretation is performed, consult CPT code 74360.	
	45305	with biopsy, single or multiple	❶
	45307	with removal of foreign body	❶ 80
	45308	with removal of single tumor, polyp, or other lesion by hot biopsy forceps or bipolar cautery	❶
	45309	with removal of single tumor, polyp, or other lesion by snare technique	❶
	45315	with removal of multiple tumors, polyps, or other lesions by hot biopsy forceps, bipolar cautery or snare technique	❶
▲	45317	with control of bleeding (eg, injection, bipolar cautery, unipolar cautery, laser, heater probe, stapler, plasma coagulator)	❶
	45320	with ablation of tumor(s), polyp(s), or other lesion(s) not amenable to removal by hot biopsy forceps, bipolar cautery or snare technique (eg, laser)	❶
	45321	with decompression of volvulus	❶
	45327	with transendoscopic stent placement (includes predilation)	
	45330	Sigmoidoscopy, flexible; diagnostic, with or without collection of specimen(s) by brushing or washing (separate procedure)	
	45331	with biopsy, single or multiple	❶
	45332	with removal of foreign body	❶
	45333	with removal of tumor(s), polyp(s), or other lesion(s) by hot biopsy forceps or bipolar cautery	❶

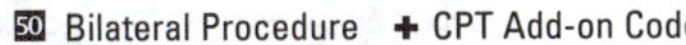

The rectum is the section of colon below the sigmoid flexure and above the anal canal. The anal canal is the terminal part of the large intestine. The pectinate line marks the division in mucosal covering, innervation, and venous drainage

---

Digestive System

45334 — 45915*

▲ 45334   **with control of bleeding (eg, injection, bipolar cautery, unipolar cautery, laser, heater probe, stapler, plasma coagulator)** ❶ 26

45337   **with decompression of volvulus, any method** ❶ 26

45338   **with removal of tumor(s), polyp(s), or other lesion(s) by snare technique** ❶ 26

45339   **with ablation of tumor(s), polyp(s), or other lesion(s) not amenable to removal by hot biopsy forceps, bipolar cautery or snare technique** ❶ 26

45341   **with endoscopic ultrasound examination** 26

Do not report 76975 when reporting CPT code 45341. For transrectal ultrasound with rigid probe device, consult CPT code 76872.

45342   **with transendoscopic ultrasound guided intramural or transmural fine needle aspiration/biopsy(s)** 26

Do not report 76975 when reporting CPT code 45342. For transrectal ultrasound with rigid probe device, consult CPT code 76872.

For the interpretation of specimen, consult CPT codes 88172-88173.

45345   **with transendoscopic stent placement (includes predilation)** 26

45355   **Colonoscopy, rigid or flexible, transabdominal via colotomy, single or multiple** ❶ 26

MCM 15038. MULTIPLE SURGERIES (CPT MODIFIER 51)

A. General. When more than one surgical service is performed on the same patient, by the same physician, and on the same day:

The fee schedule amount for a second procedure is 50 percent of the fee schedule amount that would have been otherwise applicable for that procedure; and

The fee schedule amount for the third through fifth procedures is 50 percent of the fee schedule amount that would have been otherwise applicable for that procedure. Prior to January 1, 1995, the third through fifth procedures were paid at 25 percent of the fee schedule amount. Surgical procedures beyond the fifth are priced "by report" based on documentation of the services furnished.

B. Multiple Endoscopies. For multiple endoscopic procedures, use the full value of the highest valued endoscopy plus the difference between the next highest and the base endoscopy. For example, in the course of performing a fiberoptic colonoscopy (code 45378), a physician performs a biopsy (code 45380) and removes a polyp (code 45385). Both codes 45380 and 45385 contain the values of the base endoscopy, code 45378. Use the actual value of code 45385 plus the difference between codes 45380 and 45378.

The endoscopic base codes are listed in the Physician Fee Schedule.

MCM 4180.10 AMBULATORY SURGICAL CENTER FACILITY FEE

CPT code 45378, which is used to code a diagnostic colonoscopy, is on the list of procedures approved by Medicare for payment of an ambulatory surgical center (ASC) facility fee and is currently assigned to ASC payment group 2. Code G0105 is also assigned to ASC payment group 2. The ASC facility service is the same whether the procedure is a screening or a diagnostic colonoscopy.

45378   **Colonoscopy, flexible, proximal to splenic flexure; diagnostic, with or without collection of specimen(s) by brushing or washing, with or without colon decompression (separate procedure)** ❷ 26

45379   **with removal of foreign body** ❷ 26

45380   **with biopsy, single or multiple** ❷ 26

▲ 45382   **with control of bleeding (eg, injection, bipolar cautery, unipolar cautery, laser, heater probe, stapler, plasma coagulator)** ❷ 26

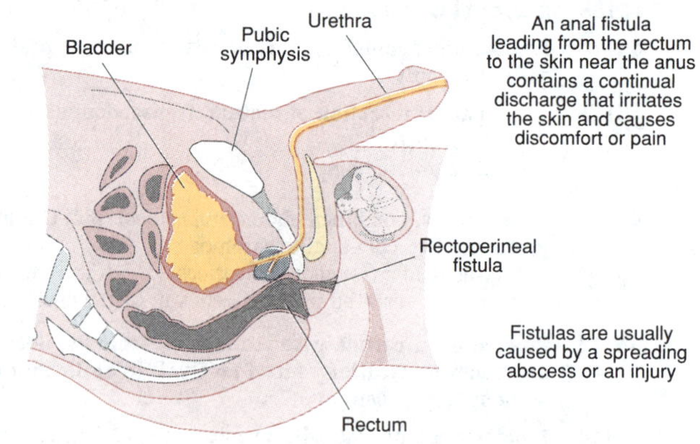

45383   **with ablation of tumor(s), polyp(s), or other lesion(s) not amenable to removal by hot biopsy forceps, bipolar cautery or snare technique** ❷ 26

45384   **with removal of tumor(s), polyp(s), or other lesion(s) by hot biopsy forceps or bipolar cautery** ❷ 26

45385   **with removal of tumor(s), polyp(s), or other lesion(s) by snare technique** ❷ 26

If a small intestine and stomal endoscopy is performed, consult CPT codes 44360-44393.

45387   **with transendoscopic stent placement (includes predilation)** 26

REPAIR

45500   **Proctoplasty; for stenosis** ❷ 80 26

45505   **for prolapse of mucous membrane** ❷ 26

45520   **Perirectal injection of sclerosing solution for prolapse** 26

45540   **Proctopexy for prolapse; abdominal approach** 80 26

45541   **perineal approach** 80 26

45550   **Proctopexy combined with sigmoid resection, abdominal approach** 80 26

   Frickman proctopexy

45560   **Repair of rectocele (separate procedure)** ❷ 80 26

If a rectocele is repaired with a posterior colporrhaphy, consult CPT code 57250.

45562   **Exploration, repair, and presacral drainage for rectal injury;** 80 26

45563   **with colostomy** 80 26

   Maydl colostomy

45800   **Closure of rectovesical fistula;** 80 26

45805   **with colostomy** 80 26

45820   **Closure of rectourethral fistula;** 80 26

45825   **with colostomy** 80 26

If a rectovaginal fistula is closed, consult CPT codes 57300-57308.

MANIPULATION

45900*   **Reduction of procidentia (separate procedure) under anesthesia** ❶ 80 26

45905*   **Dilation of anal sphincter (separate procedure) under anesthesia other than local** ❶ 26

45910   **Dilation of rectal stricture (separate procedure) under anesthesia other than local** ❶ 26

45915*   **Removal of fecal impaction or foreign body (separate procedure) under anesthesia** ❶ 26

---

26 Professional Component Only   80/80 Assist-at-Surgery Allowed/With Documentation   Unlisted   Commonly Miscoded   Not Covered

TC Technical Component Only   **MCM & CIM** Medicare References   ❶❷❸❹❺❻❼❽ ASC Group   ♂ Male Only   ♀ Female Only

OTHER PROCEDURES

45999	Unlisted procedure, rectum	80

ANUS

INCISION

● 46020 **Placement of seton** ☒
Code 46020 is not to be used with to 46060, 46280, 46600.

46030* **Removal of anal seton, other marker** ❶ 80 ☒

46040 **Incision and drainage of ischiorectal and/or perirectal abscess (separate procedure)** ❸ ☒

46045 **Incision and drainage of intramural, intramuscular or submucosal abscess, transanal, under anesthesia** ❷ ☒

46050* **Incision and drainage, perianal abscess, superficial** ❶ ☒
Consult also CPT codes 45020 and 46060.

46060 **Incision and drainage of ischiorectal or intramural abscess, with fistulectomy or fistulotomy, submuscular, with or without placement of seton** ❷ ☒
Consult also CPT code 45020.
Code 46060 is not to be used with 46020.

46070 **Incision, anal septum (infant)** N 80 ☒
If anoplasty is performed, consult CPT codes 46700-46705.

46080* **Sphincterotomy, anal, division of sphincter (separate procedure)** ❸ ☒

46083 **Incision of thrombosed hemorrhoid, external** ☒

EXCISION

46200 **Fissurectomy, with or without sphincterotomy** ❷ ☒

46210 **Cryptectomy; single** ❷ 80 ☒

46211 **multiple (separate procedure)** ❷ 80 ☒

46220 **Papillectomy or excision of single tag, anus (separate procedure)** ❶ ☒

46221 **Hemorrhoidectomy, by simple ligature (eg, rubber band)** ☒

46230 **Excision of external hemorrhoid tags and/or multiple papillae** ☒

46250 **Hemorrhoidectomy, external, complete** ❸ ☒

46255 **Hemorrhoidectomy, internal and external, simple;** ❸ ☒

46257 **with fissurectomy** ❸ ☒

46258 **with fistulectomy, with or without fissurectomy** ❸ 80 ☒

46260 **Hemorrhoidectomy, internal and external, complex or extensive;** ❸ ☒

Whitehead hemorrhoidectomy

46261 **with fissurectomy** ❹ ☒

46262 **with fistulectomy, with or without fissurectomy** ❹ ☒

46270 **Surgical treatment of anal fistula (fistulectomy/fistulotomy); subcutaneous** ❸ ☒

46275 **submuscular** ❸ ☒

46280 **complex or multiple, with or without placement of seton** ❹ ☒
Code 46280 is not to be used with to 46020.

46285 **second stage** ❶ ☒

46288 **Closure of anal fistula with rectal advancement flap** ☒

46320* **Enucleation or excision of external thrombotic hemorrhoid** ☒

INTRODUCTION

46500* **Injection of sclerosing solution, hemorrhoids** ☒

ENDOSCOPY

CIM 35-59 ENDOSCOPY

Although endoscopy is primarily a diagnostic tool, it includes certain therapeutic procedures such as removal of polyps, and endoscopic papillotomy, by which stones are removed from the bile duct. Endoscopic procedures are covered when reasonable and necessary for the individual patient.

46600 **Anoscopy; diagnostic, with or without collection of specimen(s) by brushing or washing (separate procedure)** ☒
Do not report 46600 in addition to 46020.

▲ 46604 **with dilation (eg, balloon, guide wire, bougie)** ☒

46606 **with biopsy, single or multiple** ☒

46608 **with removal of foreign body** ❶ 80 ☒

46610 **with removal of single tumor, polyp, or other lesion by hot biopsy forceps or bipolar cautery** ❶ ☒

46611 **with removal of single tumor, polyp, or other lesion by snare technique** ❶ 80 ☒

46612 **with removal of multiple tumors, polyps, or other lesions by hot biopsy forceps, bipolar cautery or snare technique** ❶ 80 ☒

▲ 46614 **with control of bleeding (eg, injection, bipolar cautery, unipolar cautery, laser, heater probe, stapler, plasma coagulator)** ☒

46615 **with ablation of tumor(s), polyp(s), or other lesion(s) not amenable to removal by hot biopsy forceps, bipolar cautery or snare technique** 80 ☒

REPAIR

46700 **Anoplasty, plastic operation for stricture; adult** ❸ ☒

46705 **infant** N 80 ☒
If a simple incision of the anal septum is performed, consult CPT code 46070.

46715 **Repair of low imperforate anus; with anoperineal fistula (cut-back procedure)** ♀ 80 ☒

46716 **with transposition of anoperineal or anovestibular fistula** ♀ 80 ☒

46730 **Repair of high imperforate anus without fistula; perineal or sacroperineal approach** 80 ☒

46735 **combined transabdominal and sacroperineal approaches** 80 ☒

46740 **Repair of high imperforate anus with rectourethral or rectovaginal fistula; perineal or sacroperineal approach** 80 ☒

Digestive System

46742 — 47100

46742	combined transabdominal and sacroperineal approaches	80 ◻
46744	Repair of cloacal anomaly by anorectovaginoplasty and urethroplasty, sacroperineal approach	♀ 80 ◻
46746	Repair of cloacal anomaly by anorectovaginoplasty and urethroplasty, combined abdominal and sacroperineal approach;	♀ 80 ◻
46748	with vaginal lengthening by intestinal graft or pedicle flaps	♀ 80 ◻

CIM 65-9 INCONTINENCE CONTROL DEVICES

Prior to collagen implant therapy, a skin test for collagen sensitivity must be administered and evaluated over a four week period. In male patients, the evaluation must include a complete history and physical examination and a simple cystometrogram to determine that the bladder fills and stores properly. The patient then is asked to stand upright with a full bladder and to cough or otherwise exert abdominal pressure on his bladder. If the patient leaks, the diagnosis of ISD is established. In female patients, the evaluation must include a complete history and physical examination (including a pelvic exam) and a simple cystometrogram to rule out abnormalities of bladder compliance and abnormalities of urethral support. Following that determination, an abdominal leak point pressure (ALLP) test is performed. If the patient has an ALLP of less than 100 cm H_2O, the diagnosis of ISD is established.

To use a collagen implant, physicians must have urology training in the use of a cystoscope and must complete a collagen implant training program. Coverage of a collagen implant, and the procedure to inject it, is limited to the following types of patients with stress urinary incontinence due to ISD:

a. Male or female patients with congenital sphincter weakness secondary to conditions such as myelomeningocele

b. Male or female patients with acquired sphincter weakness secondary to spinal cord lesions

c. Male patients following trauma, including prostatectomy and/or radiation

d. Female patients without urethral hypermobility and with abdominal leak point pressures of 100 centimeters H_2O or less

Patients whose incontinence does not improve with five injection procedures are considered treatment failures, and no further treatment of urinary incontinence by collagen implant is covered. Patients who have a reoccurrence of incontinence following successful treatment with collagen implants in the past may benefit from additional treatment sessions. Coverage of additional sessions must be supported by medical justification.

46750	Sphincteroplasty, anal, for incontinence or prolapse; adult	❸ 80 ◻
46751	child	P 80 ◻
46753	Graft (Thiersch operation) for rectal incontinence and/or prolapse	❸ ◻
46754	Removal of Thiersch wire or suture, anal canal	❷ 80 ◻
46760	Sphincteroplasty, anal, for incontinence, adult; muscle transplant	❷ 80 ◻
46761	levator muscle imbrication (Park posterior anal repair)	80 ◻
46762	implantation artificial sphincter	80 ◻

DESTRUCTION

46900*	Destruction of lesion(s), anus (eg, condyloma, papilloma, molluscum contagiosum, herpetic vesicle), simple; chemical	◻
46910*	electrodesiccation	◻
46916	cryosurgery	◻

CIM 35-52 LASER PROCEDURES

Coverage is determined on the basis that the use of lasers to alter, revise, or destroy tissue is a surgical procedure and restricted to practitioners with training in the surgical management of the disease or condition being treated.

46917	laser surgery	◻
46922	surgical excision	❶ ◻

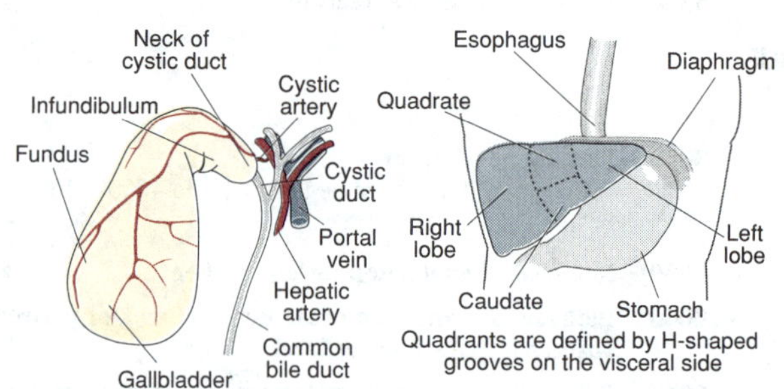

The liver is divided into four lobes for descriptive purposes, although the left and right halves are functionally separate, each receiving its own arterial supply and venous drainage. The liver is the largest gland in the body and serves many metabolic purposes including secretion of bile. The gallbladder is located on the visceral side of the quadrate lobe and stores bile between active phases of digestion; positions of the sac and its structures varies

▲	46924	Destruction of lesion(s), anus (eg, condyloma, papilloma, molluscum contagiosum, herpetic vesicle), extensive (eg, laser surgery, electrosurgery, cryosurgery, chemosurgery)	❶ ◻
	46934	Destruction of hemorrhoids, any method; internal	◻
	46935	external	◻
	46936	internal and external	◻
	46937	Cryosurgery of rectal tumor; benign	❷ 80 ◻
	46938	malignant	❷ 80 ◻
▲	46940	Curettage or cautery of anal fissure, including dilation of anal sphincter (separate procedure); initial	◻
	46942	subsequent	80 ◻

SUTURE

46945	Ligation of internal hemorrhoids; single procedure	◻
46946	multiple procedures	◻

OTHER PROCEDURES

46999	Unlisted procedure, anus	80

LIVER

INCISION

47000*	Biopsy of liver, needle; percutaneous	❶ ◻

To report imaging guidance, consult CPT codes 76003, 76360, 76393, and 76942.

+ 47001	when done for indicated purpose at time of other major procedure (List separately in addition to code for primary procedure)	

To report imaging guidance, consult CPT codes 76003, 76942.

For fine needle aspiration performed in conjunction with 47000, 47001, see 10021, 10022.

To report evaluation of fine needle aspirate, consult CPT codes 88172, 88173.

47010	Hepatotomy; for open drainage of abscess or cyst, one or two stages	80 ◻
47011	for percutaneous drainage of abscess or cyst, one or two stages	80 ◻

For radiological supervision and interpretation, consult CPT code 75989.

47015	Laparotomy, with aspiration and/or injection of hepatic parasitic (eg, amoebic or echinococcal) cyst(s) or abscess(es)	80 ◻

EXCISION

47100	Biopsy of liver, wedge	80 ◻

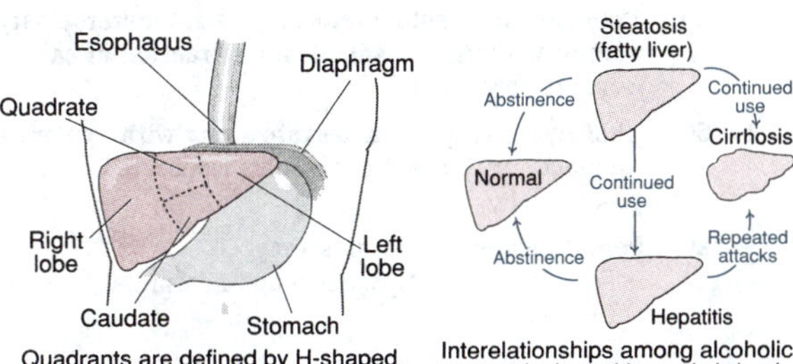

Quadrants are defined by H-shaped grooves on the visceral side

Interelationships among alcoholic steatosis, hepatitis, and cirrhosis

The liver is the largest gland in the body and serves many metabolic purposes including secretion of bile. Chronic alcohol use leads to three similar forms of alcoholic liver disease: steatosis (fatty liver), hepatitis, and cirrhosis. The conditions have many overlapping features and each may occur without involvement of alcohol. Alcoholic cirrhosis accounts for about 60 percent of all cirrhosis cases and the risk appears to rise with the amount of alcohol consumed daily. The liver tends to shrink and become fibrotic

47120	**Hepatectomy, resection of liver; partial lobectomy**	80
47122	**trisegmentectomy**	80
47125	**total left lobectomy**	80
47130	**total right lobectomy**	80
47133	**Donor hepatectomy, with preparation and maintenance of allograft; from cadaver donor**	
47134	**partial, from living donor**	80

CIM 35-53 ADULT LIVER TRANSPLANTATION
See Intermediary Manual, §3101.14 and Carriers Manual, §2300.1.

See Intermediary Manual, §3660.8 and Carriers Manual, §§2050.3, 4471, and 5249.

Adult liver transplantation when performed on beneficiaries with end stage liver disease other than hepatitis B or malignancies is covered under Medicare when performed in a facility which is approved by CMS as meeting institutional coverage criteria. Follow-up care or retransplantation required as a result of a covered liver transplant is covered. In addition, it is covered for patients who have been discharged from a hospital after receiving a noncovered liver transplant. Effective September 1, 2001, Medicare covers adult liver transplantation for hepatocellular carcinoma when the following conditions are met: 1. The patient is not a candidate for subtotal liver resection; 2. The patient's tumor(s) is less than or equal to 5 cm in diameter; 3. There is no macrovascular involvement; 4. There is no identifiable extrahepatic spread of tumor to surrounding lymph nodes, lungs, abdominal organs or bone; and 5. The transplant is furnished in a facility which is approved by CMS as meeting institutional coverage criteria for liver transplants (See 65 FR 15006).

MCM 2300.1 SERVICES RELATED TO AND REQUIRED AS A RESULT OF SERVICES WHICH ARE NOT COVERED UNDER MEDICARE
Medical and hospital services may be required to treat a condition that arises as a result of services not covered because they are not reasonable and necessary or excluded for other reasons. Services "related to" noncovered services (e.g., cosmetic surgery, noncovered organ transplants, noncovered artificial organ implants), including services related to follow-up care and complications of noncovered services that require treatment during a hospital stay when noncovered service were performed, are not covered services under Medicare. Services "not related to" noncovered services are covered under Medicare.Effective September 1, 2001, Medicare covers adult liver transplantation for hepatocellular carcinoma when the following conditions are met: 1. The patient is not a candidate for subtotal liver resection; 2. The patient's tumor(s) is less than or equal to 5 cm in diameter; 3. There is no macrovascular involvement; 4. There is no identifiable extrahepatic spread of tumor to surrounding lymph nodes, lungs, abdominal organs or bone; and 5. The transplant is furnished in a facility which is approved by CMS as meeting institutional coverage criteria for liver transplants (See 65 FR 15006).

MCM 2050.3 INCIDENT TO PHYSICIAN'S SERVICE IN CLINIC
A physician directed clinic is one where:

a. A physician (or a number of physicians) is present to perform medical (rather than administrative) services at all times the clinic is open

b. Each patient is under the care of a clinic physician

c. The nonphysician services are under medical supervision

In highly organized clinics, particularly those that are departmentalized, direct personal physician supervision may be the responsibility of several physicians as opposed to an individual attending physician. In this situation, medical management of all services provided in the clinic is assured. The physician ordering a particular service need not be the physician who is supervising the service. Supplies provided by the clinic during the course of treatment are also covered. When the auxiliary personnel perform services outside the clinic premises, the services are covered only if performed under the direct personal supervision of a clinic physician. If the clinic refers a patient for auxiliary services performed by personnel who are not employed by the clinic, such services are not incident to a physician's service.

MCM 4471.2 DETERMINATION OF ELIGIBILITY
Benefit eligibility is limited to the one-year period following the date of the beneficiary's discharge from a hospital or transplant center after a Medicare covered kidney, heart or liver transplant. The specialty carrier consults one of three alternative sources of information to determine the date of kidney transplant:

1. HCFA compiles and furnishes in hardcopy or tape format to specialty carriers a monthly listing of beneficiaries who have received kidney transplants. HCFA's system is not yet equipped to handle heart and liver transplant data. The initial listing included all beneficiaries who had received a kidney transplant since January 1, 1986. It is updated monthly.

2. Intermediaries send copies of the Part A Medicare Benefit Notice that contains the date of transplant to the specialty carriers. The specialty carriers maintain the data and release it to area carriers upon request.

3. If you are unable to locate the beneficiary's transplant information above, refer to the discharge date listed on the prescription form. The prescription form should accompany the initial claim and indicate the date of discharge. You may contact the prescribing physician for substantiation of the discharge date. If there is no other eligibility information other than the prescription regarding the discharge date, the beneficiary may pay for a one month's supply of immunosuppressive drugs based upon the discharge date listed. If the information obtained indicates transplant failure, do not approve payment for drugs in subsequent periods.

MCM 5249. PAYMENT FOR IMMUNOSUPPRESSIVE DRUGS FURNISHED TO TRANSPLANT PATIENTS
Medicare pays for FDA approved immunosuppressive drugs. This benefit is subject to the Part B deductible and coinsurance provision and is limited to the one-year period after the date of the transplant procedure. Medicare pays for immunosuppressive drugs provided outside the one-year period if the drugs are covered under some other provision of the law (e.g., when the drugs are covered as inpatient hospital services or are furnished incident to a physician's service). We interpret "1-year period after the date of the transplant procedure" to mean 365 days from the day an inpatient is discharged from the hospital; from surgery until hospital discharge, payment for these drugs is included in Medicare's Part A payment to the hospital. If the same patient receives a subsequent transplant operation within 365 days, the period for this benefit begins anew.

The physician should supply the patient with a non-refillable 30-day prescription for the immunosuppressive drugs and to the carrier the date of that patient's discharge from the hospital on the first immunosuppressive drug prescription for subsequent transplant patients. The date is used for limitation purposes because the dosage of these drugs frequently diminishes over a period of time and prescription changes.

CIM 35-53.1 PEDIATRIC LIVER TRANSPLANTATION
Liver transplantation is covered for children (under age 18) with extrahepatic biliary atresia or any other form of end stage liver disease, and when performed in a pediatric hospital that performs pediatric liver transplants. The hospital must submit an application with HCFA documenting that the

---

Digestive System

47135 — 47556

hospital's pediatric liver transplant program is operated jointly by the hospital and another facility that has been found by HCFA to meet the institutional coverage criteria in the Federal Register notice of April 12, 1991.

47135	Liver allotransplantation; orthotopic, partial or whole, from cadaver or living donor, any age	80 🔁
47136	heterotopic, partial or whole, from cadaver or living donor, any age	80 🔁

REPAIR

47300	Marsupialization of cyst or abscess of liver	80 🔁
47350	Management of liver hemorrhage; simple suture of liver wound or injury	80 🔁
47360	complex suture of liver wound or injury, with or without hepatic artery ligation	80 🔁
47361	exploration of hepatic wound, extensive debridement, coagulation and/or suture, with or without packing of liver	80 🔁
47362	re-exploration of hepatic wound for removal of packing	80 🔁

LAPAROSCOPY

Diagnostic laproscopy is included in surgical laproscopy.

- 47370 **Laparoscopy, surgical, ablation of one or more liver tumor(s); radiofrequency**
  To report imaging guidance, consult CPT code 76490.
- 47371 **cryosurgical**
  To report imaging guidance, consult CPT code 76490.
- 47379 **Unlisted laparoscopic procedure, liver** 80

OTHER PROCEDURES

- 47380 **Ablation, open, of one or more liver tumor(s); radiofrequency**
  To report imaging guidance, consult CPT code 76490.
- 47381 **cryosurgical**
- 47382 **Ablation, one or more liver tumor(s), percutaneous, radiofrequency**
  To report imaging guidance and monitoring, consult CPT codes 76362, 76394, or 76490.
- 47399 **Unlisted procedure, liver** 80

BILIARY TRACT

INCISION

47400	Hepaticotomy or hepaticostomy with exploration, drainage, or removal of calculus	80 🔁
47420	Choledochotomy or choledochostomy with exploration, drainage, or removal of calculus, with or without cholecystotomy; without transduodenal sphincterotomy or sphincteroplasty	80 🔁
47425	with transduodenal sphincterotomy or sphincteroplasty	80 🔁

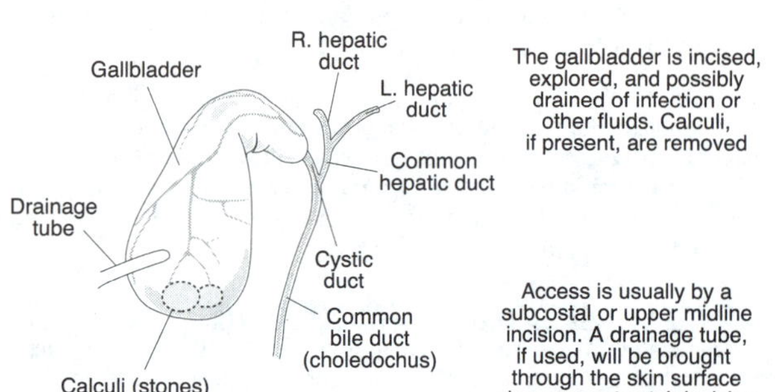

47460	Transduodenal sphincterotomy or sphincteroplasty, with or without transduodenal extraction of calculus (separate procedure)	80 🔁
47480	Cholecystotomy or cholecystostomy with exploration, drainage, or removal of calculus (separate procedure)	80 🔁
47490	Percutaneous cholecystostomy	🔁
	For radiological supervision and interpretation, consult CPT code 75989.	

INTRODUCTION

47500	Injection procedure for percutaneous transhepatic cholangiography	🔁
	For radiological supervision and interpretation, consult CPT code 74320.	
47505	Injection procedure for cholangiography through an existing catheter (eg, percutaneous transhepatic or T-tube)	80 🔁
	For radiological supervision and interpretation, consult CPT code 74305.	
47510	Introduction of percutaneous transhepatic catheter for biliary drainage	❷ 🔁
	For radiological supervision and interpretation, consult CPT code 75980.	
47511	Introduction of percutaneous transhepatic stent for internal and external biliary drainage	🔁 50
	For radiological supervision and interpretation, consult CPT code 75982.	
47525	Change of percutaneous biliary drainage catheter	❶ 🔁
	For radiological supervision and interpretation, consult CPT code 75984.	
47530	Revision and/or reinsertion of transhepatic tube	❶ 🔁
	For radiological supervision and interpretation, consult CPT code 75984.	

ENDOSCOPY

Diagnostic endoscopy is included in surgical endoscopy.

CIM 35-59 ENDOSCOPY

Although endoscopy is primarily a diagnostic tool, it includes certain therapeutic procedures such as removal of polyps, and endoscopic papillotomy, by which stones are removed from the bile duct. Endoscopic procedures are covered when reasonable and necessary for the individual patient.

+ 47550	Biliary endoscopy, intraoperative (choledochoscopy) (List separately in addition to code for primary procedure)	80
47552	Biliary endoscopy, percutaneous via T-tube or other tract; diagnostic, with or without collection of specimen(s) by brushing and/or washing (separate procedure)	❷ 🔁
47553	with biopsy, single or multiple	❸ 🔁
▲ 47554	with removal of calculus/calculi	❸ 🔁
47555	with dilation of biliary duct stricture(s) without stent	❸ 🔁
	If imaging guidance is provided, consult CPT codes 74363, 75982.	
	If an endoscopic retrograde cholangiopancreatography (ERCP) is performed, consult CPT codes 43260-43272 and 74363.	
47556	with dilation of biliary duct stricture(s) with stent	🔁
	If imaging guidance is provided, consult CPT codes 74363, 75982.	

LAPAROSCOPY

47560	Laparoscopy, surgical; with guided transhepatic cholangiography, without biopsy	80
47561	with guided transhepatic cholangiography with biopsy	❸ 80

CIM 35-91 LAPAROSCOPIC CHOLECYSTECTOMY

Laparoscopic cholecystectomy is a covered surgical procedure that removes diseased gall bladder through instruments introduced via cannulae. Vision of the operative field is maintained by high-resolution television camera-monitor system (video laparoscope). For inpatient claims, use ICD-9-CM code 51.23, Laparoscopic cholecystectomy. For all other claims, use CPT codes 49310 and 49311.

47562	cholecystectomy	80
47563	cholecystectomy with cholangiography	80
47564	cholecystectomy with exploration of common duct	80
47570	cholecystoenterostomy	80
47579	Unlisted laparoscopy procedure, biliary tract	80 50

EXCISION

47600	Cholecystectomy;	80
47605	with cholangiography	80
47610	Cholecystectomy with exploration of common duct;	80
47612	with choledochoenterostomy	80
47620	with transduodenal sphincterotomy or sphincteroplasty, with or without cholangiography	80
47630	Biliary duct stone extraction, percutaneous via T-tube tract, basket or snare (eg, Burhenne technique)	❸

For radiological supervision and interpretation, consult CPT code 74327.

47700	Exploration for congenital atresia of bile ducts, without repair, with or without liver biopsy, with or without cholangiography	80
47701	Portoenterostomy (eg, Kasai procedure)	80
47711	Excision of bile duct tumor, with or without primary repair of bile duct; extrahepatic	80
47712	intrahepatic	80

If anastomosis is performed, consult CPT codes 47760-47800.

47715	Excision of choledochal cyst	80
47716	Anastomosis, choledochal cyst, without excision	80

REPAIR

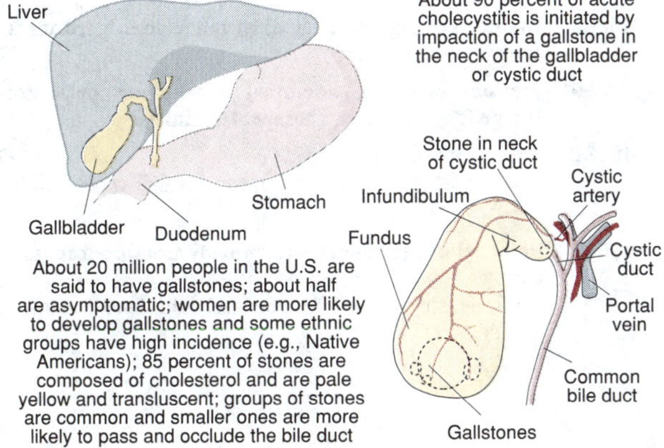

About 90 percent of acute cholecystitis is initiated by impaction of a gallstone in the neck of the gallbladder or cystic duct

About 20 million people in the U.S. are said to have gallstones; about half are asymptomatic; women are more likely to develop gallstones and some ethnic groups have high incidence (e.g., Native Americans); 85 percent of stones are composed of cholesterol and are pale yellow and translucent; groups of stones are common and smaller ones are more likely to pass and occlude the bile duct

47720	Cholecystoenterostomy; direct	80

If a laparoscopic approach is used, consult CPT code 47570.

47721	with gastroenterostomy	80
47740	Roux-en-Y	80
47741	Roux-en-Y with gastroenterostomy	80
47760	Anastomosis, of extrahepatic biliary ducts and gastrointestinal tract	80
47765	Anastomosis, of intrahepatic ducts and gastrointestinal tract	80

Longmire anastomosis

47780	Anastomosis, Roux-en-Y, of extrahepatic biliary ducts and gastrointestinal tract	80
47785	Anastomosis, Roux-en-Y, of intrahepatic biliary ducts and gastrointestinal tract	80
47800	Reconstruction, plastic, of extrahepatic biliary ducts with end-to-end anastomosis	80
47801	Placement of choledochal stent	80
47802	U-tube hepaticoenterostomy	80
47900	Suture of extrahepatic biliary duct for pre-existing injury (separate procedure)	80

OTHER PROCEDURES

47999	Unlisted procedure, biliary tract	80

PANCREAS

If peroral pancreatic endoscopic procedures are performed, consult CPT codes 43260-43272.

INCISION

48000	Placement of drains, peripancreatic, for acute pancreatitis;	80
48001	with cholecystostomy, gastrostomy, and jejunostomy	80
48005	Resection or debridement of pancreas and peripancreatic tissue for acute necrotizing pancreatitis	80
48020	Removal of pancreatic calculus	80

EXCISION

▲ 48100	Biopsy of pancreas, open (eg, fine needle aspiration, needle core biopsy, wedge biopsy)	80
48102*	Biopsy of pancreas, percutaneous needle	❶

For radiological supervision and interpretation, consult CPT codes 76003, 76360, 76393, and 76942.

To report fine needle aspiration, consult CPT code 10022.

To report evaluation of fine needle aspirate, consult CPT codes 88172, 88173.

48120	Excision of lesion of pancreas (eg, cyst, adenoma)	80

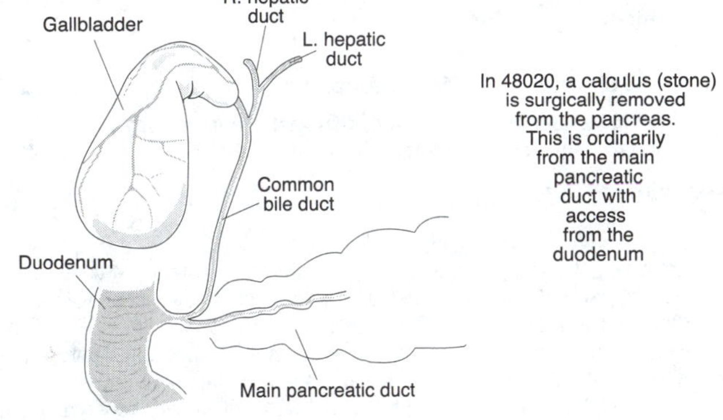

In 48020, a calculus (stone) is surgically removed from the pancreas. This is ordinarily from the main pancreatic duct with access from the duodenum

---

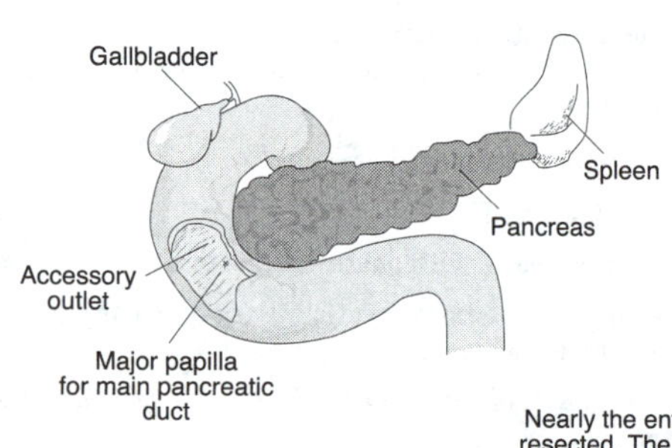

Nearly the entire pancreas is resected. The complex where the pancreatic ducts enter the duodenum is preserved (48146)

it does not contain an appropriate diagnosis code. Pancreas transplantation for diabetic patients who have not experienced end stage renal failure secondary to diabetes continues to be excluded from Medicare coverage. Medicare also excludes coverage of transplantation of partial pancreatic tissue or islet cells. There is not sufficient evidence at this time to support a determination that these procedures are reasonable and necessary.

48550 Donor pancreatectomy, with preparation and maintenance of allograft from cadaver donor, with or without duodenal segment for transplantation

48554 Transplantation of pancreatic allograft

48556 Removal of transplanted pancreatic allograft

OTHER PROCEDURES

48999 Unlisted procedure, pancreas

ABDOMEN, PERITONEUM, AND OMENTUM

INCISION

49000 Exploratory laparotomy, exploratory celiotomy with or without biopsy(s) (separate procedure)
If wound exploration due to a penetrating trauma without laparotomy is performed, consult CPT code 20102.

49002 Reopening of recent laparotomy
If re-exploration is performed of a hepatic wound for removal of packing, consult CPT code 47362.

49010 Exploration, retroperitoneal area with or without biopsy(s) (separate procedure)
If wound exploration is performed due to a penetrating trauma without a laparotomy, consult CPT code 20102.

49020 Drainage of peritoneal abscess or localized peritonitis, exclusive of appendiceal abscess; open
If an appendiceal abscess is incised and drained, consult CPT code 44900.

49021 percutaneous
For radiological supervision and interpretation, consult CPT code 75989.

49040 Drainage of subdiaphragmatic or subphrenic abscess; open

49041 percutaneous
For radiological supervision and interpretation, consult CPT code 75989.

49060 Drainage of retroperitoneal abscess; open

49061 percutaneous
If laparoscopic drainage is performed, consult CPT code 49323.
For radiological supervision and interpretation, consult CPT code 75989.

49062 Drainage of extraperitoneal lymphocele to peritoneal cavity, open

49080* Peritoneocentesis, abdominal paracentesis, or peritoneal lavage (diagnostic or therapeutic); initial

49081* subsequent
To report imaging guidance, consult CPT codes 76360, 76942.

49085 Removal of peritoneal foreign body from peritoneal cavity
If lysis is performed on intestinal adhesions, consult CPT code 44005.

48140 Pancreatectomy, distal subtotal, with or without splenectomy; without pancreaticojejunostomy

48145 with pancreaticojejunostomy

48146 Pancreatectomy, distal, near-total with preservation of duodenum (Child-type procedure)

48148 Excision of ampulla of Vater

48150 Pancreatectomy, proximal subtotal with total duodenectomy, partial gastrectomy, choledochoenterostomy and gastrojejunostomy (Whipple-type procedure); with pancreatojejunostomy

48152 without pancreatojejunostomy

48153 Pancreatectomy, proximal subtotal with near-total duodenectomy, choledochoenterostomy and duodenojejunostomy (pylorus-sparing, Whipple-type procedure); with pancreatojejunostomy

48154 without pancreatojejunostomy

48155 Pancreatectomy, total

▲ **48160** Pancreatectomy, total or subtotal, with autologous transplantation of pancreas or pancreatic islet cells

48180 Pancreaticojejunostomy, side-to-side anastomosis (Puestow-type operation)

INTRODUCTION

+ **48400** Injection procedure for intraoperative pancreatography (List separately in addition to code for primary procedure)
For radiological supervision and interpretation, consult CPT codes 74300-74305.

REPAIR

▲ **48500** Marsupialization of pancreatic cyst

48510 External drainage, pseudocyst of pancreas; open

48511 percutaneous
For radiological supervision and interpretation, consult CPT code 75989.

48520 Internal anastomosis of pancreatic cyst to gastrointestinal tract; direct

48540 Roux-en-Y

▲ **48545** Pancreatorrhaphy for injury

▲ **48547** Duodenal exclusion with gastrojejunostomy for pancreatic injury

PANCREAS TRANSPLANTATION

CIM 35-82 PANCREAS TRANSPLANTS

Medicare covers whole organ pancreas transplantation (ICD-9-CM code 52.80, or 52.82, CPT code 48554) only when it is performed simultaneous with or after a kidney transplant (ICD-9-CM code 55.69, CPT 50360, or 50365). If the pancreas transplant occurs after the kidney transplant, immunosuppressive therapy will begin with the date of discharge from the inpatient stay for the pancreas transplant. The claim will be denied for medical necessity reasons if

---

EXCISION, DESTRUCTION

49180* Biopsy, abdominal or retroperitoneal mass, percutaneous needle ❶ 🔲

> To report imaging guidance, consult CPT codes 76003, 76360, 76393, 76942.
>
> To report fine needle aspiration, consult CPT codes 10021 or 10022.
>
> To report evaluation of fine needle aspirate, consult CPT codes 88172, 88173.

49200 Excision or destruction by any method of intra-abdominal or retroperitoneal tumors or cysts or endometriomas; 80 🔲

49201 extensive 80 🔲

49215 Excision of presacral or sacrococcygeal tumor 80 🔲

MCM 2070 DIAGNOSTIC X-RAY, DIAGNOSTIC LABORATORY, AND OTHER DIAGNOSTIC TESTS

Medicare covers diagnostic x-ray, diagnostic laboratory, and other diagnostic tests, including materials and the services of technicians. Medicare covers diagnostic X-ray services performed in a facility directed by a physician or group of physicians if they are performed under the direct supervision of a physician. Certain diagnostic X-ray procedures are also covered when performed by technicians without direct personal physician supervision if the technicians' general supervision and training, as well as the maintenance of the necessary equipment and supplies, are the continuing responsibility of a physician. Covered diagnostic tests include:

Histopathology

Tissue Decalcification

Bone Marrow Biopsy

Tissue Pathology

Surgical pathology

Frozen sections

Autopsy and sections

▲ **49220** Staging laparotomy for Hodgkins disease or lymphoma (includes splenectomy, needle or open biopsies of both liver lobes, possibly also removal of abdominal nodes, abdominal node and/or bone marrow biopsies, ovarian repositioning) 80 🔲

49250 Umbilectomy, omphalectomy, excision of umbilicus (separate procedure) ❹ 🔲

49255 Omentectomy, epiploectomy, resection of omentum (separate procedure) 80 🔲

LAPAROSCOPY

Surgical laparoscopy always includes diagnostic laparoscopy.

49320 Laparoscopy, abdomen, peritoneum, and omentum, diagnostic, with or without collection of specimen(s) by brushing or washing (separate procedure) ❸ 80 🔲

49321 Laparoscopy, surgical; with biopsy (single or multiple) ❹ 80 🔲

49322 with aspiration of cavity or cyst (eg, ovarian cyst) (single or multiple) ❹ 80 🔲

49323 with drainage of lymphocele to peritoneal cavity 80 🔲

> If percutaneous or open drainage is performed, consult CPT codes 49060 and 49061.

49329 Unlisted laparoscopy procedure, abdomen, peritoneum and omentum 80 50

INTRODUCTION, REVISION, AND/OR REMOVAL

49400* Injection of air or contrast into peritoneal cavity (separate procedure) 🔲

> For radiological supervision and interpretation, consult CPT code 74190.

49420* Insertion of intraperitoneal cannula or catheter for drainage or dialysis; temporary ❶ 🔲

49421 permanent ❶ 🔲

49422 Removal of permanent intraperitoneal cannula or catheter 🔲

> If a temporary catheter/cannula is removed, use the appropriate E/M code.

49423 Exchange of previously placed abscess or cyst drainage catheter under radiological guidance (separate procedure) 80 🔲

> For radiological supervision and interpretation, consult CPT code 75984.

▲ **49424** Contrast injection for assessment of abscess or cyst via previously placed drainage catheter or tube (separate procedure) 80 🔲

> For radiological supervision and interpretation, consult CPT code 76080.

49425 Insertion of peritoneal-venous shunt ❷ 80 🔲

49426 Revision of peritoneal-venous shunt ❷ 🔲

> If a shunt patency test is performed, consult CPT code 78291.

49427 Injection procedure (eg, contrast media) for evaluation of previously placed peritoneal-venous shunt 80 🔲

> For radiological supervision and interpretation, consult CPT code 75809, 78291.

49428 Ligation of peritoneal-venous shunt 🔲

49429 Removal of peritoneal-venous shunt 🔲

REPAIR — HERNIOPLASTY, HERNIORRHAPHY, HERNIOTOMY

In CPT, the hernia repair codes are categorized by the type of hernia, depending on the site.

There are many types of hernias, such the inguinal, which occurs in the inguinal canal. Codes are also determined by the recurrence of the hernia; such as "initial" or "recurrent." Also, review the physician's description of the presentation, such as "strangulated" or "incarcerated."

If an intra-abdominal hernia is reduced and repaired, consult CPT code 44050. If debridement is performed on the abdominal wall, consult CPT codes 11042 and 11043. If these procedures are performed bilaterally, append modifier -50 to the procedural code.

● **49491** Repair, initial inguinal hernia, preterm infant (less than 37 weeks gestation at birth), performed from birth up to 50 weeks post-conceptual age, with or without hydrocelectomy; reducible N

● **49492** incarcerated or strangulated N

> Post-conceptual age equals gestational age at birth plus age of infant in weeks at the time of the repair. To report initial inguinal hernia repairs that are performed on preterm infants who are over 50 weeks postconceptual age and under age 6 months at the time of surgery, consult CPT codes 49495, 49496.

▲ **49495** Repair, initial inguinal hernia, full term infant under age 6 months, or preterm infant over 50 weeks postconceptual age and under age 6 months at the time of surgery, with or without hydrocelectomy; reducible N 80 🔲 50

> **Halsted repair**

49496 incarcerated or strangulated N 80 🔲 50

> Post-conceptual age equals gestational age at birth plus age in weeks at the time of the repair. To report initial inguinal hernia repairs that are performed on preterm infants who are under or up to 50 weeks postconceptual age but under 6 months of age since birth, consult CPT codes 49491, 49492. For inguinal hernia repairs on infants age 6 months to under 5 years, consult CPT codes 49500-49501.

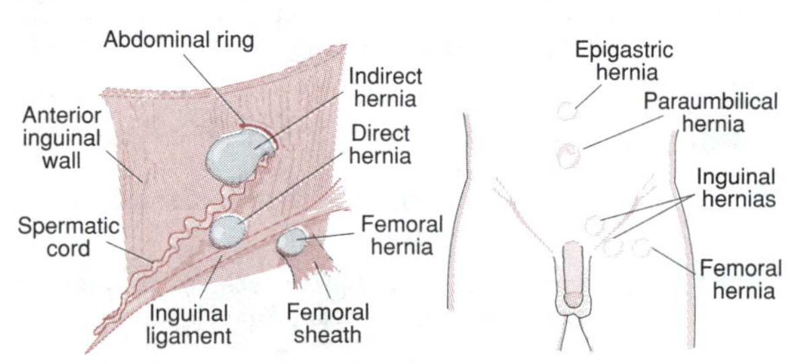

A hernia is a protrusion, usually through an abdominal wall containment. Often, hernias are congenital. Groin hernias are most common among both sexes and all age groups. In males, indirect hernias are often associated with incomplete closure of the path the testicle takes as it descends just prior to birth (the processus vaginalis). Direct hernias simply protrude through the wall. Femoral hernias occur below the inguinal ligament. Strangulation and necrosis of the protruding bowel section can occur. Umbilical hernias are often linked to incomplete closure of the umbilicus.

49500 Repair initial inguinal hernia, age 6 months to under 5 years, with or without hydrocelectomy; reducible `N/P` `80` `50`

49501 incarcerated or strangulated `N/P` `80` `50`

49505 Repair initial inguinal hernia, age 5 years or over; reducible `4` `80` `50`

MacEwen hernia repair

49507 incarcerated or strangulated `80` `50`

49520 Repair recurrent inguinal hernia, any age; reducible `7` `80` `50`

49521 incarcerated or strangulated `80` `50`

49525 Repair inguinal hernia, sliding, any age `4` `80` `50`

49540 Repair lumbar hernia `2` `80` `50`

49550 Repair initial femoral hernia, any age, reducible; `5` `80` `50`

49553 incarcerated or strangulated `80` `50`

49555 Repair recurrent femoral hernia; reducible `5` `80` `50`

49557 incarcerated or strangulated `80` `50`

49560 Repair initial incisional or ventral hernia; reducible `4` `80` `50`

49561 incarcerated or strangulated `80` `50`

49565 Repair recurrent incisional or ventral hernia; reducible `4` `80` `50`

49566 incarcerated or strangulated `80` `50`

+ **49568** Implantation of mesh or other prosthesis for incisional or ventral hernia repair (List separately in addition to code for the incisional or ventral hernia repair) `80` `50`

49570 Repair epigastric hernia (eg, preperitoneal fat); reducible (separate procedure) `4` `80` `50`

49572 incarcerated or strangulated `80` `50`

49580 Repair umbilical hernia, under age 5 years; reducible `N/P` `80`

49582 incarcerated or strangulated `N/P` `80`

49585 Repair umbilical hernia, age 5 years or over; reducible `4` `80`

Mayo hernia repair

49587 incarcerated or strangulated `80`

49590 Repair spigelian hernia `3` `80` `50`

49600 Repair of small omphalocele, with primary closure `80`

If a diaphragmatic or hiatal hernia is repaired, consult CPT codes 39502-39541.

49605 Repair of large omphalocele or gastroschisis; with or without prosthesis `80`

If a diaphragmatic or hiatal hernia is repaired, consult CPT codes 39502-39541.

If an intra-abdominal hernia is reduced and repaired, consult CPT code 44050.

49606 with removal of prosthesis, final reduction and closure, in operating room `80`

49610 Repair of omphalocele (Gross type operation); first stage `80`

49611 second stage `80`

LAPAROSCOPY

Surgical laparoscopy always includes diagnostic laparoscopy.

49650 Laparoscopy, surgical; repair initial inguinal hernia `4` `80` `50`

49651 repair recurrent inguinal hernia `7` `80` `50`

49659 Unlisted laparoscopy procedure, hernioplasty, herniorrhaphy, herniotomy `80` `50`

SUTURE

49900 Suture, secondary, of abdominal wall for evisceration or dehiscence `80`

If a ruptured diaphragm is sutured, consult CPT codes 39540 and 39541. If debridement is performed on the abdominal wall, consult CPT codes 11042 and 11043.

OTHER PROCEDURES

+ **49905** Omental flap (eg, for reconstruction of sternal and chest wall defects) (list separately in addition to code for primary procedure) `80`

49906 Free omental flap with microvascular anastomosis

Do not report 69990 in addition to 49906 as the operating microscope is considered an inclusive component of the surgery.

49999 Unlisted procedure, abdomen, peritoneum and omentum `80`

In 49525, a sliding inguinal hernia (depicted above, right) is repaired in a patient of any age.

URINARY SYSTEM

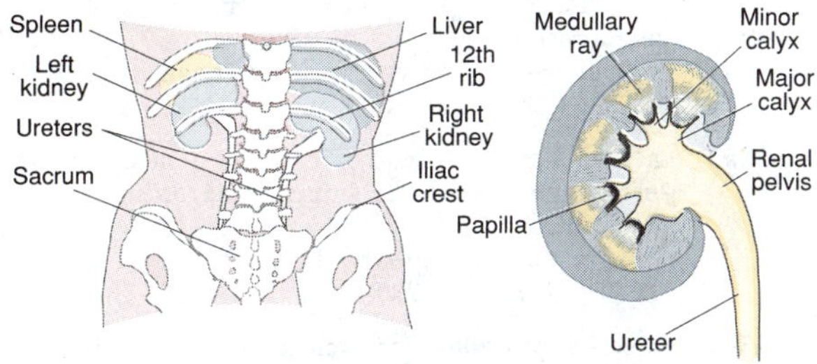

The kidneys remove waste products of protein metabolism and other excess materials and fluids from the blood. Variations in kidney anatomy are fairly common, though abnormalities can complicate procedures. "Pyelo" refers to the renal pelvis, an important access site to the inner kidney. Each kidney is imbedded in a mass of peritoneal fat that helps to enclose and position it

KIDNEY

INCISION

If retroperitoneal exploration is performed on an abscess, tumor, or cyst, consult CPT codes 49101, 49060, 49200, and 49201.

50010   **Renal exploration, not necessitating other specific procedures** 80

50020   **Drainage of perirenal or renal abscess; open** ❷

50021   **percutaneous** 80
For radiological supervision and interpretation, consult CPT code 75989.

50040   **Nephrostomy, nephrotomy with drainage** ❸

50045   **Nephrotomy, with exploration** 80
If renal endoscopy is performed in conjunction with this procedure, consult CPT codes 50570-50580.

50060   **Nephrolithotomy; removal of calculus** 80

50065   **secondary surgical operation for calculus** 80

50070   **complicated by congenital kidney abnormality** 80

50075   **removal of large staghorn calculus filling renal pelvis and calyces (including anatrophic pyelolithotomy)** 80

CIM 35-81 TREATMENT OF KIDNEY STONES

Medicare covers invasive and non-invasive lithotripsy techniques used in the surgical management of upper urinary tract kidney stones. In addition to the traditional surgical/endoscopic techniques for the treatment of kidney stones, the following lithotripsy techniques are also covered:

- Extracorporeal Shock Wave Lithotripsy (ESWL) is a non-invasive method of treating kidney stones using a device called a lithotriptor. The lithotriptor uses shock waves generated outside of the body to break up upper urinary tract stones. Medicare covers ESWL for treating upper urinary tract kidney stones

- Percutaneous lithotripsy (or nephrolithotomy) is an invasive method of treating kidney stones by using ultrasound, electrohydraulic or mechanical lithotripsy. Medicare covers percutaneous lithotripsy of kidney stones by ultrasound or by electrohydraulic or mechanical lithotripsy

- Transurethral ureteroscopic lithotripsy is a method of fragmenting and removing ureteral and renal stones through a cystoscope. Medicare covers transurethral ureteroscopic lithotripsy for the treatment of urinary tract stones of the kidney or ureter

CIM 35-59 ENDOSCOPY

Although endoscopy is primarily a diagnostic tool, it includes certain therapeutic procedures such as removal of polyps, and endoscopic papillotomy, by which stones are removed from the bile duct. Endoscopic procedures are covered when reasonable and necessary for the individual patient.

50080   **Percutaneous nephrostolithotomy or pyelostolithotomy, with or without dilation, endoscopy, lithotripsy, stenting or basket extraction; up to 2 cm**

50081   **over 2 cm** 80
If nephrostomy is established without a nephrostolithotomy, consult CPT codes 50040, 50395, and 52334. If fluoroscopic guidance is used, consult CPT codes 76000 and 76001.

50100   **Transection or repositioning of aberrant renal vessels (separate procedure)** 80

50120   **Pyelotomy; with exploration** 80
If renal endoscopy is performed in conjunction with this procedure, consult CPT codes 50570-50580.
Gol-Vernet pyelotomy

50125   **with drainage, pyelostomy** 80
If retroperitoneal exploration is performed on an abscess, tumor, or cyst, consult CPT codes 49101, 49060, 49200, and 49201.

50130   **with removal of calculus (pyelolithotomy, pelviolithotomy, including coagulum pyelolithotomy)** 80

50135   **complicated (eg, secondary operation, congenital kidney abnormality)** 80
Report 99070 for supply of anticarcinogenic agents when used, in addition to primary procedure.

EXCISION

If a retroperitoneal tumor or cyst is excised, consult CPT codes 49200 and 49201.

50200*   **Renal biopsy; percutaneous, by trocar or needle** ❶
For radiological supervision and interpretation, consult CPT codes 76003, 76360, 76393, and 76942.
To report fine needle aspiration, consult CPT code 10022.
To report evaluation of fine needle aspirate, consult CPT code 88172, 88173.

50205   **by surgical exposure of kidney** 80

▲ **50220**   **Nephrectomy, including partial ureterectomy, any open approach including rib resection;** 80

50225   **complicated because of previous surgery on same kidney** 80

50230   **radical, with regional lymphadenectomy and/or vena caval thrombectomy** 80
If vena caval resection with reconstruction is necessary, consult CPT code 37799.

50234   **Nephrectomy with total ureterectomy and bladder cuff; through same incision** 80

50236   **through separate incision** 80

50240   **Nephrectomy, partial** 80

50280   **Excision or unroofing of cyst(s) of kidney** 80
If laparoscopic ablation is performed on renal cysts, consult CPT code 50541.

50290   **Excision of perinephric cyst** 80

Urinary System

50300 — 50520

RENAL TRANSPLANTATION

If dialysis is performed, consult CPT codes 90935-90999. If laparoscopic drainage of a lymphocele to peritoneal cavity is performed, consult CPT code 49323.

If a laparoscopic donor nephrectomy is performed, consult CPT code 50547.

CIM 35-58 THORACIC DUCT DRAINAGE (TDD) IN RENAL TRANSPLANTS

Thoracic duct drainage (TDD) is performed on an inpatient basis, and the inpatient stay is covered for patients admitted for treatment in advance of a kidney transplant as well as for those receiving it post-transplant. TDD is a covered technique when furnished to a kidney transplant recipient or an individual approved to receive kidney transplantation in a hospital approved to perform kidney transplantation.

CIM 35-71 NONSELECTIVE (RANDOM) TRANSFUSIONS AND LIVING—RELATED DONOR SPECIFIC TRANSFUSIONS (DST) IN KIDNEY TRANSPLANTATION

Pretransplant transfusions are covered under Medicare without a specific limit on the number of transfusions, subject to the normal Medicare blood deductible provisions. Where blood is given directly to the transplant patient, (e.g., donor specific transfusions) the blood is considered replaced for purposes of blood deductible provisions.

50300   Donor nephrectomy, with preparation and maintenance of allograft, from cadaver donor, unilateral or bilateral

50320   Donor nephrectomy, open from living donor (excluding preparation and maintenance of allograft)

50340   Recipient nephrectomy (separate procedure)

50360   Renal allotransplantation, implantation of graft; excluding donor and recipient nephrectomy

50365   with recipient nephrectomy

CIM 45-22 LYMPHOCYTE IMMUNE GLOBULIN, ANTI-THYMOCYTE GLOBULIN (EQUINE)

The Food and Drug Administration (FDA) has approved one lymphocyte immune globulin preparation, anti-thymocyte globulin (equine). Medicare covers equine when used for managing allograft rejection episodes in renal transplantation.

CIM 50-23 HISTOCOMPATIBILITY TESTING

Histocompatibility testing is covered when it is performed on patients:

- In preparation for a kidney transplant
- In preparation for bone marrow transplantation
- In preparation for blood platelet transfusions (particularly where multiple infusions are involved)
- Who are suspected of having ankylosing spondylitis

It is covered for ankylosing spondylitis when other methods of diagnosis would not be appropriate or have yielded inconclusive results. Documentation is required.

50370   Removal of transplanted renal allograft

50380   Renal autotransplantation, reimplantation of kidney

If extra-corporeal "bench" surgery is performed, report autotransplantation as the primary procedure and then add the secondary procedure (e.g., partial nephrectomy, nephrolithotomy) and append modifier -51 or 09951.

INTRODUCTION

50390*   Aspiration and/or injection of renal cyst or pelvis by needle, percutaneous

For radiological supervision and interpretation, consult CPT codes 74425, 74470, 76003, 76360, 76393, 76942.

For evaluation of fine needle aspirate, consult CPT codes 88172, 88173.

50392   Introduction of intracatheter or catheter into renal pelvis for drainage and/or injection, percutaneous

For radiological supervision and interpretation, consult CPT codes 74475, 76360, and 76942.

50393   Introduction of ureteral catheter or stent into ureter through renal pelvis for drainage and/or injection, percutaneous

For radiological supervision and interpretation, consult CPT codes 74480, 76003, 76360, 76942.

50394   Injection procedure for pyelography (as nephrostogram, pyelostogram, antegrade pyeloureterograms) through nephrostomy or pyelostomy tube, or indwelling ureteral catheter

For radiological supervision and interpretation, consult CPT code 74425.

50395   Introduction of guide into renal pelvis and/or ureter with dilation to establish nephrostomy tract, percutaneous

If a nephrostolithotomy is performed, consult CPT codes 50080 and 50081. If a retrograde percutaneous nephrostomy is performed, consult CPT code 52334. If endoscopic surgery is performed, consult CPT codes 50551-50561.

For radiological supervision and interpretation, consult CPT codes 74475, 74480, 74485.

50396   Manometric studies through nephrostomy or pyelostomy tube, or indwelling ureteral catheter

For radiological supervision and interpretation, consult CPT codes 74425, 74475, 74480.

50398*   Change of nephrostomy or pyelostomy tube

If fluoroscopic guidance is used, consult CPT code 76000. If radiological supervision and interpretation is performed, consult CPT code 75984.

REPAIR

50400   Pyeloplasty (Foley Y-pyeloplasty), plastic operation on renal pelvis, with or without plastic operation on ureter, nephropexy, nephrostomy, pyelostomy, or ureteral splinting; simple

50405   complicated (congenital kidney abnormality, secondary pyeloplasty, solitary kidney, calycoplasty)

If a laparoscopic approach is used, consult CPT code 50544.

50500   Nephrorrhaphy, suture of kidney wound or injury

50520   Closure of nephrocutaneous or pyelocutaneous fistula

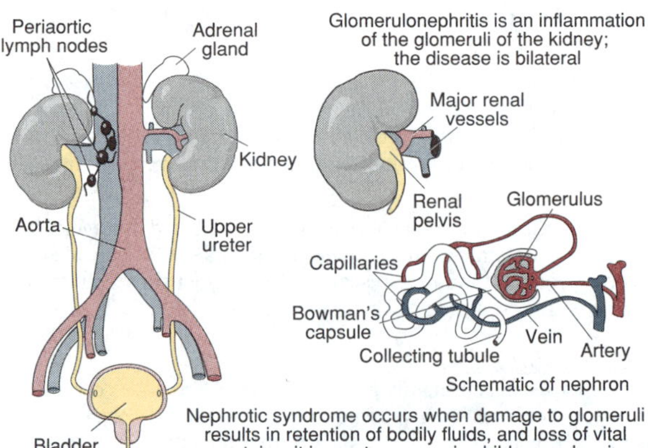

50525	Closure of nephrovisceral fistula (eg, renocolic), including visceral repair; abdominal approach [80]
50526	thoracic approach [80]
50540	Symphysiotomy for horseshoe kidney with or without pyeloplasty and/or other plastic procedure, unilateral or bilateral (one operation) [80]

LAPAROSCOPY

If laparoscopic drainage is performed of a lymphocele to the peritoneal cavity, consult CPT code 49323.

50541	Laparoscopy, surgical; ablation of renal cysts [80]
50544	pyeloplasty [80]
● 50545	radical nephrectomy (includes removal of Gerota's fascia and surrounding fatty tissue, removal of regional lymph nodes, and adrenalectomy) [80] [50] Consult CPT code 50230 for open procedure.
▲ 50546	nephrectomy, including partial ureterectomy [80] If laparoscopic drainage is performed of a lymphocele to the peritoneal cavity, consult CPT code 49323.
50547	donor nephrectomy from living donor (excluding preparation and maintenance of allograft) [80] [50] Consult CPT code 50230 for open procedure
▲ 50548	nephrectomy with total ureterectomy [80] Consult CPT codes 50234, 50236 for open procedure.
50549	Unlisted laparoscopy procedure, renal [80] [50]

ENDOSCOPY

CIM 35-59 ENDOSCOPY

Although endoscopy is primarily a diagnostic tool, it includes certain therapeutic procedures such as removal of polyps, and endoscopic papillotomy, by which stones are removed from the bile duct. Endoscopic procedures are covered when reasonable and necessary for the individual patient.

To report supplies and material, consult CPT code 99070.

50551	Renal endoscopy through established nephrostomy or pyelostomy, with or without irrigation, instillation, or ureteropyelography, exclusive of radiologic service; [O] [80] [50]
50553	with ureteral catheterization, with or without dilation of ureter [O] [50]
50555	with biopsy [O] [80] [50]
50557	with fulguration and/or incision, with or without biopsy [O] [80] [50]
50559	with insertion of radioactive substance with or without biopsy and/or fulguration [O] [80] [50]
50561	with removal of foreign body or calculus [O] [80] [50] If these procedures provide a significant identifiable service, they may be added to 50045 and 50120.
50570	Renal endoscopy through nephrotomy or pyelotomy, with or without irrigation, instillation, or ureteropyelography, exclusive of radiologic service; [O] [80] [50] If a nephrotomy is performed, consult CPT code 50045. If a pyelotomy is performed, consult CPT code 50120.
50572	with ureteral catheterization, with or without dilation of ureter [O] [80] [50]
50574	with biopsy [O] [80] [50]
50575	with endopyelotomy (includes cystoscopy, ureteroscopy, dilation of ureter and ureteral pelvic junction, incision of ureteral pelvic junction and insertion of endopyelotomy stent) [50]
50576	with fulguration and/or incision, with or without biopsy [O] [80] [50]

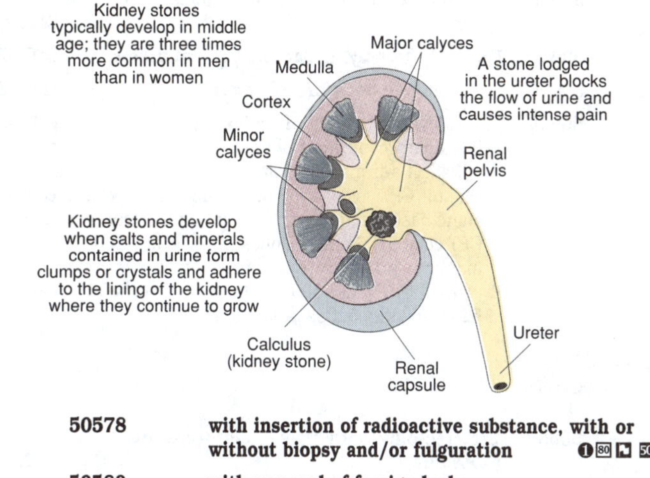

50578	with insertion of radioactive substance, with or without biopsy and/or fulguration [O] [80] [50]
50580	with removal of foreign body or calculus [O] [80] [50]

OTHER PROCEDURES

CIM 35-81 TREATMENT OF KIDNEY STONES

Medicare covers invasive and non-invasive lithotripsy techniques used in the surgical management of upper urinary tract kidney stones. In addition to the traditional surgical/endoscopic techniques for the treatment of kidney stones, the following lithotripsy techniques are also covered:

- Extracorporeal Shock Wave Lithotripsy (ESWL) is a non-invasive method of treating kidney stones using a device called a lithotriptor. The lithotriptor uses shock waves generated outside of the body to break up upper urinary tract stones. Medicare covers ESWL for treating upper urinary tract kidney stones

- Percutaneous lithotripsy (or nephrolithotomy) is an invasive method of treating kidney stones by using ultrasound, electrohydraulic or mechanical lithotripsy. Medicare covers percutaneous lithotripsy of kidney stones by ultrasound or by electrohydraulic or mechanical lithotripsy

- Transurethral ureteroscopic lithotripsy is a method of fragmenting and removing ureteral and renal stones through a cystoscope. Medicare covers transurethral ureteroscopic lithotripsy for the treatment of urinary tract stones of the kidney or ureter

50590	Lithotripsy, extracorporeal shock wave [50]

URETER

INCISION

50600	Ureterotomy with exploration or drainage (separate procedure) [80] [50] If ureteral endoscopy is performed in conjunction with this procedure, consult CPT codes 50970-50980.

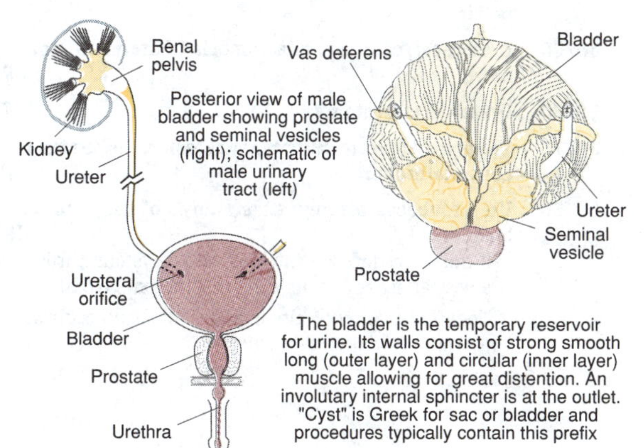

Urinary System

50605 — 50949

50605	Ureterotomy for insertion of indwelling stent, all types	80 ↰ 50
50610	Ureterolithotomy; upper one-third of ureter	80 ↰ 50
50620	middle one-third of ureter	80 ↰ 50
50630	lower one-third of ureter	80 ↰ 50

If a laparoscopic approach is used, consult CPT code 50945. If a transvesical ureterolithotomy is performed, consult CPT code 51060. If a cystotomy is performed with stone basket extraction of the ureteral calculus, consult CPT code 51065. If an endoscopic extraction or manipulation of the ureteral calculus is performed, consult CPT codes 50080, 50081, 50561, 50961, 50980, 52320-52330, 52352, and 52353.

EXCISION

For ureterocele, see 51535, 52300.

50650	Ureterectomy, with bladder cuff (separate procedure)	80 ↰
50660	Ureterectomy, total, ectopic ureter, combination abdominal, vaginal and/or perineal approach	80 ↰

INTRODUCTION

50684	Injection procedure for ureterography or ureteropyelography through ureterostomy or indwelling ureteral catheter	❶ ↰ 50

For radiological supervision and interpretation, consult CPT code 74425.

50686	Manometric studies through ureterostomy or indwelling ureteral catheter	80 ↰
50688*	Change of ureterostomy tube	❶ ↰

For imaging guidance consult CPT code 75984

50690	Injection procedure for visualization of ileal conduit and/or ureteropyelography, exclusive of radiologic service	❶ ↰

For radiological supervision and interpretation, consult CPT code 74425.

REPAIR

50700	Ureteroplasty, plastic operation on ureter (eg, stricture)	80 ↰
50715	Ureterolysis, with or without repositioning of ureter for retroperitoneal fibrosis	80 ↰ 50
50722	Ureterolysis for ovarian vein syndrome	♀ 80 ↰
50725	Ureterolysis for retrocaval ureter, with reanastomosis of upper urinary tract or vena cava	80 ↰
50727	Revision of urinary-cutaneous anastomosis (any type urostomy);	80 ↰
50728	with repair of fascial defect and hernia	80 ↰
50740	Ureteropyelostomy, anastomosis of ureter and renal pelvis	80 ↰
50750	Ureterocalycostomy, anastomosis of ureter to renal calyx	80 ↰
50760	Ureteroureterostomy	80 ↰
50770	Transureteroureterostomy, anastomosis of ureter to contralateral ureter	80 ↰
50780	Ureteroneocystostomy; anastomosis of single ureter to bladder	80 ↰ 50

If this procedure is combined with a cystourethroplasty or a vesical neck revision, consult CPT code 51820.

Note that this procedure includes minor procedures to prevent vesicoureteral reflux.

50782	anastomosis of duplicated ureter to bladder	80 ↰ 50

Note that this procedure includes minor procedures to prevent vesicoureteral reflux.

50783	with extensive ureteral tailoring	80 ↰ 50

Note that this procedure includes minor procedures to prevent vesicoureteral reflux.

50785	with vesico-psoas hitch or bladder flap	80 ↰ 50

Note that this procedure includes minor procedures to prevent vesicoureteral reflux.

50800	Ureteroenterostomy, direct anastomosis of ureter to intestine	80 ↰ 50

If these procedures 50800-50820 are performed with a cystectomy, consult CPT codes 51580-51595.

▲ **50810**	Ureterosigmoidostomy, with creation of sigmoid bladder and establishment of abdominal or perineal colostomy, including intestine anastomosis	80 ↰
▲ **50815**	Ureterocolon conduit, including intestine anastomosis	80 ↰ 50
▲ **50820**	Ureteroileal conduit (ileal bladder), including intestine anastomosis (Bricker operation)	80 ↰ 50
▲ **50825**	Continent diversion, including intestine anastomosis using any segment of small and/or large intestine (Kock pouch or Camey enterocystoplasty)	80 ↰
50830	Urinary undiversion (eg, taking down of ureteroileal conduit, ureterosigmoidostomy or ureteroenterostomy with ureteroureterostomy or ureteroneocystostomy)	80 ↰
▲ **50840**	Replacement of all or part of ureter by intestine segment, including intestine anastomosis	80 ↰ 50
50845	Cutaneous appendico-vesicostomy	80 ↰
	Mitrofanoff operation	

<u>*CIM 45-22 LYMPHOCYTE IMMUNE GLOBULIN, ANTI-THYMOCYTE GLOBULIN (EQUINE)*</u>

The Food and Drug Administration (FDA) has approved one lymphocyte immune globulin preparation, anti-thymocyte globulin (equine). Medicare covers equine when used for managing allograft rejection episodes in renal transplantation.

50860	Ureterostomy, transplantation of ureter to skin	80 ↰ 50
50900	Ureterorrhaphy, suture of ureter (separate procedure)	80 ↰
50920	Closure of ureterocutaneous fistula	80 ↰
50930	Closure of ureterovisceral fistula (including visceral repair)	80 ↰
50940	Deligation of ureter	80 ↰ 50

If ureteroplasty or ureterolysis is performed, consult CPT codes 50700-50860.

LAPAROSCOPY

50945	Laparoscopy, surgical; ureterolithotomy	80 ↰ 50
50947	ureteroneocystostomy with cystoscopy and ureteral stent placement	80 50
50948	ureteroneocystostomy without cystoscopy and ureteral stent placement	80 50
50949	Unlisted laparoscopy procedure, ureter	80 50

ENDOSCOPY

<u>*CIM 35-59 ENDOSCOPY*</u>

Although endoscopy is primarily a diagnostic tool, it includes certain therapeutic procedures such as removal of polyps, and endoscopic papillotomy, by which stones are removed from the bile duct. Endoscopic procedures are covered when reasonable and necessary for the individual patient.

26 Professional Component Only	**80/80** Assist-at-Surgery Allowed/With Documentation	Unlisted
TC Technical Component Only	**MCM & CIM** Medicare References ❶❷❸❹❺❻❼❽ ASC Group	Commonly Miscoded Not Covered
	♂ Male Only ♀ Female Only	

50951	Ureteral endoscopy through established ureterostomy, with or without irrigation, instillation, or uretero-pyelography, exclusive of radiologic service;
50953	with ureteral catheterization, with or without dilation of ureter
50955	with biopsy
50957	with fulguration and/or incision, with or without biopsy
50959	with insertion of radioactive substance, with or without biopsy and/or fulguration (not including provision of material)
50961	with removal of foreign body or calculus
50970	Ureteral endoscopy through ureterotomy, with or without irrigation, instillation, or ureteropyelography, exclusive of radiologic service;

If a ureterotomy is performed, consult CPT code 50600.

If these procedures (50970-50980) provide a significant identifiable service, they may be added to 50600.

50972	with ureteral catheterization, with or without dilation of ureter
50974	with biopsy
50976	with fulguration and/or incision, with or without biopsy
50978	with insertion of radioactive substance, with or without biopsy and/or fulguration (not including provision of material)
50980	with removal of foreign body or calculus

BLADDER

INCISION

51000*	Aspiration of bladder by needle
51005*	Aspiration of bladder; by trocar or intracatheter
51010	with insertion of suprapubic catheter

To report imaging guidance, consult CPT codes 76003, 76360, 76942.

51020	Cystotomy or cystostomy; with fulguration and/or insertion of radioactive material
51030	with cryosurgical destruction of intravesical lesion
51040	Cystostomy, cystotomy with drainage
51045	Cystotomy, with insertion of ureteral catheter or stent (separate procedure)
51050	Cystolithotomy, cystotomy with removal of calculus, without vesical neck resection
51060	Transvesical ureterolithotomy
▲ 51065	Cystotomy, with calculus basket extraction and/or ultrasonic or electrohydraulic fragmentation of ureteral calculus
51080	Drainage of perivesical or prevesical space abscess

EXCISION

51500	Excision of urachal cyst or sinus, with or without umbilical hernia repair
51520	Cystotomy; for simple excision of vesical neck (separate procedure)
51525	for excision of bladder diverticulum, single or multiple (separate procedure)
51530	for excision of bladder tumor

If transurethral resection is performed, consult CPT codes 52234-52240 and 52305.

| 51535 | Cystotomy for excision, incision, or repair of ureterocele |

If a transurethral excision is performed, consult CPT code 52300.

51550	Cystectomy, partial; simple
51555	complicated (eg, postradiation, previous surgery, difficult location)
51565	Cystectomy, partial, with reimplantation of ureter(s) into bladder (ureteroneocystostomy)
51570	Cystectomy, complete; (separate procedure)
51575	with bilateral pelvic lymphadenectomy, including external iliac, hypogastric, and obturator nodes
51580	Cystectomy, complete, with ureterosigmoidostomy or ureterocutaneous transplantations;
51585	with bilateral pelvic lymphadenectomy, including external iliac, hypogastric, and obturator nodes
▲ 51590	Cystectomy, complete, with ureteroileal conduit or sigmoid bladder, including intestine anastomosis;
51595	with bilateral pelvic lymphadenectomy, including external iliac, hypogastric, and obturator nodes
▲ 51596	Cystectomy, complete, with continent diversion, any open technique, using any segment of small and/or large intestine to construct neobladder
51597	Pelvic exenteration, complete, for vesical, prostatic or urethral malignancy, with removal of bladder and ureteral transplantations, with or without hysterectomy and/or abdominoperineal resection of rectum and colon and colostomy, or any combination thereof

If a pelvic exenteration is performed for gynecologic malignancy, consult CPT code 58240.

INTRODUCTION

CIM 50-33 UROFLOWMETRIC EVALUATIONS

Medicare covers uroflowmetric evaluations (also referred to as urodynamic voiding or urodynamic flow studies) for diagnosing various urological dysfunctions, including bladder outlet obstructions.

If bladder catheterization is performed, consult CPT codes 53670 and 53675.

| 51600* | Injection procedure for cystography or voiding urethrocystography |

For radiological supervision and interpretation, consult CPT codes 74430 and 74455.

| 51605 | Injection procedure and placement of chain for contrast and/or chain urethrocystography |

For radiological supervision and interpretation, consult CPT code 74430.

| 51610 | Injection procedure for retrograde urethrocystography |

For radiological supervision and interpretation, consult CPT code 74450.

51700*	Bladder irrigation, simple, lavage and/or instillation
51705*	Change of cystostomy tube; simple
51710*	complicated

Consult CPT code 75984 for imaging guidance.

| 51715 | Endoscopic injection of implant material into the submucosal tissues of the urethra and/or bladder neck |
| 51720 | Bladder instillation of anticarcinogenic agent (including detention time) |

URODYNAMICS

CPT codes 51725-51797 imply that ALL supplies, equipment, and technician's fees are provided by the physician. If the physician only interprets the results and/or operates the equipment, modifier -26 should be appended.

51725	Simple cystometrogram (CMG) (eg, spinal manometer)	
51726	Complex cystometrogram (eg, calibrated electronic equipment)	
51736	Simple uroflowmetry (UFR) (eg, stop-watch flow rate, mechanical uroflowmeter)	
51741	Complex uroflowmetry (eg, calibrated electronic equipment)	
51772	Urethral pressure profile studies (UPP) (urethral closure pressure profile), any technique	
	Keitzer test	
51784	Electromyography studies (EMG) of anal or urethral sphincter, other than needle, any technique	
51785	Needle electromyography studies (EMG) of anal or urethral sphincter, any technique	
51792	Stimulus evoked response (eg, measurement of bulbocavernosus reflex latency time)	
51795	Voiding pressure studies (VP); bladder voiding pressure, any technique	
51797	intra-abdominal voiding pressure (AP) (rectal, gastric, intraperitoneal)	

REPAIR

51800	Cystoplasty or cystourethroplasty, plastic operation on bladder and/or vesical neck (anterior Y-plasty, vesical fundus resection), any procedure, with or without wedge resection of posterior vesical neck	
51820	Cystourethroplasty with unilateral or bilateral ureteroneocystostomy	
51840	Anterior vesicourethropexy, or urethropexy (eg, Marshall-Marchetti-Krantz, Burch); simple	
51841	complicated (eg, secondary repair)	

If urethropexy (Pereyra type) is performed, consult CPT code 57289.

51845	Abdomino-vaginal vesical neck suspension, with or without endoscopic control (eg, Stamey, Raz, modified Pereyra)	
51860	Cystorrhaphy, suture of bladder wound, injury or rupture; simple	
51865	complicated	
51880	Closure of cystostomy (separate procedure)	
51900	Closure of vesicovaginal fistula, abdominal approach	

If a vaginal approach is used, consult CPT codes 57320-57330.

51920	Closure of vesicouterine fistula;	
51925	with hysterectomy	

If a vesicoenteric fistula is closed, consult CPT codes 44660 and 44661. If a rectovesical fistula is closed, consult CPT codes 45800-45805.

▲ 51940	Closure, exstrophy of bladder	

Consult also CPT code 54390.

▲ 51960	Enterocystoplasty, including intestinal anastomosis	
51980	Cutaneous vesicostomy	

LAPAROSCOPY

Diagnostic laparoscopy is always included in a surgical laparoscopy. For diagnostic laparoscopy only, consult CPT code 49320.

51990	Laparoscopy, surgical; urethral suspension for stress incontinence	
51992	sling operation for stress incontinence (eg, fascia or synthetic)	

Consult CPT code 57288 for open sling operation for stress incontinence. For removal or revision of sling operation consult CPT code 57287.

ENDOSCOPY-CYSTOSCOPY, URETHROSCOPY, CYSTOURETHROSCOPY

52000	Cystourethroscopy (separate procedure)	
● 52001	Cystourethroscopy with irrigation and evacuation of clots	

Do not report 52001 in conjunction with 52000.

52005	Cystourethroscopy, with ureteral catheterization, with or without irrigation, instillation, or ureteropyelography, exclusive of radiologic service;	
	Howard test	
52007	with brush biopsy of ureter and/or renal pelvis	
52010	Cystourethroscopy, with ejaculatory duct catheterization, with or without irrigation, instillation, or duct radiography, exclusive of radiologic service	

For radiological supervision and interpretation, consult CPT code 74440.

TRANSURETHRAL SURGERY, URETHRA AND BLADDER

52204	Cystourethroscopy, with biopsy	
52214	Cystourethroscopy, with fulguration (including cryosurgery or laser surgery) of trigone, bladder neck, prostatic fossa, urethra, or periurethral glands	
52224	Cystourethroscopy, with fulguration (including cryosurgery or laser surgery) or treatment of MINOR (less than 0.5 cm) lesion(s) with or without biopsy	
52234	Cystourethroscopy, with fulguration (including cryosurgery or laser surgery) and/or resection of; SMALL bladder tumor(s) (0.5 to 2.0 cm)	
52235	MEDIUM bladder tumor(s) (2.0 to 5.0 cm)	
52240	LARGE bladder tumor(s)	
52250	Cystourethroscopy with insertion of radioactive substance, with or without biopsy or fulguration	

CIM 45-23 DIMETHYL SULFOXIDE (DMSO)

Medicare covers dimethyl sulfoxide (DMSO) when reasonable and necessary for a patient in the treatment of interstitial cystitis.

52260	Cystourethroscopy, with dilation of bladder for interstitial cystitis; general or conduction (spinal) anesthesia	
52265	local anesthesia	
52270	Cystourethroscopy, with internal urethrotomy; female	
52275	male	
52276	Cystourethroscopy with direct vision internal urethrotomy	
52277	Cystourethroscopy, with resection of external sphincter (sphincterotomy)	
52281	Cystourethroscopy, with calibration and/or dilation of urethral stricture or stenosis, with or without meatotomy, with or without injection procedure for cystography, male or female	

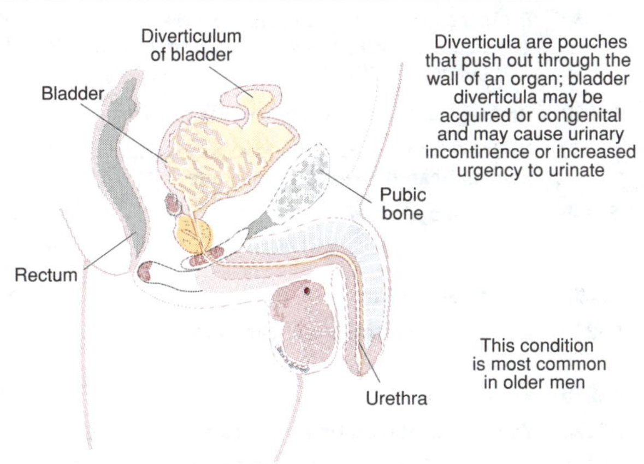

52282	Cystourethroscopy, with insertion of urethral stent	
52283	Cystourethroscopy, with steroid injection into stricture	
52285	Cystourethroscopy for treatment of the female urethral syndrome with any or all of the following: urethral meatotomy, urethral dilation, internal urethrotomy, lysis of urethrovaginal septal fibrosis, lateral incisions of the bladder neck, and fulguration of polyp(s) of urethra, bladder neck, and/or trigone	♀
52290	Cystourethroscopy; with ureteral meatotomy, unilateral or bilateral	
52300	with resection or fulguration of orthotopic ureterocele(s), unilateral or bilateral	
52301	with resection or fulguration of ectopic ureterocele(s), unilateral or bilateral	
52305	with incision or resection of orifice of bladder diverticulum, single or multiple	
52310	Cystourethroscopy, with removal of foreign body, calculus, or ureteral stent from urethra or bladder (separate procedure); simple	
52315	complicated	
52317	Litholapaxy: crushing or fragmentation of calculus by any means in bladder and removal of fragments; simple or small (less than 2.5 cm)	
52318	complicated or large (over 2.5 cm)	

URETER AND PELVIS

CPT codes 52320-52355 include the insertion and removal of a temporary stent during a therapeutic or diagnostic cystourethroscopy and should not be reported separately.

CPT codes 52320-52355 include the insertion and removal of a temporary stent during a therapeutic or diagnostic cystourethroscopy and should not be reported separately.

CPT code 52332 is considered a unilateral procedure.

52320	Cystourethroscopy (including ureteral catheterization); with removal of ureteral calculus	
52325	with fragmentation of ureteral calculus (eg, ultrasonic or electro-hydraulic technique)	
52327	with subureteric injection of implant material	
52330	with manipulation, without removal of ureteral calculus	
52332	Cystourethroscopy, with insertion of indwelling ureteral stent (eg, Gibbons or double-J type)	

52334	Cystourethroscopy with insertion of ureteral guide wire through kidney to establish a percutaneous nephrostomy, retrograde	

If percutaneous nephrolithotomy is performed, consult CPT codes 50080 and 50081. If establishment of the nephrostomy tract is performed by itself, consult CPT code 50395.

52341	Cystourethroscopy; with treatment of ureteral stricture (eg, balloon dilation, laser, electrocautery, and incision)	
52342	with treatment of ureteropelvic junction stricture (eg, balloon dilation, laser, electrocautery, and incision)	
52343	with treatment of intra-renal stricture (eg, balloon dilation, laser, electrocautery, and incision)	
52344	Cystourethroscopy with ureteroscopy; with treatment of ureteral stricture (eg, balloon dilation, laser, electrocautery, and incision)	
52345	with treatment of ureteropelvic junction stricture (eg, balloon dilation, laser, electrocautery, and incision)	
52346	with treatment of intra-renal stricture (eg, balloon dilation, laser, electrocautery, and incision)	
● 52347	Cystourethroscopy with transurethral resection or incision of ejaculatory ducts	♂
52351	Cystourethroscopy, with ureteroscopy and/or pyeloscopy; diagnostic	

For radiological supervision and interpretation, consult CPT code 74485.

Do not report CPT code 52351 when reporting 52341-52346, or 52352-52355.

52352	with removal or manipulation of calculus (ureteral catheterization is included)	

CIM 35-81 TREATMENT OF KIDNEY STONES

Medicare covers invasive and non-invasive lithotripsy techniques used in the surgical management of upper urinary tract kidney stones. In addition to the traditional surgical/endoscopic techniques for the treatment of kidney stones, the following lithotripsy techniques are also covered:

- Extracorporeal Shock Wave Lithotripsy (ESWL) is a non-invasive method of treating kidney stones using a device called a lithotriptor. The lithotriptor uses shock waves generated outside of the body to break up upper urinary tract stones. Medicare covers ESWL for treating upper urinary tract kidney stones

- Percutaneous lithotripsy (or nephrolithotomy) is an invasive method of treating kidney stones by using ultrasound, electrohydraulic or mechanical lithotripsy. Medicare covers percutaneous lithotripsy of kidney stones by ultrasound or by electrohydraulic or mechanical lithotripsy

Transurethral ureteroscopic lithotripsy is a method of fragmenting and removing ureteral and renal stones through a cystoscope. Medicare covers transurethral ureteroscopic lithotripsy for the treatment of urinary tract stones of the kidney or ureter.

52353	with lithotripsy (ureteral catheterization is included)	
52354	with biopsy and/or fulguration of lesion	
52355	with resection of tumor	

VESICAL NECK AND PROSTATE

52400	Cystourethroscopy with incision, fulguration, or re-section of congenital posterior urethral valves, or congenital obstructive hypertrophic mucosal folds	
52450	Transurethral incision of prostate	♂

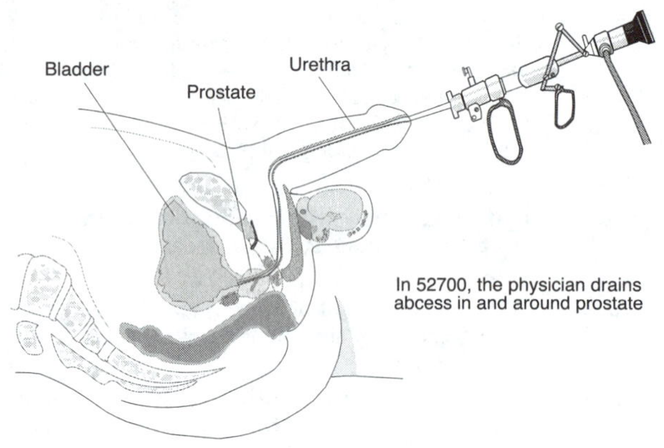

52500	Transurethral resection of bladder neck (separate procedure)	❸
▲ 52510	Transurethral balloon dilation of the prostatic urethra	♂
52601	Transurethral electrosurgical resection of prostate, including control of postoperative bleeding, complete (vasectomy, meatotomy, cystourethroscopy, urethral calibration and/or dilation, and internal urethrotomy are included)	♂❹
	If other approaches are used, consult CPT codes 55801-55845.	
52606	Transurethral fulguration for postoperative bleeding occurring after the usual follow-up time	❶
52612	Transurethral resection of prostate; first stage of two-stage resection (partial resection)	♂❷
52614	second stage of two-stage resection (resection completed)	♂❶
52620	Transurethral resection; of residual obstructive tissue after 90 days postoperative	❶
52630	of regrowth of obstructive tissue longer than one year postoperative	❷
52640	of postoperative bladder neck contracture	❷
52647	Non-contact laser coagulation of prostate, including control of postoperative bleeding, complete (vasectomy, meatotomy, cystourethroscopy, urethral calibration and/or dilation, and internal urethrotomy are included)	♂
52648	Contact laser vaporization with or without transurethral resection of prostate, including control of postoperative bleeding, complete (vasectomy, meatotomy, cystourethroscopy, urethral calibration and/or dilation, and internal urethrotomy are included)	♂
52700	Transurethral drainage of prostatic abscess	♂❷[80]

URETHRA

If an endoscopy is performed, consult cystoscopy, urethroscopy, and cystourethroscopy procedures, 52000-52700. If an injection procedure is performed for urethrocystography, consult CPT codes 51600-51610.

INCISION

53000	Urethrotomy or urethrostomy, external (separate procedure); pendulous urethra	❶
53010	perineal urethra, external	❶
53020	Meatotomy, cutting of meatus (separate procedure); except infant	❶
53025	infant	N [80]

53040	Drainage of deep periurethral abscess	❷[80]
	If a subcutaneous abscess is drained, consult CPT codes 10060 and 10061.	
53060	Drainage of Skene's gland abscess or cyst	
53080	Drainage of perineal urinary extravasation; uncomplicated (separate procedure)	
53085	complicated	[80]

EXCISION

53200	Biopsy of urethra	❶
53210	Urethrectomy, total, including cystostomy; female	♀❺[80]
53215	male	♂❺[80]
53220	Excision or fulguration of carcinoma of urethra	❷[80]
53230	Excision of urethral diverticulum (separate procedure); female	♀❷[80]
53235	male	♂❸[80]
53240	Marsupialization of urethral diverticulum, male or female	❷
53250	Excision of bulbourethral gland (Cowper's gland)	❷
53260	Excision or fulguration; urethral polyp(s), distal urethra	❷
	If an endoscopic approach is used, consult CPT codes 52214 and 52224.	
53265	urethral caruncle	❷
53270	Skene's glands	
53275	urethral prolapse	❷

REPAIR

If hypospadias is repaired, consult CPT codes 54300-54352.

53400	Urethroplasty; first stage, for fistula, diverticulum, or stricture (eg, Johannsen type)	❸[80]
53405	second stage (formation of urethra), including urinary diversion	❷[80]
53410	Urethroplasty, one-stage reconstruction of male anterior urethra	♂❷[80]
53415	Urethroplasty, transpubic or perineal, one stage, for reconstruction or repair of prostatic or membranous urethra	♂[80]
53420	Urethroplasty, two-stage reconstruction or repair of prostatic or membranous urethra; first stage	♂❸
53425	second stage	♂❷[80]
53430	Urethroplasty, reconstruction of female urethra	♀❷[80]
● 53431	Urethroplasty with tubularization of posterior urethra and/or lower bladder for incontinence (eg, Tenago, Leadbetter procedure)	❷

CIM 65-9 INCONTINENCE CONTROL DEVICES

Prior to collagen implant therapy, a skin test for collagen sensitivity must be administered and evaluated over a four week period. In male patients, the evaluation must include a complete history and physical examination and a simple cystometrogram to determine that the bladder fills and stores properly. The patient then is asked to stand upright with a full bladder and to cough or otherwise exert abdominal pressure on his bladder. If the patient leaks, the diagnosis of ISD is established. In female patients, the evaluation must include a complete history and physical examination (including a pelvic exam) and a simple cystometrogram to rule out abnormalities of bladder compliance and abnormalities of urethral support. Following that determination, an abdominal leak point pressure (ALLP) test is performed. If the patient has an ALLP of less than 100 cm H_2O, the diagnosis of ISD is established.

To use a collagen implant, physicians must have urology training in the use of a cystoscope and must complete a collagen implant training program.

Coverage of a collagen implant, and the procedure to inject it, is limited to the following types of patients with stress urinary incontinence due to ISD:

a. Male or female patients with congenital sphincter weakness secondary to conditions such as myelomeningocele

b. Male or female patients with acquired sphincter weakness secondary to spinal cord lesions

c. Male patients following trauma, including prostatectomy and/or radiation

d. Female patients without urethral hypermobility and with abdominal leak point pressures of 100 cm H_2O or less

Patients whose incontinence does not improve with 5 injection procedures are considered treatment failures, and no further treatment of urinary incontinence by collagen implant is covered. Patients who have a reoccurrence of incontinence following successful treatment with collagen implants in the past may benefit from additional treatment sessions. Coverage of additional sessions must be supported by medical justification.

53440   **Operation for correction of male urinary incontinence, with or without introduction of prosthesis**

53442   **Removal of perineal prosthesis introduced for continence`**

~~**53443**~~   ~~**Urethroplasty with tubularization of posterior urethra and/or lower bladder for incontinence (eg, Tenago, Leadbetter procedure)**~~ This code is deleted in 2002. See code 53431.

● **53444**   **Insertion of tandem cuff (dual cuff)**

▲ **53445**   **Insertion of inflatable urethral/bladder neck sphincter, including placement of pump, reservoir, and cuff**

● **53446**   **Removal of inflatable urethral/bladder neck sphincter, including pump, reservoir, and cuff**

▲ **53447**   **Removal and replacement of inflatable urethral/bladder neck sphincter including pump, reservoir, and cuff at the same operative session**

● **53448**   **Removal and replacement of inflatable urethral/bladder neck sphincter including pump, reservoir, and cuff through an infected field at the same operative session including irrigation and debridement of infected tissue**

     Do not report 11040-11043 in conjunction with code 53448.

▲ **53449**   **Repair of inflatable urethral/bladder neck sphincter, including pump, reservoir, and cuff**

53450   **Urethromeatoplasty, with mucosal advancement**

     If a meatotomy is performed, consult CPT codes 53020 and 53025.

53460   **Urethromeatoplasty, with partial excision of distal urethral segment (Richardson type procedure)**

53502   **Urethrorrhaphy, suture of urethral wound or injury, female**

53505   **Urethrorrhaphy, suture of urethral wound or injury; penile**

53510   **perineal**

53515   **prostatomembranous**

53520   **Closure of urethrostomy or urethrocutaneous fistula, male (separate procedure)**

     If a urethrovaginal fistula is closed, consult CPT code 57310. If a urethrorectal fistula is closed, consult CPT codes 45820 and 45825.

MANIPULATION

For radiological supervision and interpretation, consult CPT code 74485.

If an endoscopy is performed, consult cystoscopy, urethroscopy, and cystourethroscopy procedures, 52000-52700. If an injection procedure is performed for urethrocystography, consult CPT codes 51600-51610.

53600*   **Dilation of urethral stricture by passage of sound or urethral dilator, male; initial**

53601*   **subsequent**

53605   **Dilation of urethral stricture or vesical neck by passage of sound or urethral dilator, male, general or conduction (spinal) anesthesia**

53620*   **Dilation of urethral stricture by passage of filiform and follower, male; initial**

53621*   **subsequent**

53660*   **Dilation of female urethra including suppository and/or instillation; initial**

53661*   **subsequent**

53665   **Dilation of female urethra, general or conduction (spinal) anesthesia**

53670*   **Catheterization, urethra; simple**

53675*   **complicated (may include difficult removal of balloon catheter)**

OTHER PROCEDURES

If an endoscopy is performed, consult cystoscopy, urethroscopy, and cystourethroscopy procedures, 52000-52700. If an injection procedure is performed for urethrocystography, consult CPT codes 51600-51610.

53850   **Transurethral destruction of prostate tissue; by microwave thermotherapy**

53852   **by radiofrequency thermotherapy**

● **53853**   **by water-induced thermotherapy**

53899   **Unlisted procedure, urinary system**

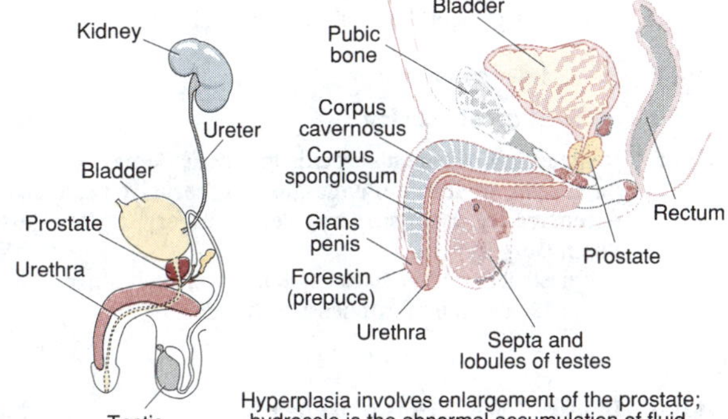

Hyperplasia involves enlargement of the prostate; hydrocele is the abnormal accumulation of fluid in the scrotum; orchitis is inflammation of a testis; balanitis is inflammation of the glans penis

Male/Female

54000 — 54250

MALE GENITAL SYSTEM

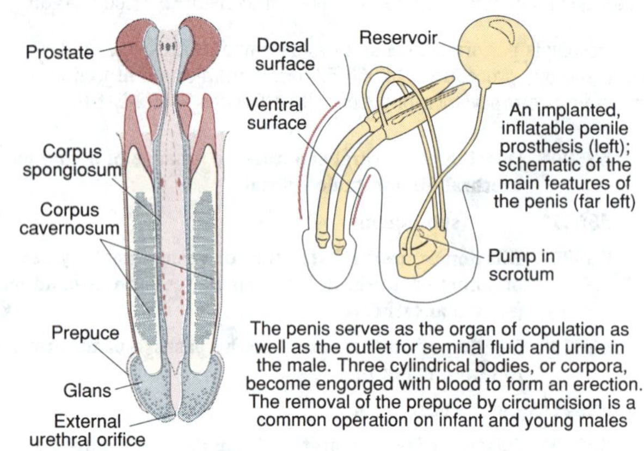

The penis serves as the organ of copulation as well as the outlet for seminal fluid and urine in the male. Three cylindrical bodies, or corpora, become engorged with blood to form an erection. The removal of the prepuce by circumcision is a common operation on infant and young males

PENIS

INCISION

54000	Slitting of prepuce, dorsal or lateral (separate procedure); newborn	N ♂ 80 ▶
54001	except newborn	♂ ❷ ▶
54015	Incision and drainage of penis, deep	♂ ❹ 80 ▶
	If a subcutaneous abscess is incised and drained, consult CPT codes 10060-10160.	

DESTRUCTION

54050*	Destruction of lesion(s), penis (eg, condyloma, papilloma, molluscum contagiosum, herpetic vesicle), simple; chemical	♂ ▶
54055*	electrodesiccation	♂ ▶
54056	cryosurgery	♂ ▶

CIM 35-52 LASER PROCEDURES

Coverage is determined on the basis that the use of lasers to alter, revise, or destroy tissue is a surgical procedure and restricted to practitioners with training in the surgical management of the disease or condition being treated.

54057	laser surgery	♂ ❶ ▶
54060	surgical excision	♂ ❶ ▶
▲ 54065	Destruction of lesion(s), penis (eg, condyloma, papilloma, molluscum contagiosum, herpetic vesicle), extensive (eg, laser surgery, electrosurgery, cryosurgery, chemosurgery)	♂ ❶ ▶
	If destruction or an excision is performed on other lesions, see the Integumentary System.	

EXCISION

54100	Biopsy of penis; (separate procedure)	♂ ❶ ▶
54105	deep structures	♂ ❶ ▶
54110	Excision of penile plaque (Peyronie disease);	♂ ❷ 80 ▶
54111	with graft to 5 cm in length	♂ 80 ▶
54112	with graft greater than 5 cm in length	♂ 80 ▶
54115	Removal foreign body from deep penile tissue (eg, plastic implant)	♂ ❶ 80 ▶
54120	Amputation of penis; partial	♂ ❷ 80 ▶
54125	complete	♂ ❷ 80 ▶
54130	Amputation of penis, radical; with bilateral inguinofemoral lymphadenectomy	♂ 80 ▶

54135	in continuity with bilateral pelvic lymphadenectomy, including external iliac, hypogastric and obturator nodes	♂ 80 ▶
	If a lymphadenectomy (separate procedure) is performed, consult CPT codes 38760-38770.	
54150	Circumcision, using clamp or other device; newborn	N ♂ 80 ▶
54152	except newborn	♂ ❶ ▶
54160	Circumcision, surgical excision other than clamp, device or dorsal slit; newborn	N ♂ ▶
54161	except newborn	♂ ❷ ▶
● 54162	Lysis or excision of penile post-circumcision adhesions	♂ ❷
● 54163	Repair incomplete circumcision	♂ ❷
● 54164	Frenulotomy of penis	♂ ❷
	Do not use in conjunction with circumcision codes 54150-54161, 54162, 54163.	

INTRODUCTION

54200*	Injection procedure for Peyronie disease;	♂ ▶
54205	with surgical exposure of plaque	♂ ❹ 80 ▶
54220	Irrigation of corpora cavernosa for priapism	♂ ❶ ▶
54230	Injection procedure for corpora cavernosography	♂ ▶
	For radiological supervision and interpretation, consult CPT code 74445.	
54231	Dynamic cavernosometry, including intracavernosal injection of vasoactive drugs (eg, papaverine, phentolamine)	♂ ▶
54235	Injection of corpora cavernosa with pharmacologic agent(s) (eg, papaverine, phentolamine)	♂ ▶

CIM 50-6 PLETHYSMOGRAPHY

Plethysmography is a noninvasive technique for diagnostic, preoperative, and postoperative evaluation of peripheral artery disease in the internal medicine or vascular surgery practice. In addition, plethysmography is used preoperative podiatric evaluation of the diabetic patient or one who has intermittent claudication or other signs or symptoms of peripheral vascular disease which bear on the patient's candidacy for foot surgery. Medicare coverage is extended to those procedures listed in Category I below when used for the accepted medical indications. The procedures in Category II are still considered experimental and are not covered.

Category I (covered)

1. Segmental Plethysmography (includes services performed with a regional plethysmograph, differential plethysmograph, recording oscillometer, and a pulse volume recorder)
2. Electrical Impedance Plethysmography
3. Ultrasonic Measurement of Blood Flow (Doppler)
4. Oculoplethysmography
5. Strain Gauge Plethysmography

Category II (not covered)

1. Inductance Plethysmography
2. Capacitance Plethysmography
3. Mechanical Oscillometry
4. Strain Gauge Plethysmography
5. Photoelectric Plethysmography

(If the physician only interprets the results and/or operates the equipment, modifier -26 should be appended to codes 54240 and 54350.)

54240	Penile plethysmography	♂ 80 ▶
54250	Nocturnal penile tumescence and/or rigidity test	♂ 80 ▶

    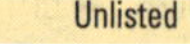 **CPT only © 2001 American Medical Association. All Rights Reserved.** *(Black Ink)*   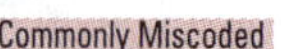 **©2001 Ingenix, Inc.** *(Blue Ink)*

REPAIR

If other urethroplasties are performed, consult CPT codes 53400-53430. If penile revascularization is performed, consult CPT code 37788.

54300 Plastic operation of penis for straightening of chordee (eg, hypospadias), with or without mobilization of urethra ♂ ❸ 80 ▣

54304 Plastic operation on penis for correction of chordee or for first stage hypospadias repair with or without transplantation of prepuce and/or skin flaps ♂ 80 ▣

54308 Urethroplasty for second stage hypospadias repair (including urinary diversion); less than 3 cm ♂ 80 ▣

54312 greater than 3 cm ♂ 80 ▣

54316 Urethroplasty for second stage hypospadias repair (including urinary diversion) with free skin graft obtained from site other than genitalia ♂ 80 ▣

54318 Urethroplasty for third stage hypospadias repair to release penis from scrotum (eg, third stage Cecil repair) ♂ 80 ▣

54322 One stage distal hypospadias repair (with or without chordee or circumcision); with simple meatal advancement (eg, Magpi, V-flap) ♂ 80 ▣

54324 with urethroplasty by local skin flaps (eg, flip-flap, prepucial flap) ♂ 80 ▣
Browne's operation

54326 with urethroplasty by local skin flaps and mobilization of urethra ♂ 80 ▣

54328 with extensive dissection to correct chordee and urethroplasty with local skin flaps, skin graft patch, and/or island flap ♂ 80 ▣

54332 One stage proximal penile or penoscrotal hypospadias repair requiring extensive dissection to correct chordee and urethroplasty by use of skin graft tube and/or island flap ♂ 80 ▣

54336 One stage perineal hypospadias repair requiring extensive dissection to correct chordee and urethroplasty by use of skin graft tube and/or island flap ♂ 80 ▣

54340 Repair of hypospadias complications (ie, fistula, stricture, diverticula); by closure, incision, or excision, simple ♂ 80 ▣

54344 requiring mobilization of skin flaps and urethroplasty with flap or patch graft ♂ 80 ▣

54348 requiring extensive dissection and urethroplasty with flap, patch or tubed graft (includes urinary diversion) ♂ 80 ▣

54352 Repair of hypospadias cripple requiring extensive dissection and excision of previously constructed structures including re-release of chordee and reconstruction of urethra and penis by use of local skin as grafts and island flaps and skin brought in as flaps or grafts ♂ 80 ▣

54360 Plastic operation on penis to correct angulation ♂ ❸ 80 ▣

54380 Plastic operation on penis for epispadias distal to external sphincter; ♂ 80 ▣
Lowsley's operation

CIM 65-9 INCONTINENCE CONTROL DEVICES

Prior to collagen implant therapy, a skin test for collagen sensitivity must be administered and evaluated over a four week period. In male patients, the evaluation must include a complete history and physical examination and a simple cystometrogram to determine that the bladder fills and stores properly. The patient then is asked to stand upright with a full bladder and to cough or otherwise exert abdominal pressure on his bladder. If the patient leaks, the diagnosis of ISD is established. In female patients, the evaluation must

include a complete history and physical examination (including a pelvic exam) and a simple cystometrogram to rule out abnormalities of bladder compliance and abnormalities of urethral support. Following that determination, an abdominal leak point pressure (ALLP) test is performed. If the patient has an ALLP of less than 100 cm H_2O, the diagnosis of ISD is established.

To use a collagen implant, physicians must have urology training in the use of a cystoscope and must complete a collagen implant training program. Coverage of a collagen implant, and the procedure to inject it, is limited to the following types of patients with stress urinary incontinence due to ISD:

a. Male or female patients with congenital sphincter weakness secondary to conditions such as myelomeningocele

b. Male or female patients with acquired sphincter weakness secondary to spinal cord lesions

c. Male patients following trauma, including prostatectomy and/or radiation

d. Female patients without urethral hypermobility and with abdominal leak point pressures of 100 cm H_2O or less

Patients whose incontinence does not improve with 5 injection procedures are considered treatment failures, and no further treatment of urinary incontinence by collagen implant is covered. Patients who have a reoccurrence of incontinence following successful treatment with collagen implants in the past may benefit from additional treatment sessions. Coverage of additional sessions must be supported by medical justification.

54385 with incontinence ♂ 80 ▣

54390 with exstrophy of bladder ♂ 80 ▣

CIM 35-24 DIAGNOSIS AND TREATMENT OF IMPOTENCE

Impotence is a failure of a body part that frequently requires medical expertise for diagnosis and treatment. Depending on the cause of the condition, treatment may be surgical (e.g., implantation of a penile prosthesis) or nonsurgical (e.g., medical or psychotherapeutic treatment). It may be necessary to request documentation of appropriateness in individual cases when abuse is suspected. If treatment is furnished to patients (other than hospital inpatients) in connection with a mental condition, apply the psychiatric service limitation described in the Carriers Manual, §2470.

54400 Insertion of penile prosthesis; non-inflatable (semi-rigid) ♂ ▣

54401 inflatable (self-contained) ♂ ▣

~~**54402** Removal or replacement of non-inflatable (semi-rigid) or inflatable (self-contained) penile prosthesis~~ This code is deleted in 2002. See codes 54415, 54416. ♂ 80 ▣

▲ **54405** Insertion of multi-component, inflatable penile prosthesis, including placement of pump, cylinders, and reservoir ♂ 80 ▣
If service is reduced, report 54405 with modifier -52.

● **54406** Removal of all components of a multi-component, inflatable penile prosthesis without replacement of prosthesis ♂
If service is reduced, report 54406 with modifier -52.

~~**54407** Removal, repair, or replacement of inflatable (multi-component) penile prosthesis, including pump and/or reservoir and/or cylinders~~ This code is deleted in 2002. See codes 54406, 54408, 54410. ♂ 80 ▣

● **54408** Repair of component(s) of a multi-component, inflatable penile prosthesis ♂

~~**54409** Surgical correction of hydraulic abnormality of inflatable (multi-component) prosthesis including pump and/or reservoir and/or cylinders~~ This code is deleted in 2002. See code 54408. 80 ▣

● **54410** Removal and replacement of all component(s) of a multi-component, inflatable penile prosthesis at the same operative session ♂

▣ CCI Comprehensive Code	80 Bilateral Procedure	✚ CPT Add-on Code

✪ Modifier -51 Exempt Code   ● New Code   ▲ Revised Code

M Maternity   N Newborn   P Pediatric   N/P Newborn/Pediatric

Male/Female

54411 — 54700

- **54411** Removal and replacement of all components of a multi-component inflatable penile prosthesis through an infected field at the same operative session, including irrigation and debridement of infected tissue ♂

    If service is reduced, report 54411 with modifier -52.

    Do not report 11040-11043 in conjunction with code 54411.

- **54415** Removal of non-inflatable (semi-rigid) or inflatable (self-contained) penile prosthesis, without replacement of prosthesis ♂

- **54416** Removal and replacement of non-inflatable (semi-rigid) or inflatable (self-contained) penile prosthesis at the same operative session ♂

- **54417** Removal and replacement of non-inflatable (semi-rigid) or inflatable (self-contained) penile prosthesis through an infected field at the same operative session, including irrigation and debridement of infected tissue ♂

    Do not report 11040-11043 in conjunction with 54417.

54420 Corpora cavernosa-saphenous vein shunt (priapism operation), unilateral or bilateral ♂ ❹ 80 ▣

54430 Corpora cavernosa-corpus spongiosum shunt (priapism operation), unilateral or bilateral ♂ 80 ▣

54435 Corpora cavernosa-glans penis fistulization (eg, biopsy needle, Winter procedure, rongeur, or punch) for priapism ♂ ❹ ▣

54440 Plastic operation of penis for injury ♂ ❹ 80 ▣

MANIPULATION

54450 Foreskin manipulation including lysis of preputial adhesions and stretching ♂ ❶ ▣

TESTIS

EXCISION

54500 Biopsy of testis, needle (separate procedure) ♂ ❶ 80 ▣ 50

    To report fine needle aspiration, consult CPT codes 10021, 10022.

    To report evaluation of fine needle aspirate, consult CPT codes 88172, 88173.

54505 Biopsy of testis, incisional (separate procedure) ♂ ❶ 80 ▣ 50

    If this procedure is combined with a vasogram, a seminal vesiculogram, or a epididymogram, consult CPT code 55300.

~~**54510** Excision of local lesion of testis~~ This code is deleted in 2002. See code 54512. ❷ 80 ▣ 50

54512 Excision of extraparenchymal lesion of testis ♂ ❷ 80 ▣ 50

CIM 35-11 STERILIZATION

Payment may be made when sterilization is a necessary part of the treatment of an illness or injury, e.g., removal of a uterus because of a tumor, removal of diseased ovaries (bilateral oophorectomy), or bilateral orchidectomy in a case of cancer of the prostate. Payers deny claims when the pathological evidence of the necessity to perform any such procedures to treat an illness or injury is absent. Medicare does not cover sterilization when performed as:

- An elective hysterectomy, tubal ligation, and vasectomy, if the stated reason for these procedures is sterilization

- A precaution when the physician believes another pregnancy would endanger the overall general health of the woman.

- As a means to prevent conception for a person with developmental delays

54520 Orchiectomy, simple (including subcapsular), with or without testicular prosthesis, scrotal or inguinal approach ♂ ❸ ▣ 50

    Huggins' orchiectomy

54522 Orchiectomy, partial` ♂ 80 50

54530 Orchiectomy, radical, for tumor; inguinal approach ♂ ❹ 80 ▣ 50

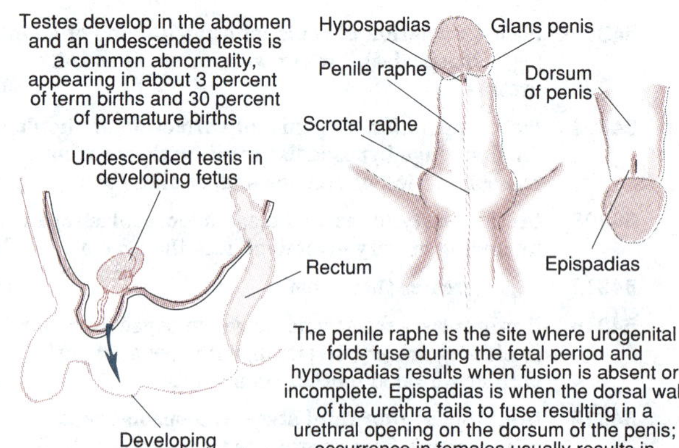

The penile raphe is the site where urogenital folds fuse during the fetal period and hypospadias results when fusion is absent or incomplete. Epispadias is when the dorsal wall of the urethra fails to fuse resulting in a urethral opening on the dorsum of the penis; occurrence in females usually results in a urethral opening into the vaginal canal

54535 with abdominal exploration ♂ 80 ▣ 50

    If an orchiectomy is performed with repair of a hernia, consult CPT codes 49505 or 49507 and 54520. If a radical retroperitoneal lymphadenectomy is performed, consult CPT code 38780.

54550 Exploration for undescended testis (inguinal or scrotal area) ♂ ❹ 80 ▣ 50

54560 Exploration for undescended testis with abdominal exploration ♂ 80 ▣ 50

REPAIR

54600 Reduction of torsion of testis, surgical, with or without fixation of contralateral testis ♂ ❹ ▣ 50

54620 Fixation of contralateral testis (separate procedure) ♂ ❸ ▣ 50

54640 Orchiopexy, inguinal approach, with or without hernia repair ♂ ❹ ▣ 50

    To report inguinal hernia repair with inguinal orchiopexy, consult CPT codes 49495-49525.

    Bevan's operation

54650 Orchiopexy, abdominal approach, for intra-abdominal testis (eg, Fowler-Stephens) ♂ 80 ▣ 50

    If a laparoscopic approach is used, consult CPT code 54692.

54660 Insertion of testicular prosthesis (separate procedure) ♂ ❷ 80 ▣ 50

54670 Suture or repair of testicular injury ♂ ❸ 80 ▣ 50

54680 Transplantation of testis(es) to thigh (because of scrotal destruction) ♂ ❸ 80 ▣ 50

LAPAROSCOPY

54690 Laparoscopy, surgical; orchiectomy ♂ 80 ▣ 50

54692 orchiopexy for intra-abdominal testis ♂ ▣ 50

54699 Unlisted laparoscopy procedure, testis 80 50

EPIDIDYMIS

INCISION

54700 Incision and drainage of epididymis, testis and/or scrotal space (eg, abscess or hematoma) ♂ ❷ ▣

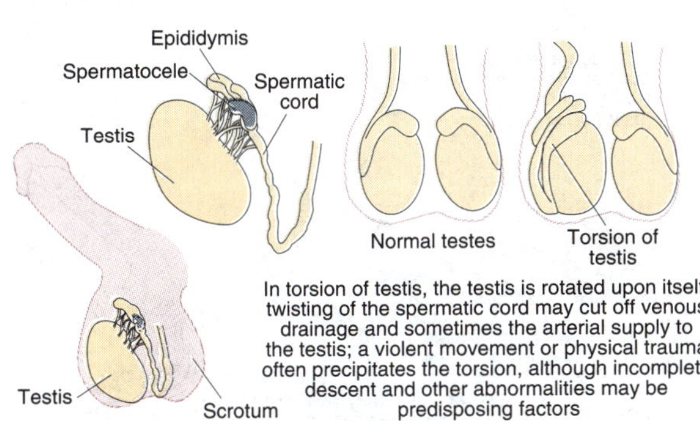

In torsion of testis, the testis is rotated upon itself; twisting of the spermatic cord may cut off venous drainage and sometimes the arterial supply to the testis; a violent movement or physical trauma often precipitates the torsion, although incomplete descent and other abnormalities may be predisposing factors

A spermatocele is a cystic accumulation of semen, usually in the spermatic cord or at the head of the epididymis

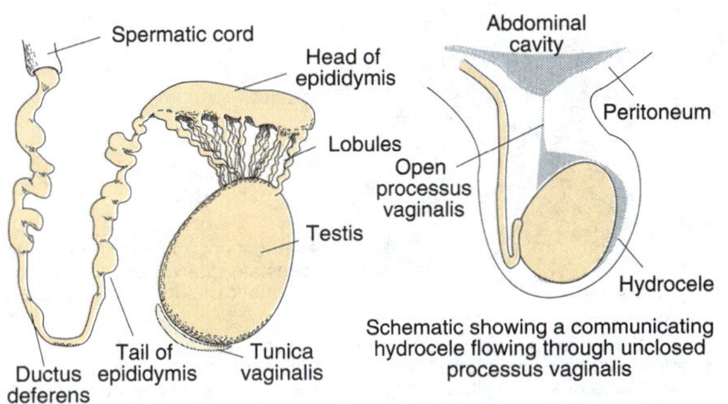

Schematic showing a communicating hydrocele flowing through unclosed processus vaginalis

The tunica vaginalis is a closed sac within the scrotum and is the lower remnant of the path taken by the testis as it descends from the abdomen just prior to birth. The presence of fluid in this pathway is called a hydrocele. The testes, or testicles, are the male reproductive organs. Each produces sperm and male sex hormones.

EXCISION

54800 **Biopsy of epididymis, needle** ♂ ❶ 80 ▣
To report fine needle aspiration, consult CPT codes 10021, 10022.

To report evaluation of fine needle aspirate, consult CPT codes 88172, 88173.

54820 **Exploration of epididymis, with or without biopsy** ♂ ❶ 80 ▣

54830 **Excision of local lesion of epididymis** ♂ ❸ 80 ▣

54840 **Excision of spermatocele, with or without epididymectomy** ♂ ❹ ▣

54860 **Epididymectomy; unilateral** ♂ ❸ ▣

54861 **bilateral** ♂ ❹ 80 ▣

REPAIR

54900 **Epididymovasostomy, anastomosis of epididymis to vas deferens; unilateral** ♂ ❹ 80 ▣

54901 **bilateral** ♂ ❹ 80 ▣
If an operating microscope is used, consult CPT code 69990.

TUNICA VAGINALIS

INCISION

55000* **Puncture aspiration of hydrocele, tunica vaginalis, with or without injection of medication** ♂ ▣

EXCISION

55040 **Excision of hydrocele; unilateral** ♂ ❸ ▣

55041 **bilateral** ♂ ❺ ▣
If this procedure is performed with hernia repair, consult CPT codes 49495-49501.

REPAIR

55060 **Repair of tunica vaginalis hydrocele (Bottle type)** ♂ ❹ 80 ▣ 50

SCROTUM

INCISION

55100* **Drainage of scrotal wall abscess** ♂ ❶ ▣
Consult also CPT code 54700.

55110 **Scrotal exploration** ♂ ❷ ▣

55120 **Removal of foreign body in scrotum** ♂ ❷ 80 ▣

EXCISION

55150 **Resection of scrotum** ♂ ❶ 80 ▣
If a local lesion on the skin of the scrotum is excised, see the Integumentary System.

REPAIR

55175 **Scrotoplasty; simple** ♂ ❶ 80 ▣

55180 **complicated** ♂ ❷ 80 ▣

VAS DEFERENS

INCISION

55200 **Vasotomy, cannulization with or without incision of vas, unilateral or bilateral (separate procedure)** ♂ ❷ 80 ▣

EXCISION

CIM 35-11 STERILIZATION
Payment may be made when sterilization is a necessary part of the treatment of an illness or injury, e.g., removal of a uterus because of a tumor, removal of diseased ovaries (bilateral oophorectomy), or bilateral orchidectomy in a case of cancer of the prostate. Payers deny claims when the pathological evidence of the necessity to perform any such procedures to treat an illness or injury is absent. Medicare does not cover sterilization when performed as:

- An elective hysterectomy, tubal ligation, and vasectomy, if the stated reason for these procedures is sterilization

- As a means to prevent conception for a person with developmental delays

55250 **Vasectomy, unilateral or bilateral (separate procedure), including postoperative semen examination(s)** ♂ ▣

INTRODUCTION

55300 **Vasotomy for vasograms, seminal vesiculograms, or epididymograms, unilateral or bilateral** ♂ 80 ▣
For radiological supervision and interpretation, consult CPT code 74440. If this procedure is combined with a biopsy of the testis, consult CPT code 54505 and append modifier -51 or 09951.

REPAIR

55400 **Vasovasostomy, vasovasorrhaphy** ♂ ❶ 80 ▣ 50
If an operating microscope is used, consult CPT code 69990.

SUTURE

55450 **Ligation (percutaneous) of vas deferens, unilateral or bilateral (separate procedure)** ♂ 80 ▣

SPERMATIC CORD

EXCISION

55500 **Excision of hydrocele of spermatic cord, unilateral (separate procedure)** ♂ ❸ 80 ▣

55520 **Excision of lesion of spermatic cord (separate procedure)** ♂ ❹ 80 ▣

55530 **Excision of varicocele or ligation of spermatic veins for varicocele; (separate procedure)** ♂ ❹ ▣

Male/Female

55535 — 55870

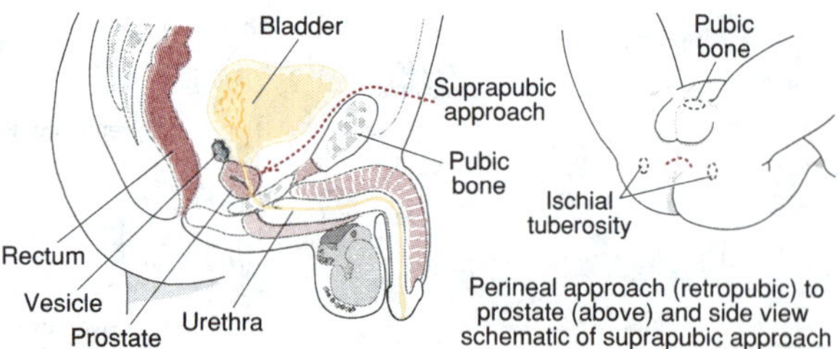

The walnut-sized prostate gland secretes a thin, milky fluid that mixes with spermatic fluids during ejaculation; its secretion constitutes about one-third of the volume of seminal fluid. The prostate is palpable via the rectum. Some procedures are via the urethra, which can be dilated to accommodate instruments. The seminal vesicles may also be palpated via the rectum. Each is a long, coiled tube which secretes a thick fluid that mixes with sperm as it passes along the ejaculatory ducts. The ejaculatory ducts are the union of the seminal vesicles and the sperm-carrying ductus deferens

55535	abdominal approach	♂ ❹ 80 ▣
55540	with hernia repair	♂ ❺ 80 ▣

LAPAROSCOPY

55550	Laparoscopy, surgical, with ligation of spermatic veins for varicocele	♂ 80 ▣ 50
55559	Unlisted laparoscopy procedure, spermatic cord	80 ▣ 50

SEMINAL VESICLES

INCISION

55600	Vesiculotomy;	♂ ❶ 80 ▣ 50
55605	complicated	♂ ❶ 80 ▣ 50

EXCISION

55650	Vesiculectomy, any approach	♂ ❶ 80 ▣ 50
55680	Excision of Mullerian duct cyst	♂ ❶ 80 ▣

If an injection procedure is performed, consult CPT codes 52010 and 55300.

PROSTATE

INCISION

55700	Biopsy, prostate; needle or punch, single or multiple, any approach	♂ ❷ ▣

To report imaging guidance, consult CPT codes 76942.

55705	incisional, any approach	♂ ❷ ▣
55720	Prostatotomy, external drainage of prostatic abscess, any approach; simple	♂ ❶ 80 ▣
55725	complicated	♂ 80 ▣

If transurethral drainage is performed, consult CPT code 52700.

EXCISION

If transurethral removal of the prostate is performed, consult CPT codes 52601-52640. If transurethral destruction of the prostate is performed, consult CPT codes 53850-53852. If a limited pelvic lymphadenectomy is performed for staging (separate procedure), consult CPT code 38562. If an independent node is dissected, consult CPT codes 38770-38780.

55801	Prostatectomy, perineal, subtotal (including control of postoperative bleeding, vasectomy, meatotomy, urethral calibration and/or dilation, and internal urethrotomy)	♂ 80 ▣
55810	Prostatectomy, perineal radical;	♂ 80 ▣
	Walsh modified radical prostatectomy	
55812	with lymph node biopsy(s) (limited pelvic lymphadenectomy)	♂ 80 ▣

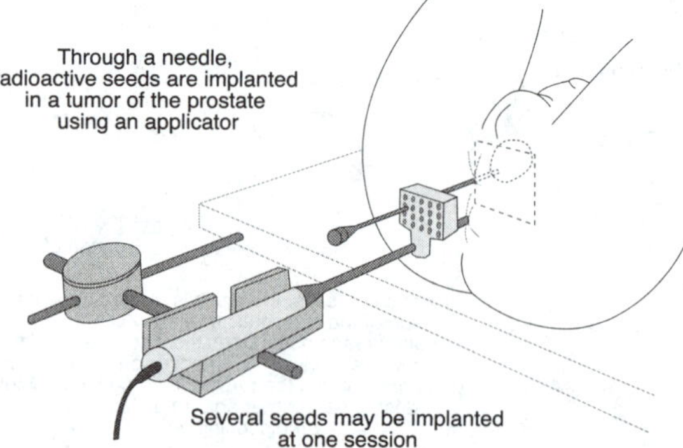

55815	with bilateral pelvic lymphadenectomy, including external iliac, hypogastric and obturator nodes	♂ 80 ▣

If this procedure is carried out on separate days, use CPT code 38770 and append modifier -50 and 55810.

55821	Prostatectomy (including control of postoperative bleeding, vasectomy, meatotomy, urethral calibration and/or dilation, and internal urethrotomy); suprapubic, subtotal, one or two stages	♂ 80 ▣
55831	retropubic, subtotal	♂ 80 ▣
55840	Prostatectomy, retropubic radical, with or without nerve sparing;	♂ 80 ▣
55842	with lymph node biopsy(s) (limited pelvic lymphadenectomy)	♂ 80 ▣
55845	with bilateral pelvic lymphadenectomy, including external iliac, hypogastric, and obturator nodes	♂ 80 ▣

If this procedure is carried out on separate days, use CPT code 38770 and append modifier -50 and 55840.

55859	Transperineal placement of needles or catheters into prostate for interstitial radioelement application, with or without cystoscopy	♂ 80 ▣

To report application of interstitial radioelement, consult CPT codes 77776–77778.

55860	Exposure of prostate, any approach, for insertion of radioactive substance;	♂ ▣

To report application of interstitial radioelement, consult CPT codes 77776–77778.

55862	with lymph node biopsy(s) (limited pelvic lymphadenectomy)	♂ 80 ▣
55865	with bilateral pelvic lymphadenectomy, including external iliac, hypogastric and obturator nodes	♂ 80 ▣

OTHER PROCEDURES

55870	Electroejaculation	♂ ▣

CIM 35-96 CRYOSURGERY OF PROSTATE

Medicare covers cryosurgery of the prostate gland, also known as cryosurgical ablation of the prostate (CSAP), which destroys prostate tissue by reducing the size of the prostate gland using extremely cold temperatures. It is safe and effective as primary treatment for patients with clinically localized prostate cancer, Stages T1-T3.(Effective for services performed after July 1, 2001) Salvage cryosurgery of the prostate for recurrent cancer is medically necessary and appropriate only for those patients with localized disease who: 1. Have failed a trial of radiation therapy as their primary treatment; and 2. Meet one of the following conditions: Stage T2B or below, Gleason score < 9, PSA < 8 ng/mL. Cryosurgery as salvage therapy is therefore not covered under Medicare after failure of other therapies as the primary treatment. Cryosurgery as salvage is only covered after the failure of a trial of radiation therapy, under the conditions noted above.

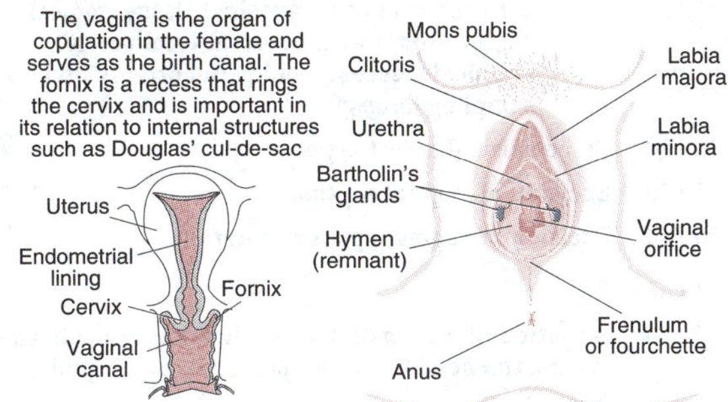

The vagina is the organ of copulation in the female and serves as the birth canal. The fornix is a recess that rings the cervix and is important in its relation to internal structures such as Douglas' cul-de-sac.

The external female genital region is collectively known as the vulva, or sometimes, the pudendum. A Bartholin's gland is located on either side of the orifice. The perineum is the space between the anus and the vagina, but is often generally defined as the entire pelvic floor and its related structures. Introitus is a general term for the vaginal entrance

55873   **Cryosurgical ablation of the prostate (includes ultrasonic guidance for interstitial cryosurgical probe placement)** ♂ ▫

55899   **Unlisted procedure, male genital system** ♂

INTERSEX SURGERY

CIM 35-61 TRANSSEXUAL SURGERY - NOT COVERED

Because of the lack of well-controlled, long-term studies of the safety and effectiveness of the surgical procedures and attendant therapies for transsexualism, the treatment is considered experimental. Moreover, there is a high rate of serious complications for these surgical procedures. For these reasons, transsexual surgery is not covered.

55970   Intersex surgery; male to female   ♂

55980   female to male   ♀

FEMALE GENITAL SYSTEM

VULVA, PERINEUM AND INTROITUS

INCISION

Consult the glossary for more terms and guidelines.

If a pelvic laparotomy is performed, consult CPT code 49000. If excision or destruction is performed of endometriomas, open method, consult CPT codes 49200 and 49201. If paracentesis is performed, consult CPT codes 49080 and 49081. If secondary closure of the abdominal wall evisceration or disruption is performed, consult CPT code 49900. If fulguration or excision of lesions is performed through a laparoscopic approach, consult CPT code 58662. If chemotherapy is needed, consult CPT codes 96400-96549.

If a sebaceous cyst, furuncle, or abscess is incised and drained, consult CPT codes 10040 and 10060.

56405*   **Incision and drainage of vulva or perineal abscess**   ♀ ❷ ▫

56420*   **Incision and drainage of Bartholin's gland abscess** ♀ ▫

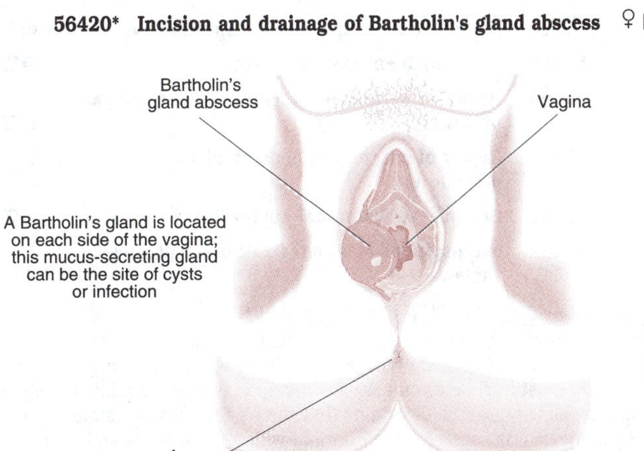

A Bartholin's gland is located on each side of the vagina; this mucus-secreting gland can be the site of cysts or infection

56440   Marsupialization of Bartholin's gland cyst   ♀ ❷ ▫

56441   Lysis of labial adhesions   ♀ ❶ 80 ▫

DESTRUCTION

If destruction is performed on a Skene's gland cyst or abscess, consult CPT code 53270. If cautery destruction of a urethral caruncle is performed, consult CPT code 53265.

▲   **56501**   **Destruction of lesion(s), vulva; simple (eg, laser surgery, electrosurgery, cryosurgery, chemosurgery)**   ♀ ▫

▲   **56515**   **extensive (eg, laser surgery, electrosurgery, cryosurgery, chemosurgery)**   ♀ ❸ ▫

EXCISION

If a local lesion is excised, consult CPT codes 11420-11426 and 11620-11626.

If a pelvic laparotomy is performed, consult CPT code 49000. If excision or destruction is performed of endometriomas, open method, consult CPT codes 49200 and 49201. If paracentesis is performed, consult CPT codes 49080 and 49081. If secondary closure of the abdominal wall evisceration or disruption is performed, consult CPT code 49900. If fulguration or excision of lesions is performed through a laparoscopic approach, consult CPT code 58662. If chemotherapy is needed, consult CPT codes 96400-96549.

56605*   **Biopsy of vulva or perineum (separate procedure); one lesion**   ♀ ❶ ▫

+   **56606***   **each separate additional lesion (List separately in addition to code for primary procedure)**   ♀

Note that 56606 is an add-on code and must be used in conjunction with 56605.

56620   Vulvectomy simple; partial   ♀ ❺ 80 ▫

56625   complete   ♀ ❼ 80 ▫

56630   Vulvectomy, radical, partial;   ♀ 80 ▫
Bassett's operation

56631   with unilateral inguinofemoral lymphadenectomy   ♀ 80 ▫
Bassett's operation

56632   with bilateral inguinofemoral lymphadenectomy   ♀ 80 ▫
Bassett's operation

56633   Vulvectomy, radical, complete;   ♀ 80 ▫
Bassett's operation

56634   with unilateral inguinofemoral lymphadenectomy   ♀ 80 ▫
Bassett's operation

56637   with bilateral inguinofemoral lymphadenectomy   ♀ 80 ▫
Bassett's operation

56640   Vulvectomy, radical, complete, with inguinofemoral, iliac, and pelvic lymphadenectomy   ♀ 80 ▫ 50

If a lymphadenectomy is performed, consult CPT codes 38760-38780.

Bassett's operation

56700   Partial hymenectomy or revision of hymenal ring   ♀ ❶ 80 ▫

56720*   Hymenotomy, simple incision   ♀ ❶ 80 ▫

56740   Excision of Bartholin's gland or cyst   ♀ ❸ ▫

If the Skene's gland is excised, consult CPT code 53270. If an excision is performed on the urethral caruncle, consult CPT code 53265. If excision or fulguration is performed on a urethral carcinoma, consult CPT code 53220. If excision or marsupialization is performed on the urethral diverticulum, consult CPT codes 53230 and 52340.

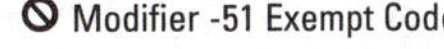

Male/Female

56800 — 57282

REPAIR

If a pelvic laparotomy is performed, consult CPT code 49000. If excision or destruction is performed of endometriomas, open method, consult CPT codes 49200 and 49201. If paracentesis is performed, consult CPT codes 49080 and 49081. If secondary closure of the abdominal wall evisceration or disruption is performed, consult CPT code 49900. If fulguration or excision of lesions is performed through a laparoscopic approach, consult CPT code 58662. If chemotherapy is needed, consult CPT codes 96400-96549.

If a repair of the urethra is performed for mucosal prolapse, consult CPT code 53275.

56800   **Plastic repair of introitus**   ♀ ❸ 80 ▣
     Emmet's operation

56805   **Clitoroplasty for intersex state**   ♀ 80 ▣

56810   **Perineoplasty, repair of perineum, non-obstetrical (separate procedure)**   ♀ ❺ 80 ▣
     Emmet's operation

     For repair of nonobstetrical recent injury, consult CPT code 57210. Consult also CPT code 56800. To report anal spincteroplasty, consult CPT codes 46750, 46751.

VAGINA

INCISION

If a pelvic laparotomy is performed, consult CPT code 49000. If excision or destruction is performed of endometriomas, open method, consult CPT codes 49200 and 49201. If paracentesis is performed, consult CPT codes 49080 and 49081. If secondary closure of the abdominal wall evisceration or disruption is performed, consult CPT code 49900. If fulguration or excision of lesions is performed through a laparoscopic approach, consult CPT code 58662. If chemotherapy is needed, consult CPT codes 96400-96549.

57000   **Colpotomy; with exploration**   ♀ ❶ 80 ▣

57010   **with drainage of pelvic abscess**   ♀ ❷ 80 ▣
     Laroyenne operation

57020*   **Colpocentesis (separate procedure)**   ♀ ❷ 80 ▣

▲ **57022**   **Incision and drainage of vaginal hematoma; obstetrical/postpartum**   ♀ 80

57023   **non-obstetrical (eg, post-trauma, spontaneous bleeding)**   ♀ 80

DESTRUCTION

▲ **57061**   **Destruction of vaginal lesion(s); simple (eg, laser surgery, electrosurgery, cryosurgery, chemosurgery)**   ♀ ▣

▲ **57065**   **extensive (eg, laser surgery, electrosurgery, cryosurgery, chemosurgery)**   ♀ ❶ ▣

EXCISION

57100*   **Biopsy of vaginal mucosa; simple (separate procedure)**   ♀ ▣

57105   **extensive, requiring suture (including cysts)**   ♀ ❷ ▣

57106   **Vaginectomy, partial removal of vaginal wall;**   ♀ 80 ▣

57107   **with removal of paravaginal tissue (radical vaginectomy)**   ♀ 80 ▣

57109   **with removal of paravaginal tissue (radical vaginectomy) with bilateral total pelvic lymphadenectomy and para-aortic lymph node sampling (biopsy)**   ♀ 80 ▣

57110   **Vaginectomy, complete removal of vaginal wall;**   ♀ 80 ▣

57111   **with removal of paravaginal tissue (radical vaginectomy)**   ♀ 80 ▣

57112   **with removal of paravaginal tissue (radical vaginectomy) with bilateral total pelvic lymphadenectomy and para-aortic lymph node sampling (biopsy)**   ♀ 80 ▣

57120   **Colpocleisis (Le Fort type)**   ♀ 80 ▣

57130   **Excision of vaginal septum**   ♀ ❷ 80 ▣

57135   **Excision of vaginal cyst or tumor**   ♀ ❷ ▣

INTRODUCTION

57150*   **Irrigation of vagina and/or application of medicament for treatment of bacterial, parasitic, or fungoid disease**   ♀ ▣

● **57155**   **Insertion of uterine tandems and/or vaginal ovoids for clinical brachytherapy**   ♀
     To report insertion of radioelement sources or ribbons, consult CPT codes 77761-77763, 77781-77784.

57160*   **Fitting and insertion of pessary or other intravaginal support device**   ♀ ▣

57170   **Diaphragm or cervical cap fitting with instructions**   ♀ 80 ▣

57180   **Introduction of any hemostatic agent or pack for spontaneous or traumatic nonobstetrical vaginal hemorrhage (separate procedure)**   ♀ ❶ ▣

REPAIR

If an anterior vesicourethropexy or urethropexy is performed (e.g., Marshall-Marchetti-Krantz type), consult CPT codes 51840 and 51841. If laparoscopic suspension is performed on the ureter, consult CPT code 51990.

If a pelvic laparotomy is performed, consult CPT code 49000. If excision or destruction is performed of endometriomas, open method, consult CPT codes 49200 and 49201. If paracentesis is performed, consult CPT codes 49080 and 49081. If secondary closure of the abdominal wall evisceration or disruption is performed, consult CPT code 49900. If fulguration or excision of lesions is performed through a laparoscopic approach, consult CPT code 58662. If chemotherapy is needed, consult CPT codes 96400-96549.

57200   **Colporrhaphy, suture of injury of vagina (nonobstetrical)**   ♀ ❶ 80 ▣

57210   **Colpoperineorrhaphy, suture of injury of vagina and/or perineum (nonobstetrical)**   ♀ ❷ 80 ▣

57220   **Plastic operation on urethral sphincter, vaginal approach (eg, Kelly urethral plication)**   ♀ ❸ 80 ▣

57230   **Plastic repair of urethrocele**   ♀ ❸ 80 ▣

57240   **Anterior colporrhaphy, repair of cystocele with or without repair of urethrocele**   ♀ ❺ 80 ▣

57250   **Posterior colporrhaphy, repair of rectocele with or without perineorrhaphy**   ♀ ❺ 80 ▣
     If rectocele is repaired without posterior colporrhaphy, consult CPT code 45560.

57260   **Combined anteroposterior colporrhaphy;**   ♀ ❺ 80 ▣

57265   **with enterocele repair**   ♀ ❼ 80 ▣

57268   **Repair of enterocele, vaginal approach (separate procedure)**   ♀ ❸ 80 ▣

57270   **Repair of enterocele, abdominal approach (separate procedure)**   ♀ 80 ▣

57280   **Colpopexy, abdominal approach**   ♀ 80 ▣

57282   **Sacrospinous ligament fixation for prolapse of vagina**   ♀ 80 ▣

CIM 65-9 INCONTINENCE CONTROL DEVICES

Prior to collagen implant therapy, a skin test for collagen sensitivity must be administered and evaluated over a four week period. In male patients, the evaluation must include a complete history and physical examination and a simple cystometrogram to determine that the bladder fills and stores properly. The patient then is asked to stand upright with a full bladder and to cough or otherwise exert abdominal pressure on his bladder. If the patient leaks, the diagnosis of ISD is established. In female patients, the evaluation must include a complete history and physical examination (including a pelvic exam) and a simple cystometrogram to rule out abnormalities of bladder compliance and abnormalities of urethral support. Following that determination, an abdominal leak point pressure (ALLP) test is performed. If the patient has an ALLP of less than 100 cm H_2O, the diagnosis of ISD is established.

To use a collagen implant, physicians must have urology training in the use of a cystoscope and must complete a collagen implant training program. Coverage of a collagen implant, and the procedure to inject it, is limited to the following types of patients with stress urinary incontinence due to ISD:

a. Male or female patients with congenital sphincter weakness secondary to conditions such as myelomeningocele

b. Male or female patients with acquired sphincter weakness secondary to spinal cord lesions

c. Male patients following trauma, including prostatectomy and/or radiation

d. Female patients without urethral hypermobility and with abdominal leak point pressures of 100 cm H_2O or less

Patients whose incontinence does not improve with 5 injection procedures are considered treatment failures, and no further treatment of urinary incontinence by collagen implant is covered. Patients who have a reoccurrence of incontinence following successful treatment with collagen implants in the past may benefit from additional treatment sessions. Coverage of additional sessions must be supported by medical justification.

57284   **Paravaginal defect repair (including repair of cystocele, stress urinary incontinence, and/or incomplete vaginal prolapse)** ♀ 80 ☐

57287   **Removal or revision of sling for stress incontinence (eg, fascia or synthetic)** ♀ 80

57288   **Sling operation for stress incontinence (eg, fascia or synthetic)** ♀ 80 ☐
    If performed via laparoscope, consult CPT code 51992.
    Millen-Read

57289   **Pereyra procedure, including anterior colporrhaphy** ♀ 80 ☐

57291   **Construction of artificial vagina; without graft** ♀ 80 ☐
    McIndoe vaginal construction

57292   **with graft** ♀ 80 ☐

57300   **Closure of rectovaginal fistula; vaginal or transanal approach** ♀ ❸ 80 ☐

57305   **abdominal approach** ♀ 80 ☐

57307   **abdominal approach, with concomitant colostomy** ♀ 80 ☐

57308   **transperineal approach, with perineal body reconstruction, with or without levator plication** ♀ 80 ☐

57310   **Closure of urethrovaginal fistula;** ♀ ❸ 80 ☐

57311   **with bulbocavernosus transplant** ♀ ❹ 80 ☐

57320   **Closure of vesicovaginal fistula; vaginal approach** ♀ ❸ 80 ☐
    If a concomitant cystostomy is performed, consult CPT codes 51005-51040.

57330   **transvesical and vaginal approach** ♀ 80 ☐
    If performed via abdominal approach, consult CPT code 51900.

57335   **Vaginoplasty for intersex state** ♀ 80 ☐

MANIPULATION

57400*   **Dilation of vagina under anesthesia** ♀ ❷ 80 ☐

57410*   **Pelvic examination under anesthesia** ♀ ❷ ☐

57415   **Removal of impacted vaginal foreign body (separate procedure) under anesthesia** ♀ 80 ☐
    If removal of an impacted vaginal foreign body is performed without anesthesia, consult the appropriate E/M code.

ENDOSCOPY

57452*   **Colposcopy (vaginoscopy); (separate procedure)** ♀ ☐

57454*   **with biopsy(s) of the cervix and/or endocervical curettage** ♀ ☐

57460   **with loop electrode excision procedure of the cervix** ♀ ☐

CERVIX UTERI

If radical surgical procedures are performed, consult CPT codes 58200-58240. If an intrauterine device is inserted, consult CPT code 58300.

If a pelvic laparotomy is performed, consult CPT code 49000. If excision or destruction is performed of endometriomas, open method, consult CPT codes 49200 and 49201. If paracentesis is performed, consult CPT codes 49080 and 49081. If secondary closure of the abdominal wall evisceration or disruption is performed, consult CPT code 49900. If fulguration or excision of lesions is performed through a laparoscopic approach, consult CPT code 58662. If chemotherapy is needed, consult CPT codes 96400-96549.

EXCISION

57500*   **Biopsy, single or multiple, or local excision of lesion, with or without fulguration (separate procedure)** ♀ ☐

57505   **Endocervical curettage (not done as part of a dilation and curettage)** ♀ ☐

▲ **57510**   **Cautery of cervix; electro or thermal** ♀ ☐

57511*   **cryocautery, initial or repeat** ♀ ☐

57513   **laser ablation** ♀ ❷ ☐

57520   **Conization of cervix, with or without fulguration, with or without dilation and curettage, with or without repair; cold knife or laser** ♀ ❷ ☐
    Consult also CPT code 58120.

57522   **loop electrode excision** ♀ ❷ ☐

57530   **Trachelectomy (cervicectomy), amputation of cervix (separate procedure)** ♀ ❸ 80 ☐

57531   **Radical trachelectomy, with bilateral total pelvic lymphadenectomy and para-aortic lymph node sampling biopsy, with or without removal of tube(s), with or without removal of ovary(s)** ♀ 80 ☐
    If radical abdominal hysterectomy is performed, consult CPT code 58210.

57540   **Excision of cervical stump, abdominal approach;** ♀ 80 ☐

57545   **with pelvic floor repair** ♀ 80 ☐

57550   **Excision of cervical stump, vaginal approach;** ♀ ❸ 80 ☐

57555   **with anterior and/or posterior repair** ♀ 80 ☐

57556   **with repair of enterocele** ♀ 80 ☐

REPAIR

57700   **Cerclage of uterine cervix, nonobstetrical** ♀ ❶ 80 ☐
    McDonald cerclage

57720   **Trachelorrhaphy, plastic repair of uterine cervix, vaginal approach** ♀ ❸ 80 ☐

MANIPULATION

57800*   **Dilation of cervical canal, instrumental (separate procedure)** ♀ ❶ ☐

57820   **Dilation and curettage of cervical stump** ♀ ❸ ☐

Male/Female

58100* — 58350*

CORPUS UTERI

EXCISION

CIM 50-10 VABRA ASPIRATOR
The VABRA aspirator collects uterine tissue for study to detect endometrial carcinoma and its is indicated where the patient exhibits clinical symptoms or signs suggestive of endometrial disease, such as irregular or heavy vaginal bleeding. Medicare does not for the aspirator or the related diagnostic services when furnished in connection with the exam of an asymptomatic patient. Payment for routine physical checkups is precluded, also.

If an endocervical curettage is performed by itself, consult CPT code 57505.

If a pelvic laparotomy is performed, consult CPT code 49000. If excision or destruction is performed of endometriomas, open method, consult CPT codes 49200 and 49201. If paracentesis is performed, consult CPT codes 49080 and 49081. If secondary closure of the abdominal wall evisceration or disruption is performed, consult CPT code 49900. If fulguration or excision of lesions is performed through a laparoscopic approach, consult CPT code 58662. If chemotherapy is needed, consult CPT codes 96400-96549.

If a postpartum curettage is performed, consult CPT code 59160.

58100* Endometrial sampling (biopsy) with or without endocervical sampling (biopsy), without cervical dilation, any method (separate procedure) ♀

58120 Dilation and curettage, diagnostic and/or therapeutic (nonobstetrical) ♀ ❷

▲ **58140** Myomectomy, excision of leiomyomata of uterus, single or multiple (separate procedure); abdominal approach ♀ 80

58145 vaginal approach ♀ ❺ 80

CIM 35-11 STERILIZATION
Payment may be made when sterilization is a necessary part of the treatment of an illness or injury, e.g., removal of a uterus because of a tumor, removal of diseased ovaries (bilateral oophorectomy), or bilateral orchidectomy in a case of cancer of the prostate. Payers deny claims when the pathological evidence of the necessity to perform any such procedures to treat an illness or injury is absent. Medicare does not cover sterilization when performed as:

- An elective hysterectomy, tubal ligation, and vasectomy, if the stated reason for these procedures is sterilization

- A precaution when the physician believes another pregnancy would endanger the overall general health of the woman

- As a means to prevent conception for a person with developmental delays

58150 Total abdominal hysterectomy (corpus and cervix), with or without removal of tube(s), with or without removal of ovary(s); ♀ 80

58152 with colpo-urethrocystopexy (eg, Marshall-Marchetti-Krantz, Burch) ♀ 80
If a urethrocystopexy is performed without a hysterectomy, consult CPT codes 51840 and 51841.

58180 Supracervical abdominal hysterectomy (subtotal hysterectomy), with or without removal of tube(s), with or without removal of ovary(s) ♀ 80

58200 Total abdominal hysterectomy, including partial vaginectomy, with para-aortic and pelvic lymph node sampling, with or without removal of tube(s), with or without removal of ovary(s) ♀ 80

58210 Radical abdominal hysterectomy, with bilateral total pelvic lymphadenectomy and para-aortic lymph node sampling (biopsy), with or without removal of tube(s), with or without removal of ovary(s) ♀ 80
If a radical hysterectomy is performed with an ovarian transposition, consult also CPT code 58825.

Wertheim hysterectomy

58240 Pelvic exenteration for gynecologic malignancy, with total abdominal hysterectomy or cervicectomy, with or without removal of tube(s), with or without removal of ovary(s), with removal of bladder and ureteral transplantations, and/or abdominoperineal resection of rectum and colon and colostomy, or any combination thereof ♀ 80
If pelvic exenteration is performed for a lower urinary tract or a male genital malignancy, consult CPT code 51597.

58260 Vaginal hysterectomy; ♀ 80

58262 with removal of tube(s), and/or ovary(s) ♀ 80

58263 with removal of tube(s), and/or ovary(s), with repair of enterocele ♀ 80

58267 with colpo-urethrocystopexy (Marshall-Marchetti-Krantz type, Pereyra type, with or without endoscopic control) ♀ 80

58270 with repair of enterocele ♀ 80
If an enterocele is repaired with removal of tubes and/or ovaries, consult CPT code 58263.

▲ **58275** Vaginal hysterectomy, with total or partial vaginectomy; ♀ 80

58280 with repair of enterocele ♀ 80

58285 Vaginal hysterectomy, radical (Schauta type operation) ♀ 80

INTRODUCTION
If implantable contraceptive capsules are inserted or removed, consult CPT codes 11975, 11976, and 11977.

If a pelvic laparotomy is performed, consult CPT code 49000. If excision or destruction is performed of endometriomas, open method, consult CPT codes 49200 and 49201. If paracentesis is performed, consult CPT codes 49080 and 49081. If secondary closure of the abdominal wall evisceration or disruption is performed, consult CPT code 49900. If fulguration or excision of lesions is performed through a laparoscopic approach, consult CPT code 58662. If chemotherapy is needed, consult CPT codes 96400-96549.

58300* Insertion of intrauterine device (IUD) ♀

58301 Removal of intrauterine device (IUD) ♀ 80

58321 Artificial insemination; intra-cervical ♀ 80

58322 intra-uterine ♀ 80

58323 Sperm washing for artificial insemination ♀ 80

58340* Catheterization and introduction of saline or contrast material for hysterosonography or hysterosalpingography ♀
For the radiological supervision and interpretation of an hysterosonography, consult CPT code 76831. For the radiological supervision and interpretation of an hysterosalpingography, consult CPT code 74740.

To report cryoblation of endometrium with ultrasonic guidance, consult CPT Category III code 0009T.

58345 Transcervical introduction of fallopian tube catheter for diagnosis and/or re-establishing patency (any method), with or without hysterosalpingography ♀ 80 50
To report radiological supervision and interpretation, consult CPT code 74742.

● **58346** Insertion of Heyman capsules for clinical brachytherapy ♀
To report radioelement sources/ribbons insertion, consult CPT codes 77761-77763, 77781-77784.

58350* Chromotubation of oviduct, including materials ♀

CIM 50-10 VABRA ASPIRATOR

The VABRA aspirator collects uterine tissue for study to detect endometrial carcinoma and its is indicated where the patient exhibits clinical symptoms or signs suggestive of endometrial disease, such as irregular or heavy vaginal bleeding. Medicare does not for the aspirator or the related diagnostic services when furnished in connection with the exam of an asymptomatic patient. Payment for routine physical checkups is precluded, also.

58353 **Endometrial ablation, thermal, without hysteroscopic guidance** ♀ 80 50

For endometrial ablation with hysteroscopy, consult CPT code 58563.

REPAIR

If a pelvic laparotomy is performed, consult CPT code 49000. If excision or destruction is performed of endometriomas, open method, consult CPT codes 49200 and 49201. If paracentesis is performed, consult CPT codes 49080 and 49081. If secondary closure of the abdominal wall evisceration or disruption is performed, consult CPT code 49900. If fulguration or excision of lesions is performed through a laparoscopic approach, consult CPT code 58662. If chemotherapy is needed, consult CPT codes 96400-96549.

58400 **Uterine suspension, with or without shortening of round ligaments, with or without shortening of sacrouterine ligaments; (separate procedure)** ♀ 80 ▣

Alexander's operation

58410 **with presacral sympathectomy** ♀ 80 ▣

Alexander's operation

58520 **Hysterorrhaphy, repair of ruptured uterus (nonobstetrical)** ♀ 80 ▣

58540 **Hysteroplasty, repair of uterine anomaly (Strassman type)** ♀ 80 ▣

If a vesicouterine fistula is closed, consult CPT code 51920.

Tompkins metroplasty

LAPAROSCOPY/HYSTEROSCOPY

If a pelvic laparotomy is performed, consult CPT code 49000. If excision or destruction is performed of endometriomas, open method, consult CPT codes 49200 and 49201. If paracentesis is performed, consult CPT codes 49080 and 49081. If secondary closure of the abdominal wall evisceration or disruption is performed, consult CPT code 49900. If fulguration or excision of lesions is performed through a laparoscopic approach, consult CPT code 58662. If chemotherapy is needed, consult CPT codes 96400-96549.

CIM 35-11 STERILIZATION

Payment may be made when sterilization is a necessary part of the treatment of an illness or injury, e.g., removal of a uterus because of a tumor, removal of diseased ovaries (bilateral oophorectomy), or bilateral orchidectomy in a case of cancer of the prostate. Payers deny claims when the pathological evidence of the necessity to perform any such procedures to treat an illness or injury is absent. Medicare does not cover sterilization when performed as:

- An elective hysterectomy, tubal ligation, and vasectomy, if the stated reason for these procedures is sterilization
- A precaution when the physician believes another pregnancy would endanger the overall general health of the woman
- As a means to prevent conception for a person with developmental delays

58550 **Laparoscopy, surgical; with vaginal hysterectomy with or without removal of tube(s), with or without removal of ovary(s) (laparoscopic assisted vaginal hysterectomy)** ♀ 80 ▣

58551 **with removal of leiomyomata (single or multiple)** ♀ 5 80 ▣

58555 **Hysteroscopy, diagnostic (separate procedure)** ♀ 1 80 ▣

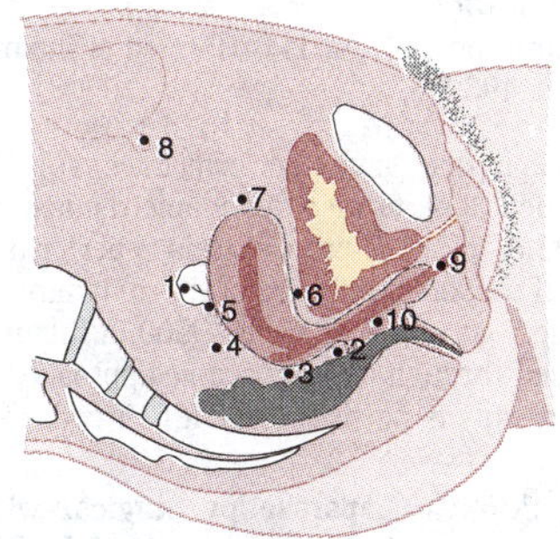

Endometriosis is a benign condition in which endometrial matter is present outside of the endometrial cavity; it is estimated that 15 percent of women have some degree of the disease; occurrence is most common in the ovaries and about 60 percent of patients will have ovarian involvement, many with cyst development

58558 **Hysteroscopy, surgical; with sampling (biopsy) of endometrium and/or polypectomy, with or without D & C** ♀ 3 ▣

58559 **with lysis of intrauterine adhesions (any method)** ♀ 2 ▣

58560 **with division or resection of intrauterine septum (any method)** ♀ 5 80 ▣

58561 **with removal of leiomyomata** ♀ 3 80 ▣

58562 **with removal of impacted foreign body** ♀ 5 ▣

▲ **58563** **with endometrial ablation (eg, endometrial resection, electrosurgical ablation, thermoablation)** ♀ 4 80 ▣

58578 **Unlisted laparoscopy procedure, uterus** 80 50

58579 **Unlisted hysteroscopy procedure, uterus** 80 50

OVIDUCT/OVARY

INCISION

If a pelvic laparotomy is performed, consult CPT code 49000. If excision or destruction is performed of endometriomas, open method, consult CPT codes 49200 and 49201. If paracentesis is performed, consult CPT codes 49080 and 49081. If secondary closure of the abdominal wall evisceration or disruption is performed, consult CPT code 49900. If fulguration or excision of lesions is performed through a laparoscopic approach, consult CPT code 58662. If chemotherapy is needed, consult CPT codes 96400-96549.

58600 **Ligation or transection of fallopian tube(s), abdominal or vaginal approach, unilateral or bilateral** ♀ 80 ▣

Madlener operation

58605 **Ligation or transection of fallopian tube(s), abdominal or vaginal approach, postpartum, unilateral or bilateral, during same hospitalization (separate procedure)** ♀ 80 ▣

If laparoscopic procedures are performed, consult CPT codes 58670 and 58371.

▲ + **58611** **Ligation or transection of fallopian tube(s) when done at the time of cesarean delivery or intra-abdominal surgery (not a separate procedure) (List separately in addition to code for primary procedure)** ♀ 80 ▣

58615 **Occlusion of fallopian tube(s) by device (eg, band, clip, Falope ring) vaginal or suprapubic approach** ♀ 80 ▣

If a laparoscopic approach is used, consult CPT code 58621.

Male/Female

58660 — 58951

LAPAROSCOPY

If a laparoscopic biopsy is performed of the ovary or fallopian tube, consult CPT code 49321.

If a pelvic laparotomy is performed, consult CPT code 49000. If excision or destruction is performed of endometriomas, open method, consult CPT codes 49200 and 49201. If paracentesis is performed, consult CPT codes 49080 and 49081. If secondary closure of the abdominal wall evisceration or disruption is performed, consult CPT code 49900. If fulguration or excision of lesions is performed through a laparoscopic approach, consult CPT code 58662. If chemotherapy is needed, consult CPT codes 96400-96549.

58660 Laparoscopy, surgical; with lysis of adhesions (salpingolysis, ovariolysis) (separate procedure) ♀ 80 ↵

58661 with removal of adnexal structures (partial or total oophorectomy and/or salpingectomy) ♀ ⑤ 80 ↵

58662 with fulguration or excision of lesions of the ovary, pelvic viscera, or peritoneal surface by any method ♀ ⑤ 80 ↵

58670 with fulguration of oviducts (with or without transection) ♀ ③ ↵

58671 with occlusion of oviducts by device (eg, band, clip, or Falope ring) ♀ ③ ↵

58672 with fimbrioplasty ♀ ⑤ 80 ↵ 50

58673 with salpingostomy (salpingoneostomy) ♀ ⑤ 80 ↵ 50

58679 Unlisted laparoscopy procedure, oviduct, ovary 80 50

EXCISION

58700 Salpingectomy, complete or partial, unilateral or bilateral (separate procedure) ♀ 80 ↵

58720 Salpingo-oophorectomy, complete or partial, unilateral or bilateral (separate procedure) ♀ 80 ↵

REPAIR

If a pelvic laparotomy is performed, consult CPT code 49000. If excision or destruction is performed of endometriomas, open method, consult CPT codes 49200 and 49201. If paracentesis is performed, consult CPT codes 49080 and 49081. If secondary closure of the abdominal wall evisceration or disruption is performed, consult CPT code 49900. If fulguration or excision of lesions is performed through a laparoscopic approach, consult CPT code 58662. If chemotherapy is needed, consult CPT codes 96400-96549.

58740 Lysis of adhesions (salpingolysis, ovariolysis) ♀ 80 ↵
If a laparoscopic approach is used, consult CPT code 58660. If excision or destruction is performed of endometriomas, open method, consult CPT codes 49200 and 49201. If fulguration or excision of lesions is performed, laparoscopic approach, consult CPT code 58662.

58750 Tubotubal anastomosis ♀ 80 ↵

58752 Tubouterine implantation ♀ 80 ↵

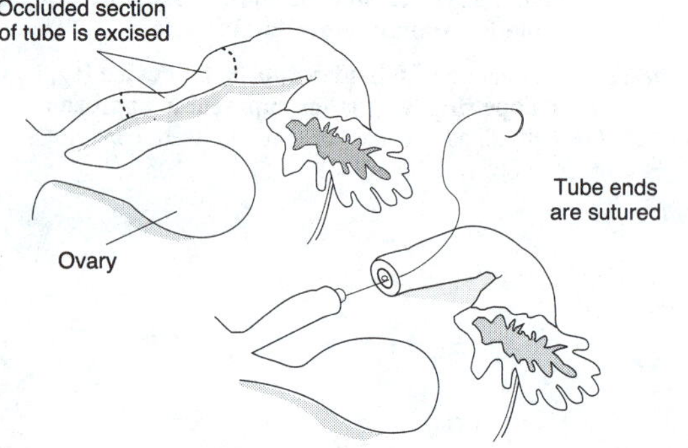

58760 Fimbrioplasty ♀ 80 ↵ 50
If a laparoscopic approach is used, consult CPT code 58672.

58770 Salpingostomy (salpingoneostomy) ♀ 80 ↵ 50
If a laparoscopic approach is used, consult CPT code 58673.

OVARY

INCISION

If a pelvic laparotomy is performed, consult CPT code 49000. If excision or destruction is performed of endometriomas, open method, consult CPT codes 49200 and 49201. If paracentesis is performed, consult CPT codes 49080 and 49081. If secondary closure of the abdominal wall evisceration or disruption is performed, consult CPT code 49900. If fulguration or excision of lesions is performed through a laparoscopic approach, consult CPT code 58662. If chemotherapy is needed, consult CPT codes 96400-96549.

58800 Drainage of ovarian cyst(s), unilateral or bilateral, (separate procedure); vaginal approach ♀ ③ ↵

58805 abdominal approach ♀ 80 ↵

58820 Drainage of ovarian abscess; vaginal approach, open ♀ ③ 80 ↵

58822 abdominal approach ♀ 80 ↵

58823 Drainage of pelvic abscess, transvaginal or transrectal approach, percutaneous (eg, ovarian, pericolic) ♀ 80 ↵
To report radiological supervision and interpretation, consult CPT code 75989.

58825 Transposition, ovary(s) ♀ 80 ↵

EXCISION

58900 Biopsy of ovary, unilateral or bilateral (separate procedure) ♀ ③ 80 ↵
If performed via laparoscope, consult CPT code 49321.

58920 Wedge resection or bisection of ovary, unilateral or bilateral ♀ 80 ↵

58925 Ovarian cystectomy, unilateral or bilateral ♀ 80 ↵

CIM 35-11 STERILIZATION

Payment may be made when sterilization is a necessary part of the treatment of an illness or injury, e.g., removal of a uterus because of a tumor, removal of diseased ovaries (bilateral oophorectomy), or bilateral orchidectomy in a case of cancer of the prostate. Payers deny claims when the pathological evidence of the necessity to perform any such procedures to treat an illness or injury is absent. Medicare does not cover sterilization when performed as:

- An elective hysterectomy, tubal ligation, and vasectomy, if the stated reason for these procedures is sterilization

- A precaution when the physician believes another pregnancy would endanger the overall general health of the woman

- As a means to prevent conception for a person with developmental delays

58940 Oophorectomy, partial or total, unilateral or bilateral; ♀ 80 ↵

58943 for ovarian, tubal or primary peritoneal malignancy, with para-aortic and pelvic lymph node biopsies, peritoneal washings, peritoneal biopsies, diaphragmatic assessments, with or without salpingectomy(s), with or without omentectomy ♀ 80 ↵

58950 Resection of ovarian, tubal or primary peritoneal malignancy with bilateral salpingo-oophorectomy and omentectomy; ♀ 80 ↵

58951 with total abdominal hysterectomy, pelvic and limited para-aortic lymphadenectomy ♀ 80 ↵

| | 58952 | with radical dissection for debulking (ie, radical excision or destruction, intra-abdominal or retroperitoneal tumors) ♀ 80 ⬛ |

- **58953** Bilateral salpingo-oophorectomy with omentectomy, total abdominal hysterectomy and radical dissection for debulking; ♀

- **58954** with pelvic lymphadenectomy and limited para-aortic lymphadenectomy ♀

58960 Laparotomy, for staging or restaging of ovarian, tubal or primary peritoneal malignancy (second look), with or without omentectomy, peritoneal washing, biopsy of abdominal and pelvic peritoneum, diaphragmatic assessment with pelvic and limited para-aortic lymphadenectomy ♀ 80 ⬛

IN VITRO FERTILIZATION

58970 Follicle puncture for oocyte retrieval, any method ♀ 80 ⬛
For radiological supervision and interpretation, consult CPT code 76948.

58974 Embryo transfer, intrauterine M ♀ 80 ⬛

58976 Gamete, zygote, or embryo intrafallopian transfer, any method M ♀ 80 ⬛

OTHER PROCEDURES

58999 Unlisted procedure, female genital system (nonobstetrical) ♀ 80

MATERNITY CARE AND DELIVERY

ANTEPARTUM SERVICES

Consult the glossary for more terms and guidelines.

To report insertion of transcervical or transvaginal fetal oximetry sensor, consult CPT Category III code 0021T.

CIM 50-7 ULTRASOUND DIAGNOSTIC PROCEDURES

Medicare coverage is extended to the procedures listed in Category I. Techniques in Category II are considered experimental and should not be covered at this time.

Category I (covered, may be adjunct to radiologic and nuclear medicine diagnostic technique)

1. Echoencephalography, (Diencephalic Midline) (A-Mode)
2. Echoencephalography, Complete (Diencephalic Midline and Ventricular Size)
3. Ocular and Orbital Echography (A-Mode) (includes determining the suitability of aphakic patients for an artificial lens implant following cataract surgery)
4. Ocular and Orbital Sonography (B-Mode)
5. Echocardiography, Pericardial Effusion (M-Mode)
6. Pericardiocentesis, by Ultrasonic Guidance
7. Echocardiography, Cardiac Valve(s) (M-Mode)
8. Echocardiography, Complete (M-Mode)
9. Echocardiography, limited (e.g., follow-up or limited study) (M-Mode)
10. Pleural Effusion Echography
11. Thoracentesis, by Ultrasonic Guidance
12. Abdominal Sonography, complete survey study (B-Scan)
13. Abdominal Sonography, limited (e.g., follow-up or limited study) (B-Scan)
14. Renal Cyst Aspiration, by Ultrasonic Guidance
15. Renal Biopsy, by Ultrasonic Guidance
16. Pancreas Sonography (B-Scan)
17. Spleen Sonography (B-Scan)
18. Abdominal Aorta Echography (A-Mode)
19. Abdominal Aorta Sonography (B-Scan)
20. Retroperitoneal Sonography (B-Scan)
21. Retroperitoneal sonography does not include planning of fields for radiation therapy.
22. Urinary Bladder Sonography (B-Scan)
23. Urinary bladder sonography does not include staging of bladder tumors.
24. Pregnancy Diagnosis sonography (B-Scan)
25. Fetal Age Determination (Biparietal Diameter) Sonography (B-Scan)
26. Fetal Growth Rate Sonography (B-Scan)
27. Placenta Localization Sonography (B-Scan)
28. Pregnancy Sonography, Complete (B-Scan)
29. Molar Pregnancy Diagnosis Sonography (B-Scan)
30. Ectopic Pregnancy Diagnosis sonography (B-Scan)
31. Passive Testing (Antepartum Monitoring of Fetal Heart Rate In the Resting Fetus)
32. Intrauterine Contraceptive Device Sonography (B-Scan)
33. Pelvic Mass Diagnosis Sonography (B-Scan)
34. Amniocentesis, by Ultrasonic Guidance
35. Arterial Flow Study, Peripheral (Doppler)
36. Venous Flow Study, Peripheral (Doppler)
37. Arterial Aneurysm, Peripheral (B-Scan)
38. Radiation Therapy Planning Sonography (B-Scan)
39. Thyroid Echography (A-Mode)
40. Thyroid Sonography (B-Scan)
41. Breast Echography (A-Mode)
42. Breast Sonography (B-Scan)
43. Hepatic Sonography (B-Scan)
44. Gallbladder Sonography
45. Renal Sonography
46. Two-Dimensional Echocardiography (B-Mode)

Category II (clinical reliability and efficacy not proven)

1. B-Scan for atherosclerotic narrowing of peripheral arteries
2. Monitoring of cardiac output (Doppler)

When appropriate, new uses for ultrasound diagnostic procedures should be forwarded to the Bureau of Eligibility, Reimbursement and Coverage, HCFA, so that revisions may be made in the coverage policy when appropriate.

▲ **59000*** **Amniocentesis; diagnostic** M ♀ ⬛
For radiological supervision and interpretation, consult CPT code 76946.

- **59001** therapeutic amniotic fluid reduction (includes ultrasound guidance) M ♀

59012 Cordocentesis (intrauterine), any method M ♀ 80 ⬛
For radiological supervision and interpretation, consult CPT code 76941.

59015 Chorionic villus sampling, any method M ♀ 80 ⬛
For radiological supervision and interpretation, consult CPT code 76945.

59020* Fetal contraction stress test M ♀ 80 ⬛
(If the physician only interprets the results and/or operates the equipment, modifier -26 should be appended to 59020.)

59025 Fetal non-stress test M ♀ 80 ⬛
(If the physician only interprets the results and/or operates the equipment, modifier -26 should be appended to 59025.)

59030* Fetal scalp blood sampling M ♀ 80 ⬛

⬛ CCI Comprehensive Code   50 Bilateral Procedure   + CPT Add-on Code   ⊘ Modifier -51 Exempt Code   ● New Code   ▲ Revised Code

M Maternity   N Newborn   P Pediatric   N/P Newborn/Pediatric

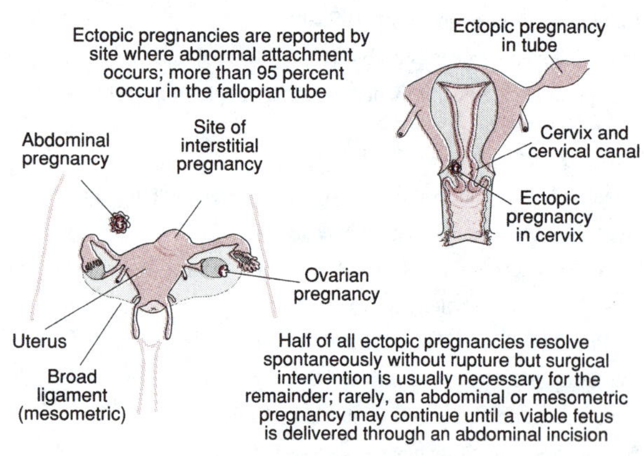

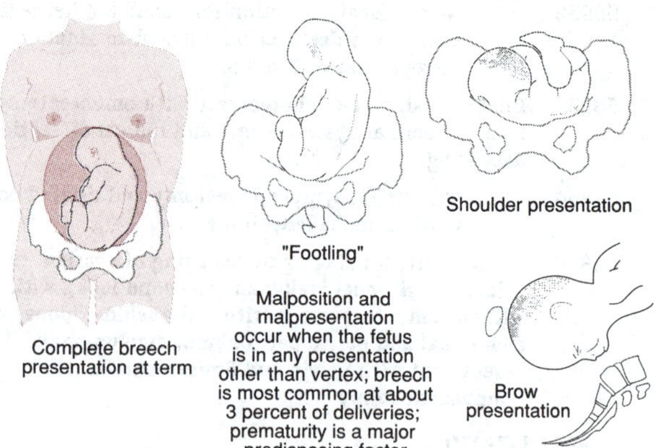

59050   **Fetal monitoring during labor by consulting physician (ie, non-attending physician) with written report; supervision and interpretation**   M ♀ 80

59051   **interpretation only**   M ♀ 80

EXCISION

59100   **Hysterotomy, abdominal (eg, for hydatidiform mole, abortion)**   M ♀ 80
       If tubal ligation is performed at the same time as the hysterotomy, consult CPT code 58611 and report in addition to 59100.

59120   **Surgical treatment of ectopic pregnancy; tubal or ovarian, requiring salpingectomy and/or oophorectomy, abdominal or vaginal approach**   M ♀ 80

59121   **tubal or ovarian, without salpingectomy and/or oophorectomy**   M ♀ 80

59130   **abdominal pregnancy**   M ♀ 80

59135   **interstitial, uterine pregnancy requiring total hysterectomy**   M ♀ 80

59136   **interstitial, uterine pregnancy with partial resection of uterus**   M ♀ 80

59140   **cervical, with evacuation**   M ♀ 80

59150   **Laparoscopic treatment of ectopic pregnancy; without salpingectomy and/or oophorectomy**   M ♀ 80

59151   **with salpingectomy and/or oophorectomy**   M ♀ 80

59160   **Curettage, postpartum**   M ♀ 80

INTRODUCTION

59200   **Insertion of cervical dilator (eg, laminaria, prostaglandin) (separate procedure)**   M ♀
       If intrauterine fetal transfusion is conducted, consult CPT code 36460. If a hypertonic solution and/or prostaglandins are introduced to initiate labor, consult CPT codes 59850-59857.

REPAIR

If tracheloplasty is performed, consult CPT code 57700.

59300   **Episiotomy or vaginal repair, by other than attending physician**   M ♀ 80

59320   **Cerclage of cervix, during pregnancy; vaginal**   M ♀ 80

59325   **abdominal**   M ♀ 80

59350   **Hysterorrhaphy of ruptured uterus**   M ♀ 80

VAGINAL DELIVERY, ANTEPARTUM AND POSTPARTUM CARE

This section addresses antepartum care, delivery, and postpartum care. Antepartum care includes monthly visits up to 28 weeks gestation, biweekly visits up to 36 weeks gestation and weekly visits until delivery. Services included are history, examinations, recording of weight, blood pressures, fetal health, urinalysis, and other examinations pertinent to the health of mother and child. Delivery services include admission, management of labor and vaginal delivery, or cesarean delivery. Postpartum care includes hospital and office visits following vaginal or cesarean section delivery.

If the physician provides all or part of the antepartum care, but doesn't perform the delivery, consult CPT codes 59425-59426. If only one to three visits are provided, consult the appropriate Evaluation and Management Codes. For postpartum care only, consult CPT code 59430.

Consult the glossary for more terms and guidelines.

To report insertion of transcervical or transvaginal fetal oximetry sensor, consult CPT Category III code 0021T.

59400   **Routine obstetric care including antepartum care, vaginal delivery (with or without episiotomy, and/or forceps) and postpartum care**   M ♀

59409   **Vaginal delivery only (with or without episiotomy and/or forceps);**   M ♀ 80

59410   **including postpartum care**   M ♀

59412   **External cephalic version, with or without tocolysis**   M ♀ 80
       Report in addition to CPT code for the delivery.

59414   **Delivery of placenta (separate procedure)**   M ♀ 80

59425   **Antepartum care only; 4-6 visits**   M ♀ 80
       If 1-3 visits for antepartum care are provided, consult the appropriate Evaluation and Management code(s).

59426   **7 or more visits**   M ♀ 80

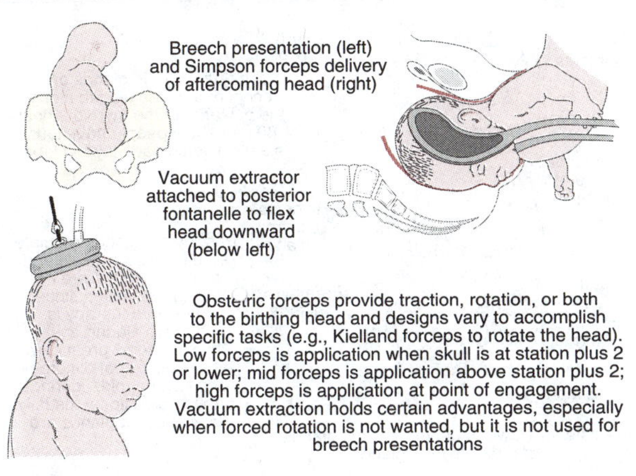

Obstetric forceps provide traction, rotation, or both to the birthing head and designs vary to accomplish specific tasks (e.g., Kielland forceps to rotate the head). Low forceps is application when skull is at station plus 2 or lower; mid forceps is application above station plus 2; high forceps is application at point of engagement. Vacuum extraction holds certain advantages, especially when forced rotation is not wanted, but it is not used for breech presentations

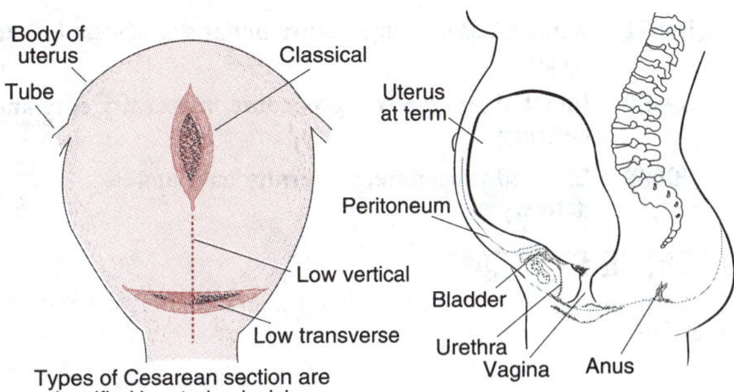

Types of Cesarean section are classified by uterine incision

Cesarean section is delivery through incisions in the anterior abdominal and uterine walls and is indicated for numerous conditions in both the fetus and the mother. Although other approaches may be warranted, low transverse is preferred to decrease chance of uterine rupture during future pregnancies

59430   Postpartum care only (separate procedure)   M ♀ ▢

CESAREAN DELIVERY

To report insertion of transcervical or transvaginal fetal oximetry sensor, consult CPT Category III code 0021T.

If a standby physician is present for an infant, consult CPT code 99360.

59510   **Routine obstetric care including antepartum care, cesarean delivery, and postpartum care**   M ♀ ▢

59514   **Cesarean delivery only;**   M ♀ 80 ▢

59515   **including postpartum care**   M ♀ ▢

+ 59525   **Subtotal or total hysterectomy after cesarean delivery (List separately in addition to code for primary procedure)**   M ♀ 80 ▢
Note that 59525 is an add-on code and must be used in conjunction with 59510, 59514, 59515, 59618, 59620, and 59622.

DELIVERY AFTER PREVIOUS CESAREAN DELIVERY

If a standby physician is present for an infant, consult CPT code 99360.

59610   **Routine obstetric care including antepartum care, vaginal delivery (with or without episiotomy, and/or forceps) and postpartum care, after previous cesarean delivery**   M ♀ 80 ▢

59612   **Vaginal delivery only, after previous cesarean delivery (with or without episiotomy and/or forceps);**   M ♀ 80 ▢

59614   **including postpartum care**   M ♀ 80 ▢

59618   **Routine obstetric care including antepartum care, cesarean delivery, and postpartum care, following attempted vaginal delivery after previous cesarean delivery**   M ♀ 80 ▢

59620   **Cesarean delivery only, following attempted vaginal delivery after previous cesarean delivery;**   M ♀ 80 ▢

59622   **including postpartum care**   M ♀ 80 ▢

ABORTION

If medical treatment is needed for a spontaneous complete abortion, any trimester, consult E/M codes 99201-99233.

59812   **Treatment of incomplete abortion, any trimester, completed surgically**   M ♀ ▢

59820   **Treatment of missed abortion, completed surgically; first trimester**   M ♀ ▢

59821   **second trimester**   M ♀ 80 ▢

59830   **Treatment of septic abortion, completed surgically**   M ♀ 80 ▢

CIM 35-99 ABORTION

Medicare covers abortions:

- If the pregnancy is the result of an act of rape or incest

- In the case where a woman suffers from a physical disorder, physical injury, or physical illness, including a life-endangering physical condition caused by or arising from the pregnancy itself, that would, as certified by a physician, place the woman in danger of death unless an abortion is performed

This restricted coverage applies to CPT codes 59840, 59841, 59850, 59851, 59852, 59855, 59856, 59857, and 59866.

59840   **Induced abortion, by dilation and curettage**   M ♀ 80 ▢

59841   **Induced abortion, by dilation and evacuation**   M ♀ 80 ▢

CIM 35-11 STERILIZATION

Payment may be made when sterilization is a necessary part of the treatment of an illness or injury, e.g., removal of a uterus because of a tumor, removal of diseased ovaries (bilateral oophorectomy), or bilateral orchidectomy in a case of cancer of the prostate. Payers deny claims when the pathological evidence of the necessity to perform any such procedures to treat an illness or injury is absent. Medicare does not cover sterilization when performed as:

- An elective hysterectomy, tubal ligation, and vasectomy, if the stated reason for these procedures is sterilization

- A precaution when the physician believes another pregnancy would endanger the overall general health of the woman

- As a means to prevent conception for a person with developmental delays

59850   **Induced abortion, by one or more intra-amniotic injections (amniocentesis-injections), including hospital admission and visits, delivery of fetus and secundines;**   M ♀ 80 ▢

59851   **with dilation and curettage and/or evacuation**   M ♀ 80 ▢

59852   **with hysterotomy (failed intra-amniotic injection)**   M ♀ 80 ▢
If a cervical dilator is inserted, consult CPT code 59200.

59855   **Induced abortion, by one or more vaginal suppositories (eg, prostaglandin) with or without cervical dilation (eg, laminaria), including hospital admission and visits, delivery of fetus and secundines;**   M ♀ 80 ▢

59856   **with dilation and curettage and/or evacuation**   M ♀ 80 ▢

59857   **with hysterotomy (failed medical evacuation)**   M ♀ 80 ▢

OTHER PROCEDURES

59866   **Multifetal pregnancy reduction(s) (MPR)**   M ♀ 80 ▢

▢ CCI Comprehensive Code   50 Bilateral Procedure   + CPT Add-on Code   Ⓢ Modifier -51 Exempt Code   ● New Code   ▲ Revised Code

M Maternity   N Newborn   P Pediatric   N/P Newborn/Pediatric

Male/Female

59870 — 60699

	59870	Uterine evacuation and curettage for hydatidiform mole　　　M ♀ 80
	59871	Removal of cerclage suture under anesthesia (other than local)　　　M ♀ 80
	59898	Unlisted laparoscopy procedure, maternity care and delivery　　　M ♀ 80 50
	59899	Unlisted procedure, maternity care and delivery　　　M ♀ 80

ENDOCRINE SYSTEM

If pituitary and pineal surgery is performed, consult the Nervous System section of CPT.

THYROID GLAND

INCISION

▲　60000*　Incision and drainage of thyroglossal duct cyst, infected　　　❶ 80

EXCISION

60001　Aspiration and/or injection, thyroid cyst

    To report fine needle aspiration, consult CPT codes 10021, 10022.

    To report imaging guidance, consult CPT codes 76360, 76942.

60100*　Biopsy thyroid, percutaneous core needle

    For imaging guidance, consult CPT codes 76003, 76360, 76393 and 76942. If fine needle aspiration is performed, consult CPT codes 10021, 10022.

60200　Excision of cyst or adenoma of thyroid, or transection of isthmus　　　❷ 80

60210　Partial thyroid lobectomy, unilateral; with or without isthmusectomy　　　80

60212　　　with contralateral subtotal lobectomy, including isthmusectomy　　　80

60220　Total thyroid lobectomy, unilateral; with or without isthmusectomy　　　❷ 80

60225　　　with contralateral subtotal lobectomy, including isthmusectomy　　　❸ 80

60240　Thyroidectomy, total or complete　　　80

60252　Thyroidectomy, total or subtotal for malignancy; with limited neck dissection　　　80

60254　　　with radical neck dissection　　　80

60260　Thyroidectomy, removal of all remaining thyroid tissue following previous removal of a portion of thyroid　　　80

▲　60270　Thyroidectomy, including substernal thyroid; sternal split or transthoracic approach　　　80

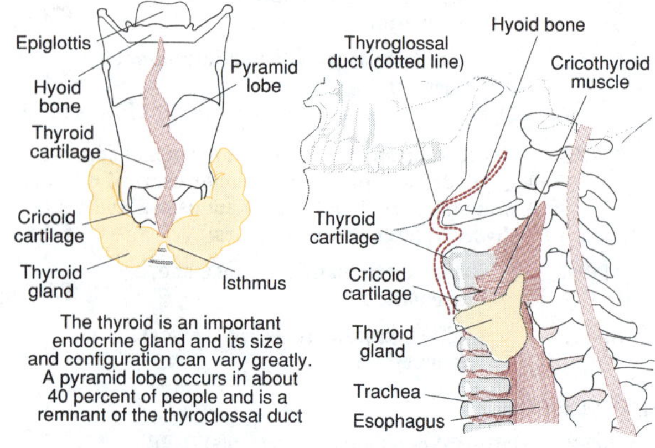

The thyroid is an important endocrine gland and its size and configuration can vary greatly. A pyramid lobe occurs in about 40 percent of people and is a remnant of the thyroglossal duct

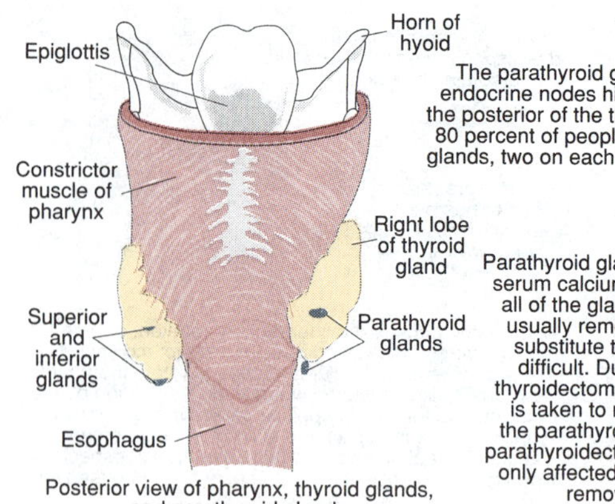

The parathyroid glands are endocrine nodes hidden along the posterior of the thyroid; about 80 percent of people have four glands, two on each thyroid lobe

Parathyroid glands regulate serum calcium levels and all of the glands are not usually removed since substitute therapy is difficult. During any thyroidectomy great care is taken to not disturb the parathyroids; during parathyroidectomy, usually only affected glands are removed

Posterior view of pharynx, thyroid glands, and parathyroid glands

60271	cervical approach	80
60280	Excision of thyroglossal duct cyst or sinus;	❹ 80
60281	recurrent	❹ 80

    If a thyroid ultrasonography is performed, consult CPT code 76536.

PARATHYROID, THYMUS, ADRENAL GLANDS, AND CAROTID BODY

60500　Parathyroidectomy or exploration of parathyroid(s);　　　80

60502　　　re-exploration　　　80

60505　　　with mediastinal exploration, sternal split or transthoracic approach　　　80

+　60512　Parathyroid autotransplantation (List separately in addition to code for primary procedure)　　　80

    Note that 60512 is an add-on code and must be used in conjunction with 60500, 60502, 60505, 60212, 60225, 60240, 60252, 60254, 60260, 60270, and 60271.

60520　Thymectomy, partial or total; transcervical approach (separate procedure)　　　80

60521　　　sternal split or transthoracic approach, without radical mediastinal dissection (separate procedure)　　　80

60522　　　sternal split or transthoracic approach, with radical mediastinal dissection (separate procedure)　　　80

60540　Adrenalectomy, partial or complete, or exploration of adrenal gland with or without biopsy, transabdominal, lumbar or dorsal (separate procedure);　　　80 50

60545　　　with excision of adjacent retroperitoneal tumor　　　80

    If a remote or disseminated pheochromocytoma is excised, consult CPT codes 49200 and 49201. If a laparoscopic approach is used, consult CPT code 60650.

60600　Excision of carotid body tumor; without excision of carotid artery　　　80

60605　　　with excision of carotid artery　　　80

LAPAROSCOPY

60650　Laparoscopy, surgical, with adrenalectomy, partial or complete, or exploration of adrenal gland with or without biopsy, transabdominal, lumbar or dorsal　　　80 50

60659　Unlisted laparoscopy procedure, endocrine system　　　80 50

OTHER PROCEDURES

60699　Unlisted procedure, endocrine system　　　80

NERVOUS SYSTEM

SKULL, MENINGES, AND BRAIN

INJECTION, DRAINAGE, OR ASPIRATION

If an injection procedure is needed for cerebral angiography, consult CPT codes 36100-36218. If an injection procedure is needed for pneumoencephalography, consult CPT code 61055. If an injection procedure is needed for ventriculography, consult CPT codes 61026, 61120, 61130.

61000*	Subdural tap through fontanelle, or suture, infant, unilateral or bilateral; initial	N ⊡
61001*	subsequent taps	N ⊡
61020*	Ventricular puncture through previous burr hole, fontanelle, suture, or implanted ventricular catheter/reservoir; without injection	❶ ⊡
▲ 61026*	with injection of medication or other substance for diagnosis or treatment	❶ ⊡
61050*	Cisternal or lateral cervical (C1-C2) puncture; without injection (separate procedure)	❶ 80 ⊡
▲ 61055*	with injection of medication or other substance for diagnosis or treatment (eg, C1-C2)	❶ ⊡

For radiological supervision and interpretation, consult the Radiology section of CPT.

61070*	Puncture of shunt tubing or reservoir for aspiration or injection procedure	❶ ⊡

For radiological supervision and interpretation, consult CPT code 75809.

TWIST DRILL, BURR HOLE(S), OR TREPHINE

61105*	Twist drill hole for subdural or ventricular puncture;	80 ⊡
⊘ 61107*	for implanting ventricular catheter or pressure recording device	⊡
61108	for evacuation and/or drainage of subdural hematoma	⊡
61120	Burr hole(s) for ventricular puncture (including injection of gas, contrast media, dye, or radioactive material)	80 ⊡
61140	Burr hole(s) or trephine; with biopsy of brain or intracranial lesion	80 ⊡
61150	with drainage of brain abscess or cyst	⊡
61151	with subsequent tapping (aspiration) of intracranial abscess or cyst	⊡
61154	Burr hole(s) with evacuation and/or drainage of hematoma, extradural or subdural	80 ⊡ 50
61156	Burr hole(s); with aspiration of hematoma or cyst, intracerebral	80 ⊡
⊘ 61210*	for implanting ventricular catheter, reservoir, EEG electrode(s) or pressure recording device (separate procedure)	⊡
61215	Insertion of subcutaneous reservoir, pump or continuous infusion system for connection to ventricular catheter	❸ ⊡

If chemotherapy is administered, consult CPT code 96450.

61250	Burr hole(s) or trephine, supratentorial, exploratory, not followed by other surgery	80 ⊡ 50
61253	Burr hole(s) or trephine, infratentorial, unilateral or bilateral	80 ⊡

If a burr hole(s) or trephine are followed by a craniotomy at the same operative session, consult CPT codes 61304-61321; do not use 61250 or 61253.

CRANIECTOMY OR CRANIOTOMY

61304	Craniectomy or craniotomy, exploratory supratentorial	80 ⊡
61305	infratentorial (posterior fossa)	80 ⊡
61312	Craniectomy or craniotomy for evacuation of hematoma, supratentorial; extradural or subdural	80 ⊡
61313	intracerebral	80 ⊡
61314	Craniectomy or craniotomy for evacuation of hematoma, infratentorial; extradural or subdural	80 ⊡
61315	intracerebellar	80 ⊡
61320	Craniectomy or craniotomy, drainage of intracranial abscess; supratentorial	80 ⊡
61321	infratentorial	80 ⊡
61330	Decompression of orbit only, transcranial approach	80 ⊡ 50

Naffziger operation

61332	Exploration of orbit (transcranial approach); with biopsy	80 ⊡
61333	with removal of lesion	80 ⊡
61334	with removal of foreign body	80 ⊡
61340	Other cranial decompression (eg, subtemporal), supratentorial	80 ⊡ 50
61343	Craniectomy, suboccipital with cervical laminectomy for decompression of medulla and spinal cord, with or without dural graft (eg, Arnold-Chiari malformation)	80 ⊡
61345	Other cranial decompression, posterior fossa	80 ⊡

If an orbital decompression is performed by a lateral wall approach, Kroenlein type, consult CPT code 67445.

61440	Craniotomy for section of tentorium cerebelli (separate procedure)	80 ⊡
61450	Craniectomy, subtemporal, for section, compression, or decompression of sensory root of gasserian ganglion	80 ⊡

Frazier-Spiller procedure

61458	Craniectomy, suboccipital; for exploration or decompression of cranial nerves	80 ⊡

Jannetta decompression

61460	for section of one or more cranial nerves	80 ⊡
61470	for medullary tractotomy	80 ⊡
61480	for mesencephalic tractotomy or pedunculotomy	80 ⊡
61490	Craniotomy for lobotomy, including cingulotomy	80 ⊡ 50
61500	Craniectomy; with excision of tumor or other bone lesion of skull	80 ⊡
61501	for osteomyelitis	80 ⊡
61510	Craniectomy, trephination, bone flap craniotomy; for excision of brain tumor, supratentorial, except meningioma	80 ⊡
61512	for excision of meningioma, supratentorial	80 ⊡
61514	for excision of brain abscess, supratentorial	80 ⊡
61516	for excision or fenestration of cyst, supratentorial	80 ⊡

If an excision is performed of a pituitary tumor or a craniopharyngioma, consult CPT codes 61545, 61546, and 61548.

61518	Craniectomy for excision of brain tumor, infratentorial or posterior fossa; except meningioma, cerebellopontine angle tumor, or midline tumor at base of skull	80 ⊡
61519	meningioma	80 ⊡
61520	cerebellopontine angle tumor	80 ⊡
61521	midline tumor at base of skull	80 ⊡

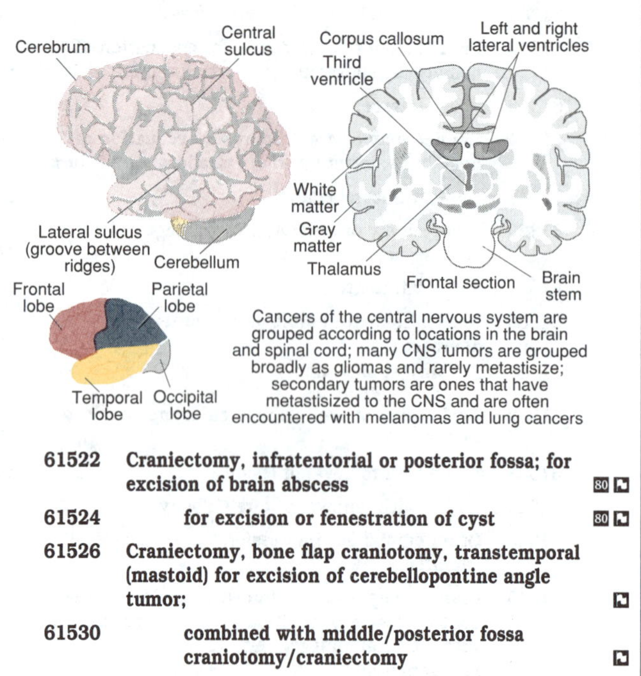

61522   **Craniectomy, infratentorial or posterior fossa; for excision of brain abscess**   80 ↻

61524   **for excision or fenestration of cyst**   80 ↻

61526   **Craniectomy, bone flap craniotomy, transtemporal (mastoid) for excision of cerebellopontine angle tumor;**   ↻

61530   **combined with middle/posterior fossa craniotomy/craniectomy**   ↻

CIM 50-40 STEREOTAXIC DEPTH ELECTRODE IMPLANTATION

Medicare covers stereotaxic depth electrode implantation prior to surgical treatment of focal epilepsy for patients unresponsive to anticonvulsant medications for diagnosing resectable seizure foci that may go undetected by conventional scalp electroencephalographs (EEGs).

By taking several readings during seizure activity, the location of the epileptic focus may be found, so that decisions can be made regarding surgical treatment.

61531   **Subdural implantation of strip electrodes through one or more burr or trephine hole(s) for long term seizure monitoring**   80 ↻

     If stereotactic implantation of electrodes is performed, consult CPT code 61760.

61533   **Craniotomy with elevation of bone flap; for subdural implantation of an electrode array, for long term seizure monitoring**   80 ↻

     If continuous EEG monitoring is needed, consult CPT codes 95950-95954.

61534   **for excision of epileptogenic focus without electrocorticography during surgery**   80 ↻

61535   **for removal of epidural or subdural electrode array, without excision of cerebral tissue (separate procedure)**   80 ↻

61536   **for excision of cerebral epileptogenic focus, with electrocorticography during surgery (includes removal of electrode array)**   80 ↻

61538   **for lobectomy with electrocorticography during surgery, temporal lobe**   80 ↻

61539   **for lobectomy with electrocorticography during surgery, other than temporal lobe, partial or total**   80 ↻

61541   **for transection of corpus callosum**   80 ↻

61542   **for total hemispherectomy**   80 ↻

61543   **for partial or subtotal hemispherectomy**   80 ↻

61544   **for excision or coagulation of choroid plexus**   80 ↻

61545   **for excision of craniopharyngioma**   80 ↻

61546   **Craniotomy for hypophysectomy or excision of pituitary tumor, intracranial approach**   80 ↻

61548   **Hypophysectomy or excision of pituitary tumor, transnasal or transseptal approach, nonstereotactic**   80 ↻

     Do not report 69990 in addition to code 61548 as the operating microscope is considered an inclusive component of the surgery.

61550   **Craniectomy for craniosynostosis; single cranial suture**   80 ↻

61552   **multiple cranial sutures**   80 ↻

     If cranial reconstruction is performed for orbital hypertelorism, consult CPT codes 21260-21263.

61556   **Craniotomy for craniosynostosis; frontal or parietal bone flap**   80 ↻

61557   **bifrontal bone flap**   80 ↻

61558   **Extensive craniectomy for multiple cranial suture craniosynostosis (eg, cloverleaf skull); not requiring bone grafts**   80 ↻

61559   **recontouring with multiple osteotomies and bone autografts (eg, barrel-stave procedure) (includes obtaining grafts)**   80 ↻

61563   **Excision, intra and extracranial, benign tumor of cranial bone (eg, fibrous dysplasia); without optic nerve decompression**   80 ↻

61564   **with optic nerve decompression**   80 ↻

     If reconstruction is required, consult CPT codes 21181-21183.

61570   **Craniectomy or craniotomy; with excision of foreign body from brain**   80 ↻

61571   **with treatment of penetrating wound of brain**   80 ↻

     If a sequestrectomy is performed for osteomyelitis, consult CPT code 61501.

61575   **Transoral approach to skull base, brain stem or upper spinal cord for biopsy, decompression or excision of lesion;**   80 ↻

61576   **requiring splitting of tongue and/or mandible (including tracheostomy)**   80 ↻

     If arthrodesis is performed, consult CPT code 22548.

SURGERY OF SKULL BASE, APPROACH PROCEDURES, ANTERIOR CRANIAL FOSSA

Many physicians participate in the removal of lesions involving the skull base. Often working simultaneous, physicians from several specialties must work quickly to avoid infection. One physician may perform the approach procedure, another may perform the definitive procedure, and another may repair or reconstruct the dura, skull, and skin. Each must report the specific procedure performed.

Consult the glossary for more terms and guidelines.

61580   **Craniofacial approach to anterior cranial fossa; extradural, including lateral rhinotomy, ethmoidectomy, sphenoidectomy, without maxillectomy or orbital exenteration**   80 50

61581   **extradural, including lateral rhinotomy, orbital exenteration, ethmoidectomy, sphenoidectomy and/or maxillectomy**   ↻ 50

61582   **extradural, including unilateral or bifrontal craniotomy, elevation of frontal lobe(s), osteotomy of base of anterior cranial fossa**   80

61583   **intradural, including unilateral or bifrontal craniotomy, elevation or resection of frontal lobe, osteotomy of base of anterior cranial fossa**   80

61584   Orbitocranial approach to anterior cranial fossa, extradural, including supraorbital ridge osteotomy and elevation of frontal and/or temporal lobe(s); without orbital exenteration   80 50

61585   with orbital exenteration   80 ⊡ 50

61586   Bicoronal, transzygomatic and/or LeFort I osteotomy approach to anterior cranial fossa with or without internal fixation, without bone graft   80 ⊡

SURGERY OF SKULL BASE, APPROACH PROCEDURES, MIDDLE CRANIAL FOSSA

61590   Infratemporal pre-auricular approach to middle cranial fossa (parapharyngeal space, infratemporal and midline skull base, nasopharynx), with or without disarticulation of the mandible, including parotidectomy, craniotomy, decompression and/or mobilization of the facial nerve and/or petrous carotid artery   80 50

61591   Infratemporal post-auricular approach to middle cranial fossa (internal auditory meatus, petrous apex, tentorium, cavernous sinus, parasellar area, infratemporal fossa) including mastoidectomy, resection of sigmoid sinus, with or without decompression and/or mobilization of contents of auditory canal or petrous carotid artery   80 ⊡ 50

61592   Orbitocranial zygomatic approach to middle cranial fossa (cavernous sinus and carotid artery, clivus, basilar artery or petrous apex) including osteotomy of zygoma, craniotomy, extra- or intradural elevation of temporal lobe   80 50

SURGERY OF SKULL BASE, APPROACH PROCEDURES, POSTERIOR CRANIAL FOSSA

61595   Transtemporal approach to posterior cranial fossa, jugular foramen or midline skull base, including mastoidectomy, decompression of sigmoid sinus and/or facial nerve, with or without mobilization\   80 50

61596   Transcochlear approach to posterior cranial fossa, jugular foramen or midline skull base, including labyrinthectomy, decompression, with or without mobilization of facial nerve and/or petrous carotid artery   80 50

61597   Transcondylar (far lateral) approach to posterior cranial fossa, jugular foramen or midline skull base, including occipital condylectomy, mastoidectomy, resection of C1-C3 vertebral body(s), decompression of vertebral artery, with or without mobilization   80 50

61598   Transpetrosal approach to posterior cranial fossa, clivus or foramen magnum, including ligation of superior petrosal sinus and/or sigmoid sinus   80

SURGERY OF SKULL BASE, DEFINITIVE PROCEDURES, BASE OF ANTERIOR CRANIAL FOSSA

61600   Resection or excision of neoplastic, vascular or infectious lesion of base of anterior cranial fossa; extradural   80

61601   intradural, including dural repair, with or without graft   80

SURGERY OF SKULL BASE, DEFINITIVE PROCEDURES, BASE OF MIDDLE CRANIAL FOSSA

61605   Resection or excision of neoplastic, vascular or infectious lesion of infratemporal fossa, parapharyngeal space, petrous apex; extradural   80

61606   intradural, including dural repair, with or without graft   80

61607   Resection or excision of neoplastic, vascular or infectious lesion of parasellar area, cavernous sinus, clivus or midline skull base; extradural   80

61608   intradural, including dural repair, with or without graft   80

\+ 61609   Transection or ligation, carotid artery in cavernous sinus; without repair (List separately in addition to code for primary procedure)   80 50

> Note that 61609-61612 are reported in addition to code(s) for primary procedure(s) 61605-61608. Report only one transection or ligation of carotid artery code per operative session.

\+ 61610   with repair by anastomosis or graft (List separately in addition to code for primary procedure)   80 50

\+ 61611   Transection or ligation, carotid artery in petrous canal; without repair (List separately in addition to code for primary procedure)   80 50

\+ 61612   with repair by anastomosis or graft (List separately in addition to code for primary procedure)   80 50

61613   Obliteration of carotid aneurysm, arteriovenous malformation, or carotid-cavernous fistula by dissection within cavernous sinus   80 ⊡ 50

SURGERY OF SKULL BASE, DEFINITIVE PROCEDURES, BASE OF POSTERIOR CRANIAL FOSSA

61615   Resection or excision of neoplastic, vascular or infectious lesion of base of posterior cranial fossa, jugular foramen, foramen magnum, or C1-C3 vertebral bodies; extradural   80

61616   intradural, including dural repair, with or without graft   80

SURGERY OF SKULL BASE, REPAIR AND/OR RECONSTRUCTION OF SURGICAL DEFECTS OF SKULL BASE

▲ 61618   Secondary repair of dura for cerebrospinal fluid leak, anterior, middle or posterior cranial fossa following surgery of the skull base; by free tissue graft (eg, pericranium, fascia, tensor fascia lata, adipose tissue, homologous or synthetic grafts)   80

61619   by local or regionalized vascularized pedicle flap or myocutaneous flap (including galea, temporalis, frontalis or occipitalis muscle)   80

ENDOVASCULAR THERAPY

Consult the glossary for more terms and guidelines.

CIM 35-35 THERAPEUTIC EMBOLIZATION

Therapeutic embolization is covered when done for hemorrhage and for other conditions amenable to treatment by the procedure. Renal embolization for the treatment of renal adenocarcinoma is covered as a type of therapeutic embolization to:

- Reduce tumor vascularity preoperatively
- Reduce tumor bulk in inoperable cases
- Palliate specific symptoms

61624   Transcatheter occlusion or embolization (eg, for tumor destruction, to achieve hemostasis, to occlude a vascular malformation), percutaneous, any method; central nervous system (intracranial, spinal cord)

> Consult also CPT code 37204. If radiological supervision and interpretation is needed, consult CPT code 75894.

61626   non-central nervous system, head or neck (extracranial, brachiocephalic branch)

> Consult also CPT code 37204. If radiological supervision and interpretation is needed, consult CPT code 75894.

⊡ CCI Comprehensive Code   50 Bilateral Procedure   + CPT Add-on Code   ⊘ Modifier -51 Exempt Code   ● New Code   ▲ Revised Code

M Maternity   N Newborn   P Pediatric   N/P Newborn/Pediatric

SURGERY FOR ANEURYSM, ARTERIOVENOUS MALFORMATION OR VASCULAR DISEASE

CPT codes 61680-61711 include craniotomy when it is appropriate for the procedure.

61680	**Surgery of intracranial arteriovenous malformation; supratentorial, simple**	80
61682	**supratentorial, complex**	80 ⤵
61684	**infratentorial, simple**	80
61686	**infratentorial, complex**	80 ⤵
61690	**dural, simple**	80
61692	**dural, complex**	80 ⤵
61697	**Surgery of complex intracranial aneurysm, intracranial approach; carotid circulation**	80

CPT codes 61697, 61698 involve aneurysms that are larger than 15mm or have calcification of the aneurysm neck, or if procedure requires temoprary vessel occlusion, trapping or cardiopulmonary bypass to successfully treat the aneurysm.

61698	**vertebrobasilar circulation**	80
▲ **61700**	**Surgery of simple intracranial aneurysm, intracranial approach; carotid circulation**	80 ⤵
61702	**vertebrobasilar circulation**	80
61703	**Surgery of intracranial aneurysm, cervical approach by application of occluding clamp to cervical carotid artery (Selverstone-Crutchfield type)**	80

If direct ligation of the carotid artery is performed through a cervical approach, consult CPT codes 37600-37606.

61705	**Surgery of aneurysm, vascular malformation or carotid-cavernous fistula; by intracranial and cervical occlusion of carotid artery**	80
61708	**by intracranial electrothrombosis**	80

If ligation or gradual occlusion is performed for a internal/common carotid artery, consult CPT codes 37605 and 37606.

61710	**by intra-arterial embolization, injection procedure, or balloon catheter**	80
61711	**Anastomosis, arterial, extracranial-intracranial (eg, middle cerebral/cortical) arteries**	80

STEREOTAXIS

61720	**Creation of lesion by stereotactic method, including burr hole(s) and localizing and recording techniques, single or multiple stages; globus pallidus or thalamus**	⤵
61735	**subcortical structure(s) other than globus pallidus or thalamus**	⤵

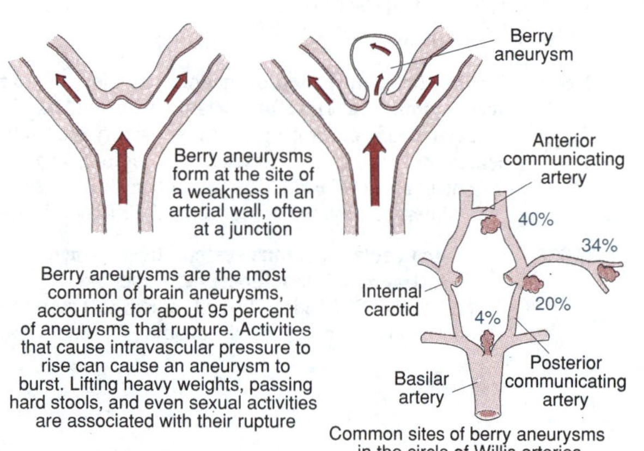

Berry aneurysms are the most common of brain aneurysms, accounting for about 95 percent of aneurysms that rupture. Activities that cause intravascular pressure to rise can cause an aneurysm to burst. Lifting heavy weights, passing hard stools, and even sexual activities are associated with their rupture.

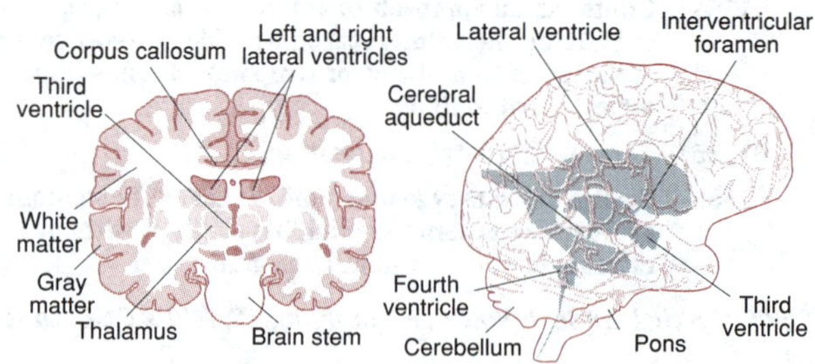

Frontal secion of the brain (left) and lateral view schematic showing the ventricular system in blue (right)

Cerebral spinal fluid (CSF) is secreted in the ventricles and flows generally from the laterals into the third ventricle via the interventricular foramina, and into the fourth ventricle via the cerebral aqueduct. Many brain disorders upset ventricular fluid pressures and shunts are employed to restore balance

CIM 35-84 STEREOTACTIC CINGULOTOMY AS A MEANS OF PSYCHOSURGERY - NOT COVERED

Cingulotomy is a psychosurgical procedure designed to interrupt the neuronal pathways of the brain to modify disturbances of behavior, thought content, or mood that are not responsive to other conventional modes of therapy. Stereotactic cingulotomy is not covered under Medicare because the procedure is considered to be investigational.

61750	**Stereotactic biopsy, aspiration, or excision, including burr hole(s), for intracranial lesion;**	⤵

CIM 35-84 STEREOTACTIC CINGULOTOMY AS A MEANS OF PSYCHOSURGERY - NOT COVERED

Cingulotomy is a psychosurgical procedure designed to interrupt the neuronal pathways of the brain to modify disturbances of behavior, thought content, or mood that are not responsive to other conventional modes of therapy. Stereotactic cingulotomy is not covered under Medicare because the procedure is considered to be investigational.

CIM 50-12 COMPUTERIZED TOMOGRAPHY

Diagnostic examinations of the head (head scans) and of other parts of the body (body scans) performed by computerized tomography (CT) scanners are covered if medical and scientific literature and opinion support the effective use of a scan for the condition.

There is no general rule that requires other diagnostic tests to be tried before CT scanning is used. However, in an individual case the contractor's medical staff may determine that a CT scan as the initial diagnostic test was not reasonable and necessary if not supported by the patient's symptoms or complaints stated on the claim form; e.g., "periodic headaches."

CT equipment must meet the following criteria:

1. Known to the Food and Drug Administration

2. In the full market release phase of development

Mobile CT scan services furnished at an ambulatory health care facility other than a hospital-based facility (e.g., a freestanding physician-directed clinic) must be performed under the direct personal supervision of a radiologist or other qualified physician. In addition, the facility must maintain a record of the attending physician's order. Bill the same as for scans performed on stationary equipment.

Medicare covers multiplanar diagnostic imaging (MPDI), known as planar image reconstruction or reformatted imaging, when performed by an entity offering covered CT scans.

CIM 50-13 MAGNETIC RESONANCE

Medicare covers magnetic resonance imaging (MRI), formerly called nuclear magnetic resonance (NMR), when furnished using MRI units with Food and Drug Administration pre-market approval. An MRI is covered when used to detect:

- To detect and stage pelvic and retroperitoneal neoplasms
- To evaluate disorders of cancellous bone and soft tissues
- To detect pericardial thickening

- To detect and monitor early-stage primary and secondary bone neoplasm and aseptic necrosis

- To detect early states of bone infections for patients with metallic prostheses, especially of the hip, to which the prothesis is attached

- Disc disease without regard to radiological imaging

In addition:

- The inherent tissue contrast resolution of MRI makes it an appropriate standard diagnostic modality for general neuroradiology

- When a clinical need exists to visualize the parenchyma of solid organs to detect anatomic disruption or neoplasia, this can be accomplished in the liver, urogenital system, adrenals, and pelvic organs without the use of radiological contrast materials

- Gating devices that eliminate distorted images caused by cardiac and respiratory movement cycles may be covered. Surface and other specialty coils may be covered, as they are used routinely for high-resolution imaging where small limited regions of the body are studied

MRI is not covered for patients with cardiac pacemakers or with metallic clips on vascular aneurysms. In addition, the long imaging time and the enclosed position of the patient may result in claustrophobia, making patients who have a history of claustrophobia unsuitable candidates for MRI procedures. Several uses of MRI have been identified as investigational and are not covered. These include measurement of blood flow and spectroscopy. In addition, MRI is not suitable for the imaging of cortical bone and calcifications and for procedures involving spatial resolution of bone or calcifications.

61751   **with computerized axial tomography and/or magnetic resonance guidance**

> If radiological supervision and interpretation of computerized tomography is needed, consult CPT codes 70450, 70460, and 70470 as appropriate. If radiological supervision and interpretation of magnetic resonance imaging is needed, consult CPT codes 70551, 70552, and 70553 as appropriate.

CIM 50-40 STEREOTAXIC DEPTH ELECTRODE IMPLANTATION

Medicare covers stereotaxic depth electrode implantation prior to surgical treatment of focal epilepsy for patients unresponsive to anticonvulsant medications for diagnosing resectable seizure foci that may go undetected by conventional scalp electroencephalographs (EEGs).

By taking several readings during seizure activity, the location of the epileptic focus may be found, so that decisions can be made regarding surgical treatment.

61760   **Stereotactic implantation of depth electrodes into the cerebrum for long term seizure monitoring**

61770   **Stereotactic localization, including burr hole(s), with insertion of catheter(s) or probe(s) for placement of radiation source**

61790   **Creation of lesion by stereotactic method, percutaneous, by neurolytic agent (eg, alcohol, thermal, electrical, radiofrequency); gasserian ganglion**

61791   **trigeminal medullary tract**

61793   **Stereotactic radiosurgery (particle beam, gamma ray or linear accelerator), one or more sessions**

> To report intensity modulated beam delivery plan and treatment, consult CPT codes 77301, 77418.

+ 61795   **Stereotactic computer assisted volumetric (navigational) procedure, intracranial, extracranial, or spinal (List separately in addition to code for primary procedure)**

NEUROSTIMULATORS (INTRACRANIAL)

Consult the glossary for more terms and guidelines.

For programming or electronic analysis of neurostimulator pulse generators, initial or subsequent, consult CPT codes 95970-95975.

CIM 35-20 TREATMENT OF MOTOR FUNCTION DISORDERS WITH ELECTRIC NERVE STIMULATION - NOT COVERED

No reimbursement may be made for electric nerve stimulation or for the services related to its implantation since this treatment cannot be considered reasonable and necessary. However, Medicare covers deep brain stimulation by implanting a stimulator device at the carrier's discretion.

CIM 65-8 ELECTRICAL NERVE STIMULATORS

Two general classifications of electrical nerve stimulators are employed to treat chronic intractable pain: peripheral nerve stimulators and central nervous system stimulators.

There are two types of implantations covered by this instruction:

- Dorsal column (spinal cord) neurostimulation.

- Depth brain neurostimulation

No payment may be made unless all of the conditions listed below have been met:

a. The implantation of the stimulator is used only as a late resort (if not a last resort) for patients with chronic intractable pain

b. Other treatment modalities (pharmacological, surgical, physical, or psychological therapies) have been tried and did not prove satisfactory, or are judged to be unsuitable or contraindicated for the given patient

c. Patients have undergone careful screening, evaluation and diagnosis by a multidisciplinary team prior to implantation. (psychological and physical evaluation)

d. All the facilities, equipment, and professional and support personnel required for the proper diagnosis, treatment training, and follow-up of the patient must be available

e. Demonstration of pain relief with a temporarily implanted electrode precedes permanent implantation

61850   **Twist drill or burr hole(s) for implantation of neurostimulator electrodes, cortical**

61860   **Craniectomy or craniotomy for implantation of neurostimulator electrodes, cerebral, cortical**

61862   **Twist drill, burr hole, craniotomy, or craniectomy for stereotactic implantation of one neurostimulator array in subcortical site (eg, thalamus, globus pallidus, subthalamic nucleus, periventricular, periaqueductal gray)**

61870   **Craniectomy for implantation of neurostimulator electrodes, cerebellar; cortical**

61875   **subcortical**

61880   **Revision or removal of intracranial neurostimulator electrodes**

61885   **Incision and subcutaneous placement of cranial neurostimulator pulse generator or receiver, direct or inductive coupling; with connection to a single electrode array**

61886   **with connection to two or more electrode arrays**

> If open placement of a cranial nerve (e.g., vagal, trigeminal) neurostimulator electrode(s) is performed, consult CPT code 64573. If percutaneous placement of a cranial nerve (eg, vagal, trigeminal) neurostimulator electrode(s) is performed, consult CPT code 65443. If revision or removal of a cranial nerve (eg, vagal, trigeminal) neurostimulator electrode(s) is performed, consult CPT code 64585.

61888   **Revision or removal of cranial neurostimulator pulse generator or receiver**

REPAIR

Consult the glossary for more terms and guidelines.

62000   **Elevation of depressed skull fracture; simple, extradural**

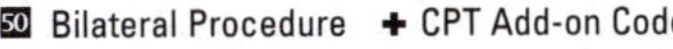 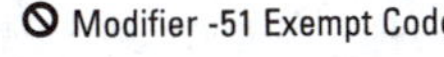

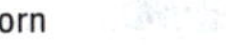 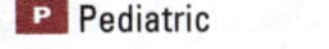

▪ CCI Comprehensive Code   **50** Bilateral Procedure   **+** CPT Add-on Code   Ⓢ Modifier -51 Exempt Code   ● New Code   ▲ Revised Code

M Maternity   **N** Newborn   **P** Pediatric   **N/P** Newborn/Pediatric

Nervous System

62005 — 62282*

62005	compound or comminuted, extradural	80
62010	with repair of dura and/or debridement of brain	80
▲ 62100	Craniotomy for repair of dural/cerebrospinal fluid leak, including surgery for rhinorrhea/otorrhea	80

If a spinal dural/CSF leak is repaired, consult CPT codes 63707 and 63709.

62115	Reduction of craniomegalic skull (eg, treated hydrocephalus); not requiring bone grafts or cranioplasty	80
62116	with simple cranioplasty	80
62117	requiring craniotomy and reconstruction with or without bone graft (includes obtaining grafts)	80
62120	Repair of encephalocele, skull vault, including cranioplasty	80
62121	Craniotomy for repair of encephalocele, skull base	80
62140	Cranioplasty for skull defect; up to 5 cm diameter	80
62141	larger than 5 cm diameter	80
62142	Removal of bone flap or prosthetic plate of skull	80
62143	Replacement of bone flap or prosthetic plate of skull	80
62145	Cranioplasty for skull defect with reparative brain surgery	80
62146	Cranioplasty with autograft (includes obtaining bone grafts); up to 5 cm diameter	80
62147	larger than 5 cm diameter	80

CSF SHUNT

62180	Ventriculocisternostomy (Torkildsen type operation)	80
62190	Creation of shunt; subarachnoid/subdural-atrial, -jugular, -auricular	
62192	subarachnoid/subdural-peritoneal, -pleural, other terminus	80
62194	Replacement or irrigation, subarachnoid/subdural catheter	❶ 80
62200	Ventriculocisternostomy, third ventricle;	80
	Dandy ventriculocisternostomy	
62201	stereotactic method	
62220	Creation of shunt; ventriculo-atrial, -jugular, -auricular	80
62223	ventriculo-peritoneal, -pleural, other terminus	80
62225	Replacement or irrigation, ventricular catheter	❶
▲ 62230	Replacement or revision of cerebrospinal fluid shunt, obstructed valve, or distal catheter in shunt system	❷ 80
▲ 62252	Reprogramming of programmable cerebrospinal shunt	80

(If the physician interprets the results and/or operates the equipment, modifer-26 should be appended to 66252)

▲ 62256	Removal of complete cerebrospinal fluid shunt system; without replacement	❷ 80
62258	with replacement by similar or other shunt at same operation	80

If percutaneous irrigation or aspiration of a shunt reservoir is performed, consult CPT code 61070.

For reprogramming of programmable CSF shunt, consult CPT code 62252.

SPINE AND SPINAL CORD

Most common agent in neonates is E. coli; Haemophilus influenzae b and streptococcus pneumoniae are common agents in adult cases

The brain and spinal cord are encased in a tough fibrous membrane known as the meninges and meningitis is an inflammation of that tissue and commonly affects the underlying central nervous system tissues and fluids; causes are numerous and classification is based on type of infection; purulent refers to forms usually caused by bacteria; chronic meningitis is usually caused by mycobacteria and fungi; aseptic or abacterial meningitis is commonly associated with a viral infection and is reported with the underlying disease. Encephalitis is inflammation of the brain and is also usually associated with a viral infection and also is reported with the underlying disease

If application of caliper or tongs is performed, consult CPT code 20660. If a fracture or dislocation of the spine is treated, consult CPT codes 22305-22327.

INJECTION, DRAINAGE, OR ASPIRATION

62263	Percutaneous lysis of epidural adhesions using solution injection (eg, hypertonic saline, enzyme) or mechanical means (eg, spring-wound catheter) including radiologic localization (includes contrast when administered)	❶
62268*	Percutaneous aspiration, spinal cord cyst or syrinx	❶

For radiological supervision and interpretation, consult CPT codes 76003, 76360, and 76942.

62269*	Biopsy of spinal cord, percutaneous needle	❶ 80

For radiological supervision and interpretation, consult CPT codes 76003, 76360, and 76942.

CPT codes 62270-62273 include the injection of contrast during fluoroscopic guidance and localization. Report CPT code 76005 for fluoroscopic guidance and localization unless a formal contrast study (e.g., arthrography, myelography, and epidurography) is performed.

62270*	Spinal puncture, lumbar, diagnostic	❶
▲ 62272*	Spinal puncture, therapeutic, for drainage of cerebrospinal fluid (by needle or catheter)	❶

CIM 45-11 AUTOGENOUS EPIDURAL BLOOD GRAFT

Medicare covers autogenous epidural blood grafts as a remedy for severe headaches that may occur after spinal anesthesia, spinal taps, or myelograms. In the procedure, blood is removed from the patient's vein and injected into the epidural space to seal the leak and stop the pain.

62273*	Injection, epidural, of blood or clot patch	❶

CPT codes 62280-62282 include the injection of contrast during fluoroscopic guidance and localization. Report CPT code 76005 for fluoroscopic guidance and localization unless a formal contrast study (e.g., arthrography, myelography, and epidurography) is performed.

62280*	Injection/infusion of neurolytic substance (eg, alcohol, phenol, iced saline solutions), with or without other therapeutic substance; subarachnoid	❶
62281*	epidural, cervical or thoracic	
62282*	epidural, lumbar, sacral (caudal)	❶

CIM 50-12 COMPUTERIZED TOMOGRAPHY

Diagnostic examinations of the head (head scans) and of other parts of the body (body scans) performed by computerized tomography (CT) scanners are covered if medical and scientific literature and opinion support the effective use of a scan for the condition.

There is no general rule that requires other diagnostic tests to be tried before CT scanning is used. However, in an individual case the contractor's medical staff may determine that a CT scan as the initial diagnostic test was not reasonable and necessary if not supported by the patient's symptoms or complaints stated on the claim form; e.g., "periodic headaches."

CT equipment must meet the following criteria:

1. Known to the Food and Drug Administration

2. In the full market release phase of development

Mobile CT scan services furnished at an ambulatory health care facility other than a hospital-based facility (e.g., a freestanding physician-directed clinic) must be performed under the direct personal supervision of a radiologist or other qualified physician. In addition, the facility must maintain a record of the attending physician's order. Bill the same as for scans performed on stationary equipment.

Medicare covers multiplanar diagnostic imaging (MPDI), known as planar image reconstruction or reformatted imaging, when performed by an entity offering covered CT scans.

62284* **Injection procedure for myelography and/or computerized axial tomography, spinal (other than C1-C2 and posterior fossa)**

If an injection procedure is performed at C1-C2, consult CPT code 61055. For radiological supervision and interpretation, consult the Radiology section of CPT.

62287 **Aspiration or decompression procedure, percutaneous, of nucleus pulposus of intervertebral disk, any method, single or multiple levels, lumbar (eg, manual or automated percutaneous diskectomy, percutaneous laser diskectomy)**

If fluoroscopic guidance is performed, consult CPT code 76003.

62290* **Injection procedure for diskography, each level; lumbar**

62291* **cervical or thoracic**

For radiological supervision and interpretation, consult CPT codes 72285 and 72295.

62292 **Injection procedure for chemonucleolysis, including diskography, intervertebral disk, single or multiple levels, lumbar**

62294 **Injection procedure, arterial, for occlusion of arteriovenous malformation, spinal**

CPT codes 62310-62319 include the injection of contrast during fluoroscopic guidance and localization. Report CPT code 76005 for fluoroscopic guidance and localization unless a formal contrast study (e.g., arthrography, myelography, and epidurography) is performed.

If a transforaminal epidural injection is performed, consult CPT codes 64479-64484.

62310 **Injection, single (not via indwelling catheter), not including neurolytic substances, with or without contrast (for either localization or epidurography), of diagnostic or therapeutic substance(s) (including anesthetic, antispasmodic, opioid, steroid, other solution), epidural or subarachnoid; cervical or thoracic**

62311 **lumbar, sacral (caudal)**

62318 **Injection, including catheter placement, continuous infusion or intermittent bolus, not including neurolytic substances, with or without contrast (for either localization or epidurography), of diagnostic or therapeutic substance(s) (including anesthetic, antispasmodic, opioid, steroid, other solution), epidural or subarachnoid; cervical or thoracic**

62319 **lumbar, sacral (caudal)**

CATHETER IMPLANTATION

If an implantable reservoir or infusion pump is refilled and maintained, consult CPT code 96530. If an intrathecal or epidural is placed percutaneously, consult CPT codes 62270-62273, 62280-62284, and 62310-62319.

If application of caliper or tongs is performed, consult CPT code 20660. If a fracture or dislocation of the spine is treated, consult CPT codes 22305-22327.

62350 **Implantation, revision or repositioning of tunneled intrathecal or epidural catheter, for long-term medication administration via an external pump or implantable reservoir/infusion pump; without laminectomy**

62351 **with laminectomy**

62355 **Removal of previously implanted intrathecal or epidural catheter**

RESERVOIR/PUMP IMPLANTATION

62360 **Implantation or replacement of device for intrathecal or epidural drug infusion; subcutaneous reservoir**

62361 **non-programmable pump**

62362 **programmable pump, including preparation of pump, with or without programming**

62365 **Removal of subcutaneous reservoir or pump, previously implanted for intrathecal or epidural infusion**

62367 **Electronic analysis of programmable, implanted pump for intrathecal or epidural drug infusion (includes evaluation of reservoir status, alarm status, drug prescription status); without reprogramming**

(If the physician interprets the results and/or operates the equipment, modifer-26 should be appended to 62367).

62368 **with reprogramming**

If an implantable pump or reservoir is refilled, consult CPT code 96530.

(If the physician interprets the results and/or operates the equipment, modifer-26 should be appended to 62368).

POSTERIOR EXTRADURAL LAMINOTOMY OR LAMINECTOMY FOR EXPLORATION/DECOMPRESSION OF NEURAL ELEMENTS OR EXCISION OF HERNIATED INTERVERTEBRAL DISKS

If application of caliper or tongs is performed, consult CPT code 20660. If a fracture or dislocation of the spine is treated, consult CPT codes 22305-22327.

If these procedures are followed by arthrodesis, consult CPT codes 22590-22614.

63001 **Laminectomy with exploration and/or decompression of spinal cord and/or cauda equina, without facetectomy, foraminotomy or diskectomy, (eg, spinal stenosis), one or two vertebral segments; cervical**

63003 **thoracic**

63005 **lumbar, except for spondylolisthesis**

63011 **sacral**

63012 **Laminectomy with removal of abnormal facets and/or pars inter-articularis with decompression of cauda equina and nerve roots for spondylolisthesis, lumbar (Gill type procedure)**

63015 **Laminectomy with exploration and/or decompression of spinal cord and/or cauda equina, without facetectomy, foraminotomy or diskectomy, (eg, spinal stenosis), more than 2 vertebral segments; cervical**

63016 **thoracic**

63017 **lumbar**

63020 **Laminotomy (hemilaminectomy), with decompression of nerve root(s), including partial facetectomy, foraminotomy and/or excision of herniated intervertebral disk; one interspace, cervical**

63030   one interspace, lumbar (including open or endoscopically-assisted approach)   80 50

+ 63035   each additional interspace, cervical or lumbar (List separately in addition to code for primary procedure)   80 50
> Note that 63035 is an add-on code and must be used in conjunction with 63020-63030.

63040   Laminotomy (hemilaminectomy), with decompression of nerve root(s), including partial facetectomy, foraminotomy and/or excision of herniated intervertebral disk, reexploration, single interspace; cervical   80 50

63042   lumbar   80 50

● + 63043   each additional cervical interspace (List separately in addition to code for primary procedure)
> Note that CPT code 63043 is an add-on code and must be used in conjunction with 63040.

● + 63044   each additional lumbar interspace (List separately in addition to code for primary procedure)
> Note taht 63044 is an add-on code and must be used in conjunction with 63042.

63045   Laminectomy, facetectomy and foraminotomy (unilateral or bilateral with decompression of spinal cord, cauda equina and/or nerve root(s), (eg, spinal or lateral recess stenosis), single vertebral segment; cervical   80

63046   thoracic   80

63047   lumbar   80

+ 63048   each additional segment, cervical, thoracic, or lumbar (List separately in addition to code for primary procedure)   80
> Note that 63048 is an add-on code and must be used in conjunction with 63045-63047.

TRANSPEDICULAR OR COSTOVERTEBRAL APPROACH FOR POSTEROLATERAL EXTRADURAL EXPLORATION/DECOMPRESSION

If application of caliper or tongs is performed, consult CPT code 20660. If a fracture or dislocation of the spine is treated, consult CPT codes 22305-22327.

63055   Transpedicular approach with decompression of spinal cord, equina and/or nerve root(s) (eg, herniated intervertebral disk), single segment; thoracic   80

63056   lumbar (including transfacet, or lateral extraforaminal approach) (eg, far lateral herniated intervertebral disk)   80

+ 63057   each additional segment, thoracic or lumbar (List separately in addition to code for primary procedure)   80
> Note that 63057 is an add-on code and must be used in conjunction with 63055, 63056.

63064   Costovertebral approach with decompression of spinal cord or nerve root(s), (eg, herniated intervertebral disk), thoracic; single segment   80

+ 63066   each additional segment (List separately in addition to code for primary procedure)   80
> Note that 63066 is an add-on code and must be used in conjunction with 63064.

ANTERIOR OR ANTEROLATERAL APPROACH FOR EXTRADURAL EXPLORATION/DECOMPRESSION

Do not report 69990 in addition to codes 63075-63078 as the operating microscope is considered an inclusive component of these procedures.

If application of caliper or tongs is performed, consult CPT code 20660. If a fracture or dislocation of the spine is treated, consult CPT codes 22305-22327.

63075   Diskectomy, anterior, with decompression of spinal cord and/or nerve root(s), including osteophytectomy; cervical, single interspace   80

+ 63076   cervical, each additional interspace (List separately in addition to code for primary procedure)   80
> Note that 63076 is an add-on code and must be used in conjunction with 63075.

63077   thoracic, single interspace   80

+ 63078   thoracic, each additional interspace (List separately in addition to code for primary procedure)   80
> Note that 63078 is an add-on code and must be used in conjunction with 63077.

If application of caliper or tongs is performed, consult CPT code 20660. If a fracture or dislocation of the spine is treated, consult CPT codes 22305-22327.

Note that 63081-63091 include diskectomy above and/or below vertebral segment. If these procedures are followed by arthrodesis, consult CPT codes 22554-22812. If the spine is reconstructed, use the appropriate vertebral corpectomy (63081-63091), bone graft codes (20930-20938), arthrodesis codes (22548-22812), and spinal instrumentation codes (22840-22855). If resection of the sternocleidomastoid muscle is performed, consult CPT code 21720.

63081   Vertebral corpectomy (vertebral body resection), partial or complete, anterior approach with decompression of spinal cord and/or nerve root(s); cervical, single segment   80

+ 63082   cervical, each additional segment (List separately in addition to code for primary procedure)   80
> Note that 63082 is an add-on code and must be used in conjunction with 63081.
>
> If a transoral approach is used, consult CPT codes 61575 and 61576.

63085   Vertebral corpectomy (vertebral body resection), partial or complete, transthoracic approach with decompression of spinal cord and/or nerve root(s); thoracic, single segment   80

+ 63086   thoracic, each additional segment (List separately in addition to code for primary procedure)   80
> Note that 63086 is an add-on code and must be used in conjunction with 63085.

63087   Vertebral corpectomy (vertebral body resection), partial or complete, combined thoracolumbar approach with decompression of spinal cord, cauda equina or nerve root(s), lower thoracic or lumbar; single segment   80

+ **63088**   each additional segment (List separately in
                   addition to code for primary procedure)   80
          Note that 63088 is an add-on code and must be used in
          conjunction with 63087.

63090   Vertebral corpectomy (vertebral body resection), partial
            or complete, transperitoneal or retroperitoneal approach
            with decompression of spinal cord, cauda equina or
            nerve root(s), lower thoracic, lumbar, or sacral; single
            segment   80 ▣

+ **63091**   each additional segment (List separately in
                   addition to code for primary procedure)   80
          Note that 63091 is an add-on code and must be used in
          conjunction with 63090.

INCISION

If application of caliper or tongs is performed, consult CPT code 20660. If a
fracture or dislocation of the spine is treated, consult CPT codes 22305-
22327.

63170	Laminectomy with myelotomy (eg, Bischof or DREZ type), cervical, thoracic or thoracolumbar	80 ▣
63172	Laminectomy with drainage of intramedullary cyst/syrinx; to subarachnoid space	80 ▣
63173	to peritoneal space	80 ▣
63180	Laminectomy and section of dentate ligaments, with or without dural graft, cervical; one or two segments	80 ▣
63182	more than two segments	80 ▣
63185	Laminectomy with rhizotomy; one or two segments	80 ▣
	Dana rhizotomy	
63190	more than two segments	80 ▣
63191	Laminectomy with section of spinal accessory nerve	80 ▣ 50
	If resection of the sternocleidomastoid muscle is performed, consult CPT code 21720.	
63194	Laminectomy with cordotomy, with section of one spinothalamic tract, one stage; cervical	80 ▣
63195	thoracic	80 ▣
63196	Laminectomy with cordotomy, with section of both spinothalamic tracts, one stage; cervical	80 ▣
63197	thoracic	80 ▣
63198	Laminectomy with cordotomy with section of both spinothalamic tracts, two stages within 14 days; cervical	80 ▣
	Keen laminectomy	
63199	thoracic	80 ▣
63200	Laminectomy, with release of tethered spinal cord, lumbar	80 ▣

EXCISION BY LAMINECTOMY OF LESION OTHER THAN HERNIATED DISK

63250	Laminectomy for excision or occlusion of arteriovenous malformation of spinal cord; cervical	80 ▣
63251	thoracic	80 ▣
63252	thoracolumbar	80 ▣
63265	Laminectomy for excision or evacuation of intraspinal lesion other than neoplasm, extradural; cervical	80 ▣
63266	thoracic	80 ▣
63267	lumbar	80 ▣
63268	sacral	80 ▣
63270	Laminectomy for excision of intraspinal lesion other than neoplasm, intradural; cervical	80 ▣
63271	thoracic	80 ▣

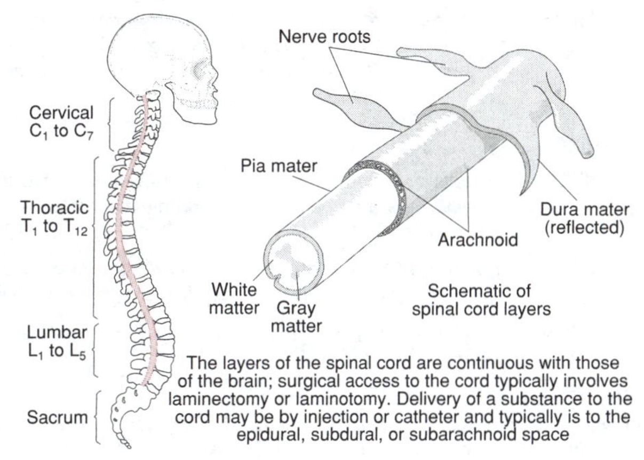

63272	lumbar	80 ▣
63273	sacral	80 ▣
63275	Laminectomy for biopsy/excision of intraspinal neoplasm; extradural, cervical	80 ▣
63276	extradural, thoracic	80 ▣
63277	extradural, lumbar	80 ▣
63278	extradural, sacral	80 ▣
63280	intradural, extramedullary, cervical	80 ▣
63281	intradural, extramedullary, thoracic	80 ▣
63282	intradural, extramedullary, lumbar	80 ▣
63283	intradural, sacral	80 ▣
63285	intradural, intramedullary, cervical	80 ▣
63286	intradural, intramedullary, thoracic	80 ▣
63287	intradural, intramedullary, thoracolumbar	80 ▣
63290	combined extradural-intradural lesion, any level	80 ▣
	For an intramedullary cyst/syrinx is drained, consult CPT codes 63172 and 63173.	

EXCISION, ANTERIOR OR ANTEROLATERAL APPROACH, INTRASPINAL LESION

If application of caliper or tongs is performed, consult CPT code 20660. If a
fracture or dislocation of the spine is treated, consult CPT codes 22305-
22327.

If arthrodesis is performed, consult CPT codes 22548-22585. If the spine is
reconstructed, consult CPT codes 20930-20938.

63300	Vertebral corpectomy (vertebral body resection), partial or complete, for excision of intraspinal lesion, single segment; extradural, cervical	80 ▣
63301	extradural, thoracic by transthoracic approach	80 ▣
63302	extradural, thoracic by thoracolumbar approach	80 ▣
63303	extradural, lumbar or sacral by transperitoneal or retroperitoneal approach	80 ▣
63304	intradural, cervical	80 ▣
63305	intradural, thoracic by transthoracic approach	80 ▣
63306	intradural, thoracic by thoracolumbar approach	80 ▣
63307	intradural, lumbar or sacral by transperitoneal or retroperitoneal approach	80 ▣

+ **63308** each additional segment (List separately in addition to codes for single segment) `80`
Note that 63308 is an add-on code and must be used in conjunction with 63300-63307.

STEREOTAXIS

63600 Creation of lesion of spinal cord by stereotactic method, percutaneous, any modality (including stimulation and/or recording) `❷ 80`

63610 Stereotactic stimulation of spinal cord, percutaneous, separate procedure not followed by other surgery `❶ 80`

63615 Stereotactic biopsy, aspiration, or excision of lesion, spinal cord

NEUROSTIMULATORS (SPINAL)

For programming or electronic analysis of neurostimulator pulse generators, initial or subsequent, consult CPT codes 95970-95975.

Consult the glossary for more terms and guidelines.

CIM 35-20 TREATMENT OF MOTOR FUNCTION DISORDERS WITH ELECTRIC NERVE STIMULATION - NOT COVERED

No reimbursement may be made for electric nerve stimulation or for the services related to its implantation since this treatment cannot be considered reasonable and necessary. However, Medicare covers deep brain stimulation by implanting a stimulator device at the carrier's discretion.

CIM 65-8 ELECTRICAL NERVE STIMULATORS

Two general classifications of electrical nerve stimulators are employed to treat chronic intractable pain: peripheral nerve stimulators and central nervous system stimulators.

There are two types of implantations covered by this instruction:

- Dorsal column (spinal cord) neurostimulation.
- Depth brain neurostimulation

No payment may be made unless all of the conditions listed below have been met:

a. The implantation of the stimulator is used only as a late resort (if not a last resort) for patients with chronic intractable pain

b. Other treatment modalities (pharmacological, surgical, physical, or psychological therapies) have been tried and did not prove satisfactory, or are judged to be unsuitable or contraindicated for the given patient

c. Patients have undergone careful screening, evaluation and diagnosis by a multidisciplinary team prior to implantation. (psychological and physical evaluation)

d. All the facilities, equipment, and professional and support personnel required for the proper diagnosis, treatment training, and follow-up of the patient must be available

e. Demonstration of pain relief with a temporarily implanted electrode precedes permanent implantation

63650 Percutaneous implantation of neurostimulator electrode array, epidural `❷`

63655 Laminectomy for implantation of neurostimulator electrodes, plate/paddle, epidural `80`

63660 Revision or removal of spinal neurostimulator electrode percutaneous array(s) or plate/paddle(s) `❶`

63685 Incision and subcutaneous placement of spinal neurostimulator pulse generator or receiver, direct or inductive coupling `❷ 80`

63688 Revision or removal of implanted spinal neurostimulator pulse generator or receiver `❶`

REPAIR

63700 Repair of meningocele; less than 5 cm diameter `80`

63702 larger than 5 cm diameter `80`

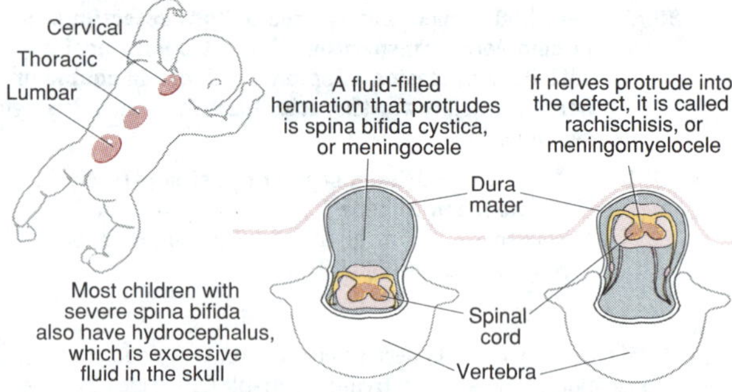

63704 Repair of myelomeningocele; less than 5 cm diameter `80`

63706 larger than 5 cm diameter `80`
If this procedure involves complex skin closure, consult the Integumentary System section of CPT.

▲ **63707** Repair of dural/cerebrospinal fluid leak, not requiring laminectomy `80`

▲ **63709** Repair of dural/cerebrospinal fluid leak or pseudomeningocele, with laminectomy `80`

63710 Dural graft, spinal `80`
If a cervical laminectomy and section of dentate ligaments are performed, with or without a dural graft, consult CPT codes 63180 and 63182.

SHUNT, SPINAL CSF

63740 Creation of shunt, lumbar, subarachnoid-peritoneal, -pleural, or other; including laminectomy `80`

63741 percutaneous, not requiring laminectomy `80`

63744 Replacement, irrigation or revision of lumbosubarachnoid shunt `❸ 80`

63746 Removal of entire lumbosubarachnoid shunt system without replacement `❷ 80`

EXTRACRANIAL NERVES, PERIPHERAL NERVES, AND AUTONOMIC NERVOUS SYSTEM

To report intracranial surgery on cranial nerves, consult CPT codes 61450, 61460, 61790.

INTRODUCTION/INJECTION OF ANESTHETIC AGENT (NERVE BLOCK), DIAGNOSTIC, OR THERAPEUTIC, SOMATIC NERVES

64400* Injection, anesthetic agent; trigeminal nerve, any division or branch

64402* facial nerve

64405* greater occipital nerve

64408* vagus nerve `80`

64410* phrenic nerve `❶ 80`

64412* spinal accessory nerve

64413* cervical plexus

64415* brachial plexus `❶`

64417* axillary nerve `❶`

64418* suprascapular nerve

64420* intercostal nerve, single `❶`

64421* intercostal nerves, multiple, regional block `❶`

64425* ilioinguinal, iliohypogastric nerves

64430* pudendal nerve `❶`

| 64435* | paracervical (uterine) nerve | ♀ |
| 64445* | sciatic nerve | |

CIM 35-46 ASSESSING PATIENT'S SUITABILITY FOR ELECTRICAL NERVE STIMULATION THERAPY

Electrical nerve stimulation assesses a patient's suitability for ongoing treatment with a transcutaneous or an implanted nerve stimulator. Accordingly, program payment may be made for the following techniques when used to determine the potential therapeutic usefulness of an electrical nerve stimulator:

- Transcutaneous Electrical Nerve Stimulation (TENS) - technique involves attaching a transcutaneous nerve stimulator to the surface of the skin over the peripheral nerve to be stimulated. If TENS significantly alleviates pain, it may be considered as primary treatment. If it produces no relief or greater discomfort than the original pain electrical nerve stimulation therapy is ruled out. However, where TENS produces incomplete relief, further evaluation with percutaneous electrical nerve stimulation may be considered to determine whether an implanted peripheral nerve stimulator would provide significant relief from pain.

- Percutaneous Electrical Nerve Stimulation (PENS) - diagnostic procedure involves stimulating peripheral nerves by a needle electrode inserted through the skin and is performed only in a physician's office, clinic, or hospital outpatient department. If pain is controlled by percutaneous stimulation, implantation of electrodes is warranted. The medical necessity for such diagnostic services furnished beyond the first month must be documented.

| 64450* | other peripheral nerve or branch | |

If phenol destruction is performed, consult CPT codes 64622-64627. If a subarachnoid or subdural injection is administered, consult CPT codes 62280, 62310-62319. If an epidural or a caudal injection is administered, consult CPT codes 62273, 62281-62282, 62310-62319.

64470 Injection, anesthetic agent and/or steroid, paravertebral facet joint or facet joint nerve; cervical or thoracic, single level

If fluoroscopic guidance and localization for needle placement and injection is performed in conjunction with 64470-64484, consult CPT code 76005.

+ **64472** cervical or thoracic, each additional level (List separately in addition to code for primary procedure)

Note taht 64472 is an add-on code and must be used in conjunction with 64470.

64475 lumbar or sacral, single level

+ **64476** lumbar or sacral, each additional level (List separately in addition to code for primary procedure)

Note that 64476 is an add-on code and must be used in conjunction with 64475.

64479 Injection, anesthetic agent and/or steroid, transforaminal epidural; cervical or thoracic, single level

+ **64480** cervical or thoracic, each additional level (List separately in addition to code for primary procedure)

Note that 64480 is an add-on code and must be used in conjunction with 64479.

64483 lumbar or sacral, single level

+ **64484** lumbar or sacral, each additional level (List separately in addition to code for primary procedure)

Note that 64484 is an add-on code and must be used in conjunction with 64483.

INTRODUCTION/INJECTION OF ANESTHETIC AGENT (NERVE BLOCK), DIAGNOSTIC, OR THERAPEUTIC, SYMPATHETIC NERVES

64505*	Injection, anesthetic agent; sphenopalatine ganglion	
64508*	carotid sinus (separate procedure)	
64510*	stellate ganglion (cervical sympathetic)	
64520*	lumbar or thoracic (paravertebral sympathetic)	
64530*	celiac plexus, with or without radiologic monitoring	

NEUROSTIMULATORS (PERIPHERAL NERVE)

CIM 35-20 TREATMENT OF MOTOR FUNCTION DISORDERS WITH ELECTRIC NERVE STIMULATION - NOT COVERED

No reimbursement may be made for electric nerve stimulation or for the services related to its implantation since this treatment cannot be considered reasonable and necessary. However, Medicare covers deep brain stimulation by implanting a stimulator device at the carrier's discretion.

CIM 35-46 ASSESSING PATIENT'S SUITABILITY FOR ELECTRICAL NERVE STIMULATION THERAPY

Electrical nerve stimulation assesses a patient's suitability for ongoing treatment with a transcutaneous or an implanted nerve stimulator. Accordingly, program payment may be made for the following techniques when used to determine the potential therapeutic usefulness of an electrical nerve stimulator:

- Transcutaneous Electrical Nerve Stimulation (TENS) - technique involves attaching a transcutaneous nerve stimulator to the surface of the skin over the peripheral nerve to be stimulated. If TENS significantly alleviates pain, it may be considered as primary treatment. If it produces no relief or greater discomfort than the original pain electrical nerve stimulation therapy is ruled out. However, where TENS produces incomplete relief, further evaluation with percutaneous electrical nerve stimulation may be considered to determine whether an implanted peripheral nerve stimulator would provide significant relief from pain.

- Percutaneous Electrical Nerve Stimulation (PENS) - diagnostic procedure involves stimulating peripheral nerves by a needle electrode inserted through the skin and is performed only in a physician's office, clinic, or hospital outpatient department. If pain is controlled by percutaneous stimulation, implantation of electrodes is warranted. The medical necessity for such diagnostic services furnished beyond the first month must be documented.

CIM 45-19 TRANSCUTANEOUS ELECTRICAL NERVE STIMULATION (TENS) FOR ACUTE POST-OPERATIVE PAIN

Medicare covers the use of transcutaneous electrical nerve stimulation (TENS) for the relief of acute post-operative pain. TENS may be covered whether used as an adjunct to the use of drugs, or as an alternative to drugs, in the treatment of acute pain resulting from surgery. When used for the purpose of treating acute post-operative pain, TENS devices may be hospital supplies furnished inpatients (covered under Part A) or supplies incident to a physician's service when furnished with outpatient surgery (covered under Part B). In cases when TENS is used for longer than 30-day periods, TENS coverage may be covered as durable medical equipment for treating chronic pain.

CIM 45-25 SUPPLIES USED IN THE DELIVERY OF TRANSCUTANEOUS ELECTRICAL NERVE STIMULATION (TENS) AND NEUROMUSCULAR ELECTRICAL STIMULATION (NMES)

There are times patients receiving Transcutaneous Electrical Nerve Stimulation (TENS) and/or Neuromuscular Electrical Stimulation (NMES) treatment may need to use adhesive tapes and lead wires, a form-fitting conductive garment. A form-fitting conductive garment (and medically necessary related supplies) may be covered under the program when:

1. It has received permission or approval for marketing by the Food and Drug Administration (FDA)

2. It has been prescribed by a physician for use in delivering covered TENS or NMES treatment

3. One of the medical indications outlined below is met:

- Patient cannot manage without the conductive garment due to the large area or number of areas requiring stimulation

- Patient cannot manage without the conductive garment because the areas or sites to be stimulated are inaccessible with the use of conventional methods

- Patient has a documented medical condition such as skin problems that preclude the application of conventional devices

- Patient requires electrical stimulation beneath a cast either to treat disuse atrophy or to treat chronic intractable pain

- Patient has a medical need for rehabilitation strengthening (pursuant to a written plan of rehabilitation) following an injury

A conductive garment is covered for use with a TENS device during the trial period when:

1. Patient has a documented skin problem prior to the start of the trial period

2. Carrier's medical consultants are satisfied that use is medically necessary

For programming or electronic analysis of neurostimulator pulse generators, initial or subsequent, consult CPT codes 95970-95975.

Consult the glossary for more terms and guidelines.

64550	**Application of surface (transcutaneous) neurostimulator**	▢

CIM 65-8 ELECTRICAL NERVE STIMULATORS

Two general classifications of electrical nerve stimulators are employed to treat chronic intractable pain: peripheral nerve stimulators and central nervous system stimulators.

There are two types of implantations covered by this instruction:

- Dorsal column (spinal cord) neurostimulation.

- Depth brain neurostimulation

No payment may be made unless all of the conditions listed below have been met:

a. The implantation of the stimulator is used only as a late resort (if not a last resort) for patients with chronic intractable pain

b. Other treatment modalities (pharmacological, surgical, physical, or psychological therapies) have been tried and did not prove satisfactory, or are judged to be unsuitable or contraindicated for the given patient

c. Patients have undergone careful screening, evaluation and diagnosis by a multidisciplinary team prior to implantation. (psychological and physical evaluation)

d. All the facilities, equipment, and professional and support personnel required for the proper diagnosis, treatment training, and follow-up of the patient must be available

e. Demonstration of pain relief with a temporarily implanted electrode precedes permanent implantation

	64553	**Percutaneous implantation of neurostimulator electrodes; cranial nerve**	80 ▢

If this procedure involves open placement of a cranial nerve (e.g., vagal, trigeminal) neurostimulator pulse generator or receiver, consult CPT codes 61885 and 61886, as appropriate.

▲	**64555**	**peripheral nerve (excludes sacral nerve)**	
	64560	**autonomic nerve**	80 ▢
●	**64561**	**sacral nerve (transforaminal placement)**	

NEUROSTIMULATORS (PERIPHERAL NERVE)

For programming or electronic analysis of neurostimulator pulse generators, initial or subsequent, consult CPT codes 95970-95975.

Consult the glossary for more terms and guidelines.

CIM 35-77 NEUROMUSCULAR ELECTRICAL STIMULATION (NMES) IN THE TREATMENT OF DISUSE ATROPHY

Coverage of Neuromuscular electrical stimulation (NMES) is limited to the treatment of disuse atrophy where nerve supply to the muscle is intact, including brain, spinal cord and peripheral nerves, and other non-neurological reasons for disuse are causing atrophy. Some examples would be casting or splinting of a limb, contracture due to scarring of soft tissue as in burn lesions, and hip replacement surgery (until orthotic training begins).

64565	**neuromuscular**	▢

CIM 60-22 VAGUS NERVE STIMULATION FOR TREATMENT OF SEIZURES

Medicare covers vagus nerve stimulation for patients with medically refractory partial onset seizures for whom surgery is not recommended or for whom surgery has failed. This policy is in accordance with the FDA-labelled usage for the device. The neurostimulator pulse generator is implanted subcutaneously below the left clavicle and the lead is attached to the vagus nerve in the neck. The procedure is performed in the hospital and usually requires an overnight stay. The procedure is usually coded using CPT codes 64573 (lead placement), and 64590 (generator implantation).

The ICD-9-CM for implantation of a neurostimulator into the vagus nerve is 04.92. The diagnosis codes for intractable epilepsy are 345.01, 345.11, 345.41, 345.51, and 345.91. Infrequently contractors might see the diagnosis code for convulsions, 780.3, used to identify eligible patients.

	64573	**Incision for implantation of neurostimulator electrodes; cranial nerve**	80 ▢

If this procedure involves open placement of a cranial nerve neurostimulator pulse generator or receiver, consult CPT codes 61885, 61886.

▲	**64575**	**peripheral nerve (excludes sacral nerve)**	❶ ▢
	64577	**autonomic nerve**	▢
	64580	**neuromuscular**	80 ▢
●	**64581**	**sacral nerve (transforaminal placement)**	
	64585	**Revision or removal of peripheral neurostimulator electrodes**	80 ▢
	64590	**Incision and subcutaneous placement of peripheral neurostimulator pulse generator or receiver, direct or inductive coupling**	❷ 80 ▢
	64595	**Revision or removal of peripheral neurostimulator pulse generator or receiver**	❶ ▢

DESTRUCTION BY NEUROLYTIC AGENT (EG, CHEMICAL, THERMAL, ELECTRICAL, RADIOFREQUENCY), SOMATIC NERVES

	64600	**Destruction by neurolytic agent, trigeminal nerve; supraorbital, infraorbital, mental, or inferior alveolar branch**	❶ ▢
	64605	**second and third division branches at foramen ovale**	❶ 80 ▢

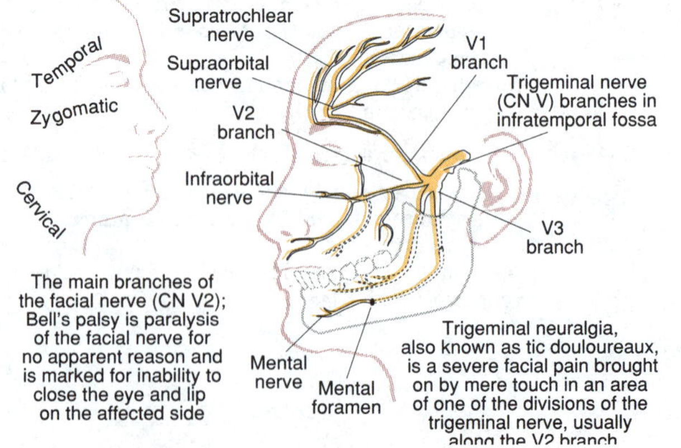

64610	second and third division branches at foramen ovale under radiologic monitoring
64612	Chemodenervation of muscle(s); muscle(s) innervated by facial nerve (eg, for blepharospasm, hemifacial spasm)
64613	cervical spinal muscle(s) (eg, for spasmodic torticollis)

CIM 45-17 TRANSFER FACTOR FOR TREATMENT OF MULTIPLE SCLEROSIS

Transfer factor, the dialysate of an extract from sensitized leukocytes that increases cellular immune activity, is not covered for treating multiple sclerosis because its use is experimental.

| 64614 | extremity(s) and/or trunk muscle(s) (eg, for dystonia, cerebral palsy, multiple sclerosis) |

If chemodenervation is performed for strabismus involving the extraocular muscles, consult CPT code 67345.

64620	Destruction by neurolytic agent, intercostal nerve
64622	Destruction by neurolytic agent, paravertebral facet joint nerve; lumbar or sacral, single level
+ 64623	lumbar or sacral, each additional level (List separately in addition to code for primary procedure)

Note that 64623 is an add-on code and must be used in conjunction with 64622.

| 64626 | cervical or thoracic, single level |
| + 64627 | cervical or thoracic, each additional level (List separately in addition to code for primary procedure) |

Note that 64627 is an add-on code and must be used in conjunction with 64626.

| 64630 | Destruction by neurolytic agent; pudendal nerve |
| 64640 | other peripheral nerve or branch |

DESTRUCTION BY NEUROLYTIC AGENT (EG, CHEMICAL, THERMAL, ELECTRICAL, RADIOFREQUENCY), SYMPATHETIC NERVES

| 64680 | Destruction by neurolytic agent, celiac plexus, with or without radiologic monitoring |

NEUROPLASTY (EXPLORATION, NEUROLYSIS OR NERVE DECOMPRESSION)

If facial nerve decompression is performed, consult CPT code 69720.

If internal neurolysis is performed and requires the use of an operating microscope, consult CPT code 64727.

64702	Neuroplasty; digital, one or both, same digit
64704	nerve of hand or foot
64708	Neuroplasty, major peripheral nerve, arm or leg; other than specified
64712	sciatic nerve
64713	brachial plexus
64714	lumbar plexus
64716	Neuroplasty and/or transposition; cranial nerve (specify)
64718	ulnar nerve at elbow
64719	ulnar nerve at wrist
64721	median nerve at carpal tunnel
64722	Decompression; unspecified nerve(s) (specify)
64726	plantar digital nerve

| + 64727 | Internal neurolysis, requiring use of operating microscope (list separately in addition to code for neuroplasty) (Neuroplasty includes external neurolysis) |

Do not report 69990 in addition to code 64727 as the operating microscope is considered an inclusive component of the surgery.

TRANSECTION OR AVULSION

| 64732 | Transection or avulsion of; supraorbital nerve |
| 64734 | infraorbital nerve |

CIM 35-17 INDUCED LESIONS OF NERVE TRACTS

Surgically induced lesions of nerve tracts, which involve destroying nerve tissue, control the chronic or acute pain arising from conditions such as terminal cancer or lumbar degenerative arthritis. Induced lesions of nerve tracts may be produced by surgical cutting of the nerve (rhizolysis), chemical destruction of the nerve, or by creation of a radio-frequency lesion (electrocautery). Accordingly, program payment may be made for these denervation procedures when used in selected cases (concurred in by contractor's medical staff) to treat chronic pain.

64736	mental nerve
64738	inferior alveolar nerve by osteotomy
64740	lingual nerve
64742	facial nerve, differential or complete
64744	greater occipital nerve
64746	phrenic nerve

If section of a recurrent laryngeal nerve is performed, consult CPT code 31595.

| 64752 | vagus nerve (vagotomy), transthoracic |
| ▲ 64755 | vagus nerves limited to proximal stomach (selective proximal vagotomy, proximal gastric vagotomy, parietal cell vagotomy, supra- or highly selective vagotomy) |

If a laparoscopic approach is used, consult CPT code 43652.

| 64760 | vagus nerve (vagotomy), abdominal |

If a laparoscopic approach is used, consult CPT code 43651.

64761	pudendal nerve
64763	Transection or avulsion of obturator nerve, extrapelvic, with or without adductor tenotomy
64766	Transection or avulsion of obturator nerve, intrapelvic, with or without adductor tenotomy
64771	Transection or avulsion of other cranial nerve, extradural
64772	Transection or avulsion of other spinal nerve, extradural

If an excision is performed on a tender scar, skin, and subcutaneous tissue, with or without tiny neuroma, consult CPT codes 11400-11446 and 13100-13153.

EXCISION, SOMATIC NERVES

If a Morton Neurectomy is performed, consult CPT code 28080.

64774	Excision of neuroma; cutaneous nerve, surgically identifiable
64776	digital nerve, one or both, same digit
+ 64778	digital nerve, each additional digit (List separately in addition to code for primary procedure)

Note that 64778 is an add-on code and must be used in conjunction with 64776.

| 64782 | hand or foot, except digital nerve |

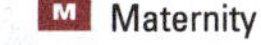 CCI Comprehensive Code   50 Bilateral Procedure   + CPT Add-on Code   ⊘ Modifier -51 Exempt Code   ● New Code   ▲ Revised Code

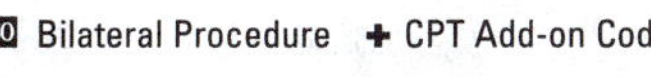 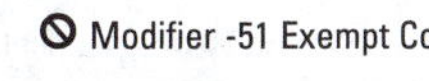

M Maternity   **N** Newborn   **P** Pediatric   **N/P** Newborn/Pediatric

| + | 64783 | hand or foot, each additional nerve, except same digit (List separately in addition to code for primary procedure) ❷ | |
| | | Note that 64783 is an add-on code and must be used in conjunction with 64782. | |

| | 64784 | major peripheral nerve, except sciatic | ❸ 80 ↻ |
| | 64786 | sciatic nerve | ❸ 80 ↻ |

| + | 64787 | Implantation of nerve end into bone or muscle (list separately in addition to neuroma excision) ❷ 80 | |
| | | Note that 64787 is an add-on code and must be used in conjunction with 64774-64786. | |

	64788	Excision of neurofibroma or neurolemmoma; cutaneous nerve	❸ ↻
	64790	major peripheral nerve	❸ 80 ↻
	64792	extensive (including malignant type)	❸ 80 ↻
	64795	Biopsy of nerve	❷ ↻

EXCISION, SYMPATHETIC NERVES

	64802	Sympathectomy, cervical	❷ 80 ↻ 50
	64804	Sympathectomy, cervicothoracic	80 ↻ 50
	64809	Sympathectomy, thoracolumbar	80 ↻ 50
		Leriche sympathectomy	
	64818	Sympathectomy, lumbar	80 ↻ 50
▲	64820	Sympathectomy; digital arteries, each digit	↻
		Code 69990 should not be reported in addition to 64820.	
●	64821	radial artery	
		Code 69990 should not be reported in addition to 64821.	
●	64822	ulnar artery	
		Code 69990 should not be reported in addition to 64822.	
●	64823	superficial palmar arch	
		Code 69990 should not be reported in addition to 64823.	

NEURORRHAPHY

	64831	Suture of digital nerve, hand or foot; one nerve	❹ ↻
+	64832	each additional digital nerve (List separately in addition to code for primary procedure) ❶ 80	
		Note that 64832 is an add-on code and must be used in conjunction with 64831.	
	64834	Suture of one nerve, hand or foot; common sensory nerve	❷ 80 ↻
	64835	median motor thenar	❸ 80 ↻
	64836	ulnar motor	❸ 80 ↻
+	64837	Suture of each additional nerve, hand or foot (List separately in addition to code for primary procedure) ❶ 80	
		Note that 64837 is an add-on code and must be used in conjunction with 64834-64836.	
	64840	Suture of posterior tibial nerve	❷ 80 ↻
	64856	Suture of major peripheral nerve, arm or leg, except sciatic; including transposition	❷ ↻
	64857	without transposition	❷ 80 ↻
	64858	Suture of sciatic nerve	❷ 80 ↻
+	64859	Suture of each additional major peripheral nerve (List separately in addition to code for primary procedure) ❶ 80	
		Note that 64859 is an add-on code and must be used in conjunction with 64856 and 64857.	
	64861	Suture of; brachial plexus	❸ 80 ↻
	64862	lumbar plexus	❸ 80 ↻
	64864	Suture of facial nerve; extracranial	❸ 80 ↻
	64865	infratemporal, with or without grafting	❹ 80 ↻

	64866	Anastomosis; facial-spinal accessory	80 ↻
	64868	facial-hypoglossal	80 ↻
		Korte-Ballance anastomosis	
	64870	facial-phrenic	❹ 80 ↻
+	64872	Suture of nerve; requiring secondary or delayed suture (list separately in addition to code for primary neurorrhaphy) ❷ 80	
		Note that 64872 is an add-on code and must be used in conjunction with 64831-64865.	
+	64874	requiring extensive mobilization, or transposition of nerve (list separately in addition to code for nerve suture) ❸ 80	
		Note that 64874 is an add-on code and must be used in conjunction with 64831-64865.	
+	64876	requiring shortening of bone of extremity (list separately in addition to code for nerve suture) ❸ 80	
		Note that 64876 is an add-on code and must be used in conjunction with 64831-64865.	

NEURORRHAPHY WITH NERVE GRAFT

	64885	Nerve graft (includes obtaining graft), head or neck; up to 4 cm in length	80 ↻
	64886	more than 4 cm in length	80 ↻
	64890	Nerve graft (includes obtaining graft), single strand, hand or foot; up to 4 cm length	❷ 80 ↻
	64891	more than 4 cm length	❷ 80 ↻
	64892	Nerve graft (includes obtaining graft), single strand, arm or leg; up to 4 cm length	❷ 80 ↻
	64893	more than 4 cm length	❷ 80 ↻
	64895	Nerve graft (includes obtaining graft), multiple strands (cable), hand or foot; up to 4 cm length	❸ 80 ↻
	64896	more than 4 cm length	❸ 80 ↻
	64897	Nerve graft (includes obtaining graft), multiple strands (cable), arm or leg; up to 4 cm length	❸ 80 ↻
	64898	more than 4 cm length	❸ 80 ↻
+	64901	Nerve graft, each additional nerve; single strand (List separately in addition to code for primary procedure) ❷ 80	
		Note that 64901 is an add-on code and must be used in conjunction with 64885-64893.	
+	64902	multiple strands (cable) (List separately in addition to code for primary procedure) ❷ 80	
		Note that 64902 is an add-on code and must be used in conjunction with 64885, 64886, and 64895-64898.	
	64905	Nerve pedicle transfer; first stage	❷ 80 ↻
	64907	second stage	❶ 80 ↻

OTHER PROCEDURES

| | 64999 | Unlisted procedure, nervous system | 80 |

EYE AND OCULAR ADNEXA

EYEBALL

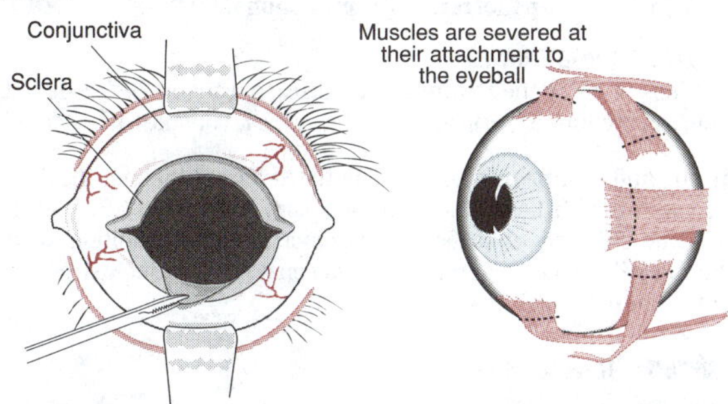

Evisceration involves removal of the contents of the eyeball: the vitreous; retina; choroid; lens; iris; and ciliary muscle. Only the scleral shell remains. A temporary or permanent implant is usually inserted

Enucleation involves severing the extraorbital muscles and optic nerve with removal of the eyeball. An implant is usually inserted and, if permanent, may involve attachment to the severed extraorbital muscles

REMOVAL OF EYE

If a diagnostic and treatment program is initiated for ophthalmological services, consult the Medicine and Ophthalmology sections of CPT and CPT code 92002 and subsequent codes. Do not report 69990 in addition to codes 65091-68850 as the operating microscope is considered an inclusive component of these procedures.

65091   Evisceration of ocular contents; without implant ❸ 80 ⬌ 50

65093   with implant ❸ ⬌ 50

65101   Enucleation of eye; without implant ❸ ⬌ 50

65103   with implant, muscles not attached to implant ❸ ⬌ 50

65105   with implant, muscles attached to implant ❹ 80 ⬌ 50

If a conjunctivoplasty is performed after enucleation, consult CPT codes 68320 and subsequent codes.

65110   Exenteration of orbit (does not include skin graft), removal of orbital contents; only ❺ 80 ⬌ 50

65112   with therapeutic removal of bone ❼ 80 ⬌ 50

65114   with muscle or myocutaneous flap ❼ 80 ⬌ 50

If a split skin graft is performed on the orbit, consult CPT codes 15120 and 15121. If a full thickness graft, free, is performed, consult CPT codes 15260 and 15261. If an eyelid, involving more than skin, is repaired, consult CPT codes 67930 and subsequent codes.

SECONDARY IMPLANT(S) PROCEDURES

Consult the glossary for more terms and guidelines.

If a diagnostic and treatment program is initiated for ophthalmological services, consult the Medicine and Ophthalmology sections of CPT and CPT code 92002 and subsequent codes. Do not report 69990 in addition to codes 65091-68850 as the operating microscope is considered an inclusive component of these procedures.

65125   Modification of ocular implant with placement or replacement of pegs (eg, drilling receptacle for prosthesis appendage) (separate procedure) ⬌ 50

65130   Insertion of ocular implant secondary; after evisceration, in scleral shell ❸ ⬌ 50

65135   after enucleation, muscles not attached to implant ❷ ⬌ 50

65140   after enucleation, muscles attached to implant ❸ ⬌ 50

65150   Reinsertion of ocular implant; with or without conjunctival graft ❷ 80 ⬌ 50

65155   with use of foreign material for reinforcement and/or attachment of muscles to implant ❸ ⬌ 50

65175   Removal of ocular implant ❶ ⬌ 50

If an orbital implant (implant outside muscle cone) is inserted, consult CPT code 67550. If the implant is removed, consult CPT code 67560.

REMOVAL OF FOREIGN BODY

If a diagnostic and treatment program is initiated for ophthalmological services, consult the Medicine and Ophthalmology sections of CPT and CPT code 92002 and subsequent codes. Do not report 69990 in addition to codes 65091-68850 as the operating microscope is considered an inclusive component of these procedures.

If implanted material is removed, consult the following CPT codes: ocular implant, see 56175; anterior segment implant, see 65920; posterior segment implant, see 67120; and orbital implant, see 67560. If a diagnostic x-ray is taken for a foreign body, consult CPT code 70030. If a diagnostic echography is needed for a foreign body, consult CPT code 76529. If a foreign body is removed from the orbit, consult the following CPT codes: frontal approach, see 67413; lateral approach, see 67430; and transcranial approach, see 61334. If an embedded foreign body is removed from the eyelid, consult CPT code 67938. If a foreign body is removed from the lacrimal system, consult CPT code 68530.

65205*   Removal of foreign body, external eye; conjunctival superficial ⬌ 50

65210*   conjunctival embedded (includes concretions), subconjunctival, or scleral nonperforating ⬌ 50

65220*   corneal, without slit lamp ⬌ 50

65222*   corneal, with slit lamp ⬌ 50

▲ **65235**   Removal of foreign body, intraocular; from anterior chamber of eye or lens ❷ 80 ⬌ 50

65260   from posterior segment, magnetic extraction, anterior or posterior route ❸ 80 ⬌ 50

65265   from posterior segment, nonmagnetic extraction ❹ 80 ⬌ 50

REPAIR OF LACERATION

If a diagnostic and treatment program is initiated for ophthalmological services, consult the Medicine and Ophthalmology sections of CPT and CPT code 92002 and subsequent codes. Do not report 69990 in addition to codes 65091-68850 as the operating microscope is considered an inclusive component of these procedures.

If the orbit is fractured, consult CPT code 21385 and subsequent codes. If a wound on the skin of the eyelid is repaired, linear, simple, consult CPT codes 12011-12018; intermediate, layered closure, consult CPT codes 12051-12057; linear, complex, consult CPT codes 13150-13153; and other, consult CPT codes 67930 and 67935. If a wound of the lacrimal system is repaired, consult CPT code 68700. If an operative wound is repaired, consult CPT code 66250.

65270*   Repair of laceration; conjunctiva, with or without nonperforating laceration sclera, direct closure ❷ 80 ⬌ 50

65272   conjunctiva, by mobilization and rearrangement, without hospitalization ❷ ⬌ 50

65273   conjunctiva, by mobilization and rearrangement, with hospitalization ⬌ 50

65275   cornea, nonperforating, with or without removal foreign body ❹ 80 ⬌ 50

65280   cornea and/or sclera, perforating, not involving uveal tissue ❹ 80 ⬌ 50

65285   cornea and/or sclera, perforating, with reposition or resection of uveal tissue ❹ 80 ⬌ 50

65286   application of tissue glue, wounds of cornea and/or sclera ⬌ 50

| 65290 | Repair of wound, extraocular muscle, tendon and/or Tenon's capsule | ❸ ⬚ 50 |

ANTERIOR SEGMENT

If a diagnostic and treatment program is initiated for ophthalmological services, consult the Medicine and Ophthalmology sections of CPT and CPT code 92002 and subsequent codes. Do not report 69990 in addition to codes 65091-68850 as the operating microscope is considered an inclusive component of these procedures.

CORNEA, EXCISION

65400	Excision of lesion, cornea (keratectomy, lamellar, partial), except pterygium	❶ ⬚ 50
65410*	Biopsy of cornea	❷ 80 ⬚ 50
65420	Excision or transposition of pterygium; without graft	❷ ⬚ 50
65426	with graft	❺ ⬚ 50

CORNEA, REMOVAL OR DESTRUCTION

65430*	Scraping of cornea, diagnostic, for smear and/or culture	⬚ 50
65435*	Removal of corneal epithelium; with or without chemocauterization (abrasion, curettage	⬚ 50
65436	with application of chelating agent (eg, EDTA)	⬚ 50
65450	Destruction of lesion of cornea by cryotherapy, photocoagulation or thermocauterization	⬚ 50
65600	Multiple punctures of anterior cornea (eg, for corneal erosion, tattoo)	⬚ 50

CORNEA, KERATOPLASTY

Corneal transplant procedures include the use of preserved or fresh grafts and the preparation of the donor material.

If refractive dermatoplasty procedures are performed in conjunction with this procedure, consult CPT codes 65760, 65765, and 65767.

If a diagnostic and treatment program is initiated for ophthalmological services, consult the Medicine and Ophthalmology sections of CPT and CPT code 92002 and subsequent codes. Do not report 69990 in addition to codes 65091-68850 as the operating microscope is considered an inclusive component of these procedures.

CIM 35-54 REFRACTIVE KERATOPLASTY- NOT COVERED

The use of radial keratotomy and/or keratoplasty for the purpose of refractive error compensation is considered a substitute or alternative to eye glasses or contact lenses, which are specifically excluded (except in certain cases in connection with cataract surgery). Keratoplasty that treats specific lesions of the cornea deals with an abnormality of the eye and is not cosmetic surgery and may be covered. Ophthalmalgic surgery coverage is restricted to practitioners who have completed an approved training program.

| 65710 | Keratoplasty (corneal transplant); lamellar | ❼ 80 ⬚ 50 |

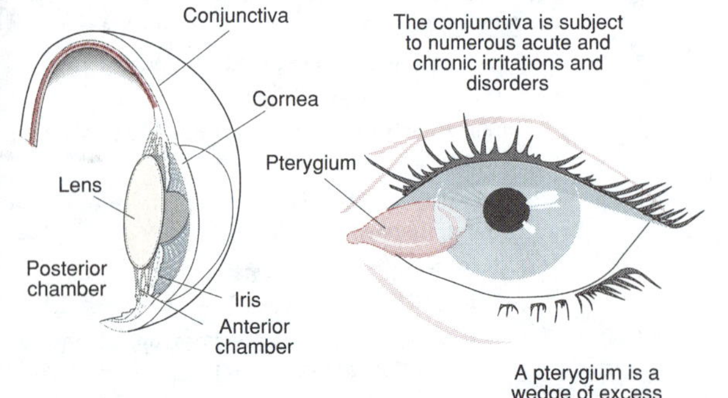

Keratitis is an often painful inflammation of the cornea, the clear membrane covering the anterior segment of the eye

A pterygium is a wedge of excess tissue extending from the medial canthus toward the cornea

65730	penetrating (except in aphakia)	❼ 80 ⬚ 50
65750	penetrating (in aphakia)	❼ 80 ⬚ 50
65755	penetrating (in pseudophakia)	❼ 80 ⬚ 50

CORNEA, OTHER PROCEDURES

If a contact lens is fit for the treatment of a disease, consult CPT code 92070. If an unlisted procedure is performed on the cornea, consult CPT code 66999.

If a diagnostic and treatment program is initiated for ophthalmological services, consult the Medicine and Ophthalmology sections of CPT and CPT code 92002 and subsequent codes. Do not report 69990 in addition to codes 65091-68850 as the operating microscope is considered an inclusive component of these procedures.

65760	Keratomileusis	
65765	Keratophakia	
65767	Epikeratoplasty	
65770	Keratoprosthesis	❼ 80 ⬚ 50
65771	Radial keratotomy	
65772	Corneal relaxing incision for correction of surgically induced astigmatism	⬚ 50
65775	Corneal wedge resection for correction of surgically induced astigmatism	⬚ 50

ANTERIOR CHAMBER, INCISION

If a diagnostic and treatment program is initiated for ophthalmological services, consult the Medicine and Ophthalmology sections of CPT and CPT code 92002 and subsequent codes. Do not report 69990 in addition to codes 65091-68850 as the operating microscope is considered an inclusive component of these procedures.

65800*	Paracentesis of anterior chamber of eye (separate procedure); with diagnostic aspiration of aqueous	❶ ⬚ 50
65805*	with therapeutic release of aqueous	❶ ⬚ 50
65810	with removal of vitreous and/or discission of anterior hyaloid membrane, with or without air injection	❸ ⬚ 50
65815	with removal of blood, with or without irrigation and/or air injection	❷ ⬚ 50

If an injection is needed, consult CPT codes 66020-66030.

| 65820 | Goniotomy | 80 ⬚ 50 |

Barkan's operation

| 65850 | Trabeculotomy ab externo | ❹ ⬚ 50 |
| 65855 | Trabeculoplasty by laser surgery, one or more sessions (defined treatment series) | ⬚ 50 |

If re-treatment is necessary after several months because of disease progression, a new treatment or treatment series should be reported with a modifier to indicate lesser or greater complexity. If a trabeculectomy is performed, consult CPT code 66170.

| 65860 | Severing adhesions of anterior segment, laser technique (separate procedure) | 80 ⬚ 50 |

ANTERIOR CHAMBER, OTHER PROCEDURES

If a diagnostic and treatment program is initiated for ophthalmological services, consult the Medicine and Ophthalmology sections of CPT and CPT code 92002 and subsequent codes. Do not report 69990 in addition to codes 65091-68850 as the operating microscope is considered an inclusive component of these procedures.

| 65865 | Severing adhesions of anterior segment of eye, incisional technique (with or without injection of air or liquid) (separate procedure); goniosynechiae | ❶ ⬚ 50 |

If trabeculoplasty is performed by laser surgery, consult CPT code 65855.

| 65870 | anterior synechiae, except goniosynechiae | ❹ ⬚ 50 |

65875	posterior synechiae	❹ ▣ 50
65880	corneovitreal adhesions	❹ ▣ 50

If laser surgery is performed, consult CPT code 66821.

▲ **65900**   **Removal of epithelial downgrowth, anterior chamber of eye** ❺ 80 ▣ 50

▲ **65920**   **Removal of implanted material, anterior segment of eye** ❼ ▣ 50

▲ **65930**   **Removal of blood clot, anterior segment of eye** ❺ ▣ 50

▲ **66020**   **Injection, anterior chamber of eye (separate procedure); air or liquid** ❶ ▣ 50

   66030*   medication   ❶ ▣ 50

If the procedure performed on the anterior segment is unlisted, consult CPT code 66999.

ANTERIOR SCLERA, EXCISION

If a diagnostic and treatment program is initiated for ophthalmological services, consult the Medicine and Ophthalmology sections of CPT and CPT code 92002 and subsequent codes. Do not report 69990 in addition to codes 65091-68850 as the operating microscope is considered an inclusive component of these procedures.

If an intraocular foreign body is removed, consult CPT code 65235. If an operation is performed on the posterior sclera, consult CPT codes 67250 and 67255.

66130   **Excision of lesion, sclera**   ❼ 80 ▣ 50

66150   **Fistulization of sclera for glaucoma; trephination with iridectomy** ❹ ▣ 50

   66155   thermocauterization with iridectomy   ❹ ▣ 50

   66160   sclerectomy with punch or scissors, with iridectomy ❷ ▣ 50

     Knapp's operation

   66165   iridencleisis or iridotasis   ❹ 80 ▣ 50

   66170   trabeculectomy ab externo in absence of previous surgery ❹ 80 ▣ 50

If a trabeculotomy ab externo is performed, consult CPT code 65850. If an operative wound is repaired, consult CPT code 66250.

   66172   trabeculectomy ab externo with scarring from previous ocular surgery or trauma (includes injection of antifibrotic agents) ❹ 80 ▣ 50

66180   **Aqueous shunt to extraocular reservoir (eg, Molteno, Schocket, Denver-Krupin)** ❺ 80 ▣ 50

66185   **Revision of aqueous shunt to extraocular reservoir** ❷ 80 ▣ 50

If an implanted shunt is removed, consult CPT code 67120.

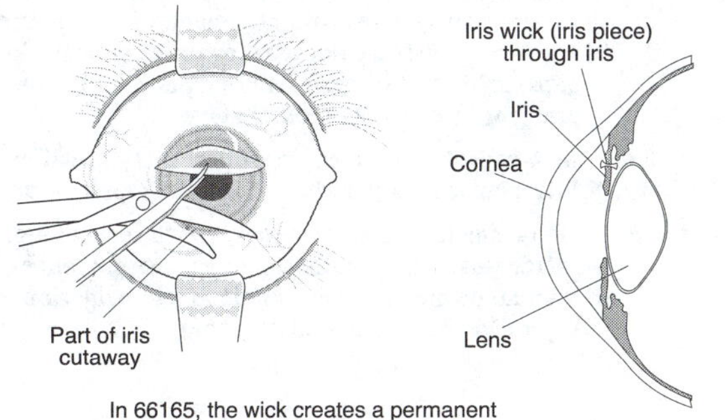

In 66165, the wick creates a permanent drainage route for the anterior chamber

ANTERIOR SCLERA, REPAIR OR REVISION

If a diagnostic and treatment program is initiated for ophthalmological services, consult the Medicine and Ophthalmology sections of CPT and CPT code 92002 and subsequent codes. Do not report 69990 in addition to codes 65091-68850 as the operating microscope is considered an inclusive component of these procedures.

If scleral procedures are performed in retinal surgery, consult CPT code 67101 and subsequent codes.

66220	Repair of scleral staphyloma; without graft	❸ 80 ▣ 50
66225	with graft	❹ 80 ▣ 50

If scleral reinforcement is needed, consult CPT codes 67250 and 67255.

66250   **Revision or repair of operative wound of anterior segment, any type, early or late, major or minor procedure** ❷ ▣ 50

IRIS, CILIARY BODY, INCISION

If a diagnostic and treatment program is initiated for ophthalmological services, consult the Medicine and Ophthalmology sections of CPT and CPT code 92002 and subsequent codes. Do not report 69990 in addition to codes 65091-68850 as the operating microscope is considered an inclusive component of these procedures.

If an "iridotomy" is performed by photocoagulation, consult CPT code 66761.

66500   **Iridotomy by stab incision (separate procedure); except transfixion** ❶ ▣ 50

   66505   with transfixion as for iris bombe   ❶ ▣ 50

IRIS, CILIARY BODY, EXCISION

If a diagnostic and treatment program is initiated for ophthalmological services, consult the Medicine and Ophthalmology sections of CPT and CPT code 92002 and subsequent codes. Do not report 69990 in addition to codes 65091-68850 as the operating microscope is considered an inclusive component of these procedures.

If "coreoplasty" is performed by photocoagulation, consult CPT code 66762.

66600   **Iridectomy, with corneoscleral or corneal section; for removal of lesion** ❸ ▣ 50

   66605   with cyclectomy   ❸ ▣ 50

   66625   peripheral for glaucoma (separate procedure) ❸ ▣ 50

   66630   sector for glaucoma (separate proedure) ❸ ▣ 50

   66635   optical (separate procedure)   ❸ ▣ 50

IRIS, CILIARY BODY, REPAIR

If a diagnostic and treatment program is initiated for ophthalmological services, consult the Medicine and Ophthalmology sections of CPT and CPT code 92002 and subsequent codes. Do not report 69990 in addition to codes 65091-68850 as the operating microscope is considered an inclusive component of these procedures.

If uveal tissue is repositioned or resected because of a perforating wound of the cornea or the sclera, consult CPT code 65285.

66680   **Repair of iris, ciliary body (as for iridodialysis)** ❸ ▣ 50

66682   **Suture of iris, ciliary body (separate procedure) with retrieval of suture through small incision (eg, McCannel suture)** ❷ ▣ 50

IRIS, CILIARY BODY, DESTRUCTION

66700   **Ciliary body destruction; diathermy** ❷ 80 ▣ 50

     Heine's operation

   66710   cyclophotocoagulation   ❷ ▣ 50

   66720   cryotherapy   ❷ ▣ 50

   66740   cyclodialysis   ❷ ▣ 50

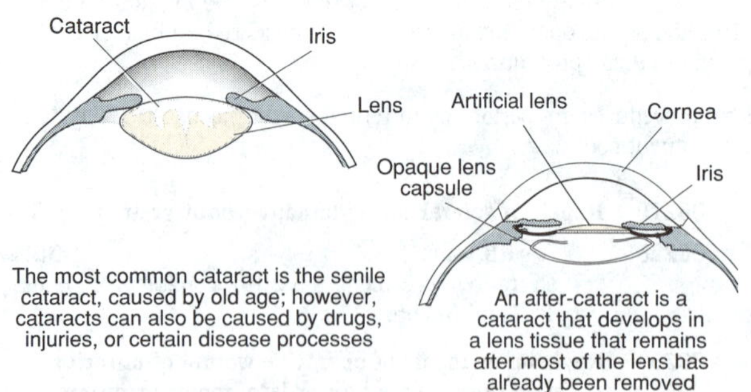

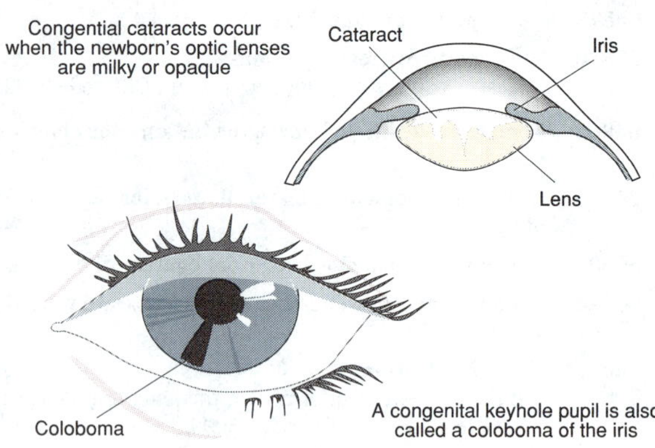

66761	**Iridotomy/iridectomy by laser surgery (eg, for glaucoma) (one or more sessions)**	50
66762	**Iridoplasty by photocoagulation (one or more sessions) (eg, for improvement of vision, for widening of anterior chamber angle)**	50
66770	**Destruction of cyst or lesion iris or ciliary body (nonexcisional procedure)**	50

If an iridectomy is performed for removal of a lesion, with corneoscleral or corneal section, consult CPT codes 66600 and 66605. If an epithelial downgrowth is removed from the anterior chamber of the eye, consult CPT code 65900. If a procedure performed on the iris or ciliary body is unlisted, consult CPT code 66999.

LENS, INCISION

If a diagnostic and treatment program is initiated for ophthalmological services, consult the Medicine and Ophthalmology sections of CPT and CPT code 92002 and subsequent codes. Do not report 69990 in addition to codes 65091-68850 as the operating microscope is considered an inclusive component of these procedures.

66820	**Discission of secondary membranous cataract (opacified posterior lens capsule and/or anterior hyaloid); stab incision technique (Ziegler or Wheeler knife)**	50
66821	**laser surgery (eg, YAG laser) (one or more stages)**	50
66825	**Repositioning of intraocular lens prosthesis, requiring an incision (separate procedure)**	80 50

LENS, REMOVAL CATARACT

If a diagnostic and treatment program is initiated for ophthalmological services, consult the Medicine and Ophthalmology sections of CPT and CPT code 92002 and subsequent codes. Do not report 69990 in addition to codes 65091-68850 as the operating microscope is considered an inclusive component of these procedures.

Anterior and/or posterior capsulotomy, iridotomy, iridectomy, lateral canthotomy, use of viscoelastic agents, enzymatic zonulysis, or the use of other pharmacologic agents, subconjunctival or sub-tenon injections, are all included as part of the CPT code(s) for extraction of lens.

66830	**Removal of secondary membranous cataract (opacified posterior lens capsule and/or anterior hyaloid) with corneo-scleral section, with or without iridectomy (iridocapsulotomy, iridocapsulectomy)**	50

If an implanted material from the anterior segment is removed, consult CPT code 65920.

Daviel's operation

66840	**Removal of lens material; aspiration technique, one or more stages**	50

If an implanted material from the anterior segment is removed, consult CPT code 65920.

Fukala's operation

66850	**phacofragmentation technique (mechanical or ultrasonic) (eg, phacoemulsification), with aspiration**	50

CIM 35-16 VITRECTOMY

Vitrectomy may be considered reasonable and necessary for the following conditions:

- Vitreous loss incident to cataract surgery
- Vitreous opacities due to vitreous hemorrhage or other causes
- Retinal detachments secondary to vitreous strands
- Proliferative retinopathy

The CPT codes for vitrectomy services are 67005, 67010, 67036, 67038, 67039, and 67040.

66852	**pars plana approach, with or without vitrectomy**	80 50
66920	**intracapsular**	80 50
66930	**intracapsular, for dislocated lens**	80 50
66940	**extracapsular (other than 66840, 66850, 66852)**	80 50

If an intralenticular foreign body is removed without lens extraction, consult CPT code 65235. If an operative wound is repaired, consult CPT code 66250.

LENS

CIM 35-9 PHACO-EMULSIFICATION PROCEDURE - CATARACT EXTRACTION

Medicare reimburses necessary services furnished in connection with cataract extraction utilizing the phaco-emulsification procedure.

▲ **66982**	**Extracapsular cataract removal with insertion of intraocular lens prosthesis (one stage procedure), manual or mechanical technique (eg, irrigation and aspiration or phacoemulsification), complex, requiring devices or techniques not generally used in routine cataract surgery (eg, iris expansion device, suture support for intraocular lens, or primary posterior capsulorrhexis) or performed on patients in the amblyogenic developmental stage**	50
66983	**Intracapsular cataract extraction with insertion of intraocular lens prosthesis (one stage procedure)**	50
66984	**Extracapsular cataract removal with insertion of intraocular lens prosthesis (one stage procedure), manual or mechanical technique (eg, irrigation and aspiration or phacoemulsification)**	50

66985 Insertion of intraocular lens prosthesis (secondary implant), not associated with concurrent cataract removal ⑥ ⌧ 50

    If an implant is performed at the time of a concurrent cataract surgery, consult CPT code 66982, 66983 or 66984. If a secondary fixation (separate procedure) is performed, consult CPT code 66682.

66986 Exchange of intraocular lens ⑥ ⌧ 50

OTHER PROCEDURES

66999 Unlisted procedure, anterior segment of eye 80 50

POSTERIOR SEGMENT

VITREOUS

If a diagnostic and treatment program is initiated for ophthalmological services, consult the Medicine and Ophthalmology sections of CPT and CPT code 92002 and subsequent codes. Do not report 69990 in addition to codes 65091-68850 as the operating microscope is considered an inclusive component of these procedures.

CIM 35-16 VITRECTOMY

Vitrectomy may be considered reasonable and necessary for the following conditions:

- Vitreous loss incident to cataract surgery
- Vitreous opacities due to vitreous hemorrhage or other causes
- Retinal detachments secondary to vitreous strands
- Proliferative retinopathy

The CPT codes for vitrectomy services are 67005, 67010, 67036, 67038, 67039, and 67040.

67005 Removal of vitreous, anterior approach (open sky technique or limbal incision); partial removal ④ ⌧ 50

67010   subtotal removal with mechanical vitrectomy ④ 80 ⌧ 50

    If a procedure performed on the vitreous is unlisted, consult CPT code 67299.

    If paracentesis is performed on the anterior chamber of the eye, with removal of the vitreous, consult CPT code 65810. If corneovitreal adhesions are removed, consult CPT code 65880.

67015 Aspiration or release of vitreous, subretinal or choroidal fluid, pars plana approach (posterior sclerotomy) ① ⌧ 50

67025 Injection of vitreous substitute, pars plana or limbal approach, (fluid-gas exchange), with or without aspiration (separate procedure) ① ⌧ 50

67027 Implantation of intravitreal drug delivery system (eg, ganciclovir implant), includes concomitant removal of vitreous 80 ⌧ 50

    If the implant is removed, consult CPT code 67121.

67028 Intravitreal injection of a pharmacologic agent (separate procedure) ⌧ 50

67030 Discission of vitreous strands (without removal), pars plana approach ① 80 ⌧ 50

67031 Severing of vitreous strands, vitreous face adhesions, sheets, membranes or opacities, laser surgery (one or more stages) ② ⌧ 50

67036 Vitrectomy, mechanical, pars plana approach; ④ 80 ⌧ 50

67038   with epiretinal membrane stripping ⑤ 80 ⌧ 50

67039   with focal endolaser photocoagulation ⑦ 80 ⌧ 50

67040   with endolaser panretinal photocoagulation ⑦ 80 ⌧ 50

    If an associated lensectomy is performed, consult CPT code 66850. If the retinal detachment surgery includes a vitrectomy, consult CPT code 67108. If a foreign body is removed, consult CPT codes 65260 and 65265.

RETINA OR CHOROID, REPAIR

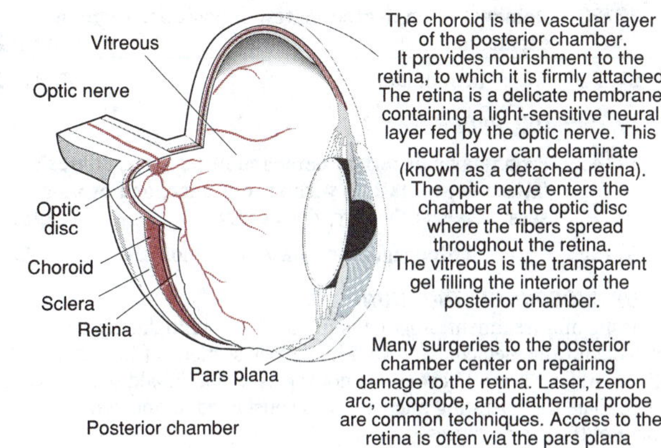

If a diagnostic and treatment program is initiated for ophthalmological services, consult the Medicine and Ophthalmology sections of CPT and CPT code 92002 and subsequent codes. Do not report 69990 in addition to codes 65091-68850 as the operating microscope is considered an inclusive component of these procedures.

If diathermy, cryotherapy, and/or photocoagulation are combined, report the procedure under the principal modality used.

67101 Repair of retinal detachment, one or more sessions; cryotherapy or diathermy, with or without drainage of subretinal fluid ⌧ 50

67105   photocoagulation, with or without drainage of subretinal fluid ⌧ 50

67107 Repair of retinal detachment; scleral buckling (such as lamellar scleral dissection, imbrication or encircling procedure), with or without implant, with or without cryotherapy, photocoagulation, and drainage of subretinal fluid ⑤ 80 ⌧ 50

    Gonin's operation

67108   with vitrectomy, any method, with or without air or gas tamponade, focal endolaser photocoagulation, cryotherapy, drainage of subretinal fluid, scleral buckling, and/or removal of lens by same technique ⑦ 80 ⌧ 50

67110   by injection of air or other gas (eg, pneumatic retinopexy) ⌧ 50

67112   by scleral buckling or vitrectomy, on patient having previous ipsilateral retinal detachment repair(s) using scleral buckling or vitrectomy techniques ⑦ 80 ⌧ 50

    If subretinal or subchoroidal fluid is aspirated or drained, consult CPT code 67015.

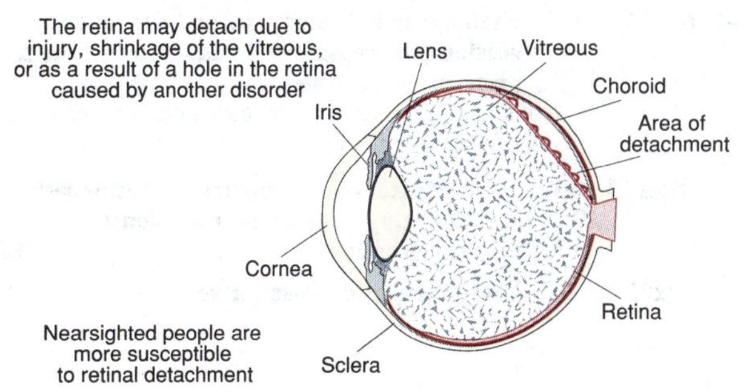

| 67115 | Release of encircling material (posterior segment) | ❷ TC 50 |

| 67120 | Removal of implanted material, posterior segment; extraocular | ❷ TC 50 |

| 67121 | intraocular | ❷ 80 TC 50 |

RETINA OR CHOROID, PROPHYLAXIS

| 67141 | Prophylaxis of retinal detachment (eg, retinal break, lattice degeneration) without drainage, one or more sessions; cryotherapy, diathermy | ❷ TC 50 |

| 67145 | photocoagulation (laser or xenon arc) | TC 50 |

RETINA OR CHOROID, DESTRUCTION

If a diagnostic and treatment program is initiated for ophthalmological services, consult the Medicine and Ophthalmology sections of CPT and CPT code 92002 and subsequent codes. Do not report 69990 in addition to codes 65091-68850 as the operating microscope is considered an inclusive component of these procedures.

If a procedure performed on the retina is unlisted, consult CPT code 67299.

| 67208 | Destruction of localized lesion of retina (eg, macular edema, tumors), one or more sessions; cryotherapy, diathermy | TC 50 |

| 67210 | photocoagulation | TC 50 |

| 67218 | radiation by implantation of source (includes removal of source) | ❺ TC 50 |

| 67220 | Destruction of localized lesion of choroid (eg, choroidal neovascularization); photocoagulation (eg, laser), one or more sessions | TC 50 |

> To report destruction of macular drusen, photocoagulation, consult CPT Category III code 0017T.
>
> To report destruction of localized lesion of choroid by transpupillary thermotherapy, consult CPT Category III code 0016T.

CIM 35-100 PHOTODYNAMIC THERAPY

Photodynamic therapy is a medical procedure that involves the infusion of a photosensitive (light-activated) drug with a very specific absorption peak. Once introduced to the body, the drug accumulates and is retained in diseased tissue to a greater degree than in normal tissue. Infusion is followed by the targeted irradiation of this tissue with a non-thermal laser, calibrated to emit light at a wavelength that corresponds to the drug's absorption peak. The drug then becomes active and locally treats the diseased tissue. Ocular photodynamic therapy (OPT) is used in the treatment of ophthalmologic diseases. Effective July 1, 2001, OPT (CPT code 67221) is only covered when used in conjunction with verteporfin. For patients with age-related macular degeneration, OPT is only covered with a diagnosis of neovascular age-related macular degeneration (ICD-9-CM 362.52) with predominately classic subfoveal choroidal neovascular (CNV) lesions (where the area of classic CNV occupies = 50% of the area of the entire lesion) at the initial visit as determined by a fluorescein angiogram (CPT code 92235).

| 67221 | photodynamic therapy (includes intravenous infusion) | TC |

| ● + 67225 | photodynamic therapy, second eye, at single session (List separately in addition to code for primary eye treatment) | |

> Note that 67225 is an add-on code and must be used in conjunction with 67221.

| 67227 | Destruction of extensive or progressive retinopathy (eg, diabetic retinopathy), one or more sessions; cryotherapy, diathermy | ❶ TC 50 |

| 67228 | photocoagulation (laser or xenon arc) | TC 50 |

SCLERA, REPAIR

If a diagnostic and treatment program is initiated for ophthalmological services, consult the Medicine and Ophthalmology sections of CPT and CPT code 92002 and subsequent codes. Do not report 69990 in addition to codes 65091-68850 as the operating microscope is considered an inclusive component of these procedures.

If a procedure performed on the retina is unlisted, consult CPT code 67299.

| 67250 | Scleral reinforcement (separate procedure); without graft | ❸ TC 50 |

| 67255 | with graft | ❸ 80 TC 50 |

> If a scleral staphyloma is repaired, consult CPT codes 66220 and 66225.

OTHER PROCEDURES

| 67299 | Unlisted procedure, posterior segment | 80 50 |

OCULAR ADNEXA

EXTRAOCULAR MUSCLES

If adjustable sutures are used, consult CPT code 67335 in addition to primary procedure (67311-67334) used that reflects the number of muscles operated on.

If a diagnostic and treatment program is initiated for ophthalmological services, consult the Medicine and Ophthalmology sections of CPT and CPT code 92002 and subsequent codes. Do not report 69990 in addition to codes 65091-68850 as the operating microscope is considered an inclusive component of these procedures.

| 67311 | Strabismus surgery, recession or resection procedure; one horizontal muscle | ❸ TC 50 |

| 67312 | two horizontal muscles | ❹ TC 50 |

| 67314 | one vertical muscle (excluding superior oblique) | ❹ TC 50 |

| 67316 | two or more vertical muscles (excluding superior oblique) | ❹ 80 TC 50 |

| 67318 | Strabismus surgery, any procedure, superior oblique muscle | ❹ TC 50 |

| + 67320 | Transposition procedure (eg, for paretic extraocular muscle), any extraocular muscle (specify) (List separately in addition to code for primary procedure) | ❹ TC 50 |

> Note that 67320 is an add-on code and must be used in conjunction with 67311-67318.

| + 67331 | Strabismus surgery on patient with previous eye surgery or injury that did not involve the extraocular muscles (List separately in addition to code for primary procedure) | ❹ TC 50 |

> Note that 67331 is an add-on code and must be used in conjunction with 67311-67318.

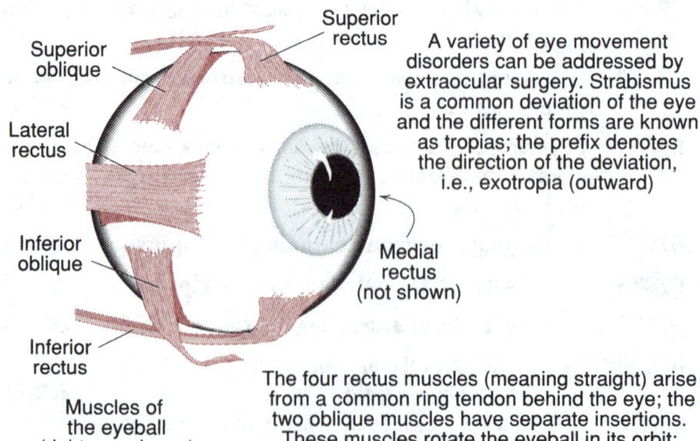

+ **67332** Strabismus surgery on patient with scarring of extraocular muscles (eg, prior ocular injury, strabismus or retinal detachment surgery) or restrictive myopathy (eg, dysthyroid ophthalmopathy) (List separately in addition to code for primary procedure)
> Note that 67332 is an add-on code and must be used in conjunction with 67311-67318.

+ **67334** Strabismus surgery by posterior fixation suture technique, with or without muscle recession (List separately in addition to code for primary procedure)
> Note that 67334 is an add-on code and must be used in conjunction with 67311-67318.

+ **67335** Placement of adjustable suture(s) during strabismus surgery, including postoperative adjustment(s) of suture(s) (List separately in addition to code for specific strabismus surgery)
> Note that 67335 is an add-on code and must be used in conjunction with 67311-67334.

+ **67340** Strabismus surgery involving exploration and/or repair of detached extraocular muscle(s) (List separately in addition to code for primary procedure)
> Note that 67340 is an add-on code and must be used in conjunction with 67311-67334.

> **Hummelshein operation**

67343 Release of extensive scar tissue without detaching extraocular muscle (separate procedure)
> Report 67343 in conjunction with 67311-67340, when performed other than on the affected muscle.

67345 Chemodenervation of extraocular muscle
> If chemodenervation is performed for blepharospasm and other neurological disorders, consult CPT codes 64612 and 64613.

OTHER PROCEDURES

67350 Biopsy of extraocular muscle
> If a wound of the extraocular muscle, tendon, and/or Tenon's capsule is repaired, consult CPT code 65290.

67399 Unlisted procedure, ocular muscle

ORBIT, EXPLORATION, EXCISION, DECOMPRESSION

If an orbitotomy is performed through a transcranial approach, consult CPT codes 61330-61334. If an orbital implant is inserted, consult CPT codes 67550 and 67560. If an eyeball is removed or repaired after removal, consult CPT codes 65091-65175.

If a diagnostic and treatment program is initiated for ophthalmological services, consult the Medicine and Ophthalmology sections of CPT and CPT code 92002 and subsequent codes. Do not report 69990 in addition to codes 65091-68850 as the operating microscope is considered an inclusive component of these procedures.

67400 Orbitotomy without bone flap (frontal or transconjunctival approach); for exploration, with or without biopsy

67405 with drainage only

67412 with removal of lesion

67413 with removal of foreign body

67414 with removal of bone for decompression

67415 Fine needle aspiration of orbital contents
> If exenteration, enucleation, and repair are performed, consult CPT code 65101 and subsequent codes. If optic nerve decompression is performed, consult CPT code 67570.

67420 Orbitotomy with bone flap or window, lateral approach (eg, Kroenlein); with removal of lesion

67430 with removal of foreign body

67440 with drainage

67445 with removal of bone for decompression
> If optic nerve sheath decompression is performed, consult CPT codes 67570.

67450 for exploration, with or without biopsy

ORBIT, OTHER PROCEDURES

If a diagnostic and treatment program is initiated for ophthalmological services, consult the Medicine and Ophthalmology sections of CPT and CPT code 92002 and subsequent codes. Do not report 69990 in addition to codes 65091-68850 as the operating microscope is considered an inclusive component of these procedures.

67500* Retrobulbar injection; medication (separate procedure, does not include supply of medication)

67505 alcohol

▲ **67515*** Injection of medication or other substance into Tenon's capsule
> If a subconjunctival injection is needed, consult CPT code 68200.

67550 Orbital implant (implant outside muscle cone); insertion
> If an ocular implant is needed (implant inside muscle cone), consult CPT codes 65093-65105 and 65130-65175. If treatment is needed for fractures of the malar area or orbit, consult CPT codes 21355 and subsequent codes.

67560 removal or revision
> If an ocular implant is needed (implant inside muscle cone), consult CPT codes 65093-65105 and 65130-65175. If treatment is needed for fractures of the malar area or orbit, consult CPT code 21355 and subsequent codes.

67570 Optic nerve decompression (eg, incision or fenestration of optic nerve sheath)

67599 Unlisted procedure, orbit

EYELIDS, INCISION

67700* Blepharotomy, drainage of abscess, eyelid

67710* Severing of tarsorrhaphy

67715* Canthotomy (separate procedure)
> If canthoplasty is performed, consult CPT code 67950. If a division of the symblepharon is performed, consult CPT code 68340.

EYELIDS, EXCISION

These codes include the lid margin, palpebral conjunctiva, and tarsus.

If a diagnostic and treatment program is initiated for ophthalmological services, consult the Medicine and Ophthalmology sections of CPT and CPT code 92002 and subsequent codes. Do not report 69990 in addition to codes 65091-68850 as the operating microscope is considered an inclusive component of these procedures.

If a lesion involving mainly the skin of the eyelid is removed, consult CPT codes 11310-11313, 11400-11446, 11640-11646, and 17000-17004.

67800 Excision of chalazion; single

67801 multiple, same lid

67805 multiple, different lids

67808 under general anesthesia and/or requiring hospitalization, single or multiple

67810* Biopsy of eyelid

67820* Correction of trichiasis; epilation, by forceps only

67825* epilation by other than forceps (eg, by electrosurgery, cryotherapy, laser surgery)

67830 incision of lid margin

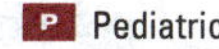

Eye and Ocular Adnexa

67835 — 67975

67835	incision of lid margin, with free mucous membrane graft	❷ 80 ↵

67840* Excision of lesion of eyelid (except chalazion) without closure or with simple direct closure   ↵

If an eyelid is excised and repaired by reconstructive surgery, consult CPT codes 67961 and 67966.

67850* Destruction of lesion of lid margin (up to 1 cm)   ↵

If Mohs micrographic surgery is performed, consult CPT codes 17304-17310.

EYELIDS, TARSORRHAPHY

If a diagnostic and treatment program is initiated for ophthalmological services, consult the Medicine and Ophthalmology sections of CPT and CPT code 92002 and subsequent codes. Do not report 69990 in addition to codes 65091-68850 as the operating microscope is considered an inclusive component of these procedures.

67875 Temporary closure of eyelids by suture (eg, Frost suture)   ↵

67880 Construction of intermarginal adhesions, median tarsorrhaphy, or canthorrhaphy;   ❸ ↵

67882 with transposition of tarsal plate   ❸ ↵

If severing of the tarsorrhaphy occurs, consult CPT code 67710. If canthoplasty is performed for reconstruction of the canthus, consult CPT code 67950. If a canthotomy is performed, consult CPT code 67715.

EYELIDS, REPAIR (BROW PTOSIS, BLEPHAROPTOSIS, LID RETRACTION, ECTROPION, ENTROPION)

If a diagnostic and treatment program is initiated for ophthalmological services, consult the Medicine and Ophthalmology sections of CPT and CPT code 92002 and subsequent codes. Do not report 69990 in addition to codes 65091-68850 as the operating microscope is considered an inclusive component of these procedures.

If a rhytidectomy is performed on the forehead, consult CPT code 15824.

67900 Repair of brow ptosis (supraciliary, mid-forehead or coronal approach)   ↵

67901 Repair of blepharoptosis; frontalis muscle technique with suture or other material   ❺ ↵ 50

67902 frontalis muscle technique with fascial sling (includes obtaining fascia)   ❺ ↵ 50

67903 (tarso)levator resection or advancement, internal approach   ❹ ↵ 50

67904 (tarso)levator resection or advancement, external approach   ❹ ↵ 50

Everbusch's operation

67906 superior rectus technique with fascial sling (includes obtaining fascia)   ❺ ↵ 50

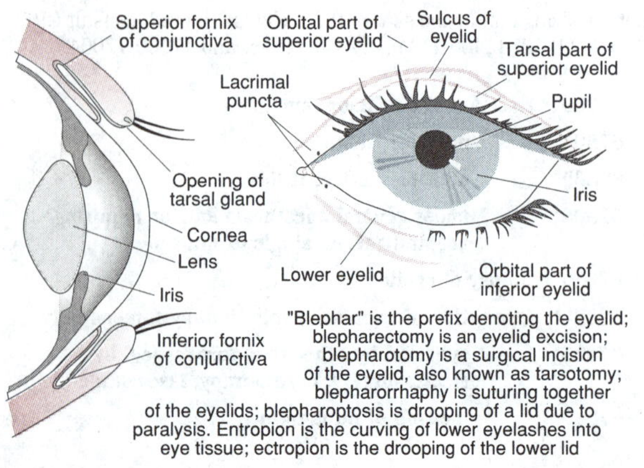

"Blephar" is the prefix denoting the eyelid; blepharectomy is an eyelid excision; blepharotomy is a surgical incision of the eyelid, also known as tarsotomy; blepharorrhaphy is suturing together of the eyelids; blepharoptosis is drooping of a lid due to paralysis. Entropion is the curving of lower eyelashes into eye tissue; ectropion is the drooping of the lower lid

67908 conjunctivo-tarso-Muller's muscle-levator resection (eg, Fasanella-Servat type)   ❹ ↵ 50

67909 Reduction of overcorrection of ptosis   ❹ ↵ 50

67911 Correction of lid retraction   ❸ ↵ 50

If obtaining autogenous graft materials, consult CPT codes 20920 and 20922 or 20926. If a mucous membrane graft corrects trichiasis, consult CPT code 67835.

67914 Repair of ectropion; suture   ❸ ↵ 50

67915 thermocauterization   ↵ 50

67916 blepharoplasty, excision tarsal wedge   ❹ ↵ 50

67917 blepharoplasty, extensive (eg, Kuhnt-Szymanowski or tarsal strip operations)   ❹ ↵ 50

If an everted punctum is corrected, consult CPT code 68705.

67921 Repair of entropion; suture   ❸ ↵ 50

67922 thermocauterization   ↵ 50

67923 blepharoplasty, excision tarsal wedge   ❹ ↵ 50

67924 blepharoplasty, extensive (eg, Wheeler operation)   ❹ ↵ 50

If a cicatricial ectropion or an entropion requiring scar excision or skin graft is repaired, consult also CPT code 67961 and subsequent codes.

EYELIDS, RECONSTRUCTION

These codes include the lid margin, palpebral conjunctiva, and tarsus.

If a diagnostic and treatment program is initiated for ophthalmological services, consult the Medicine and Ophthalmology sections of CPT and CPT code 92002 and subsequent codes. Do not report 69990 in addition to codes 65091-68850 as the operating microscope is considered an inclusive component of these procedures.

If the skin of the eyelid is repaired, consult CPT codes 12011-12018, 12051-12057, 13150, and 13153. If tarsorrhaphy or canthorrhaphy is performed, consult CPT codes 67880 and 67882. If blepharoptosis and lid retraction is repaired, consult CPT codes 6790

67930 Suture of recent wound, eyelid, involving lid margin, tarsus, and/or palpebral conjunctiva direct closure; partial thickness   ↵

67935 full thickness   ❷ ↵

67938 Removal of embedded foreign body, eyelid   ↵

67950 Canthoplasty (reconstruction of canthus)   ❷ ↵

67961 Excision and repair of eyelid, involving lid margin, tarsus, conjunctiva, canthus, or full thickness, may include preparation for skin graft or pedicle flap with adjacent tissue transfer or rearrangement; up to one-fourth of lid margin   ❸ 80 ↵

If a canthoplasty is performed, consult CPT code 67950. If free skin grafts are performed, consult CPT codes 15120, 15121, 15260, and 15261. If a tubed pedicle flap is prepared, consult CPT code 15576; if delayed, consult CPT code 15630; if attached, consult CPT code 15630.

67966 over one-fourth of lid margin   ❸ ↵

67971 Reconstruction of eyelid, full thickness by transfer of tarsoconjunctival flap from opposing eyelid; up to two-thirds of eyelid, one stage or first stage   ❸ 80 ↵

Dupuy-Dutemp reconstruction

67973 total eyelid, lower, one stage or first stage   ❸ 80 ↵

67974 total eyelid, upper, one stage or first stage   ❸ 80 ↵

Landboldt's operation

67975 second stage   ❸ ↵

Landboldt's operation

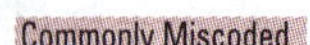

EYELIDS, OTHER PROCEDURES

67999   Unlisted procedure, eyelids   [80]

CONJUNCTIVA

If a foreign body is removed, consult CPT code 65205 and subsequent codes.

If a diagnostic and treatment program is initiated for ophthalmological services, consult the Medicine and Ophthalmology sections of CPT and CPT code 92002 and subsequent codes. Do not report 69990 in addition to codes 65091-68850 as the operating microscope is considered an inclusive component of these procedures.

INCISION AND DRAINAGE

68020   Incision of conjunctiva, drainage of cyst

68040   Expression of conjunctival follicles, eg, for trachoma

EXCISION AND/OR DESTRUCTION

If a diagnostic and treatment program is initiated for ophthalmological services, consult the Medicine and Ophthalmology sections of CPT and CPT code 92002 and subsequent codes. Do not report 69990 in addition to codes 65091-68850 as the operating microscope is considered an inclusive component of these procedures.

68100   Biopsy of conjunctiva

68110   Excision of lesion, conjunctiva; up to 1 cm

68115   over 1 cm

68130   with adjacent sclera

68135*   Destruction of lesion, conjunctiva

INJECTION

68200*   Subconjunctival injection
If an injection is made into the Tenon's capsule or if a retrobulbar injection is needed, consult CPT codes 67500-67515.

CONJUNCTIVOPLASTY

If a diagnostic and treatment program is initiated for ophthalmological services, consult the Medicine and Ophthalmology sections of CPT and CPT code 92002 and subsequent codes. Do not report 69990 in addition to codes 65091-68850 as the operating microscope is considered an inclusive component of these procedures.

If a wound is repaired, consult CPT codes 65270-65273.

68320   Conjunctivoplasty; with conjunctival graft or extensive rearrangement

68325   with buccal mucous membrane graft (includes obtaining graft)

68326   Conjunctivoplasty, reconstruction cul-de-sac; with conjunctival graft or extensive rearrangement

68328   with buccal mucous membrane graft (includes obtaining graft)

68330   Repair of symblepharon; conjunctivoplasty, without graft

68335   with free graft conjunctiva or buccal mucous membrane (includes obtaining graft)

68340   division of symblepharon, with or without insertion of conformer or contact lens

OTHER PROCEDURES

68360   Conjunctival flap; bridge or partial (separate procedure)

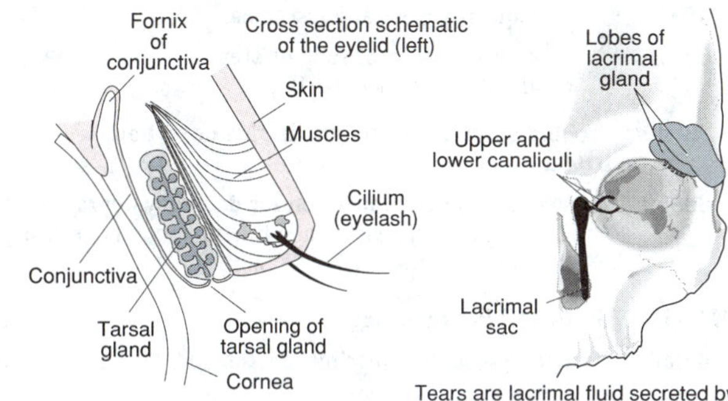

The eyelid is a moveable fold covered by skin externally and highly vascularized conjunctiva internally. The tarsal glands secrete lubricant to the edges of the eyelid

Tears are lacrimal fluid secreted by the almond-sized lacrimal gland through ducts into the fornix of the conjunctiva; fluid is drained through the puncta and into the lacrimal sac and into the nose

68362   total (such as Gunderson thin flap or purse string flap)
If a conjunctival flap is used for a perforating injury, consult CPT codes 65280 and 65285. If an operative wound is repaired, consult CPT code 66250. If a conjunctival foreign body is removed, consult CPT codes 65205 and 65210.

68399   Unlisted procedure, conjunctiva   [80]

LACRIMAL SYSTEM, INCISION

68400   Incision, drainage of lacrimal gland

68420   Incision, drainage of lacrimal sac (dacryocystotomy or dacryocystostomy)

68440*   Snip incision of lacrimal punctum

LACRIMAL SYSTEM, EXCISION

68500   Excision of lacrimal gland (dacryoadenectomy), except for tumor; total

68505   partial

68510   Biopsy of lacrimal gland

68520   Excision of lacrimal sac (dacryocystectomy)

68525   Biopsy of lacrimal sac

68530   Removal of foreign body or dacryolith, lacrimal passages
     Meller's excision

68540   Excision of lacrimal gland tumor; frontal approach

68550   involving osteotomy

LACRIMAL SYSTEM, REPAIR

68700   Plastic repair of canaliculi

68705   Correction of everted punctum, cautery

68720   Dacryocystorhinostomy (fistulization of lacrimal sac to nasal cavity)

68745   Conjunctivorhinostomy (fistulization of conjunctiva to nasal cavity); without tube

68750   with insertion of tube or stent

68760   Closure of the lacrimal punctum; by thermocauterization, ligation, or laser surgery

68761   by plug, each

68770   Closure of lacrimal fistula (separate procedure)

LACRIMAL SYSTEM, PROBING AND/OR RELATED PROCEDURES

68801*   Dilation of lacrimal punctum, with or without irrigation

68810*   Probing of nasolacrimal duct, with or without irrigation;

[CCI] CCI Comprehensive Code   [50] Bilateral Procedure   + CPT Add-on Code   ⊘ Modifier -51 Exempt Code   ● New Code   ▲ Revised Code

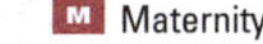 Maternity   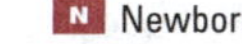 Newborn   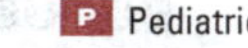 Pediatric   N/P Newborn/Pediatric

| 68811 | requiring general anesthesia | ❷ ☐ 50 |
| 68815 | with insertion of tube or stent | ❷ ☐ 50 |

Consult also CPT code 92018.

| 68840* | Probing of lacrimal canaliculi, with or without irrigation | ☐ |
| 68850* | Injection of contrast medium for dacryocystography | ☐ |

If radiological supervision and interpretation is needed, consult CPT codes 70170, 78660.

LACRIMAL SYSTEM, OTHER PROCEDURES

| 68899 | Unlisted procedure, lacrimal system | 80 |

AUDITORY SYSTEM

EXTERNAL EAR

If diagnostic services are performed (e.g., audiometry, vestibular tests), consult CPT code 92502 and subsequent codes.

INCISION

69000*	Drainage external ear, abscess or hematoma; simple	☐
69005	complicated	☐
69020*	Drainage external auditory canal, abscess	☐
69090	Ear piercing	

EXCSISION

69100	Biopsy external ear	☐
69105	Biopsy external auditory canal	☐
69110	Excision external ear; partial, simple repair	❶ ☐
69120	complete amputation	❷ ☐

If the ear is reconstructed, consult CPT code 15120 and subsequent codes.

69140	Excision exostosis(es), external auditory canal	❷ 80 ☐
69145	Excision soft tissue lesion, external auditory canal	❷ ☐
69150	Radical excision external auditory canal lesion; without neck dissection	❸ ☐
69155	with neck dissection	80 ☐

If skin grafting is necessary, consult CPT codes 15000-15261.

If the temporal bone is resected, consult CPT code 69535.

REMOVAL OF FOREIGN BODY

If diagnostic services are performed (e.g., audiometry, vestibular tests), consult CPT code 92502 and subsequent codes.

| 69200 | Removal foreign body from external auditory canal; without general anesthesia | ☐ |
| 69205 | with general anesthesia | ❶ ☐ |

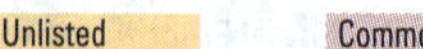

The external ear, or auricle, is a single elastic cartilage covered by skin and normal adnexal features (hair follicles, sweat glands, and sebaceous glands). The ridged nature of the auricle contributes to channeling sounds into the acoustic meatus. The semi-circular depression leading into the middle ear is named the concha, Latin for shell.

Coronal cutaway schematic of left ear and meatus

69210	Removal impacted cerumen (separate procedure), one or both ears	☐
69220	Debridement, mastoidectomy cavity, simple (eg, routine cleaning)	☐ 50
69222	Debridement, mastoidectomy cavity, complex (eg, with anesthesia or more than routine cleaning)	☐ 50

REPAIR

If a wound or injury of the external ear is sutured, consult CPT codes 12011-14300.

If diagnostic services are performed (e.g., audiometry, vestibular tests), consult CPT code 92502 and subsequent codes.

69300	Otoplasty, protruding ear, with or without size reduction	80 ☐
▲ 69310	Reconstruction of external auditory canal (meatoplasty) (eg, for stenosis due to injury, infection) (separate procedure)	❸ ☐
69320	Reconstruction external auditory canal for congenital atresia, single stage	❼ 80 ☐

If combination surgery is needed for middle ear reconstruction, consult CPT codes 69631 and 69641. If other reconstructive procedures are performed with grafts (e.g., skin, cartilage, bone), consult CPT codes 13150-15760 and 21230-21235.

OTHER PROCEDURES

If diagnostic services are performed (e.g., audiometry, vestibular tests), consult CPT code 92502 and subsequent codes.

If otoscopy is performed under general anesthesia, consult CPT code 92502.

| 69399 | Unlisted procedure, external ear | 80 |

MIDDLE EAR

INTRODUCTION

69400	Eustachian tube inflation, transnasal; with catheterization	☐
69401	without catheterization	☐
69405	Eustachian tube catheterization, transtympanic	80 ☐
69410	Focal application of phase control substance, middle ear (baffle technique)	80 ☐

INCISION

69420*	Myringotomy including aspiration and/or eustachian tube inflation	☐ 50
69421*	Myringotomy including aspiration and/or eustachian tube inflation requiring general anesthesia	❸ ☐ 50
69424	Ventilating tube removal when originally inserted by another physician	❶ ☐ 50
69433*	Tympanostomy (requiring insertion of ventilating tube), local or topical anesthesia	☐ 50
69436	Tympanostomy (requiring insertion of ventilating tube), general anesthesia	❸ ☐ 50
69440	Middle ear exploration through postauricular or ear canal incision	❸ ☐

If an atticotomy is performed, consult CPT code 69601 and subsequent codes.

| 69450 | Tympanolysis, transcanal | ❶ 80 ☐ |

EXCSISION

69501	Transmastoid antrotomy (simple mastoidectomy)	❼ ☐
69502	Mastoidectomy; complete	❼ 80 ☐
69505	modified radical	❼ 80 ☐

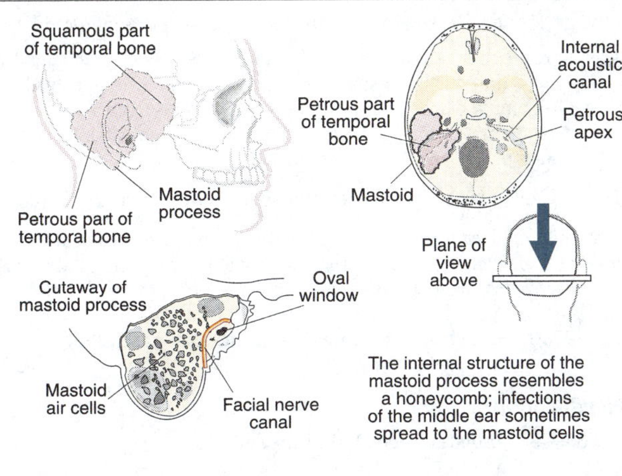

The internal structure of the mastoid process resembles a honeycomb; infections of the middle ear sometimes spread to the mastoid cells

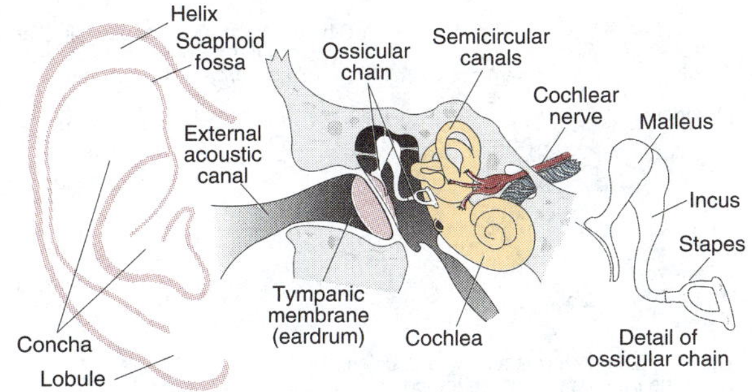

The tympanic membrane is a thin, sensitive tissue and is the gateway to the middle ear; the membrane vibrates in response to sound waves and the movement is transmitted via the ossicular chain to the internal ear. Many surgeries to the middle ear involve repair to the tympanic membrane and reconstruction to the various components of the ossicular chain

69511   radical   ❼ 80 ▣
If a skin graft is needed, consult CPT code 15000 and subsequent codes. If debridement is performed on the mastoidectomy cavity, consult CPT codes 69220 and 69222.

69530 Petrous apicectomy including radical mastoidectomy   ❼ 80 ▣

69535 Resection temporal bone, external approach   ▣
If a middle fossa approach is used, consult CPT codes 69950-69970.

69540 Excision aural polyp   ▣

69550 Excision aural glomus tumor; transcanal   ❺ 80 ▣

69552   transmastoid   ❼ 80 ▣

69554   extended (extratemporal)   80 ▣

REPAIR

69601 Revision mastoidectomy; resulting in complete mastoidectomy   ❼ 80 ▣

69602   resulting in modified radical mastoidectomy   ❼ 80 ▣

69603   resulting in radical mastoidectomy   ❼ 80 ▣

69604   resulting in tympanoplasty   ❼ ▣
If a secondary tympanoplasty is planned after mastoidectomy, consult CPT codes 69631 and 69632.

69605   with apicectomy   ❼ 80 ▣
If a skin graft is performed, consult CPT codes 15120, 15121, 15260, and 15261.

69610 Tympanic membrane repair, with or without site preparation or perforation for closure, with or without patch   ▣

69620 Myringoplasty (surgery confined to drumhead and donor area)   ❷ ▣

69631 Tympanoplasty without mastoidectomy (including canalplasty, atticotomy and/or middle ear surgery), initial or revision; without ossicular chain reconstruction   ❺ ▣

69632   with ossicular chain reconstruction (eg, postfenestration)   ❺ ▣

69633   with ossicular chain reconstruction and synthetic prosthesis (eg, partial ossicular replacement prosthesis, (PORP), total ossicular replacement prosthesis (TORP))   ❺ ▣

69635 Tympanoplasty with antrotomy or mastoidotomy (including canalplasty, atticotomy, middle ear surgery, and/or tympanic membrane repair); without ossicular chain reconstruction   ❼ ▣

69636   with ossicular chain reconstruction   ❼ 80 ▣

69637   with ossicular chain reconstruction and synthetic prosthesis (eg, partial ossicular replacement prosthesis, (PORP), total ossicular replacement prosthesis (TORP))   ❼ 80 ▣

69641 Tympanoplasty with mastoidectomy (including canalplasty, middle ear surgery, tympanic membrane repair); without ossicular chain reconstruction   ❼ ▣

69642   with ossicular chain reconstruction   ❼ ▣

69643   with intact or reconstructed wall, without ossicular chain reconstruction   ❼ ▣

69644   with intact or reconstructed canal wall, with ossicular chain reconstruction   ❼ ▣

69645   radical or complete, without ossicular chain reconstruction   ❼ ▣

69646   radical or complete, with ossicular chain reconstruction   ❼ 80 ▣

69650   Stapes mobilization   ❼ ▣

69660 Stapedectomy or stapedotomy with reestablishment of ossicular continuity, with or without use of foreign material;   ❺ ▣

69661   with footplate drill out   ❺ 80 ▣

69662 Revision of stapedectomy or stapedotomy   ❺ ▣

69666 Repair oval window fistula   ❹ 80 ▣

69667 Repair round window fistula   ❹ 80 ▣

69670 Mastoid obliteration (separate procedure)   ❸ 80 ▣

69676 Tympanic neurectomy   ❸ ▣ 50

OTHER PROCEDURES

69700 Closure postauricular fistula, mastoid (separate procedure)   ❸ ▣

69710 Implantation or replacement of electromagnetic bone conduction hearing device in temporal bone
The replacement procedure includes the removal of the old device.

69711 Removal or repair of electromagnetic bone conduction hearing device in temporal bone   ❶ 80 ▣

69714 Implantation, osseointegrated implant, temporal bone, with percutaneous attachment to external speech processor/cochlear stimulator; without mastoidectomy

69715   with mastoidectomy

69717 Replacement (including removal of existing device), osseointegrated implant, temporal bone, with percutaneous attachment to external speech processor/cochlear stimulator; without mastoidectomy

69718   with mastoidectomy

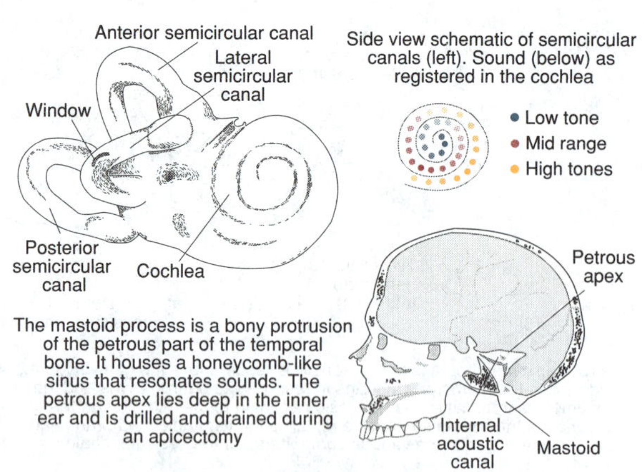

The mastoid process is a bony protrusion of the petrous part of the temporal bone. It houses a honeycomb-like sinus that resonates sounds. The petrous apex lies deep in the inner ear and is drilled and drained during an apicectomy

69720	**Decompression facial nerve, intratemporal; lateral to geniculate ganglion**	⑤ 80 ↻
69725	**including medial to geniculate ganglion**	⑤ 80 ↻
69740	**Suture facial nerve, intratemporal, with or without graft or decompression; lateral to geniculate ganglion**	⑤ 80 ↻
69745	**including medial to geniculate ganglion**	⑤ 80 ↻

If an extracranial suture of facial nerve is performed, consult CPT code 64864.

69799	**Unlisted procedure, middle ear**	80

INNER EAR

INCISION AND/OR DESTRUCTION

69801	**Labyrinthotomy, with or without cryosurgery including other nonexcisional destructive procedures or perfusion of vestibuloactive drugs (single or multiple perfusions); transcanal**	⑤ 80 ↻

This procedure includes all of the required infusions performed on initial and subsequent days of treatment.

69802	**with mastoidectomy**	⑦ 80 ↻
69805	**Endolymphatic sac operation; without shunt**	⑦ 80 ↻
69806	**with shunt**	⑦ ↻
69820	**Fenestration semicircular canal**	⑤ 80 ↻
	Lempert's fenestration	
69840	**Revision fenestration operation**	⑤ 80 ↻

EXCISION

69905	**Labyrinthectomy; transcanal**	⑦ ↻
69910	**with mastoidectomy**	⑦ 80 ↻
69915	**Vestibular nerve section, translabyrinthine approach**	⑦ 80 ↻

If a transcranial approach is used, consult CPT code 69950.

INTRODUCTION

CIM 65-14 COCHLEAR IMPLANTATION

Medicare coverage is provided only for those patients who meet all of the following guidelines:

- Diagnosis of bilateral severe-to-profound sensorineural hearing impairment with limited benefit from appropriate hearing (or vibrotactile) aids

- Cognitive ability to use auditory clues and a willingness to undergo an extended program of rehabilitation

- Freedom from middle ear infection, an accessible cochlear lumen that is structurally suited to implantation, and freedom from lesions in the auditory nerve and acoustic areas of the central nervous system

- No contraindications to surgery

- The device must be used in accordance withe the FDA-approved labeling

Cochlear implants may be covered for adults (over age 18) for prelinguistically, perilinguistically, and postlinguistically deafened adults. Postlinguistically deafened adults must demonstrate test scores of 30 percent or less on sentence recognition scores from tape-recorded tests in the patient's best listening condition.

Cochlear implants may be covered for prelinguistically and postlinguistically

deafened children aged 2 through 17. Bilateral profound sensorineural deafness must be demonstrated by the inability to improve on age appropriate closed-set word identification tasks with amplification.

69930	**Cochlear device implantation, with or without mastoidectomy**	⑦ 80 ↻

OTHER PROCEDURES

69949	**Unlisted procedure, inner ear**	80

TEMPORAL BONE

MIDDLE FOSSA APPROACH

If an external approach is used, consult CPT code 69535.

69950	**Vestibular nerve section, transcranial approach**	80 ↻
69955	**Total facial nerve decompression and/or repair (may include graft)**	80 ↻
69960	**Decompression internal auditory canal**	80 ↻
69970	**Removal of tumor, temporal bone**	80 ↻

MIDDLE FOSSA APPROACH, OTHER PROCEDURES

69979	**Unlisted procedure, temporal bone, middle fossa approach**	80

OPERATING MICROSCOPE

▲ + 69990	**Microsurgical techniques, requiring use of operating microscope (List separately in addition to code for primary procedure)**	80

RADIOLOGY SERVICES

CPT Expert is not intended to replace the AMA's CPT manual. It does not include the AMA's official rules and guidelines, and Ingenix recommends you use this in conjunction with the AMA's 2002 CPT book.

CODING INFORMATION

Radiology services regularly employ imaging, diagnostic, and therapeutic technologies developed only a few decades ago. Consequently, the radiology section (70010-79999) is under constant review to reflect current standards of service.

Radiological procedures are divided into four subsections in the CPT book: diagnostic radiology, including computerized tomography (CT), magnetic resonance imaging (MRI), and interventional radiology procedures; diagnostic ultrasound; radiation oncology; and diagnostic and therapeutic nuclear medicine. Codes are ordered according to anatomic site (head, chest, abdomen), and body system (gastrointestinal, aorta, and arteries). The subject listings in the radiology section may be reported when a physician either performs or supervises the services.

Procedures are described by type of service (modality), specific body site, and are followed by additional information regarding the use of contrast material and the complexity of the procedure.

Procedures frequently performed by radiologists may be found outside the radiology section, such as Noninvasive Vascular Diagnostic Studies (93875-93990). Services involving the invasive or interventional component of interventional radiology services are found in the surgery section. These include percutaneous biopsies, injection procedures, and transcatheter procedures.

TECHNICAL AND PROFESSIONAL COMPONENTS

Radiology procedures are comprised of two components: technical and professional. The technical component includes the provision of the equipment, supplies, technical personnel, and costs attendant to the performance of the procedure other than the professional services. The professional component encompasses the physician's work in providing the service, including supervision, interpretation, and report of the procedure. Education, malpractice insurance, and other expenses incident to maintaining a practice are also part of the professional component.

A common division for reimbursement of routine diagnostic procedures is 60 percent for the technical component and 40 percent for the professional component.

Coding radiology services has been difficult due to the technical component inherent to this area of medicine. The advent of freestanding medical facilities including physician offices capable of offering imaging services, catheterizations, and other diagnostic and therapeutic radiology services poses a challenge in securing reimbursement for both components. The CPT book reports the physician component of services rather than the technical. Coders will not find a modifier in CPT to reflect technical services. HCPCS Level II provides the modifier -TC specifically for reporting the technical component. Unless instructed otherwise by payers, the professional component should be reported with modifier -26, the technical component with modifier -TC.

GLOBAL SERVICE

A global service may be reported when one physician provides both components of the radiology procedure, such as owning the equipment, employing the technologist, and providing a written interpretation of the examination.

TYPES OF RADIOLOGY SERVICES

The Radiology section of CPT is divided into four subsections. These are:

Diagnostic Radiology

Diagnostic Ultrasound

Radiation Oncology

Nuclear Medicine

DIAGNOSTIC RADIOLOGY

Procedures in Diagnostic Radiology section establish a diagnosis or follow the progression or remission of a disease process. However, also included in this section are procedures that are therapeutic. These therapeutic procedures are often referred to as interventional or invasive radiology services. Codes in this chapter of the CPT book report the radiological supervision and interpretation of these interventional and invasive procedures.

Diagnostic radiology uses different modalities, including x-rays, fluoroscopy, computerized tomography (CT), and Magnetic Resonance Imaging (MRI). Procedures in the diagnostic radiology section are ordered by anatomic site and described by type of service (modality), specific body site, number of views, and use of contrast materials.

TERMS AND INSTRUCTIONS

A **radiological examination** refers to plain films of specific sites. Other terms used to describe plain films include standard or conventional films. Services employing other modalities and additional techniques are described as such (i.e., radiography with fluoroscopy, computerized axial tomography, or magnetic resonance imaging).

Computerized Axial Tomography (CT or CAT scan) is a type of imaging that employs basic tomographic technique enhanced by computer imaging. Computer enhancement synthesizes the images obtained from different directions in a given plane, effectively reconstructing a cross-sectional plane of the body.

Computerized Tomography Angiography (CTA) provides multiple rapid thin section CT scans, a series of x-ray beams taken from different angles to create cross-sectional images of organs, bones, and tissues.

Magnetic Resonance Imaging (MRI) involves the application of an external magnetic field that forces a uniform alignment of hydrogen atom nuclei in the soft tissue. The nuclei emit radiofrequency signals that are converted into sets of tomographic images and displayed on a computer screen for three-dimensional visualization of the soft tissue structure.

Views describe the patient's position in relation to the camera. A code may specify a position, as in 71010 that describes a single frontal view of the chest. Other codes do not specify a position, but designate the number of views, as in 73610 that specifies a minimum of three views of the ankle.

Procedures performed with contrast material often do not specify the type of contrast, as in 74160 that reports computerized axial tomography of the abdomen with contrast. However, other codes are more specific. Radiologic examination of the colon using barium enema contrast is reported with 74270. An air contrast with specific high-density barium is reported with 74280.

The radiological supervision and interpretation of many interventional and invasive procedures are reported with codes from Diagnostic Radiology. Interventional/invasive codes may be used to report procedures that are diagnostic in nature, such as fluoroscopic localization 76003. Or, the codes may be used to report therapeutic procedures, such as radiologic supervision and interpretation of transcatheter embolization 75894.

DIAGNOSTIC ULTRASOUND

Procedures in Diagnostic Ultrasound are organized by anatomic site. However, when the ultrasound is part of an interventional radiology procedure for localization purposes, the procedure is listed under Ultrasonic Guidance Procedures.

Codes for ultrasounds performed for diagnostic purposes are selected based on the technique or type of study (A-mode, B-scan), the extent of the study (limited, complete, follow-up), and additional services performed with certain ultrasounds (intraocular lens power calculation).

TECHNIQUE

A-mode (a-scan) is an ultrasonic scanning procedure providing one-dimensional measurement.

M-mode is an ultrasonic scanning procedure that measures the amplitude and velocity of moving echo-producing structures to allow one-dimensional viewing.

B-scan is a two-dimensional ultrasonic scanning procedure providing a two-dimensional display.

Real-time is a two-dimensional scanning procedure that displays both structure and movement in time.

Doppler is an ultrasonic scanning procedure that measures the velocity of moving objects and often applied in the study of blood flow.

EXTENT

Complete defines a complete procedure that implies a scan of the entire body area.

Limited defines a limited procedure that involves scanning a single organ, quadrant, or completing a partial examination.

Follow-up/Repeat implies performing a limited study on an area previously scanned.

Ultrasound procedures may be found in other sections of the CPT book. For example, echocardiography procedures are in the Medicine Section under Cardiovascular Services. Color mapping in conjunction with fetal echocardiography (76825-76826) is reported with 93325 in the Medicine Section. Duplex scans and Doppler studies of the Vascular system are found in the Medicine Section under the heading Noninvasive Vascular Diagnostic Studies.

RADIATION ONCOLOGY

Radiation oncology is a therapeutic method as opposed to a diagnostic service. The radiologist manages and prescribes treatment for patients who have malignant neoplasms responsive to radiation therapy.

Radiation oncology involves the following services: consultation, clinical treatment, planning, medical radiation physics, and treatment delivery and management.

Consultation codes from the Evaluation and Management (E/M) section of CPT report consultations conducted by radiation oncologists and the E/M guidelines must be followed when applying these codes. Office/outpatient consultations are reported with codes 99241-99245; codes 99251-99263 are reported for inpatient consultations.

Clinical treatment planning consists of two services, planning and simulation to determine the best course of treatment. Planning is reported with codes 77261-77263, depending on the extent or complexity of the process. Simulation is reported with codes 77280-77295, depending on the extent or complexity of the service.

- Report 77261 for simple planning that requires assessment of a single treatment area. No interpretation of special tests is required. The treatment site can be in a single port or simple parallel opposed ports with simple or no blocking.

- Report 77262 for an intermediate level of planning that requires interpretation of tests performed for tumor localization. The radiation oncologist may need to assess two separate treatment areas or protect sensitive organs.

- Report 77263 for the interpretation of complex testing procedures, including CT and MR localization and/or special laboratory tests. Planning requires complex blocks and/or custom shielding blocks for the protection of sensitive normal structures. Tangential ports may be required. Three or more areas may require treatment. In addition, complex treatment planning often involves a combination of modalities such as brachytherapy, hyperthermia, chemotherapy and surgery.

- Simulation sets the treatment portals to specific treatment volumes. Simulation should be reported only once per time of set-up procedure.

- Simple simulation (77280) involves a single port or single pair of parallel ports on a single treatment area.

- Intermediate simulation (77285) involves three or more ports directed at a single treatment area. It also is required when two separate treatment areas are involved.

- Complex simulation (77290) involves a combination of multiple treatment areas, complex blocking rotation or arc therapy, multiple modalities, and use of contrast materials.

- Three-dimensional simulation (77295) involves computer-generated three-dimensional reconstruction of the tumor and surrounding critical structures.

- Medical radiation physics involves dosimetry calculation, the design and construction of treatment devices, and special services as defined below:

- Dosimetry calculation is the process a facility-based physicist uses to select the proper energy and modality to be used for each portal.

- Design and construction involves fabricating devices for the blocks. The physician must be involved in the design, selection, and placement of the devices and must document the involvement.

- Special services include hyperthermia or brachytherapy.

Treatment delivery and management (77401-77499) involves the delivery of radiation therapy and care of the patient during the course of therapy. While a nonphysician may deliver the treatment, the physician is responsible for checking and documenting the accuracy of the treatment. In addition, the physician responds to any adverse reactions to treatment and monitors the effects of the treatment on the tumor and surrounding tissues. Ongoing patient examinations are part of this service and not reported separately.

NUCLEAR MEDICINE

Nuclear medicine relies on radium or other radioelements for either diagnostic imaging or radiopharmaceutical therapy. Radiopharmaceutical therapy destroys diseased tissues, usually malignant neoplasms, using radioelements. This subsection is organized first by the nature of the procedure, diagnostic or therapeutic. The diagnostic codes are organized by body system and defined by the extent or complexity of the service.

Procedures in nuclear medicine are independent services. Diagnostic work-up or follow-up care is reported separately, except when specifically noted as included in the service. These services do not include the provision of radium or other radioelements. Report 78990 for diagnostic radiopharmaceuticals and 79900 for therapeutic radiopharmaceuticals.

SPECIAL CODING SITUATIONS

INTERVENTIONAL RADIOLOGY

Interventional Radiology services involve both an invasive component (such as a biopsy or injection) and a radiological component (radiological supervision and interpretation of the procedure). The invasive component, which may be either a diagnostic or therapeutic service, is reported with codes from the surgery section. Examples of the invasive component include Injection procedure for shoulder arthrography (23350), Percutaneous renal biopsy (50200*), and Transcatheter occlusion of a vascular malformation (61624-61626). The radiology component for supervision and interpretation is reported with codes from the Diagnostic Radiology and Diagnostic Ultrasound subsections.

Component coding was developed for services that can be performed by a single physician, usually an interventional radiologist or by two physicians, a surgeon and a radiologist. Whether performed by one or two physicians, an interventional radiology procedure must be documented as thoroughly as a surgical procedure. When two physicians perform an invasive procedure, each physician documents the portion of the service provided and references the other's involvement in the written report. Each physician reports only the CPT code for the portion of the service the respective physician provided.

NONINVASIVE VASCULAR DIAGNOSTIC STUDIES

A description of noninvasive vascular diagnostic services (93875-93990) are mentioned here since radiologists frequently perform them also. Vascular study procedures are comprised of the following services: patient care required during performance of the study, supervision of the study, written interpretation of study results, a hard copy of output, and analysis of all data.

RADIOLOGY

MODIFIERS

As in other specialties, modifiers in radiology denote circumstances that affect the performance of services and procedures. Radiologists most frequently apply -26, which reports the physician (professional) component of a service separately from the technical portion. Other modifiers for radiology include, but are not limited to:

- -22 Unusual procedural services
- -52 Reduced services
- -59 Distinct procedural service
- -76 Repeat procedure by same physician
- -77 Repeat procedure by another physician

X-RAY CONSULTATIONS

Code 76140 *Consultation on x-ray examination made elsewhere, written report* is used by a physician providing a second interpretation and report on a radiologic procedure. The previous interpretation is usually from a source outside of the physician's practice and is provided at the request of another physician. Both written reports must be maintained as part of the patient's medical record. The initial report and the consultation must document the specific procedure reviewed and the complexity of the procedure, such as the number of views. Do not report 76140 for outside films that are reviewed in conjunction with evaluation and management services. The medical decision making component of E/M codes includes "amount and/or complexity of data to be reviewed."

DOCUMENTING RADIOLOGY SERVICES

Diagnostic coding is critical in establishing medical necessity, even though the radiologist may not have the information necessary to assign a definitive diagnosis. For example, many radiological services are performed to rule out a particular problem. Tests that are normal effectively rule out the suspected condition; however, the radiologist must be given sufficient information about the patient's clinical history to justify medical necessity. In instances of a rule-out diagnosis, the physician must provide the radiologist with information, regarding the patient's symptoms, signs, or complaints.

PHYSICIAN REQUIREMENTS

In general, the patient's physician orders the study and a radiologist performs and/or interprets the procedure. The radiologist sends a report to the referring physician who includes it in the overall assessment of the patient. For coding and reimbursement purposes, the radiologist's portion of the service is reported as a complete procedure or as the professional component of the study. The ordering physician evaluates the results of the study for consideration in the medical decision making but does not file a claim for any portion of the radiological study.

REQUESTING PHYSICIAN RESPONSIBILITIES

The physician should sign or initial the radiologist's report as evidence the information was reviewed and considered in medical decision making. While the actual film may be stored elsewhere, a written report should be incorporated into the patient's medical record to prove the study was medically necessary.

RADIOLOGIST RESPONSIBILITIES

Radiologists must complete a written report for every service claimed. The specific name or title of the study must appear on the report; for example, "Chest x-ray, PA and lateral." In addition to reporting the number and type of views taken, reports also must indicate any other circumstances that may affect the exam such as, a patient's state of fasting for a bowel study. Documentation should also include:

- Quality of the study (clear or blurry)
- Pertinent positive findings (abnormal)
- Pertinent negative findings (normal)
- Other aspects of the film such as incidental findings in other areas
- Radiologist's impression and diagnosis
- Recommendations for further studies or treatment
- Signature

Although the ordering physician must indicate the medical necessity, the radiologist must indicate the reason in the report. The complexity of the study dictates the depth of the radiology statement. Results from radiological studies done for urgent, acute problems must be communicated verbally by the radiologist to the physician as soon as they are available (and, also, documented later in the patient record).

REPORTS

Radiology reports are almost universally transcribed. For that reason, precautions must be taken to keep the patient's record current. Whenever possible, apply the rules for dictated operative reports to radiology reports. For example, a handwritten summary of the study should be placed in the chart until the transcription is available. The radiologist should read the transcription for accuracy and sign it before it is sent to the ordering physician or placed permanently in the patient's record.

Dictated reports should include the number and type of views taken, whether the study required a contrast medium, and the type and amount of contrast medium or radionuclide. This information plus other pertinent documentation is necessary to support CPT code selection and eliminate any extra time that could be necessary for verification.

Document all additional views beyond the usual number. Report with modifier -22 (unusual procedural services) added to the CPT code that may qualify the service for higher reimbursement.

SECOND READINGS

The requesting physician may interpret a radiological study following the radiologist's interpretation. A second interpretation cannot be billed since it is part of the overall patient assessment. If the physician disagrees with the radiologist's findings, it should not be recorded in the patient chart. The physician should discuss any differences of opinion with the radiologist and if a change in interpretation is made, a final corrected statement should be made in the chart. A brief note stating the reason for the change should be included. This clarifies the final diagnostic interpretation of the service that simplifies the process of assigning accurate codes.

ADDITIONAL STUDIES

Findings from a routine x-ray exam may warrant further studies. For example, a radiologist may elect to do tomograms on a patient whose chest x-ray revealed a mass. The documentation must indicate that the existence of the mass establishes the medical necessity for further studies. In such a situation, the radiologist usually is not required to check with the ordering physician before proceeding with additional studies.

Steps for Accurate Coding and Documentation (level 1)

The following procedures should be followed for complete and accurate coding and documentation:

1. Obtain sufficient history from the ordering physician to assign an accurate diagnosis code.

2. Document the exam in sufficient detail to allow complete and accurate procedure coding.

3. If the report is dictated, review the transcribed report for accuracy. Correct any error on the transcribed report and return to the transcriptionist to generate new and corrected hard copy.

DIAGNOSTIC RADIOLOGY (DIAGNOSTIC IMAGING)

HEAD AND NECK

70010	Myelography, posterior fossa, radiological supervision and interpretation	80 ▢
70015	Cisternography, positive contrast, radiological supervision and interpretation	80 ▢
70030	Radiologic examination, eye, for detection of foreign body	80
70100	Radiologic examination, mandible; partial, less than four views	80
70110	complete, minimum of four views	80 ▢
70120	Radiologic examination, mastoids; less than three views per side	80
70130	complete, minimum of three views per side	80 ▢
70134	Radiologic examination, internal auditory meati, complete	80
70140	Radiologic examination, facial bones; less than three views	80
70150	complete, minimum of three views	80 ▢
70160	Radiologic examination, nasal bones, complete, minimum of three views	80
70170	Dacryocystography, nasolacrimal duct, radiological supervision and interpretation	80
70190	Radiologic examination; optic foramina	80
70200	orbits, complete, minimum of four views	80
70210	Radiologic examination, sinuses, paranasal, less than three views	80
70220	Radiologic examination, sinuses, paranasal, complete, minimum of three views	80 ▢
70240	Radiologic examination, sella turcica	80
70250	Radiologic examination, skull; less than four views, with or without stereo	80
70260	complete, minimum of four views, with or without stereo	80 ▢
70300	Radiologic examination, teeth; single view	80
70310	partial examination, less than full mouth	80 ▢
70320	complete, full mouth	80 ▢
70328	Radiologic examination, temporomandibular joint, open and closed mouth; unilateral	80
70330	bilateral	80 ▢
70332	Temporomandibular joint arthrography, radiological supervision and interpretation	80

Code 76003 should not be used in addition to 70332.

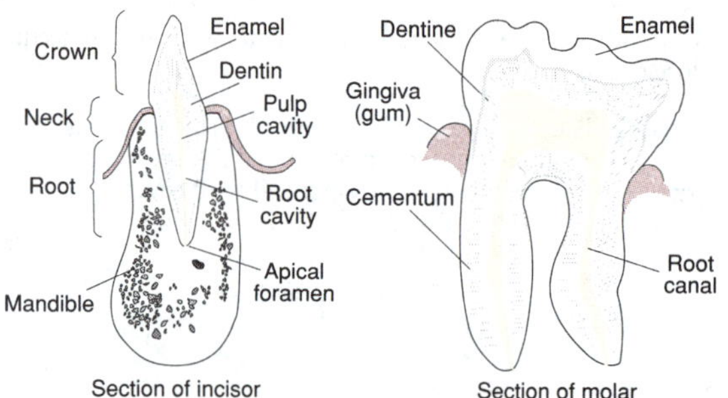

Normal dentition numbers 16 teeth in each jaw: two incisors, two canines, four premolars, and six molars. A common tooth eruption problem occurs with the third molars (wisdom teeth) which may be malposed and become impacted. Caries means "rotten" and is a decalcification of tooth enamel and sometimes penetration into the dentin and pulp. Disease processes may cause resorption of the dentin and cementum

CIM 50-13 MAGNETIC RESONANCE

Medicare covers magnetic resonance imaging (MRI), formerly called nuclear magnetic resonance (NMR), when furnished using MRI units with Food and Drug Administration pre-market approval. An MRI is covered when used to detect:

- To detect and stage pelvic and retroperitoneal neoplasms
- To evaluate disorders of cancellous bone and soft tissues
- To detect pericardial thickening
- To detect and monitor early-stage primary and secondary bone neoplasm and aseptic necrosis
- To detect early states of bone infections for patients with metallic prostheses, especially of the hip, to which the prothesis is attached
- Disc disease without regard to radiological imaging

In addition:

- The inherent tissue contrast resolution of MRI makes it an appropriate standard diagnostic modality for general neuroradiology
- When a clinical need exists to visualize the parenchyma of solid organs to detect anatomic disruption or neoplasia, this can be accomplished in the liver, urogenital system, adrenals, and pelvic organs without the use of radiological contrast materials
- Gating devices that eliminate distorted images caused by cardiac and respiratory movement cycles may be covered. Surface and other specialty coils may be covered, as they are used routinely for high-resolution imaging where small limited regions of the body are studied

MRI is not covered for patients with cardiac pacemakers or with metallic clips on vascular aneurysms. In addition, the long imaging time and the enclosed position of the patient may result in claustrophobia, making patients who have a history of claustrophobia unsuitable candidates for MRI procedures. Several uses of MRI have been identified as investigational and are not covered. These include measurement of blood flow and spectroscopy. In addition, MRI is not suitable for the imaging of cortical bone and calcifications and for procedures involving spatial resolution of bone or calcifications.

70336	Magnetic resonance (eg, proton) imaging, temporomandibular joint(s)	80
70350	Cephalogram, orthodontic	80
70355	Orthopantogram	80
70360	Radiologic examination; neck, soft tissue	80
70370	pharynx or larynx, including fluoroscopy and/or magnification technique	80 ▢
70371	Complex dynamic pharyngeal and speech evaluation by cine or video recording	80
70373	Laryngography, contrast, radiological supervision and interpretation	80 ▢
70380	Radiologic examination, salivary gland for calculus	80
70390	Sialography, radiological supervision and interpretation	80

CIM 50-12 COMPUTERIZED TOMOGRAPHY

Diagnostic examinations of the head (head scans) and of other parts of the body (body scans) performed by computerized tomography (CT) scanners are covered if medical and scientific literature and opinion support the effective use of a scan for the condition.

There is no general rule that requires other diagnostic tests to be tried before CT scanning is used. However, in an individual case the contractor's medical staff may determine that a CT scan as the initial diagnostic test was not reasonable and necessary if not supported by the patient's symptoms or complaints stated on the claim form; e.g., "periodic headaches."

CT equipment must meet the following criteria:

1. Known to the Food and Drug Administration

2. In the full market release phase of development

Mobile CT scan services furnished at an ambulatory health care facility other than a hospital-based facility (e.g., a freestanding physician-directed clinic)

---

must be performed under the direct personal supervision of a radiologist or other qualified physician. In addition, the facility must maintain a record of the attending physician's order. Bill the same as for scans performed on stationary equipment.

Medicare covers multiplanar diagnostic imaging (MPDI), known as planar image reconstruction or reformatted imaging, when performed by an entity offering covered CT scans.

70450   Computerized axial tomography, head or brain; without contrast material   80

70460   with contrast material(s)   80

70470   without contrast material, followed by contrast material(s) and further sections   80
     If performed with coronal, sagittal, and/or oblique sections, consult CPT code 76375.

70480   Computerized axial tomography, orbit, sella, or posterior fossa or outer, middle, or inner ear; without contrast material   80

70481   with contrast material(s)   80

70482   without contrast material, followed by contrast material(s) and further sections   80
     If performed with coronal, sagittal, and/or oblique sections, consult CPT code 76375.

70486   Computerized axial tomography, maxillofacial area; without contrast material   80

70487   with contrast material(s)   80

70488   without contrast material, followed by contrast material(s) and further sections   80
     If performed with coronal, sagittal, and/or oblique sections, consult CPT code 76375.

70490   Computerized axial tomography, soft tissue neck; without contrast material   80

70491   with contrast material(s)   80

70492   without contrast material followed by contrast material(s) and further sections   80
     If performed with coronal, sagittal, and/or oblique sections, consult CPT code 76375. If computerized axial tomography is performed on the cervical spine, consult CPT codes 72125 and 72126.

70496   Computed tomographic angiography, head, without contrast material(s), followed by contrast material(s) and further sections, including image post-processing   80

70498   Computed tomographic angiography, neck, without contrast material(s), followed by contrast material(s) and further sections, including image post-processing   80

70540   Magnetic resonance (eg, proton) imaging, orbit, face, and neck; without contrast material(s)   80

70542   with contrast material(s)   80

70543   without contrast material(s), followed by contrast material(s) and further sequences   80

70544   Magnetic resonance angiography, head; without contrast material(s)   80

70545   with contrast material(s)   80

70546   without contrast material(s), followed by contrast material(s) and further sequences   80

70547   Magnetic resonance angiography, neck; without contrast material(s)   80

70548   with contrast material(s)   80

70549   without contrast material(s), followed by contrast material(s) and further sequences   80

70551   Magnetic resonance (eg, proton) imaging, brain (including brain stem); without contrast material   80

70552   with contrast material(s)   80

70553   without contrast material, followed by contrast material(s) and further sequences   80
     If magnetic spectroscopy is performed, consult CPT code 76390.

CHEST

71010   Radiologic examination, chest; single view, frontal   80
     If chest x-ray, single view, frontal is performed as part of critical care services (99291-99292) do not report separately.

71015   stereo, frontal   80

71020   Radiologic examination, chest, two views, frontal and lateral;   80
     If chest x-ray, two views, frontal and lateral is performed as part of critical care services (99291-99292) do not report separately.

71021   with apical lordotic procedure   80

71022   with oblique projections   80

71023   with fluoroscopy   80

71030   Radiologic examination, chest, complete, minimum of four views;   80

71034   with fluoroscopy   80
     If a separate chest fluoroscopy is performed, consult CPT code 76000.

71035   Radiologic examination, chest, special views (eg, lateral decubitus, Bucky studies)   80

71040   Bronchography, unilateral, radiological supervision and interpretation   80

71060   Bronchography, bilateral, radiological supervision and interpretation   80

71090   Insertion pacemaker, fluoroscopy and radiography, radiological supervision and interpretation   80
     To report procedure, see appropriate CPT code.

71100   Radiologic examination, ribs, unilateral; two views   80

71101   including posteroanterior chest, minimum of three views   80

71110   Radiologic examination, ribs, bilateral; three views   80

71111   including posteroanterior chest, minimum of four views   80

71120   Radiologic examination; sternum, minimum of two views   80

71130   sternoclavicular joint or joints, minimum of three views   80

71250   Computerized axial tomography, thorax; without contrast material   80

71260   with contrast material(s)   80

71270   without contrast material, followed by contrast material(s) and further sections   80
     If performed with coronal, sagittal, and/or oblique sections, consult CPT code 76375.

71275   Computed tomographic angiography, chest, without contrast material(s), followed by contrast material(s) and further sections, including image post-processing   80

71550   Magnetic resonance (eg, proton) imaging, chest (eg, for evaluation of hilar and mediastinal lymphadenopathy); without contrast material(s)   80

71551   with contrast material(s)   80

☑ CCI Comprehensive Code   50 Bilateral Procedure   ✛ CPT Add-on Code   ⦸ Modifier -51 Exempt Code   ● New Code   ▲ Revised Code

M Maternity   N Newborn   P Pediatric   N/P Newborn/Pediatric

71552 — 72285

| 71552 | without contrast material(s), followed by contrast material(s) and further sequences 80 |

If a breast MRI is needed, consult CPT codes 76093 and 76094.

71555 Magnetic resonance angiography, chest (excluding myocardium), with or without contrast material(s) 80

SPINE AND PELVIS

72010 Radiologic examination, spine, entire, survey study, anteroposterior and lateral 80

72020 Radiologic examination, spine, single view, specify level 80

72040 Radiologic examination, spine, cervical; two or three views 80

72050 minimum of four views 80

72052 complete, including oblique and flexion and/or extension studies 80

72069 Radiologic examination, spine, thoracolumbar, standing (scoliosis) 80

72070 Radiologic examination, spine; thoracic, two views 80

72072 thoracic, three views 80

72074 thoracic, minimum of four views 80

72080 thoracolumbar, two views 80

72090 scoliosis study, including supine and erect studies 80

72100 Radiologic examination, spine, lumbosacral; two or three views 80

72110 minimum of four views 80

72114 complete, including bending views 80

72120 Radiologic examination, spine, lumbosacral, bending views only, minimum of four views 80

Contrast material in CT of spine is performed by either an intrathecal or an intravenous injection. For intrathecal injection, consult CPT code 61055 or 62284. IV injection of contrast material is included as part of this procedure. If this procedure is performed for coronal, sagittal, and/or oblique sections, consult CPT code 76375.

72125 Computerized axial tomography, cervical spine; without contrast material 80

72126 with contrast material 80

72127 without contrast material, followed by contrast material(s) and further sections 80

72128 Computerized axial tomography, thoracic spine; without contrast material 80

72129 with contrast material 80

72130 without contrast material, followed by contrast material(s) and further sections 80

72131 Computerized axial tomography, lumbar spine; without contrast material 80

72132 with contrast material 80

72133 without contrast material, followed by contrast material(s) and further sections 80

If performed with coronal, sagittal, and/or oblique sections, consult CPT code 76375.

72141 Magnetic resonance (eg, proton) imaging, spinal canal and contents, cervical; without contrast material 80

72142 with contrast material(s) 80

If cervical spine canal imaging is performed first without contrast material followed by contrast material, consult CPT code 72156.

72146 Magnetic resonance (eg, proton) imaging, spinal canal and contents, thoracic; without contrast material 80

72147 with contrast material(s) 80

If thoracic spinal canal imaging is performed first without contrast material followed by contrast material, consult CPT code 72157.

72148 Magnetic resonance (eg, proton) imaging, spinal canal and contents, lumbar; without contrast material 80

72149 with contrast material(s) 80

If lumbar spinal canal imaging is performed first without contrast material followed by contrast material, consult CPT code 72158.

72156 Magnetic resonance (eg, proton) imaging, spinal canal and contents, without contrast material, followed by contrast material(s) and further sequences; cervical 80

72157 thoracic 80

72158 lumbar 80

72159 Magnetic resonance angiography, spinal canal and contents, with or without contrast material(s)

72170 Radiologic examination, pelvis; one or two views 80

72190 complete, minimum of three views 80

If pelvimetry is performed, consult CPT code 74710.

72191 Computed tomographic angiography, pelvis, without contrast material(s), followed by contrast material(s) and further sections, including image post-processing 80

For CTA aorto-iliofemoral runoff, consult CPT code 75635.

72192 Computerized axial tomography, pelvis; without contrast material 80

72193 with contrast material(s) 80

72194 without contrast material, followed by contrast material(s) and further sections 80

If performed with coronal, sagittal, and/or oblique sections, consult CPT code 76375.

72195 Magnetic resonance (eg, proton) imaging, pelvis; without contrast material(s) 80

72196 with contrast material(s) 80

72197 without contrast material(s), followed by contrast material(s) and further sequences 80

72198 Magnetic resonance angiography, pelvis, with or without contrast material(s)

72200 Radiologic examination, sacroiliac joints; less than three views 80

72202 three or more views 80

72220 Radiologic examination, sacrum and coccyx, minimum of two views 80

72240 Myelography, cervical, radiological supervision and interpretation 80

72255 Myelography, thoracic, radiological supervision and interpretation 80

72265 Myelography, lumbosacral, radiological supervision and interpretation 80

72270 Myelography, entire spinal canal, radiological supervision and interpretation 80

72275 Epidurography, radiological supervision and interpretation

For the injection procedure, consult CPT codes 62280-62282, 62310-62319, and 64479-64484.

72285 Diskography, cervical or thoracic, radiological supervision and interpretation 80

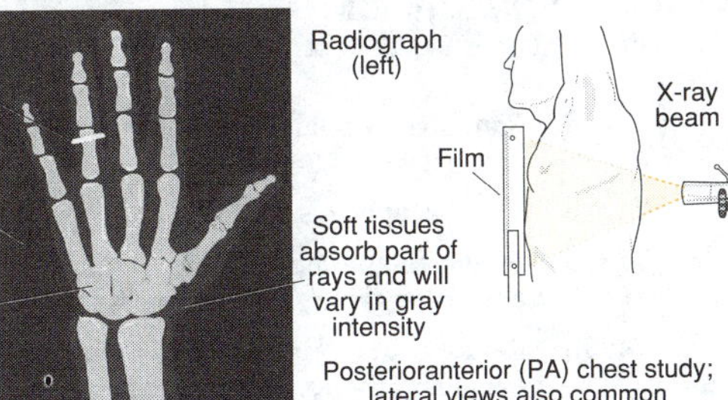

Traditional diagnostic radiography is defined by the x-ray. Radiographs, or x-rays, are "shadowgrams" of body structures and tissues and show radiopaque matter, such as bone, to be whiter and radiolucent substances, such as air, to be blacker. Each study is oriented by the direction path of the x-ray beam: e.g., PA, the most common, means the beam travels from posterior to anterior. Contrast agents are commonly used to highlight particular areas or structures

72295 Diskography, lumbar, radiological supervision and interpretation

UPPER EXTREMITIES

If a radiological examination of stress views is performed, any joint, consult CPT code 76006.

73000 Radiologic examination; clavicle, complete

73010 scapula, complete

73020 Radiologic examination, shoulder; one view

73030 complete, minimum of two views

73040 Radiologic examination, shoulder, arthrography, radiological supervision and interpretation
Code 76003 should not be used in addition to 73040.

73050 Radiologic examination; acromioclavicular joints, bilateral, with or without weighted distraction

73060 humerus, minimum of two views

73070 Radiologic examination, elbow; two views

73080 complete, minimum of three views

73085 Radiologic examination, elbow, arthrography, radiological supervision and interpretation
Code 76003 should not be used in addition to 73085.

73090 Radiologic examination; forearm, two views

73092 upper extremity, infant, minimum of two views

73100 Radiologic examination, wrist; two views

73110 complete, minimum of three views

73115 Radiologic examination, wrist, arthrography, radiological supervision and interpretation
Code 76003 should not be used in addition to 73115.

73120 Radiologic examination, hand; two views

73130 minimum of three views

73140 Radiologic examination, finger(s), minimum of two views

73200 Computerized axial tomography, upper extremity; without contrast material

73201 with contrast material(s)

73202 without contrast material, followed by contrast material(s) and further sections
If performed with coronal, sagittal, and/or oblique sections, consult CPT code 76375.

73206 Computed tomographic angiography, upper extremity, without contrast material(s), followed by contrast material(s) and further sections, including image post-processing

73218 Magnetic resonance (eg, proton) imaging, upper extremity, other than joint; without contrast material(s)

73219 with contrast material(s)

73220 without contrast material(s), followed by contrast material(s) and further sequences

73221 Magnetic resonance (eg, proton) imaging, any joint of upper extremity; without contrast material(s)

73222 with contrast material(s)

73223 without contrast material(s), followed by contrast material(s) and further sequences

73225 Magnetic resonance angiography, upper extremity, with or without contrast material(s)

LOWER EXTREMITIES

If a radiological examination of stress views is performed, any joint, consult CPT code 76006.

73500 Radiologic examination, hip unilateral; one view

73510 complete, minimum of two views

73520 Radiologic examination, hips, bilateral, minimum of two views of each hip, including anteroposterior view of pelvis

73525 Radiologic examination, hip, arthrography, radiological supervision and interpretation
Code 76003 should not be used in addition to 73525.

73530 Radiologic examination, hip, during operative procedure

73540 Radiologic examination, pelvis and hips, infant or child, minimum of two views

73542 Radiological examination, sacroiliac joint arthrography, radiological supervision and interpretation
Code 76003 should not be used in addition to 73542.
For procedure, use 27096. If formal arthrography is not performed, recorded, and a formal radiologic report is not issued, use 76005 for fluoroscopic guidance for sacroiliac joint injections.

73550 Radiologic examination, femur, two views

73560 Radiologic examination, knee; one or two views

73562 three views

73564 complete, four or more views

73565 both knees, standing, anteroposterior

73580 Radiologic examination, knee, arthrography, radiological supervision and interpretation
Code 76003 should not be used in addition to 73580.

73590 Radiologic examination; tibia and fibula, two views

73592 lower extremity, infant, minimum of two views

73600 Radiologic examination, ankle; two views

73610 complete, minimum of three views

73615 Radiologic examination, ankle, arthrography, radiological supervision and interpretation
Code 76003 should not be used in addition to 73615.

73620 Radiologic examination, foot; two views

73630 complete, minimum of three views

73650 Radiologic examination; calcaneus, minimum of two views

73660 toe(s), minimum of two views

CCI Comprehensive Code   **50** Bilateral Procedure   **+** CPT Add-on Code   Modifier -51 Exempt Code   ● New Code   ▲ Revised Code

M Maternity   **N** Newborn   **P** Pediatric   **N/P** Newborn/Pediatric

73700 — 74327

73700	Computerized axial tomography, lower extremity; without contrast material	80
73701	with contrast material(s)	80 TC
73702	without contrast material, followed by contrast material(s) and further sections	80 TC
	If performed with coronal, sagittal, and/or oblique sections, consult CPT code 76375.	
73706	Computed tomographic angiography, lower extremity, without contrast material(s), followed by contrast material(s) and further sections, including image post-processing	80 TC
	To report CTA aorto-iliofemoral runoff, consult CPT code 75635.	
73718	Magnetic resonance (eg, proton) imaging, lower extremity other than joint; without contrast material(s)	80
73719	with contrast material(s)	80
73720	without contrast material(s), followed by contrast material(s) and further sequences	80 TC
73721	Magnetic resonance (eg, proton) imaging, any joint of lower extremity; without contrast material	80
73722	with contrast material(s)	80
73723	without contrast material(s), followed by contrast material(s) and further sequences	80
73725	Magnetic resonance angiography, lower extremity, with or without contrast material(s)	80 TC

ABDOMEN

74000	Radiologic examination, abdomen; single anteroposterior view	80
74010	anteroposterior and additional oblique and cone views	80 TC
74020	complete, including decubitus and/or erect views	80 TC
74022	complete acute abdomen series, including supine, erect, and/or decubitus views, upright PA chest	80 TC
74150	Computerized axial tomography, abdomen; without contrast material	80 TC
74160	with contrast material(s)	80 TC
74170	without contrast material, followed by contrast material(s) and further sections	80 TC
	If performed with coronal, sagittal, and/or oblique sections, consult CPT code 76375.	
74175	Computed tomographic angiography, abdomen, without contrast material(s), followed by contrast material(s) and further sections, including image post-processing	80 TC
	To report CTA aorto-iliofemoral runoff, consult CPT code 75635.	
74181	Magnetic resonance (eg, proton) imaging, abdomen; without contrast material(s)	80
74182	with contrast material(s)	80
74183	without contrast material(s), followed by with contrast material(s) and further sequences	80
74185	Magnetic resonance angiography, abdomen, with or without contrast material(s)	80 TC
74190	Peritoneogram (eg, after injection of air or contrast), radiological supervision and interpretation	80
	If air or contrast is injected into the peritoneal cavity, consult CPT code 49400. If computerized axial tomography is performed on the pelvis, consult CPT code 72192 or 74150.	

GASTROINTESTINAL TRACT

If the gastrostomy tube is placed percutaneously, consult CPT code 43750.

	74210	Radiologic examination; pharynx and/or cervical esophagus	80
	74220	esophagus	80 TC
▲	74230	Swallowing function, with cineradiography/videoradiography	80 26
	74235	Removal of foreign body(s), esophageal, with use of balloon catheter, radiological supervision and interpretation	80
		For esophagoscopy or upper gastrointestinal endoscopy procedure with removal of a foreign body, consult CPT codes 43215 and 43247.	
	74240	Radiologic examination, gastrointestinal tract, upper; with or without delayed films, without KUB	80 TC
	74241	with or without delayed films, with KUB	80 TC
▲	74245	with small intestine, includes multiple serial films	80 TC
	74246	Radiological examination, gastrointestinal tract, upper, air contrast, with specific high density barium, effervescent agent, with or without glucagon; with or without delayed films, without KUB	80 TC
		Moynihan test	
	74247	with or without delayed films, with KUB	80 TC
▲	74249	with small intestine follow-through	80 TC
▲	74250	Radiologic examination, small intestine, includes multiple serial films;	80 TC
	74251	via enteroclysis tube	80 TC
	74260	Duodenography, hypotonic	80
	74270	Radiologic examination, colon; barium enema, with or without KUB	80 TC
	74280	air contrast with specific high density barium, with or without glucagon	80 TC
	74283	Therapeutic enema, contrast or air, for reduction of intussusception or other intraluminal obstruction (eg, meconium ileus)	80
	74290	Cholecystography, oral contrast;	80
	74291	additional or repeat examination or multiple day examination	80
	74300	Cholangiography and/or pancreatography; intraoperative, radiological supervision and interpretation	80 TC
+	74301	additional set intraoperative, radiological supervision and interpretation (List separately in addition to code for primary procedure)	80 TC
		Note that 74301 is an add-on code and must be used in conjunction with 74300.	
▲	74305	through existing catheter, radiological supervision and interpretation	80 TC 26
		For procedure performed, consult CPT codes 47505, 47560-47561, 47563, and 48400. If a biliary duct stone extraction is performed percutaneously, consult CPT codes 47630 and 74327.	
	74320	Cholangiography, percutaneous, transhepatic, radiological supervision and interpretation	80 TC
▲	74327	Postoperative biliary duct calculus removal, percutaneous via T-tube tract, basket, or snare (eg, Burhenne technique), radiological supervision and interpretation	80
		If a biliary duct stone extraction is performed percutaneously, consult CPT code 47630.	

74328 **Endoscopic catheterization of the biliary ductal system, radiological supervision and interpretation** 80

For endoscopic retrograde cholangiopancreatography (ECRP) procedure, consult CPT codes 43260-43272 as appropriate.

74329 **Endoscopic catheterization of the pancreatic ductal system, radiological supervision and interpretation** 80

For endoscopic retrograde cholangiopancreatography (ECRP) procedure, consult CPT codes 43260-43272 as appropriate.

74330 **Combined endoscopic catheterization of the biliary and pancreatic ductal systems, radiological supervision and interpretation** 80

For endoscopic retrograde cholangiopancreatography (ECRP) procedure, consult CPT codes 43260-43272 as appropriate.

74340 **Introduction of long gastrointestinal tube (eg, Miller-Abbott), including multiple fluoroscopies and films, radiological supervision and interpretation** 80

If tube placement is performed, consult CPT code 44500.

74350 **Percutaneous placement of gastrostomy tube, radiological supervision and interpretation** 80

74355 **Percutaneous placement of enteroclysis tube, radiological supervision and interpretation** 80

74360 **Intraluminal dilation of strictures and/or obstructions (eg, esophagus), radiological supervision and interpretation** 80

▲ **74363** **Percutaneous transhepatic dilation of biliary duct stricture with or without placement of stent, radiological supervision and interpretation** 80

If a transhepatic catheter/stent is introduced percutaneously, consult CPT codes 47510 and 47511. If a biliary endoscopy is performed percutaneously via a T-tube or other tract with dilation of the biliary duct stricture(s), consult CPT codes 47555 and 47556.

URINARY TRACT

74400 **Urography (pyelography), intravenous, with or without KUB, with or without tomography;** 80

74410 **Urography, infusion, drip technique and/or bolus technique;** 80

74415 **with nephrotomography** 80

74420 **Urography, retrograde, with or without KUB** 80

74425 **Urography, antegrade, (pyelostogram, nephrostogram, loopogram), radiological supervision and interpretation** 80

74430 **Cystography, minimum of three views, radiological supervision and interpretation** 80

74440 **Vasography, vesiculography, or epididymography, radiological supervision and interpretation** ♂ 80

74445 **Corpora cavernosography, radiological supervision and interpretation** ♂ 80

74450 **Urethrocystography, retrograde, radiological supervision and interpretation** 80

CIM 50-33 UROFLOWMETRIC EVALUATIONS

Medicare covers uroflowmetric evaluations (also referred to as urodynamic voiding or urodynamic flow studies) for diagnosing various urological dysfunctions, including bladder outlet obstructions.

74455 **Urethrocystography, voiding, radiological supervision and interpretation** 80

74470 **Radiologic examination, renal cyst study, translumbar, contrast visualization, radiological supervision and interpretation** 80

74475 **Introduction of intracatheter or catheter into renal pelvis for drainage and/or injection, percutaneous, radiological supervision and interpretation** 80

74480 **Introduction of ureteral catheter or stent into ureter through renal pelvis for drainage and/or injection, percutaneous, radiological supervision and interpretation** 80

For surgical procedure performed consult CPT codes 50392-50398 as appropriate. If transurethral surgery (ureter and pelvis) is performed, consult CPT codes 52320-52355.

74485 **Dilation of nephrostomy, ureters, or urethra, radiological supervision and interpretation** 80

If the ureter is dilated without radiological guidance, consult CPT codes 52341, 52344. If a nephrostomy or pyelostomy tube is changed, consult CPT code 50398.

GYNECOLOGICAL AND OBSTETRICAL

If radiological examination is performed on the abdomen and pelvis, consult CPT codes 72170-72190, 74000-74170.

74710 **Pelvimetry, with or without placental localization** ♀ 80

74740 **Hysterosalpingography, radiological supervision and interpretation** ♀ 80

If saline or contrast is introduced for hysterosalpingography, see 58340.

74742 **Transcervical catheterization of fallopian tube, radiological supervision and interpretation** ♀ 80

For hysterosalpingography procedure, consult CPT code 58345.

74775 **Perineogram (eg, vaginogram, for sex determination or extent of anomalies)** M ♀ 80

HEART

CIM 50-13 MAGNETIC RESONANCE

Medicare covers magnetic resonance imaging (MRI), formerly called nuclear magnetic resonance (NMR), when furnished using MRI units with Food and Drug Administration pre-market approval. An MRI is covered when used to detect:

- To detect and stage pelvic and retroperitoneal neoplasms
- To evaluate disorders of cancellous bone and soft tissues
- To detect pericardial thickening
- To detect and monitor early-stage primary and secondary bone neoplasm and aseptic necrosis
- To detect early states of bone infections for patients with metallic prostheses, especially of the hip, to which the prothesis is attached
- Disc disease without regard to radiological imaging

In addition:

- The inherent tissue contrast resolution of MRI makes it an appropriate standard diagnostic modality for general neuroradiology
- When a clinical need exists to visualize the parenchyma of solid organs to detect anatomic disruption or neoplasia, this can be accomplished in the liver, urogenital system, adrenals, and pelvic organs without the use of radiological contrast materials
- Gating devices that eliminate distorted images caused by cardiac and respiratory movement cycles may be covered. Surface and other specialty coils may be covered, as they are used routinely for high-resolution imaging where small limited regions of the body are studied

MRI is not covered for patients with cardiac pacemakers or with metallic clips on vascular aneurysms. In addition, the long imaging time and the enclosed position of the patient may result in claustrophobia, making patients who have a history of claustrophobia unsuitable candidates for MRI procedures. Several uses of MRI have been identified as investigational and are not covered. These include measurement of blood flow and spectroscopy. In addition, MRI is not suitable for the imaging of cortical bone and calcifications and for procedures involving spatial resolution of bone or calcifications.

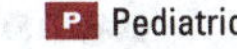

⬚ CCI Comprehensive Code	80 Bilateral Procedure + CPT Add-on Code ⊘ Modifier -51 Exempt Code ● New Code ▲ Revised Code
M Maternity	N Newborn P Pediatric N/P Newborn/Pediatric

75552   Cardiac magnetic resonance imaging for morphology; without contrast material   80 ↻

75553   with contrast material   80 ↻

75554   Cardiac magnetic resonance imaging for funciton, with or without morphology; complete study   80 ↻

75555   limited study   80 ↻

75556   Cardiac magnetic resonance imaging for velocity flow mapping

AORTA AND ARTERIES

Includes introduction and all lesser order catheterization used in the approach. Additional order catheterization within the same family of arteries should be reported using codes in the 36000 range.

75600   Aortography, thoracic, without serialography, radiological supervision and interpretation   80 ↻

75605   Aortography, thoracic, by serialography, radiological supervision and interpretation   80 ↻

75625   Aortography, abdominal, by serialography, radiological supervision and interpretation   80 ↻

75630   Aortography, abdominal plus bilateral iliofemoral lower extremity, catheter, by serialography, radiological supervision and interpretation   80 ↻

75635   Computed tomographic angiography, abdominal aorta and bilateral iliofemoral lower extremity runoff, radiological supervision and interpretation, without contrast material(s), followed by contrast material(s) and further sections, including image post-processing   80 ↻

75650   Angiography, cervicocerebral, catheter, including vessel origin, radiological supervision and interpretation   80 ↻

75658   Angiography, brachial, retrograde, radiological supervision and interpretation   80 ↻

75660   Angiography, external carotid, unilateral, selective, radiological supervision and interpretation   80 ↻

75662   Angiography, external carotid, bilateral, selective, radiological supervision and interpretation   80 ↻

75665   Angiography, carotid, cerebral, unilateral, radiological supervision and interpretation   80 ↻

75671   Angiography, carotid, cerebral, bilateral, radiological supervision and interpretation   80 ↻

75676   Angiography, carotid, cervical, unilateral, radiological supervision and interpretation   80 ↻

75680   Angiography, carotid, cervical, bilateral, radiological supervision and interpretation   80 ↻

75685   Angiography, vertebral, cervical, and/or intracranial, radiological supervision and interpretation   80 ↻

75705   Angiography, spinal, selective, radiological supervision and interpretation   80 ↻

75710   Angiography, extremity, unilateral, radiological supervision and interpretation   80 ↻

75716   Angiography, extremity, bilateral, radiological supervision and interpretation   80 ↻

75722   Angiography, renal, unilateral, selective (including flush aortogram), radiological supervision and interpretation   80 ↻

75724   Angiography, renal, bilateral, selective (including flush aortogram), radiological supervision and interpretation   80 ↻

75726   Angiography, visceral, selective or supraselective, (with or without flush aortogram), radiological supervision and interpretation   80 ↻

> If selective angiography is performed, each additional visceral vessel studied after basic examination, consult CPT code 75774.

75731   Angiography, adrenal, unilateral, selective, radiological supervision and interpretation   80 ↻

75733   Angiography, adrenal, bilateral, selective, radiological supervision and interpretation   80 ↻

75736   Angiography, pelvic, selective or supraselective, radiological supervision and interpretation   80 ↻

75741   Angiography, pulmonary, unilateral, selective, radiological supervision and interpretation   80 ↻

> For injection procedure during cardiac catheterization for pulmonary angiography, consult CPT code 93541.

75743   Angiography, pulmonary, bilateral, selective, radiological supervision and interpretation   80 ↻

> For an injection procedure during cardiac catheterization for pulmonary angiography, consult CPT code 93541.

75746   Angiography, pulmonary, by nonselective catheter or venous injection, radiological supervision and interpretation   80 ↻

> For an injection procedure during cardiac catheterization for pulmonary angiography, consult CPT code 93541. For catheter introduction, injection procedure, consult CPT codes 93501-93533, 93539, 93540, 93545, and 93556.
>
> If an intravenous procedure is performed, consult CPT codes 36000-36013, 36400-36425, and 36100-36248 for an intra-arterial procedure.

75756   Angiography, internal mammary, radiological supervision and interpretation   80 ↻

> For catheter introduction, injection procedure, consult CPT codes 93501-93533, 93545, and 93556.
>
> If an intravenous procedure is performed, consult CPT codes 36000-36013, 36400-36425, and 36100-36248 for an intra-arterial procedure.

+ 75774   Angiography, selective, each additional vessel studied after basic examination, radiological supervision and interpretation (List separately in addition to code for primary procedure)   80 ↻

> Use 75774 in addition to code for specific initial vessel studies.
>
> For angiography, see code 75600-75790.
>
> For catheterizations, see codes 36215-36248.
>
> For introduction of catheter, injection procedure, see 93501-93533, 93545, 93555, 93556.

75790   Angiography, arteriovenous shunt (eg, dialysis patient), radiological supervision and interpretation   80 ↻

> For catheter introduction, consult CPT codes 36140, 36145, 36215-36217, and 36245-36247.

VEINS AND LYMPHATICS

If injection procedure is performed for the lymphatic system, consult CPT code 38790. If injection procedure is performed for the venous system, consult CPT codes 36000-36015 and 36400-36510.

75801   Lymphangiography, extremity only, unilateral, radiological supervision and interpretation   80

75803   Lymphangiography, extremity only, bilateral, radiological supervision and interpretation   80 ↻

75805   Lymphangiography, pelvic/abdominal, unilateral, radiological supervision and interpretation   80

75807   Lymphangiography, pelvic/abdominal, bilateral, radiological supervision and interpretation   80 ↻

75809 Shuntogram for investigation of previously placed indwelling nonvascular shunt (eg, LeVeen shunt, ventriculoperitoneal shunt, indwelling infusion pump), radiological supervision and interpretation 80
> If an injection procedure is performed for the evaluation of a previously placed peritoneovenous shunt, consult CPT code 49427. For puncture of shunt tubing or reservoir for aspiration or injection procedure, consult CPT code 61070.

75810 Splenoportography, radiological supervision and interpretation 80 CCI

75820 Venography, extremity, unilateral, radiological supervision and interpretation 80 CCI

75822 Venography, extremity, bilateral, radiological supervision and interpretation 80 CCI

75825 Venography, caval, inferior, with serialography, radiological supervision and interpretation 80 CCI

75827 Venography, caval, superior, with serialography, radiological supervision and interpretation 80 CCI

75831 Venography, renal, unilateral, selective, radiological supervision and interpretation 80 CCI

75833 Venography, renal, bilateral, selective, radiological supervision and interpretation 80 CCI

75840 Venography, adrenal, unilateral, selective, radiological supervision and interpretation 80 CCI

75842 Venography, adrenal, bilateral, selective, radiological supervision and interpretation 80 CCI

75860 Venography, sinus or jugular, catheter, radiological supervision and interpretation 80 CCI

75870 Venography, superior sagittal sinus, radiological supervision and interpretation 80 CCI

75872 Venography, epidural, radiological supervision and interpretation 80 CCI

75880 Venography, orbital, radiological supervision and interpretation 80 CCI

75885 Percutaneous transhepatic portography with hemodynamic evaluation, radiological supervision and interpretation 80 CCI

75887 Percutaneous transhepatic portography without hemodynamic evaluation, radiological supervision and interpretation 80 CCI

75889 Hepatic venography, wedged or free, with hemodynamic evaluation, radiological supervision and interpretation 80 CCI

75891 Hepatic venography, wedged or free, without hemodynamic evaluation, radiological supervision and interpretation 80 CCI

75893 Venous sampling through catheter, with or without angiography (eg, for parathyroid hormone, renin), radiological supervision and interpretation 80 CCI
> If venous catheterization is performed for selective organ blood sampling, consult CPT code 36500.

TRANSCATHETER PROCEDURES

CIM 35-35 THERAPEUTIC EMBOLIZATION
Therapeutic embolization is covered when done for hemorrhage and for other conditions amenable to treatment by the procedure. Renal embolization for the treatment of renal adenocarcinoma is covered as a type of therapeutic embolization to:

- Reduce tumor vascularity preoperatively
- Reduce tumor bulk in inoperable cases
- Palliate specific symptoms

75894 Transcatheter therapy, embolization, any method, radiological supervision and interpretation 80 CCI

75896 Transcatheter therapy, infusion, any method (eg, thrombolysis other than coronary), radiological supervision and interpretation 80 CCI
> For injection procedure performed consult CPT codes 37201, 37202, If coronary thrombolysis is performed, consult CPT codes 92975 and 92977.

▲ **75898** Angiography through existing catheter for follow-up study for transcatheter therapy, embolization or infusion 80 CCI

75900 Exchange of a previously placed arterial catheter during thrombolytic therapy with contrast monitoring, radiological supervision and interpretation 80 CCI
> If a previously placed arterial catheter is exchanged during thrombolytic therapy, consult CPT code 37209.

75940 Percutaneous placement of IVC filter, radiological supervision and interpretation 80 CCI

CIM 50-7 ULTRASOUND DIAGNOSTIC PROCEDURES
Medicare coverage is extended to the procedures listed in Category I. Techniques in Category II are considered experimental and should not be covered at this time.

Category I (covered, may be adjunct to radiologic and nuclear medicine diagnostic technique)

1. Echoencephalography, (Diencephalic Midline) (A-Mode)
2. Echoencephalography, Complete (Diencephalic Midline and Ventricular Size)
3. Ocular and Orbital Echography (A-Mode) (includes determining the suitability of aphakic patients for an artificial lens implant following cataract surgery)
4. Ocular and Orbital Sonography (B-Mode)
5. Echocardiography, Pericardial Effusion (M-Mode)
6. Pericardiocentesis, by Ultrasonic Guidance
7. Echocardiography, Cardiac Valve(s) (M-Mode)
8. Echocardiography, Complete (M-Mode)
9. Echocardiography, limited (e.g., follow-up or limited study) (M-Mode)
10. Pleural Effusion Echography
11. Thoracentesis, by Ultrasonic Guidance
12. Abdominal Sonography, complete survey study (B-Scan)
13. Abdominal Sonography, limited (e.g., follow-up or limited study) (B-Scan)
14. Renal Cyst Aspiration, by Ultrasonic Guidance
15. Renal Biopsy, by Ultrasonic Guidance
16. Pancreas Sonography (B-Scan)
17. Spleen Sonography (B-Scan)
18. Abdominal Aorta Echography (A-Mode)
19. Abdominal Aorta Sonography (B-Scan)
20. Retroperitoneal Sonography (B-Scan)
21. Retroperitoneal sonography does not include planning of fields for radiation therapy.
22. Urinary Bladder Sonography (B-Scan)
23. Urinary bladder sonography does not include staging of bladder tumors.
24. Pregnancy Diagnosis sonography (B-Scan)
25. Fetal Age Determination (Biparietal Diameter) Sonography (B-Scan)
26. Fetal Growth Rate Sonography (B-Scan)
27. Placenta Localization Sonography (B-Scan)
28. Pregnancy Sonography, Complete (B-Scan)
29. Molar Pregnancy Diagnosis Sonography (B-Scan)
30. Ectopic Pregnancy Diagnosis sonography (B-Scan)

CCI Comprehensive Code   50 Bilateral Procedure   + CPT Add-on Code   Ø Modifier -51 Exempt Code   ● New Code   ▲ Revised Code

M Maternity   N Newborn   P Pediatric   N/P Newborn/Pediatric

31. Passive Testing (Antepartum Monitoring of Fetal Heart Rate In the Resting Fetus)

32. Intrauterine Contraceptive Device Sonography (B-Scan)

33. Pelvic Mass Diagnosis Sonography (B-Scan)

34. Amniocentesis, by Ultrasonic Guidance

35. Arterial Flow Study, Peripheral (Doppler)

36. Venous Flow Study, Peripheral (Doppler)

37. Arterial Aneurysm, Peripheral (B-Scan)

38. Radiation Therapy Planning Sonography (B-Scan)

39. Thyroid Echography (A-Mode)

40. Thyroid Sonography (B-Scan)

41. Breast Echography (A-Mode)

42. Breast Sonography (B-Scan)

43. Hepatic Sonography (B-Scan)

44. Gallbladder Sonography

45. Renal Sonography

46. Two-Dimensional Echocardiography (B-Mode)

Category II (clinical reliability and efficacy not proven)

1. B-Scan for atherosclerotic narrowing of peripheral arteries

2. Monitoring of cardiac output (Doppler)

When appropriate, new uses for ultrasound diagnostic procedures should be forwarded to the Bureau of Eligibility, Reimbursement and Coverage, HCFA, so that revisions may be made in the coverage policy when appropriate.

75945   **Intravascular ultrasound (non-coronary vessel), radiological supervision and interpretation; initial vessel**

+ **75946**   **each additional non-coronary vessel (List separately in addition to code for primary procedure)**

For placement of catheter, consult CPT codes 36215-36248. If transcatheter therapies are performed, consult CPT codes 37200-37208, 61624, and 61626. If an intravascular ultrasound is performed during a diagnostic evaluation and/or a therapeutic intervention, consult CPT codes 37250 and 37251.

Note that 75946 is an add-on code and must be used in conjunction with 75945.

75952   **Endovascular repair of infrarenal abdominal aortic aneurysm or dissection, radiological supervision and interpretation**

To report implantation of endovascular grafts, consult CPT codes 38400-38408.

75953   **Placement of proximal or distal extension prosthesis for endovascular repair of infrarenal abdominal aortic aneurysm, radiological supervision and interpretation**

To report implantation of endovascular extension prstheses, consult CPT codes 34825 and 34826.

75960   **Transcatheter introduction of intravascular stent(s), (non-coronary vessel), percutaneous and/or open, radiological supervision and interpretation, each vessel**

For procedure, consult CPT codes 37205-37208.

To report radiologic supervision and interpretation of transcatheter placement of extracranial cerebrovascular artery stent(s), consult CPT Category III code 0007T.

75961   **Transcatheter retrieval, percutaneous, of intravascular foreign body (eg, fractured venous or arterial catheter), radiological supervision and interpretation**

For procedure consult CPT code 37203.

75962   **Transluminal balloon angioplasty, peripheral artery, radiological supervision and interpretation**

For transluminal balloon angioplasty procedure, see 35450-35460 or 35470-35476.

+ **75964**   **Transluminal balloon angioplasty, each additional peripheral artery, radiological supervision and interpretation (List separately in addition to code for primary procedure)**

Note that 75964 is an add-on code and must be used in conjunction with 75962.

75966   **Transluminal balloon angioplasty, renal or other visceral artery, radiological supervision and interpretation**

For transluminal balloon angioplasty procedure see 35450-35460 or 35470-35476.

+ **75968**   **Transluminal balloon angioplasty, each additional visceral artery, radiological supervision and interpretation (List separately in addition to code for primary procedure)**

Note that 75968 is an add-on code and must be used in conjunction with 75966. If a percutaneous transluminal coronary angioplasty is performed, consult CPT codes 92982-92984.

75970   **Transcatheter biopsy, radiological supervision and interpretation**

If an injection procedure is performed for transcatheter therapy or for a biopsy, consult CPT codes 36100-36299. If a transcatheter renal and ureteral biopsy is performed, consult CPT code 52007. If a biopsy of the pancreas is performed through a percutaneous needle, consult CPT code 48102. If a biopsy of the abdominal or retroperitoneal mass is performed, consult CPT code 49180.

75978   **Transluminal balloon angioplasty, venous (eg, subclavian stenosis), radiological supervision and interpretation**

For procedures performed, consult CPT codes 35460 and 35476.

75980   **Percutaneous transhepatic biliary drainage with contrast monitoring, radiological supervision and interpretation**

For introduction procedure of percutaneous transhepatic catheter for bilary damage, consult CPT code 47510.

75982   **Percutaneous placement of drainage catheter for combined internal and external biliary drainage or of a drainage stent for internal biliary drainage in patients with an inoperable mechanical biliary obstruction, radiological supervision and interpretation**

For procedures performed, consult CPT codes 47511 or 47556.

75984   **Change of percutaneous tube or drainage catheter with contrast monitoring (eg, gastrointestinal system, genitourinary system, abscess), radiological supervision and interpretation**

For procedure performed consult CPT codes 43760, 47525, 47530, 50398, 50688, 51705, 51710.

If a nephrostomy or pyelostomy tube is changed, consult CPT code 50398. If a percutaneous nephrostolithotomy or pyelostolithotomy is performed, consult CPT codes 50080 and 50081. For percutaneous cholecystostomy, consult CPT code 47490.

For introduction procedure only for percutaneous biliary drainage, consult CPT codes 47510 and 47511. For change of percutaneous biliary drainage catheter only, consult CPT code 47525.

▲ **75989** Radiological guidance for percutaneous drainage of abscess, or specimen collection (ie, fluoroscopy, ultrasound, or computed axial tomography), with placement of indwelling catheter, radiological supervision and interpretation [80]

TRANSLUMINAL ATHERECTOMY

CIM 50-16 HEMORRHEOGRAPH
Medicare covers the use of hemorrheograph for services performed for preoperative and postoperative diagnostic evaluation of suspected peripheral artery disease.

75992 Transluminal atherectomy, peripheral artery, radiological supervision and interpretation [80] [▯]
For procedure performed, consult CPT codes 35481-35485, 35491-35495.

+ **75993** Transluminal atherectomy, each additional peripheral artery, radiological supervision and interpretation (List separately in addition to code for primary procedure) [80] [▯]
Note that 75993 is an add-on code and must be used in conjunction with 75992. If an open or a percutaneous transluminal peripheral atherectomy is performed, consult CPT codes 35481-35485 and 35491-35495.

75994 Transluminal atherectomy, renal, radiological supervision and interpretation [80] [▯]
For an open transluminal peripheral artherectomy consult CPT code 35480. For a percutaneous transluminal peripheral atherectomy, consult CPT code 35490.

75995 Transluminal atherectomy, visceral, radiological supervision and interpretation [80] [▯]

+ **75996** Transluminal atherectomy, each additional visceral artery, radiological supervision and interpretation (List separately in addition to code for primary procedure) [80] [▯]
Note that 75996 is an add-on code and must be used in conjunction with 75995.

OTHER PROCEDURES
If an arthrography is performed of shoulder, consult CPT code 73040; elbow, consult CPT code 73085; wrist, consult CPT code 73115; hip, consult CPT code 73525; knee, consult CPT code 73580; and ankle, consult CPT code 73615.

76000 Fluoroscopy (separate procedure), up to one hour physician time, other than 71023 or 71034 (eg, cardiac fluoroscopy) [80] [▯]

76001 Fluoroscopy, physician time more than one hour, assisting a non-radiologic physician (eg, nephrostolithotomy, ERCP, bronchoscopy, transbronchial biopsy) [80] [▯]

▲ **76003** Fluoroscopic guidance for needle placement (eg, biopsy, aspiration, injection, localization device) [80]
Report the appropriate surgical code for the procedure.
Fluoroscopy 76003 is all inclusive of all radiographic arthrography except for of supervision and interpretation for CT and MR arthrography.
Code 76003 in should not be used in addition to 70332, 73040, 73085, 73115, 73525, 73580, 73615.
Fluoroscopy 76003 specific radiological supervision and interpretation procedures 74320, 74350, 74355, 74445, 74470, 74475, 75809, 75810, 75885, 75887, 75980, 75982, 75989.

76005 Fluoroscopic guidance and localization of needle or catheter tip for spine or paraspinous diagnostic or therapeutic injection procedures (epidural, transforaminal epidural, subarachnoid, paravertebral facet joint, paravertebral facet joint nerve or sacroiliac joint), including neurolytic agent destruction [▯]
Note that contrast injected during fluoroscopic guidance and localization is an inclusive component of CPT codes 62270-62273, 62280-62282, and 62310-62319. Note that fluoroscopic guidance of a subarachnoid puncture for diagnostic radiographic myelography is included in supervision and interpretation codes 72240, 72255, 72265, and 72270. If an epidural subarachnoid needle or catheter is placed and an injection is made, consult CPT codes 62270-62273, 62280-62282, and 62310-62319. If arthrography is performed on the sacroiliac joint, consult CPT codes 27096 and 73542. If formal arthrography is not performed, recorded, and a formal radiographic report is not issued, consult CPT code 76005 for fluoroscopic guidance for sacroiliac joint injections. If a paravertebral facet joint is injected, consult CPT codes 64470-64476. If a transforaminal epidural needle is placed and an injection made, consult CPT codes 64479-64484. If destruction is performed by a neurolytic agent, consult CPT codes 64600-64680.

76006 Radiologic examination, stress view(s), any joint, stress applied by a physician (includes comparison views) [26] [80] [▯]

76010 Radiologic examination from nose to rectum for foreign body, single view, child [P] [80] [▯]

76012 Radiological supervision and interpretation, percutaneous vertebroplasty, per vertebral body; under fluoroscopic guidance [26] [80] [▯]

76013 under CT guidance [26] [80] [▯]
For percutaneous vertebroplasty consult CPT codes 22520, 22522.

76020 Bone age studies [80]

76040 Bone length studies (orthoroentgenogram, scanogram) [80]

76061 Radiologic examination, osseous survey; limited (eg, for metastases) [80]

76062 complete (axial and appendicular skeleton) [80] [▯]

76065 Radiologic examination, osseous survey, infant [N] [80]

▲ **76066** Joint survey, single view, one or more joints (specify) [80] [▯]

CIM 50-44 BONE (MINERAL) DENSITY STUDIES
Medicare covers the following bone (mineral) density studies

1. Single Photon Absorptiometry - A non-invasive radiological technique that provides a quantitative measurement of the bone mineral of cortical and trabecular bone, and is used in assessing an individual's treatment response at appropriate intervals. Medicare covers when used in assessing changes in bone density of patients with osteodystrophy or osteoporosis performed on the same individual at intervals of 6 to 12 months.

2. Bone Biopsy - A physiologic test used in ascertaining a differential diagnosis of bone disorders and is used primarily to differentiate osteomalacia from osteoporosis. Bone biopsy is covered under Medicare when used for the qualitative evaluation of bone no more than four times per patient, unless there is special justification given.

3. Photodensitometry (radiographic absorptiometry) - A noninvasive radiological procedure that provides a quantitative measurement of the bone mineral of cortical bone, and is used for monitoring gross bone change.

▲   **76070**   **Computerized axial tomography bone density study, one or more sites**

76075   **Dual energy x-ray absorptiometry (DEXA), bone density study, one or more sites; axial skeleton (eg, hips, pelvis, spine)**   80

76076   **appendicular skeleton (peripheral) (eg, radius, wrist, heel)**   80

▲   **76078**   **Radiographic absorptiometry (eg, photodensitometry, radiogrammetry), one or more sites**   80

76080   **Radiologic examination, abscess, fistula or sinus tract study, radiological supervision and interpretation**   80

● +   **76085**   **Digitization of film radiographic images with computer analysis for lesion detection and further physician review for interpretation, screening mammography (List separately in addition to code for primary procedure)**
     Note that 76085 is an add-on code and must be used in conjunction with 76092.

76086   **Mammary ductogram or galactogram, single duct, radiological supervision and interpretation**   80

76088   **Mammary ductogram or galactogram, multiple ducts, radiological supervision and interpretation**   80

CIM 50-21 MAMMOGRAMS

A radiological mammogram is a covered diagnostic test under the following conditions:

- A patient has distinct signs and symptoms for which a mammogram is indicated
- A patient has a history of breast cancer
- A patient is asymptomatic but, on the basis of the patient's history and other factors the physician considers significant, the physician's judgment is that a mammogram is appropriate

Use of mammograms in routine screening of (1) asymptomatic women aged 50 and over, and (2) asymptomatic women aged 40 or over whose mothers or sisters have had the disease, is considered medically appropriate, but would not be covered for Medicare purposes.

MCM 4601 SCREENING MAMMOGRAPHY AND DIAGNOSTIC MAMMOGRAPHY

The payment limitation for screening mammography no longer applies for claims with dates of service on or after January 1, 2002. Diagnostic mammography and screening mammography can both be paid when performed on the same day when provided to the same beneficiary. The Medicare payment for the service is 80 percent of the allowed charge. Coinsurance is made at 20 percent of the lower of the actual charge or the MPFS amount. For screening mammography, part B deductible is waived and co-pay applies. As with other MPFS services, the non-participation provider reduction and the limiting charge provisions apply to all mammography tests (including screening mammography).

Medicare allows additional films to be done without an additional order from the treating physician. When submitting a claim for a screening mammography and a diagnostic mammography for the same patient on the same day, attach Modifier GG to the diagnostic mammography.

CPT code 76085 has been established as an add-on code that can be billed only in conjunction with the primary service screening mammography code 76092. Payment will be made under the MPFS. HCPCS Level II code G0236 has been created as an add-on code to be billed in conjunction with a regular diagnostic mammogram (codes 76090 or 76091).

ICD-9 Code V76.12 - Diagnosis code for screening mammography

ICD-9 codes for diagnostic mammography will vary according to diagnosis.

NOTE: Plug in code V76.12 if a claim comes in for screening mammography with no ICD-9 code and the carrier file data shows this is appropriate. If there are other diagnosis codes on the claim, but not code V76.12, add it. (Do not change or overlay code V76.12 but ADD it). At a minimum, edit for age, frequency, and place of service (POS).

E. Claims with dates of service prior to January 1, 2002, are subject specific calculations

(payment limitation). The calculations do not apply to claims with dates of service on or after January 1, 2002.

- The professional portion of the screening mammography limit. The amount for 2001 is $22.15 ($21.69 in 2000, $21.19 in 1999 and $20.71 in 1998), determined by multiplying the screening mammography limit by 32 percent.

- The technical portion of the screening mammography limit. The amount for 2001 is $47.08 ($46.12 in 2000, $45.03 in 1999 and $44.02 in 1998), determined by multiplying the screening mammography limit by 68 percent.

- The limit for the procedure. The amount for 2001 is $ 69.23 ($67.81 in 2000, $66.22 in 1999 and $64.73 in 1998).

MCM 2070 DIAGNOSTIC X-RAY, DIAGNOSTIC LABORATORY, AND OTHER DIAGNOSTIC TESTS

Medicare covers diagnostic x-ray, diagnostic laboratory, and other diagnostic tests, including materials and the services of technicians. Medicare covers diagnostic X-ray services performed in a facility directed by a physician or group of physicians if they are performed under the direct supervision of a physician. Certain diagnostic X-ray procedures are also covered when performed by technicians without direct personal physician supervision if the technicians' general supervision and training, as well as the maintenance of the necessary equipment and supplies, are the continuing responsibility of a physician. Covered diagnostic tests include:

601 Histopathology

Tissue decalcification

Bone marrow biopsy

Tissue pathology

Surgical pathology

Frozen sections

Autopsy and sections

76090   **Mammography; unilateral**   80

76091   **bilateral**   80

76092   **Screening mammography, bilateral (two view film study of each breast)**   ♀
     To report computer aided detection applied to a screening mammogram, consult also CPT code 76085.

CIM 50-13 MAGNETIC RESONANCE

Medicare covers magnetic resonance imaging (MRI), formerly called nuclear magnetic resonance (NMR), when furnished using MRI units with Food and Drug Administration pre-market approval. An MRI is covered when used to detect:

- To detect and stage pelvic and retroperitoneal neoplasms
- To evaluate disorders of cancellous bone and soft tissues
- To detect pericardial thickening
- To detect and monitor early-stage primary and secondary bone neoplasm and aseptic necrosis
- To detect early states of bone infections for patients with metallic prostheses, especially of the hip, to which the prothesis is attached
- Disc disease without regard to radiological imaging

In addition:

- The inherent tissue contrast resolution of MRI makes it an appropriate standard diagnostic modality for general neuroradiology
- When a clinical need exists to visualize the parenchyma of solid organs to detect anatomic disruption or neoplasia, this can be accomplished in the liver, urogenital system, adrenals, and pelvic organs without the use of radiological contrast materials
- Gating devices that eliminate distorted images caused by cardiac and respiratory movement cycles may be covered. Surface and other

specialty coils may be covered, as they are used routinely for high-resolution imaging where small limited regions of the body are studied

MRI is not covered for patients with cardiac pacemakers or with metallic clips on vascular aneurysms. In addition, the long imaging time and the enclosed position of the patient may result in claustrophobia, making patients who have a history of claustrophobia unsuitable candidates for MRI procedures. Several uses of MRI have been identified as investigational and are not covered. These include measurement of blood flow and spectroscopy. In addition, MRI is not suitable for the imaging of cortical bone and calcifications and for procedures involving spatial resolution of bone or calcifications.

76093   **Magnetic resonance imaging, breast, without and/or with contrast material(s); unilateral** [80]

76094   **bilateral** [80] [CCI]

76095   **Stereotactic localization guidance for breast biopsy or needle placement (eg, for wire localization or for injection), each lesion, radiological supervision and interpretation** [80] [CCI]

     Report the appropriate procedure with one of the following CPT codes 10022, 19000, 19001, 19102, 19103, 19290, 19291.

     To report injection for sentinel node localization without lymphoscintigraphy, report CPT code 38792.

76096   **Mammographic guidance for needle placement, breast (eg, for wire localization or for injection), each lesion, radiological supervision and interpretation** [80]

     For reporting the procedure, consult CPT codes 10022, 19000, 19102, 19103.

     For needle localization wire placement, consult CPT codes 19290 and 19291.

     To report injection for sentinel node localization without lymphoscintigraphy, report CPT code 38792.

76098   **Radiological examination, surgical specimen** [80]

76100   **Radiologic examination, single plane body section (eg, tomography), other than with urography** [80] [CCI]

76101   **Radiologic examination, complex motion (ie, hypercycloidal) body section (eg, mastoid polytomography), other than with urography; unilateral** [80]

76102   **bilateral** [80] [CCI]

     If a nephrotomography is performed, consult CPT code 74415.

▲   **76120**   **Cineradiography/videoradiography, except where specifically included** [80]

▲ +   **76125**   **Cineradiography/videoradiography to complement routine examination (List separately in addition to code for primary procedure)** [80]

76140   **Consultation on x-ray examination made elsewhere, written report**

76150   **Xeroradiography** [TC] [80]

     Note that 76150 is to be used only for non-mammographic studies.

CIM 50-43 DIGITAL SUBTRACTION ANGIOGRAPHY

Medicare covers digital subtraction angiography (DSA) as a diagnostic imaging technique that applies computer technology to fluoroscopy for visualizing the same vascular structures observable with conventional angiography. However, reimbursement for DSA should not exceed, and may be less than, that being paid for conventional angiographic techniques.

76350   **Subtraction in conjunction with contrast studies** [TC] [80]

CIM 50-12 COMPUTERIZED TOMOGRAPHY

Diagnostic examinations of the head (head scans) and of other parts of the body (body scans) performed by computerized tomography (CT) scanners are covered if medical and scientific literature and opinion support the effective use of a scan for the condition.

There is no general rule that requires other diagnostic tests to be tried before CT scanning is used. However, in an individual case the contractor's medical staff may determine that a CT scan as the initial diagnostic test was not reasonable and necessary if not supported by the patient's symptoms or complaints stated on the claim form; e.g., "periodic headaches."

CT equipment must meet the following criteria:

1. Known to the Food and Drug Administration

2. In the full market release phase of development

Mobile CT scan services furnished at an ambulatory health care facility other than a hospital-based facility (e.g., a freestanding physician-directed clinic) must be performed under the direct personal supervision of a radiologist or other qualified physician. In addition, the facility must maintain a record of the attending physician's order. Bill the same as for scans performed on stationary equipment.

Medicare covers multiplanar diagnostic imaging (MPDI), known as planar image reconstruction or reformatted imaging, when performed by an entity offering covered CT scans.

▲   **76355**   **Computerized axial tomographic guidance for stereotactic localization** [80]

▲   **76360**   **Computerized axial tomographic guidance for needle biopsy, radiological supervision and interpretation** [80]

●   **76362**   **Computerized axial tomographic guidance for, and monitoring of, tissue ablation**

     To report percutaneous radifrequency ablation, consult CPT code 47382.

▲   **76370**   **Computerized axial tomographic guidance for placement of radiation therapy fields** [80]

▲   **76375**   **Coronal, sagittal, multiplanar, oblique, 3-dimensional and/or holographic reconstruction of computerized axial tomography, magnetic resonance imaging, or other tomographic modality** [80]

     Note that 76375 must be used in addition to the procedural code used for imaging.

▲   **76380**   **Computerized axial tomography, limited or localized follow-up study** [80]

76390   **Magnetic resonance spectroscopy** [80]

     If magnetic resonance imaging is performed, consult the appropriate MRI body site code.

76393   **Magnetic resonance guidance for needle placement (eg, for biopsy, needle aspiration, injection, or placement of localization device) radiological supervision and interpretation** [80]

     To report procedure, see appropriate organ or site.

●   **76394**   **Magnetic resonance guidance for, and monitoring of, tissue ablation**

     To report percutaneous radiofrequency ablation, consult CPT code 47382.

76400   **Magnetic resonance (eg, proton) imaging, bone marrow blood supply** [80]

●   **76490**   **Ultrasound guidance for, and monitoring of, tissue ablation**

     Code 76490 should not be used in addition to 76986.

     To report ablation, consult CPT codes 47370-47382.

76499   **Unlisted diagnostic radiologic procedure** [80]

76506 — 76800

DIAGNOSTIC ULTRASOUND
Consult the glossary for more terms and guidelines.

HEAD AND NECK
To report determination of corneal thickness with interpretation and report, bilateral, consult CPT Category III code 0025T.

CIM 50-7 ULTRASOUND DIAGNOSTIC PROCEDURES
Medicare coverage is extended to the procedures listed in Category I. Techniques in Category II are considered experimental and should not be covered at this time.

Category I (covered, may be adjunct to radiologic and nuclear medicine diagnostic technique)

1. Echoencephalography, (Diencephalic Midline) (A-Mode)

2. Echoencephalography, Complete (Diencephalic Midline and Ventricular Size)

3. Ocular and Orbital Echography (A-Mode) (includes determining the suitability of aphakic patients for an artificial lens implant following cataract surgery)

4. Ocular and Orbital Sonography (B-Mode)

5. Echocardiography, Pericardial Effusion (M-Mode)

6. Pericardiocentesis, by Ultrasonic Guidance

7. Echocardiography, Cardiac Valve(s) (M-Mode)

8. Echocardiography, Complete (M-Mode)

9. Echocardiography, limited (e.g., follow-up or limited study) (M-Mode)

10. Pleural Effusion Echography

11. Thoracentesis, by Ultrasonic Guidance

12. Abdominal Sonography, complete survey study (B-Scan)

13. Abdominal Sonography, limited (e.g., follow-up or limited study) (B-Scan)

14. Renal Cyst Aspiration, by Ultrasonic Guidance

15. Renal Biopsy, by Ultrasonic Guidance

16. Pancreas Sonography (B-Scan)

17. Spleen Sonography (B-Scan)

18. Abdominal Aorta Echography (A-Mode)

19. Abdominal Aorta Sonography (B-Scan)

20. Retroperitoneal Sonography (B-Scan)

21. Retroperitoneal sonography does not include planning of fields for radiation therapy.

22. Urinary Bladder Sonography (B-Scan)

23. Urinary bladder sonography does not include staging of bladder tumors.

24. Pregnancy Diagnosis sonography (B-Scan)

25. Fetal Age Determination (Biparietal Diameter) Sonography (B-Scan)

26. Fetal Growth Rate Sonography (B-Scan)

27. Placenta Localization Sonography (B-Scan)

28. Pregnancy Sonography, Complete (B-Scan)

29. Molar Pregnancy Diagnosis Sonography (B-Scan)

30. Ectopic Pregnancy Diagnosis sonography (B-Scan)

31. Passive Testing (Antepartum Monitoring of Fetal Heart Rate In the Resting Fetus)

32. ntrauterine Contraceptive Device Sonography (B-Scan)

33. Pelvic Mass Diagnosis Sonography (B-Scan)

34. Amniocentesis, by Ultrasonic Guidance

35. Arterial Flow Study, Peripheral (Doppler)

36. Venous Flow Study, Peripheral (Doppler)

37. Arterial Aneurysm, Peripheral (B-Scan)

38. Radiation Therapy Planning Sonography (B-Scan)

39. Thyroid Echography (A-Mode)

40. Thyroid Sonography (B-Scan)

41. Breast Echography (A-Mode)

42. Breast Sonography (B-Scan)

43. Hepatic Sonography (B-Scan)

44. Gallbladder Sonography

45. Renal Sonography

46. Two-Dimensional Echocardiography (B-Mode)

Category II (clinical reliability and efficacy not proven)

1. B-Scan for atherosclerotic narrowing of peripheral arteries

2. Monitoring of cardiac output (Doppler)

When appropriate, new uses for ultrasound diagnostic procedures should be forwarded to the Bureau of Eligibility, Reimbursement and Coverage, HCFA, so that revisions may be made in the coverage policy when appropriate.

76506   **Echoencephalography, B-scan and/or real time with image documentation (gray scale) (for determination of ventricular size, delineation of cerebral contents and detection of fluid masses or other intracranial abnormalities), including A-mode encephalography as secondary component where indicated** [80]

76511   **Ophthalmic ultrasound, echography, diagnostic; A-scan only, with amplitude quantification** [80]

76512   **contact B-scan (with or without simultaneous A-scan)** [80]

76513   **anterior segment ultrasound, immersion (water bath) B-scan or high resolution biomicroscopy** [80]

76516   **Ophthalmic biometry by ultrasound echography, A-scan;** [80]

76519   **with intraocular lens power calculation** [80]
To report partial coherence interferometry, consult CPT code 92136.

76529   **Ophthalmic ultrasonic foreign body localization** [80]

▲ **76536**   **Ultrasound, soft tissues of head and neck (eg, thyroid, parathyroid, parotid), B-scan and/or real time with image documentation** [80]

CHEST

▲ **76604**   **Ultrasound, chest, B-scan (includes mediastinum) and/or real time with image documentation** [80]

▲ **76645**   **Ultrasound, breast(s) (unilateral or bilateral), B-scan and/or real time with image documentation** [80]

ABDOMEN AND RETROPERITONEUM

▲ **76700**   **Ultrasound, abdominal, B-scan and/or real time with image documentation; complete** [80]

76705   **limited (eg, single organ, quadrant, follow-up)** [80]

▲ **76770**   **Ultrasound, retroperitoneal (eg, renal, aorta, nodes), B-scan and/or real time with image documentation; complete** [80]

76775   **limited** [80]

▲ **76778**   **Ultrasound, transplanted kidney, B-scan and/or real time with image documentation, with or without duplex Doppler study** [80]

SPINAL CANAL

▲ **76800**   **Ultrasound, spinal canal and contents** [80]

PELVIS

▲ 76805 Ultrasound, pregnant uterus, B-scan and/or real time with image documentation; complete (complete fetal and maternal evaluation)

76810 complete (complete fetal and maternal evaluation), multiple gestation, after the first trimester

76815 limited (fetal size, heart beat, placental location, fetal position, or emergency in the delivery room)

76816 follow-up or repeat

76818 Fetal biophysical profile; with non-stress testing

▲ 76819 without non-stress testing

To report fetal biophysical profile assessments for any additional fetuses, modifier -51 should be appended.

For amniotic fluid index without non-stress test, consult CPT code 76815.

76825 Echocardiography, fetal, cardiovascular system, real time with image documentation (2D) with or without M-mode recording;

76826 follow-up or repeat study

76827 Doppler echocardiography, fetal, cardiovascular system, pulsed wave and/or continuous wave with spectral display; complete

76828 follow-up or repeat study

If color mapping is performed, consult CPT code 93325.

▲ 76830 Ultrasound, transvaginal

76831 Hysterosonography, with or without color flow Doppler

If saline or contrast is introduced for a hysterosonography, consult CPT code 58340.

▲ 76856 Ultrasound, pelvic (nonobstetric), B-scan and/or real time with image documentation; complete

76857 limited or follow-up (eg, for follicles)

GENITALIA

▲ 76870 Ultrasound, scrotum and contents

76872 Echography, transrectal;

76873 prostate volume study for brachytherapy treatment planning (separate procedure)

EXTREMITIES

▲ 76880 Ultrasound, extremity, non-vascular, B-scan and/or real time with image documentation

▲ 76885 Ultrasound, infant hips, real time with imaging documentation; dynamic (requiring physician manipulation)

▲ 76886 limited, static (not requiring physician manipulation)

ULTRASONIC GUIDANCE PROCEDURES

76930 Ultrasonic guidance for pericardiocentesis, imaging supervision and interpretation

76932 Ultrasonic guidance for endomyocardial biopsy, imaging supervision and interpretation

76936 Ultrasound guided compression repair of arterial pseudo-aneurysm or arteriovenous fistulae (includes diagnostic ultrasound evaluation, compression of lesion and imaging)

76941 Ultrasonic guidance for intrauterine fetal transfusion or cordocentesis, imaging supervision and interpretation

For fetal intrauterine transfusion procedure, consult CPT code 36460. If cordocentesis is performed, consult CPT code 59012.

76942 Ultrasonic guidance for needle placement (eg, biopsy, aspiration, injection, localization device), imaging supervision and interpretation

76945 Ultrasonic guidance for chorionic villus sampling, imaging supervision and interpretation

For chorionic villus sampling, consult CPT code 59015.

76946 Ultrasonic guidance for amniocentesis, imaging supervision and interpretation

76948 Ultrasonic guidance for aspiration of ova, imaging supervision and interpretation

76950 Ultrasonic guidance for placement of radiation therapy fields

76965 Ultrasonic guidance for interstitial radioelement application

OTHER PROCEDURES

76970 Ultrasound study follow-up (specify)

76975 Gastrointestinal endoscopic ultrasound, supervision and interpretation

For upper gastrointestinal endoscopy, consult CPT code 43259.

76977 Ultrasound bone density measurement and interpretation, peripheral site(s), any method

76986 Ultrasonic guidance, intraoperative

Code 76986 should not be used in addition to 47370-47382.

For ultrasound guidance for open and laparoscopic radiofrequency tissue ablation, use 76490.

76999 Unlisted ultrasound procedure

RADIATION ONCOLOGY

CLINICAL TREATMENT PLANNING (EXTERNAL AND INTERNAL SOURCES)

The codes in this section provide for brachytherapy and teletherapy to include the initial consultation, clinical treatment planning, dosimetry, radiation physics, treatment devices and treatment management services. These codes also include follow-up care for up to three months following completion. Identify preliminary consultation and patient evaluation performed by the therapeutic radiologist by the evaluation and management code. Consult the glossary for more terms and guidelines.

77261 Therapeutic radiology treatment planning; simple

77262 intermediate

77263 complex

77280 Therapeutic radiology simulation-aided field setting; simple

77285 intermediate

77290 complex

77295 three-dimensional

77299 Unlisted procedure, therapeutic radiology clinical treatment planning

---

MEDICAL RADIATION PHYSICS, DOSIMETRY, TREATMENT DEVICES, AND SPECIAL SERVICES

▲ **77300** **Basic radiation dosimetry calculation, central axis depth dose calculation, TDF, NSD, gap calculation, off axis factor, tissue inhomogeneity factors, calculation of non-ionizing radiation surface and depth dose, as required during course of treatment, only when prescribed by the treating physician** [80] [☐]

● **77301** **Intensity modulated radiotherapy plan, including dose-volume histograms for target and critical structure partial tolerance specifications**

Dose plan is optimized using inverse or forward planning technique for modulated beam delivery (eg, binary, dynamic MLC) to create highly conformal dose distribution. Computer plan distribution must be verified for positional accuracy based on dosimetric verification of the intensity map with verification of treatment set up and interpretation of verification methodology.

77305 **Teletherapy, isodose plan (whether hand or computer calculated); simple (one or two parallel opposed unmodified ports directed to a single area of interest)** [80] [☐]

77310 **intermediate (three or more treatment ports directed to a single area of interest)** [80] [☐]

77315 **complex (mantle or inverted Y, tangential ports, the use of wedges, compensators, complex blocking, rotational beam, or special beam considerations)** [80] [☐]

Note that only one teletherapy isodose plan may be reported for a given course of therapy to a specific treatment area.

77321 **Special teletherapy port plan, particles, hemibody, total body** [80] [☐]

77326 **Brachytherapy isodose calculation; simple (calculation made from single plane, one to four sources/ribbon application, remote afterloading brachytherapy, 1 to 8 sources)** [80] [☐]

77327 **intermediate (multiplane dosage calculations, application involving five to ten sources/ribbons, remote afterloading brachytherapy, 9 to 12 sources)** [80] [☐]

77328 **complex (multiplane isodose plan, volume implant calculations, over 10 sources/ribbons used, special spatial reconstruction, remote after-loading brachytherapy, over 12 sources)** [80] [☐]

77331 **Special dosimetry (eg, TLD, microdosimetry) (specify), only when prescribed by the treating physician** [80] [☐]

77332 **Treatment devices, design and construction; simple (simple block, simple bolus)** [80] [☐]

77333 **intermediate (multiple blocks, stents, bite blocks, special bolus)** [80] [☐]

77334 **complex (irregular blocks, special shields, compensators, wedges, molds or casts)** [80] [☐]

77336 **Continuing medical physics consultation, including assessment of treatment parameters, quality assurance of dose delivery, and review of patient treatment documentation in support of the radiation oncologist, reported per week of therapy** [TC] [80] [☐]

77370 **Special medical radiation physics consultation** [TC] [80] [☐]

77399 **Unlisted procedure, medical radiation physics, dosimetry and treatment devices, and special services** [80]

RADIATION TREATMENT DELIVERY

77401 **Radiation treatment delivery, superficial and/or ortho voltage** [TC] [80] [☐]

77402 **Radiation treatment delivery, single treatment area, single port or parallel opposed ports, simple blocks or no blocks; up to 5 MeV** [TC] [80] [☐]

77403 **6-10 MeV** [TC] [80] [☐]

77404 **11-19 MeV** [TC] [80] [☐]

77406 **20 MeV or greater** [TC] [80] [☐]

77407 **Radiation treatment delivery, two separate treatment areas, three or more ports on a single treatment area, use of multiple blocks; up to 5 MeV** [TC] [80] [☐]

77408 **6-10 MeV** [TC] [80] [☐]

77409 **11-19 MeV** [TC] [80] [☐]

77411 **20 MeV or greater** [TC] [80] [☐]

77412 **Radiation treatment delivery, three or more separate treatment areas, custom blocking, tangential ports, wedges, rotational beam, compensators, special particle beam (eg, electron or neutrons); up to 5 MeV** [TC] [80] [☐]

77413 **6-10 MeV** [TC] [80] [☐]

77414 **11-19 MeV** [TC] [80] [☐]

77416 **20 MeV or greater** [TC] [80] [☐]

77417 **Therapeutic radiology port film(s)** [TC] [80] [☐]

● **77418** **Intensity modulated treatment delivery, single or multiple fields/arcs, via narrow spatially and temporally modulated beams (eg, binary, dynamic MLC), per treatment session**

To report intensity modulated treatment planning, consult CPT code 77301.

RADIATION TREATMENT MANAGEMENT

The codes in this section provide for brachytherapy and teletherapy to include the initial consultation, clinical treatment planning, dosimetry, radiation physics, treatment devices and treatment management services. These codes also include follow-up care for up to three months following completion. Identify preliminary consultation and patient evaluation performed by the therapeutic radiologist by the evaluation and management code. Consult the glossary for more terms and guidelines.

For radiation treatment management, the professional services usually furnished consist of review of patient treatment setup, port films, dosimetry, dose delivery and treatment parameters, and medical evaluation and management services.

Report radiation treatment management in units of five treatment sessions; this is not reflective of the actual time period in which the treatment are furnished. Treatment management consists of review of dosimetry, dose delivery, and treatment parameters; review of port films; review of treatment set-up; and examination of patient for medical evaluation and management.

77427 **Radiation treatment management, five treatments** [26] [☐]

77431 **Radiation therapy management with complete course of therapy consisting of one or two fractions only** [26] [80] [☐]

Note that 77431 is not to be used to fill in the last week of a long course of therapy.

77432 **Stereotactic radiation treatment management of cerebral lesion(s) (complete course of treatment consisting of one session)** [26] [80] [☐]

77470 **Special treatment procedure (eg, total body irradiation, hemibody radiation, per oral, endocavitary or intraoperative cone irradiation)** [80] [☐]

Note that 77470 assumes that this procedure is performed one or more times during the course of therapy, in addition to daily or weekly patient management.

77499 **Unlisted procedure, therapeutic radiology treatment management** [80]

PROTON BEAM TREATMENT DELIVERY

The codes in this section provide for brachytherapy and teletherapy to include the initial consultation, clinical treatment planning, dosimetry, radiation physics, treatment devices and treatment management services. These codes also include follow-up care for up to three months following completion. Identify preliminary consultation and patient evaluation performed by the therapeutic radiologist by the evaluation and management code. Consult the glossary for more terms and guidelines.

77520	**Proton treatment delivery; simple, without compensation**	TC
77522	**simple, with compensation**	TC
77523	**intermediate**	TC
77525	**complex**	TC

HYPERTHERMIA

The codes in this section provide for brachytherapy and teletherapy to include the initial consultation, clinical treatment planning, dosimetry, radiation physics, treatment devices and treatment management services. These codes also include follow-up care for up to three months following completion. Identify preliminary consultation and patient evaluation performed by the therapeutic radiologist by the evaluation and management code. Consult the glossary for more terms and guidelines.

Microwaves, ultrasound, probes, and radiofrequencies may be used in concert with radiation therapy to provide external, interstitial, and intracavitary hyperthermia. Include the management and follow-up care in the following codes; physics planning and insertion of the sources are also included.

Local hyperthermia is covered under Medicare when used in connection with radiation therapy for the treatment of primary or metastatic cutaneous or subcutaneous superficial malignancies. It is not covered when used alone or in connection with chemotherapy.

77600	**Hyperthermia, externally generated; superficial (ie, heating to a depth of 4 cm or less)**	80
77605	**deep (ie, heating to depths greater than 4 cm)**	80
77610	**Hyperthermia generated by interstitial probe(s); 5 or fewer interstitial applicators**	80
77615	**more than 5 interstitial applicators**	80

CLINICAL INTRACAVITARY HYPERTHERMIA

77620	**Hyperthermia generated by intracavitary probe(s)**	80

CLINICAL BRACHYTHERAPY

The codes in this section provide for brachytherapy and teletherapy to include the initial consultation, clinical treatment planning, dosimetry, radiation physics, treatment devices and treatment management services. These codes also include follow-up care for up to three months following completion. Identify preliminary consultation and patient evaluation performed by the therapeutic radiologist by the evaluation and management code. Consult the glossary for more terms and guidelines.

Man-made or natural radioactive elements are placed in or around the treatment field by a radiotherapist. CPT codes 77750-77799 include hospital admission and daily visits.

77750	**Infusion or instillation of radioelement solution**	80
77761	**Intracavitary radiation source application; simple**	80
77762	**intermediate**	80
77763	**complex**	80
77776	**Interstitial radiation source application; simple**	80
77777	**intermediate**	80
77778	**complex**	80

Make a separate payment for supplies furnished in connection with a procedure only when one of the two following conditions exists:

A. HCPCS codes A4550, A4200, and A4263 are billed in conjunction with the appropriate procedure in the Medicare Physician Fee Schedule Data Base (place of service is physician's office); or

B. The supply is a pharmaceutical or radiopharmaceutical diagnostic imaging agent (including codes A4641 through A4647); pharmacologic stressing agent (code J1245); or therapeutic radionuclide (CPT code 79900). The procedures performed are:

Diagnostic radiologic procedures (including diagnostic nuclear medicine) requiring pharmaceutical or radiopharmaceutical contrast media and/or pharmocological stressing agent,

Other diagnostic tests requiring a pharmacological stressing agent,

Clinical brachytherapy procedures (other than remote afterloading high intensity brachytherapy procedures (CPT codes 77781 through 77784) for which the expendable source is included in the TC RVUs), or

Therapeutic nuclear medicine procedures.

77781	**Remote afterloading high intensity brachytherapy; 1-4 source positions or catheters**	80
77782	**5-8 source positions or catheters**	80
77783	**9-12 source positions or catheters**	80
77784	**over 12 source positions or catheters**	80
77789	**Surface application of radiation source**	80
77790	**Supervision, handling, loading of radiation source**	80
77799	**Unlisted procedure, clinical brachytherapy**	80

NUCLEAR MEDICINE

In Nuclear Medicine, the procedures can be listed separately or as part of the overall medical care of the patient. The provision of radium or other radioelements is not included in CPT codes 78000-79999. These materials should be reported separately.

DIAGNOSTIC

ENDOCRINE SYSTEM

Medicare covers nuclear radiology procedures, including nuclear examinations performed with mobile radiological equipment, if reasonable and necessary for the individual patient.

78000	**Thyroid uptake; single determination**	80
78001	**multiple determinations**	80
78003	**stimulation, suppression or discharge (not including initial uptake studies)**	80
78006	**Thyroid imaging, with uptake; single determination**	80

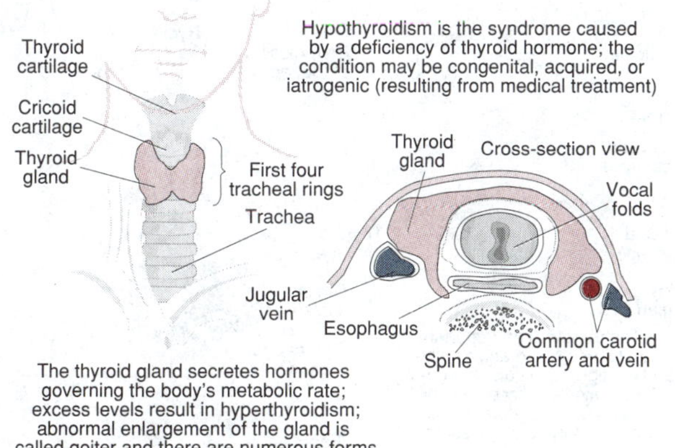

The thyroid gland secretes hormones governing the body's metabolic rate; excess levels result in hyperthyroidism; abnormal enlargement of the gland is called goiter and there are numerous forms

---

▢ CCI Comprehensive Code	50 Bilateral Procedure	✚ CPT Add-on Code	⊘ Modifier -51 Exempt Code	● New Code	▲ Revised Code
M Maternity	N Newborn	P Pediatric	N/P Newborn/Pediatric		

78007	multiple determinations	80
78010	Thyroid imaging; only	80
78011	with vascular flow	80
78015	Thyroid carcinoma metastases imaging; limited area (eg, neck and chest only)	80
78016	with additional studies (eg, urinary recovery)	80
78018	whole body	80

For total triiodothyronine T3 (TT3), consult CPT code 84480. For calcitonin, consult CPT code 82308. For free triiodothyronine T3, consult CPT code 84481. For total thyroxine, consult CPT code 84436. For thyroxine requiring elution (e.g., neonatal), consult CPT code 84437. For thyroxine, free, consult CPT code 84439.

+ **78020 Thyroid carcinoma metastases uptake (List separately in addition to code for primary procedure)** 80

Note that 78020 is an add-on code and must be used in conjunction with 78018.

78070 Parathyroid imaging 80

For parathormone (parathyroid hormone), consult CPT code 83970.

78075 Adrenal imaging, cortex and/or medulla 80

For cortisol, free or total, consult CPT code 82533. For aldosterone, consult CPT code 82088. For total ketosteroids, 17- (17-KS)17-ketosteroids, consult CPT code 83586. For insulin, total, consult CPT code 83525. For insulin antibodies, consult CPT code 86337. For proinsulin, consult CPT code 84206. For glucagon, consult CPT code 82943. For adrenocorticotropic hormone (ACTH), consult CPT code 82024. For human growth hormone (HGH), (somatotropin), consult CPT code 83003. For human growth hormone antibody, consult CPT code 86277. For thyroglobulin antibody, consult CPT code 86800. For microsomal antibodies (e.g., thyroid or liver-kidney), consult CPT code 86376. For thyrotropin releasing hormone (TRH) stimulation panel, consult CPT codes 80438 and 80439. For thyroid stimulating hormone (TSH), consult CPT code 84443. For thyroid stimulating immunoglobulins (TSI), consult CPT code 84445. For gonadotropin, follicle stimulating hormone (FSH), consult CPT code 83001. For gonadotropin, luteinizing hormone (LH), consult CPT code 83002. For luteinizing releasing factor (LRH), consult CPT code 83727. For prolactin level, consult CPT code 84146. For vasopressin level (antidiuretic hormone, ADH), consult CPT code 84588. For estradiol, consult CPT code 82670. For progesterone, consult CPT code 84144. For testosterone, total, consult CPT code 84403. For etiocholanolone, consult CPT code 82696.

78099 Unlisted endocrine procedure, diagnostic nuclear medicine 80

If a chemical analysis is needed, consult the Chemistry section of CPT.

The thyroid is an important endocrine gland and its size and configuration can vary greatly. A pyramid lobe occurs in about 40 percent of people and is a remnant of the thyroglossal duct

HEMATOPOIETIC, RETICULOENDOTHELIAL AND LYMPHATIC SYSTEM

78102	Bone marrow imaging; limited area	80
78103	multiple areas	80
78104	whole body	80
78110	Plasma volume, radiopharmaceutical volume-dilution technique (separate procedure); single sampling	80
78111	multiple samplings	80
78120	Red cell volume determination (separate procedure); single sampling	80
78121	multiple samplings	80
78122	Whole blood volume determination, including separate measurement of plasma volume and red cell volume (radiopharmaceutical volume-dilution technique)	80
78130	Red cell survival study;	80
78135	differential organ/tissue kinetics, (eg, splenic and/or hepatic sequestration)	80
78140	Labeled red cell sequestration, differential organ/tissue, (eg, splenic and/or hepatic)	80
78160	Plasma radioiron disappearance (turnover) rate	80
78162	Radioiron oral absorption	80
78170	Radioiron red cell utilization	80
78172	Chelatable iron for estimation of total body iron	80

For hemosiderin, quantitative, consult CPT code 83071. For intrinsic factor antibodies, consult CPT code 86340. For cyanocobalamin (Vitamin B-12), consult CPT code 82607. For folic acid, serum, consult CPT code 82746. For hepatitis B antigen (HBsAg) or hepatitis Be antigen (HBeAg), consult CPT codes 87340 and 87350. For hepatitis A antibody (HAAb), consult CPT codes 86708 and 86709. For hepatitis B core antibody (HBcAb), consult CPT codes 86704 and 86705. For hepatitis B surface antigen (HBsAb), consult CPT code 87340. For hepatitis B surface antibody (HBsAb), consult CPT code 86706. For hepatitis Be antigen (HBeAg), consult CPT code 87350. For hepatitis Be antibody (HBeAb), consult CPT code 86707.

| 78185 | Spleen imaging only, with or without vascular flow | 80 |

If this procedure is combined with a liver study, consult CPT codes 78215 and 78216.

78190	Kinetics, study of platelet survival, with or without differential organ/tissue localization	80
78191	Platelet survival study	80
▲ 78195	Lymphatics and lymph nodes imaging	80

If sentinel node identification is performed without scintigraphy imaging, consult CPT code 38792. If the sentinel node is excised, consult CPT codes 38500-38542.

78199 Unlisted hematopoietic, reticuloendothelial and lymphatic procedure, diagnostic nuclear medicine 80

If chemical analysis is needed, consult the Chemistry section of CPT.

GASTROINTESTINAL SYSTEM

| 78201 | Liver imaging; static only | 80 |
| 78202 | with vascular flow | 80 |

If spleen imaging is performed by itself, consult CPT code 78185.

78205	Liver imaging (SPECT)	80
78206	with vascular flow	80
78215	Liver and spleen imaging; static only	80
78216	with vascular flow	80

78220	**Liver function study with hepatobiliary agents, with serial images**	80 ☐
78223	**Hepatobiliary ductal system imaging, including gallbladder, with or without pharmacologic intervention, with or without quantitative measurement of gallbladder function**	80 ☐
78230	**Salivary gland imaging;**	80 ☐
78231	**with serial images**	80 ☐
78232	**Salivary gland function study**	80 ☐
78258	**Esophageal motility**	80 ☐
78261	**Gastric mucosa imaging**	80 ☐
78262	**Gastroesophageal reflux study**	80 ☐
78264	**Gastric emptying study**	80 ☐
78267	**Urea breath test, C-14; acquisition for analysis**	☐
78268	**analysis**	☐
78270	**Vitamin B-12 absorption study (eg, Schilling test); without intrinsic factor**	80 ☐
78271	**with intrinsic factor**	80 ☐
78272	**Vitamin B-12 absorption studies combined, with and without intrinsic factor**	80 ☐
78278	**Acute gastrointestinal blood loss imaging**	80 ☐
78282	**Gastrointestinal protein loss**	80 ☐

For gastrin, consult CPT code 82941. For intrinsic factor level, consult CPT code 83528. For carcinoembryonic antigen level (CEA), consult CPT code 82378.

▲ **78290**	**Intestine imaging (eg, ectopic gastric mucosa, Meckels localization, volvulus)**	80 ☐
78291	**Peritoneal-venous shunt patency test (eg, for LeVeen, Denver shunt)**	80 ☐

To report injection procedure, consult CPT code 49427.

78299	**Unlisted gastrointestinal procedure, diagnostic nuclear medicine**	80

If chemical analysis is needed, consult the Chemistry section of CPT.

MUSCULOSKELETAL SYSTEM

In Nuclear Medicine, the procedures can be listed separately or as part of the overall medical care of the patient. The provision of radium or other radioelements is not included in CPT codes 78000-79999. These materials should be reported separately.

This type of imaging is often performed to determine sites of neoplasm or other inflammatory conditions in the bones and joints.

78300	**Bone and/or joint imaging; limited area**	80 ☐
78305	**multiple areas**	80 ☐
78306	**whole body**	80 ☐
78315	**three phase study**	80 ☐
78320	**tomographic (SPECT)**	80 ☐

CIM 50-44 BONE (MINERAL) DENSITY STUDIES
Medicare covers the following bone (mineral) density studies

1. Single Photon Absorptiometry - A non-invasive radiological technique that provides a quantitative measurement of the bone mineral of cortical and trabecular bone, and is used in assessing an individual's treatment response at appropriate intervals. Medicare covers when used in assessing changes in bone density of patients with osteodystrophy or osteoporosis performed on the same individual at intervals of 6 to 12 months.

2. Bone Biopsy - A physiologic test used in ascertaining a differential diagnosis of bone disorders and is used primarily to differentiate osteomalacia from osteoporosis. Bone biopsy is covered under Medicare when used for the qualitative evaluation of bone no more than four times per patient, unless there is special justification given.

3. Photodensitometry (radiographic absorptiometry) - A noninvasive radiological procedure that provides a quantitative measurement of the bone mineral of cortical bone, and is used for monitoring gross bone change.

78350	**Bone density (bone mineral content) study, one or more sites; single photon asorptiometry**	80
78351	**dual photon absorptiometry, one or more sites**	

If radiographic bone density (photodensitometry) is performed, consult CPT code 76078.

78399	**Unlisted musculoskeletal procedure, diagnostic nuclear medicine**	80

CARDIOVASCULAR SYSTEM

In Nuclear Medicine, the procedures can be listed separately or as part of the overall medical care of the patient. The provision of radium or other radioelements is not included in CPT codes 78000-79999. These materials should be reported separately.

Use stress testing codes from the 93015 series when the following procedures are performed during exercise or medication-induced stress. Infusion and blood pool imaging can be performed at rest or during stress.

78414	**Determination of central c-v hemodynamics (non-imaging) (eg, ejection fraction with probe technique) with or without pharmacologic intervention or exercise, single or multiple determinations**	80 ☐
78428	**Cardiac shunt detection**	80 ☐
78445	**Non-cardiac vascular flow imaging (ie, angiography, venography)**	80 ☐
78455	**Venous thrombosis study (eg, radioactive fibrinogen)**	80 ☐
78456	**Acute venous thrombosis imaging, peptide**	☐
78457	**Venous thrombosis imaging, venogram; unilateral**	80 ☐
78458	**bilateral**	80 ☐
78459	**Myocardial imaging, positron emission tomography (PET), metabolic evaluation**	

If a myocardial perfusion study is performed, consult CPT codes 78491-78492.

78460	**Myocardial perfusion imaging; (planar) single study, at rest or stress (exercise and/or pharmacologic), with or without quantification**	80 ☐
78461	**multiple studies, (planar) at rest and/or stress (exercise and/or pharmacologic), and redistribution and/or rest injection, with or without quantification**	80 ☐
78464	**tomographic (SPECT), single study at rest or stress (exercise and/or pharmacologic), with or without quantification**	80 ☐
78465	**tomographic (SPECT), multiple studies, at rest and/or stress (exercise and/or pharmacologic) and redistribution and/or rest injection, with or without quantification**	80 ☐
78466	**Myocardial imaging, infarct avid, planar; qualitative or quantitative**	80 ☐
78468	**with ejection fraction by first pass technique**	80 ☐
78469	**tomographic SPECT with or without quantification**	80 ☐
78472	**Cardiac blood pool imaging, gated equilibrium; planar, single study at rest or stress (exercise and/or pharmacologic), wall motion study plus ejection fraction, with or without additional quantitative processing**	80 ☐

If cardiac function is assessed by a first pass technique, consult CPT code 78496.

	78473	multiple studies, wall motion study plus ejection fraction, at rest and stress (exercise and/or pharmacologic), with or without additional quantification [80]
+	78478	Myocardial perfusion study with wall motion, qualitative or quantitative study (List separately in addition to code for primary procedure) [80]

Note that 78478 is an add-on code and must be used in conjunction with 78460, 78461, 78464, and 78465.

+	78480	Myocardial perfusion study with ejection fraction (List separately in addition to code for primary procedure) [80]

Note that 78480 is an add-on code and must be used in conjunction with 78460, 78461, 78464, and 78465.

	78481	Cardiac blood pool imaging, (planar), first pass technique; single study, at rest or with stress (exercise and/or pharmacologic), wall motion study plus ejection fraction, with or without quantification [80]
	78483	multiple studies, at rest and with stress (exercise and/or pharmacologic), wall motion study plus ejection fraction, with or without quantification [80]

For digoxin, consult CPT code 80162. If a cerebral blood flow study is conducted, consult CPT code 78615.

	78491	Myocardial imaging, positron emission tomography (PET), perfusion; single study at rest or stress
	78492	multiple studies at rest and/or stress
	78494	Cardiac blood pool imaging, gated equilibrium, SPECT, at rest, wall motion study plus ejection fraction, with or without quantitative processing [80]
+	78496	Cardiac blood pool imaging, gated equilibrium, single study, at rest, with right ventricular ejection fraction by first pass technique (List separately in addition to code for primary procedure) [80]

Note that 78496 is an add-on code and must be used in conjunction with 78472.

	78499	Unlisted cardiovascular procedure, diagnostic nuclear medicine [80]

If chemical analysis is needed, consult the Chemistry section of CPT.

RESPIRATORY SYSTEM

In Nuclear Medicine, the procedures can be listed separately or as part of the overall medical care of the patient. The provision of radium or other radioelements is not included in CPT codes 78000-79999. These materials should be reported separately.

CIM 50-27 XENON SCAN

Medicare covers perfusion lung imaging with 133 xenon, unless there is evidence of abuse such as inappropriate sequence or an excessive number of procedures used in the care of patients.

	78580	Pulmonary perfusion imaging, particulate [80]
	78584	Pulmonary perfusion imaging, particulate, with ventilation; single breath [80]
	78585	rebreathing and washout, with or without single breath [80]
	78586	Pulmonary ventilation imaging, aerosol; single projection [80]
	78587	multiple projections (eg, anterior, posterior, lateral views) [80]
	78588	Pulmonary perfusion imaging, particulate, with ventilation imaging, aerosol, one or multiple projections [80]
	78591	Pulmonary ventilation imaging, gaseous, single breath, single projection [80]

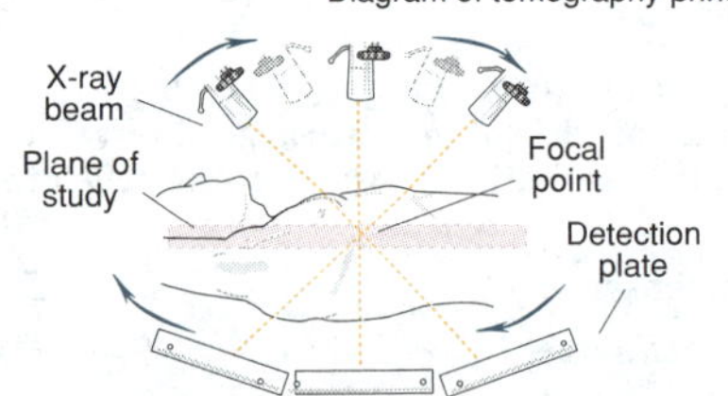

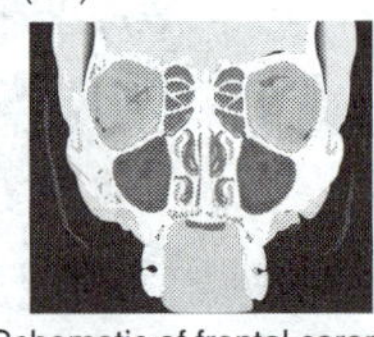

Schematic of frontal coronal CT section of skull

Tomogram is a general term for radiographic studies that focus on a single body plane, unimpeded by shadows cast by surrounding tissues and structures. The x-ray tube and the film are rotated around the patient during exposure of the focal point. Computed tomography (CT) offers a "slice" view of the study area and information is typically digitized and viewed on monitors. Magnetic resonance imaging (MRI) places a patient within the field of a powerful magnet while radio waves pass through the body; as with CT studies, views are usually of a "slice" of tissue. Ultrasound and nuclear imaging are other common radiological approaches

	78593	Pulmonary ventilation imaging, gaseous, with rebreathing and washout with or without single breath; single projection [80]
	78594	multiple projections (eg, anterior, posterior, lateral views) [80]
	78596	Pulmonary quantitative differential function (ventilation/perfusion) study [80]
	78599	Unlisted respiratory procedure, diagnostic nuclear medicine [80]

NERVOUS SYSTEM

	78600	Brain imaging, limited procedure; static [80]
	78601	with vascular flow [80]
	78605	Brain imaging, complete study; static [80]
	78606	with vascular flow [80]
	78607	tomographic (SPECT) [80]
	78608	Brain imaging, positron emission tomography (PET); metabolic evaluation
	78609	perfusion evaluation
	78610	Brain imaging, vascular flow only [80]
▲	78615	Cerebral vascular flow [80]
	78630	Cerebrospinal fluid flow, imaging (not including introduction of material); cisternography [80]

If an injection procedure is performed, consult CPT codes 61000-61070 and 62270-62319.

CIM 35-75 INTRAOPERATIVE VENTRICULAR MAPPING

The intraoperative ventricular mapping procedure is covered under Medicare only for the uses and medical conditions described:

- Localize accessory pathways associated with the Wolff-Parkinson-White (WPW) and other preexcitation syndromes

- Map the sequence of atrial and ventricular activation for drug-resistant supraventricular tachycardias

- Delineate the anatomical course of His bundle and/or bundle branches during corrective cardiac surgery for congenital heart diseases

- Direct the surgical treatment of patients with refractory ventricular tachyarrhythmias

	78635	ventriculography [80]

If an injection procedure is performed, consult CPT codes 61000-61070 and 62270-62294.

	78645	shunt evaluation [80]
	78647	tomographic (SPECT) [80]
▲	78650	Cerebrospinal fluid leakage detection and localization [80]

If an injection procedure is performed, consult CPT codes 61000-61070 and 62270-62294. For myelin basic protein, CSF, consult CPT code 83873.

78660	**Radiopharmaceutical dacryocystography**	80

78699 **Unlisted nervous system procedure, diagnostic nuclear medicine** 80

GENITOURINARY SYSTEM

78700 **Kidney imaging; static only** 80

78701 **with vascular flow** 80

78704 **with function study (ie, imaging renogram)** 80

78707 **Kidney imaging with vascular flow and function; single study without pharmacological intervention** 80

78708 **single study, with pharmacological intervention (eg, angiotensin converting enzyme inhibitor and/or diuretic** 80

78709 **multiple studies, with and without pharmacological intervention (eg, angiotensin converting enzyme inhibitor and/or diuretic)** 80

If a radioactive substance is introduced in association with renal endoscopy, consult CPT codes 50559 and 50578.

78710 **Kidney imaging, tomographic (SPECT)** 80

78715 **Kidney vascular flow only** 80

78725 **Kidney function study, non-imaging radioisotopic study** 80

For renin, consult CPT code 84244. For beta-2 microglobulin, consult CPT code 82232.

78730 **Urinary bladder residual study** 80

For radioactive substance is introduction in association with a cystotomy or a cystostomy, consult CPT code 51020. If a radioactive substance is introduced in association with a cystourethroscopy, consult CPT code 52250.

CIM 50-33 UROFLOWMETRIC EVALUATIONS

Medicare covers uroflowmetric evaluations (also referred to as urodynamic voiding or urodynamic flow studies) for diagnosing various urological dysfunctions, including bladder outlet obstructions.

78740 **Ureteral reflux study (radiopharmaceutical voiding cystogram)** 80

For catheterization, consult CPT codes 53670, 53675.

78760 **Testicular imaging;** ♂ 80

78761 **with vascular flow** ♂ 80

For total testosterone, consult CPT code 84403. For lactogen, human placental (HPL) human chorionic somatomammotropin, consult CPT code 83632. For chorionic gonadotropin, (HCG), consult CPT codes 84702 and 84703. For pregnanediol, consult CPT code 84135. For pregnanetriol, consult CPT code 84138.

78799 **Unlisted genitourinary procedure, diagnostic nuclear medicine** 80

If chemistry analysis is needed, consult the Chemistry section of CPT.

OTHER PROCEDURES

78800 **Radiopharmaceutical localization of tumor; limited area** 80

78801 **multiple areas** 80

78802 **whole body** 80

78803 **tomographic (SPECT)** 80

▲ 78805 **Radiopharmaceutical localization of inflammatory process; limited area** 80

For bone and/or joint imaging, consult CPT codes 78300, 78305, and 78306.

78806 **whole body** 80

78807 **tomographic (SPECT)** 80

For Rast, consult CPT codes 82785, 83518, 86003, and 86005. For gammaglobulin, IgE, consult CPT code 82785. For gammaglobulin, IgA, IgD, IgG, or IgM, consult CPT code 82784. For alpha-1 antitrypsin, consult CPT codes 82103 and 82014. For alpha-1 fetoprotein, consult CPT codes 82105 and 82106. For amikacin, consult CPT code 80150. For amitriptyline, consult CPT code 80152. For theophylline, consult CPT code 80198. For amphetamine or methamphetamine, consult CPT code 82145. For phenothiazine, consult CPT code 84022. For benzodiazepines, consult CPT code 80154. For cocaine or metabolite, consult CPT code 82520. For dihydromorphinone, consult CPT code 82649. For phenytoin, consult CPT code 80185. For gentamicin, consult CPT code 80170. For lactate dehydrogenase, consult CPT code 83615. For tobramycin, consult CPT code 80200.

CIM 50-36 POSITRON EMISSION TOMOGRAPHY (PET) SCANS

The following indications may be covered for PET under certain circumstances.

- Solitary Pulmonary Nodules (SPNs)
- Lung Cancer (Non Small Cell) January 1, 1998 Initial staging
- Lung Cancer (Non Small Cell) July 1, 2001 Diagnosis, staging and restaging
- Esophageal Cancer July 1, 2001 Diagnosis, staging and restaging
- Colorectal Cancer July 1, 1999 Determining location of tumors if rising
- CEA level suggests recurrence
- Colorectal Cancer July 1, 2001 Diagnosis, staging and restaging
- Lymphoma July 1, 1999 Staging and restaging only when used as an alternative to Gallium scan
- Lymphoma July 1, 2001 Diagnosis, staging and restaging
- Melanoma July 1, 1999 Evaluating recurrence prior to surgery as an alternative to a Gallium scan
- Melanoma July 1, 2001 Diagnosis, staging and restaging Head and Neck Cancers (excluding CNS and thyroid)
- July 1, 2001 Diagnosis, staging and restaging
- Myocardial Viability July 1, 2001 Covered only following inconclusive
- SPECT
- Refractory Seizures July 1, 2001 Covered for pre-surgical evaluation only
- Perfusion of the heart using Rubidium 82* tracer
- March 14, 1995 Covered for noninvasive imaging of the perfusion of the heart

In order to be covered by the Medicare program, PET scans must be performed using a camera that has either been approved or cleared for marketing by the FDA to image radionuclides in the body. For indications covered beginning July 1, 2001, scans performed with dedicated full-ring scanners will be covered.

78810 **Tumor imaging, positron emission tomography (PET), metabolic evaluation**

78890 **Generation of automated data: interactive process involving nuclear physician and/or allied health professional personnel; simple manipulations and interpretation, not to exceed 30 minutes**

78891 **complex manipulations and interpretation, exceeding 30 minutes**

Note that 78890 and 78891 must be used in addition to a primary procedure.

78990 **Provision of diagnostic radiopharmaceutical(s)**

⬘ CCI Comprehensive Code   50 Bilateral Procedure   ✚ CPT Add-on Code   ⊘ Modifier -51 Exempt Code   ● New Code   ▲ Revised Code

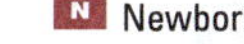 Maternity   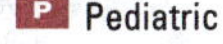 Newborn   P Pediatric   N/P Newborn/Pediatric

| 78999 | Unlisted miscellaneous procedure, diagnostic nuclear medicine 80 |

THERAPEUTIC

| 79000 | Radiopharmaceutical therapy, hyperthyroidism; initial, including evaluation of patient 80 ☑ |
| 79001 | subsequent, each therapy 80 ☑ |

If a follow-up visit is needed, consult CPT codes 99211-99215.

79020	Radiopharmaceutical therapy, thyroid suppression (euthyroid cardiac disease), including evaluation of patient 80 ☑
79030	Radiopharmaceutical ablation of gland for thyroid carcinoma 80 ☑
79035	Radiopharmaceutical therapy for metastases of thyroid carcinoma 80 ☑
79100	Radiopharmaceutical therapy, polycythemia vera, chronic leukemia, each treatment 80 ☑
79200	Intracavitary radioactive colloid therapy 80 ☑
79300	Interstitial radioactive colloid therapy 80 ☑
79400	Radiopharmaceutical therapy, nonthyroid, nonhematologic 80 ☑
79420	Intravascular radiopharmaceutical therapy, particulate 80 ☑
79440	Intra-articular radiopharmaceutical therapy 80 ☑

MCM 15030. SUPPLIES

Make a separate payment for supplies furnished in connection with a procedure only when one of the two following conditions exists:

A. HCPCS codes A4550, A4200, and A4263 are billed in conjunction with the appropriate procedure in the Medicare Physician Fee Schedule Data Base (place of service is physician's office); or

B. The supply is a pharmaceutical or radiopharmaceutical diagnostic imaging agent (including codes A4641 through A4647); pharmacologic stressing agent (code J1245); or therapeutic radionuclide (CPT code 79900). The procedures performed are:

Diagnostic radiologic procedures (including diagnostic nuclear medicine) requiring pharmaceutical or radiopharmaceutical contrast media and/or pharmocological stressing agent,

Other diagnostic tests requiring a pharmacological stressing agent,

Clinical brachytherapy procedures (other than remote afterloading high intensity brachytherapy procedures (CPT codes 77781 through 77784) for which the expendable source is included in the TC RVUs), or

Therapeutic nuclear medicine procedures.

| 79900 | Provision of therapeutic radiopharmaceutical(s) TC 80 ☑ |
| 79999 | Unlisted radiopharmaceutical therapeutic procedure 80 |

PATHOLOGY AND LABORATORY

CPT Expert **is not intended to replace the AMA's CPT manual. It does not include the AMA's official rules and guidelines, and Ingenix recommends you use this in conjunction with the AMA's 2002 CPT book.**

CODING INFORMATION

ORGANIZATION

The pathology and laboratory (80048-89399) section of CPT is divided into 14 subsections. Subsections are as follows:

Organ or Disease Oriented Panels

Drug Testing

Therapeutic Drug Assays

Evocative/Suppression Testing

Consultations (Clinical Pathology)

Urinalysis

Chemistry

Hematology and Coagulation

Immunology

Transfusion Medicine

Microbiology

Anatomic Pathology

Cytopathology

Cytogenetic Studies

Surgical Pathology

Transcutaneous Procedures

Other Procedures

GUIDELINES

Inpatient coders are not required to code pathology or laboratory tests since they are not necessary in the assignment of Diagnosis Related Groups (DRGs). However, pathology and laboratory codes are itemized on chargemasters for reporting services and supplies to patients.

Outpatient coders frequently code pathology and laboratory tests. Coding instructions include listing each laboratory procedure separately, unless it is part of a panel. Never use modifier -51 for multiple procedures in pathology or laboratory coding.

Many lab tests can be performed by different methods. To choose the correct code, carefully review code descriptions as well as any notes. When in doubt, request information from the physician or laboratory for clarification, or consult an authoritative reference.

Pathology and laboratory services are provided by the physician or by technologists under the supervision of a physician. The majority of the codes represent a technical component only, but certain codes represent a global service - a combination of professional and technical components. If the pathologist reviews a test result or renders an opinion of a test that is represented by a global code, the code selected should be identified with modifier -26 to indicate that only the professional component was provided.

SUBSECTIONS

ORGAN OR DISEASE-ORIENTED PANELS

Ten codes (80048-80090) report panels listing definitive test components: basic metabolic; general health; electrolyte; comprehensive metabolic; obstetric; hepatic function; hepatitis; lipid; toxoplasma, rubella, cytomegalovirus, herpes simplex (TORCH) antibody screen; thyroid; and thyroid with thyroid-stimulating hormone (TSH). The arthritis panel (80072) was deleted from CPT 2002 and coders are instructed to report 84550, 85651, 86255, and 86430 in place of the panel. These panels neither specify clinical parameters nor do they preclude performance of other tests. Tests performed in addition to the procedures defined in a panel can be reported separately. However, panel tests should not be reported separately on the same day as

single test codes listed as part of the panel. For example, a hepatic function panel code 80076 includes codes 82040 (albumin), 82247 (bilirubin, total), 82248 (bilirubin, direct), 84075 (phosphatase, alkaline), 84155 (protein, total), 84460 (transferase, alanine amino (ALT) (SGBT), and 84450 (transferase, aspartate amino (AST) (SGOT).

DRUG TESTING

The drug testing subsection lists codes (80100-80103) for qualitative screens that are usually confirmed by a second technique. Thirteen drugs or classes of drugs are listed as examples of commonly assayed qualitative screens: alcohols; amphetamines; barbiturates; opiates; benzodiazepines; cocaine and metabolites; methadones; methaqualones; phencyclidines; phenothiazines; propoxyphenes; tetrahydrocannabinoids; and tricyclic antidepressants.

REPORTING DRUG SCREENS

Qualitative screens should be reported when a provider is testing for the presence of a particular substance or substances. Coding for qualitative screening tests is based on procedure, not method or analyte. For example, if confirmation of five drugs requires three procedures, 80102 *Drug confirmation, each procedure* is identified three times. Drugs that have been confirmed through qualitative testing may also be quantitated. Use codes from the chemistry section (82000-84999) or therapeutic drug assay section (80150-80299) to report quantitative testing.

THERAPEUTIC DRUG ASSAYS

The therapeutic drug assays subsection (80150-80299) lists codes for quantitative assays. Several of these codes were found in the chemistry and toxicology subsection in past editions of the CPT book and reported as either qualitative or quantitative tests.

CODING FOR DRUG ASSAYS

Codes listed under therapeutic drug assays or under chemistry are used when a drug is quantitated, or measured. Screening may be used to detect a substance, but it is not a prerequisite for quantitation. For example, screening is not necessary when a known drug has been overdosed. Coding for quantitative assays is based on the substance tested. Unless the code description notes otherwise, the examination material may be from any source.

EVOCATIVE/SUPPRESSION TESTING

These procedures (80400-80440) measure the effects of administered evocative (stimulating) or suppressive agents upon the patient and represent the technical component of the service. These panels measure levels of multiple constituents or the same constituent multiple times after administering the stimulating or suppressing agent. Most of these tests are performed to evaluate specific conditions stated in the code narrative. For example, 80400 ACTH stimulation panel (adrenocorticotropic hormone) is performed for adrenal insufficiency. The physician's administration of the agent is reported separately using 90780-90799. Supplies and drugs are reported separately, (99070 or HCPCS Level II codes). To report physician attendance and monitoring during the tests, refer to the appropriate evaluation and management codes. Prolonged physician care codes may be reported separately, except when testing is performed by prolonged infusion (90780-90781).

CONSULTATION (CLINICAL PATHOLOGY)

Two consultation codes (80500 and 80502) are reserved for the pathologist to indicate a service, not a test. The pathology consultation is performed at the request of an attending physician and requires a written report. Code 80500 is a limited service without review of the patient's history and medical records. Code 80502 is a comprehensive service for a complex diagnostic problem, with review of the patient's history and medical records.

URINALYSIS

Codes 81000-81099 are used for specific analysis of one or more components of the urine. Select the appropriate code based on method (e.g., dip stick, tablet reagent, qualitative, semiquantitative) purpose (e.g., pregnancy test, timed-volume, bacteriuria screen) and specific constituents evaluated (e.g., bilirubin, glucose, pH). Not all urine analyses are listed in this section. For other tests, see appropriate section. For example, urine chloride can be found in the chemistry section.

CHEMISTRY

Chemistry codes (82000-84999) report only quantitative tests unless the description specifies otherwise, as is the case with the chromatography codes (82486-82489). Qualitative screens are reported by the four drug testing codes (80100-80103).

An individual code or a series of codes may be required for appropriate reporting. Glucose testing is an example:

82947	**Glucose; quantitative, blood (except reagent strip)**
82948	**blood, reagent strip**
82950	**post glucose dose (includes glucose)**
82951	**tolerance test (GTT), three specimens (includes glucose)**
82952	**tolerance test, each additional beyond three specimens**

Code 82951 reports a three-specimen glucose tolerance test (GTT). This code includes obtaining the fasting blood sample, supplying and administering the oral glucose dose, and obtaining the next two samples (e.g., at one-half hour and one hour). Code 82952 reports additional samples beyond the first three. Report 82951 once and 82952 twice for a three-hour GTT in which specimens are obtained at zero, one-half, one, two, and three hours.

Multiple specimens from different sources as well as specimens obtained at different times should be reported separately. For example, total bilirubin levels (82247) obtained in the morning and afternoon would be reported twice on that date of service.

MOLECULAR DIAGNOSTICS

Tests in these series (83890-83912, 87470-87799) are reported by procedure rather than analyte and should be coded separately for each procedure used in an analysis.

HEMATOLOGY AND COAGULATION

The infectious agent antibodies subsection (85002-85999) lists those laboratory procedures specific to blood and blood-forming organs, including complete blood counts (CBC), clotting factors, clotting inhibitors, prothrombin and thrombin time, platelets, and sickling.

When 85025 *Blood count; hemogram and platelet count, automated, and automated complete differential WBC count (CBC)*, is performed on the same day as a 85007 *Blood count; manual differential WBC count (includes RBC morphology and platelet estimation)*, both codes should be reported. These two tests are sometimes performed on the same date of service because a flag (abnormal value) has been identified during the automated procedure (85025), and further testing is required. A visual microscopic examination of the blood slide (85007) for immature, atypical, or clumped cells is a component of 85007, but is not included in 85025.

Codes for bone marrow aspiration, biopsy, and smear interpretation (85097-85102) are found in this subsection. However, when reporting interpretation services read procedure descriptions carefully as cell block interpretations and bone marrow biopsy interpretations should be reported with 88305.

IMMUNOLOGY

The immunology subsection (86000-86849) identifies codes for antigen and antibody studies. Detection of antibodies to infectious agents using multiple step qualitative or semiquantitative immunoassays should be reported with codes 86602-86804.

Specific tissue typing procedures are also found in the immunology subsection, see 86805-86822.

High-volume procedures include cardiolipin antibody; antigen complement; deoxyribonucleic acid antibody; hepatitis C antibody; delta agent hepatitis; heterophile antibodies; and streptococcus screening.

TRANSFUSION MEDICINE

Once listed in immunology, most blood bank codes are now grouped together under the transfusion medicine subsection (86850-86999). Since more blood bank procedures are likely to be performed on an outpatient basis, this subsection may expand in the future.

Be aware that the present codes do not report the supply of blood or blood products, and their cost may not be covered by insurance. Payers usually cover antibody screening, autologous blood or component collection, processing and storage, blood typing, and blood praeparata. Some payers require blood to be replaced (when the unit given is replaceable) instead of paid. Some payers will not cover the cost of blood components, such as albumin, plasma, or plasmanate. There may also be restrictions on procedures involving pheresis.

MICROBIOLOGY

These microbiology codes (87001-87999) identify services related to cultures, organism identification, and sensitivity studies. Many of the narratives are similar to those in the immunology section, so it is important to pay close attention to technique. Infectious agents identified by antigen detection, nucleic acid probe, or fluorescence microscopy is reported with codes 87260-87999 from microbiology. Infectious agents identified by antibody detection are reported with codes 86602-86804 from immunology. For example, cytomegalovirus (CMV) identified by infectious agent antigen detection by enzyme immunoassay technique, qualitative or semiquantitative, multiple step method is reported with 87332 from microbiology. However, CMV antibody detection by qualitative or semiquantitative immunoassay, multiple step method is reported with 86644.

ANATOMIC PATHOLOGY

Anatomic pathology (88000-88099) includes postmortem examinations (e.g., necropsy, autopsy), cytopathology (e.g., fluids, washing or brushing, Pap smears, fine needle aspirations, flow cytometry, etc.) and cytogenetic studies (e.g., tissue cultures for chromosome studies, etc.). Postmortem examination procedures report only the physician portion of the service. To report outside laboratory services, append modifier -90.

CYTOPATHOLOGY

Codes for reporting cervical and vaginal screening (Pap smears) (88141-88155, 88164-88167) have undergone considerable revision and expansion in recent years. Codes 88142-88145 report cervical or vaginal specimens collected in a preservative fluid using automated twin layer preparation. These specimens may then be examined by either Bethesda or non-Bethesda reporting systems. Codes 88150-88154 report cervical or vaginal specimens (Pap smears) prepared on slides and examined using non-Bethesda reporting systems. Codes 88164-88167 report cervical or vaginal specimens (Pap smears) prepared on slides and examined using Bethesda reporting systems. All of the above codes report manual screening and rescreening using various techniques under physician supervision. Cervical or vaginal cytopathology services requiring physician interpretation are reported separately with code 88141. Definitive hormonal evaluation is also reported separately with code 88155.

CYTOGENETIC STUDIES

Codes in this section (88230-88299) are related to the branch of genetics that studies cellular (cyto) structure and function as it relates to heredity (genetics). White blood cells, specifically T-lymphocytes, are the most commonly used specimen for chromosome analysis (88245-88289). Chromosome analysis for breakage syndromes (88245-88248) may be requested by the name of the specific syndrome being investigated, such as Fragile X, Xeroderma pigmentosum (XP), Ataxia-telangiectasia (A-T), and Fanconi anemia (FA), while 88249 reports a specific technique for the analysis of breakage syndromes involving clastogen stress. Other codes in this section include chromosome analysis for the presence of mosaicism (88263), malignant neoplasms (88264), and possible genetic abnormalities detectable within the cells of amniotic fluid (88269). Tissue and skin biopsies are reported separately using codes from the CPT surgical section. Physician interpretation and report are also reported separately, with 88291 from the cytogenetic studies section.

SURGICAL PATHOLOGY

The primary surgical pathology codes (88300-88309) describe gross and microscopic examination of specimens submitted for pathologic evaluation.

The specimen is the unit of service to report for surgical pathology. A specimen is defined as each tissue or tissues submitted for individual and separate evaluation. Each separate specimen requires individual examination and pathologic diagnosis. When two or more individual specimens are submitted from the same patient, each specimen is assigned an individual CPT code that should reflect the proper level of service.

The type of exam and the type of tissue define the level of service. CPT code 88300 should be reported for specimens requiring only gross examination. All other surgical pathology services require both gross and microscopic examination of the tissue and are defined by the type of specimen. The type of specimen included in each level is listed in the code description. For example, tissue submitted labeled "synovium knee" is examined by the pathologist and determined to be a synovial cyst. The surgical pathology code reported is 88304 because "bursa/synovial cyst" is listed under CPT code 88304.

Codes listed in 88300-88309 do not include any of the special services described by procedures 88311-88399. Procedures 88311-88399 describe additional services which should be reported separately and include the following: special stains, histochemistry, immunocytochemistry, immunofluorescent studies, electron microscopy, nerve teasing preparations, protein analysis by the western blot method, and pathology consultations during surgery.

TRANSCUTANEOUS PROCEDURES

This section (code 88400) describes the procedure to test bilirubin using a transdermal approach such as in a patch form applied to the skin.

OTHER PROCEDURES

Codes in this subsection (89050-89399) describe such procedures as crystal identification by light microscopy, duodenal intubation and aspiration, gastric intubation and aspiration, and nasal smear for eosinophils—and reproductive services such as culture and fertilization of oocytes and sperm evaluation.

LABORATORY CODING

Verify that all services performed have a signed physician order, are medically necessary and each is coded correctly, and supported by documentation in the medical record. Maintaining a current chargemaster or fee schedule is critical. Laboratories, (physician/clinic-based, hospital-based, or free-standing) must update their chargemasters and fee schedule annually and verify that the codes and descriptors match the services performed. Never report a service with a code that appears to be "close enough" to the actual service performed. If the descriptor does not match the service performed, review the CPT book to identify a more specific code. If a code cannot be identified, assign an unlisted procedure code and supply supporting documentation with the claim.

To avoid unbundling become familiar with the following subsections: Organ and Disease Oriented Panels (80048-80090), and Evocative/Suppression Testing (80400-80440). Do not report individual codes when the individual laboratory procedures are included in a panel.

ORGAN OR DISEASE ORIENTED PANELS

80048   Basic metabolic panel
This panel must include the following: Calcium (82310) Carbon dioxide (82374) Chloride (82435) Creatinine (82565) Glucose (82947) Potassium (84132) Sodium (84295) Urea Nitrogen (BUN) (84520)

80050   General health panel
This panel must include the following: Comprehensive metabolic panel (80053) Hemogram, automated, and manual differential WBC count (CBC) (85022) OR Hemogram and platelet count, automated, and automated complete differential WBC count (CBC) (85025) Thyroid stimulating hormone (TSH) (84443)

80051   Electrolyte panel
This panel must include the following: carbon dioxide (82374), chloride (82435), potassium (84132), sodium (84295)

80053   Comprehensive metabolic panel
This panel must include the following: Albumin (82040) Bilirubin, total (82247) Calcium (82310) Carbon dioxide (bicarbonate) (82374) Chloride (82435) Creatinine (82565) Glucose (82947) Phosphatase, alkaline (84075) Potassium (84132) Protein, total (84155) Sodium (84295) Transferase, alanine amino (ALT) (SGPT) (84460) Transferase, aspartate amino (AST) (SGOT) (84450) Urea Nitrogen (BUN) (84520)

Note that 80053 cannot be used in addition to CPT codes 80048 and 80076.

80055   Obstetric panel
This panel must include the following: Hemogram, automated, and manual differential WBC count (CBC) (85022) OR Hemogram and platelet count, automated, and automated complete differential WBC count (CBC) (85025) Hepatitis B surface antigen (HBsAg) (87340) Antibody, rubella (86762) Syphilis test, qualitative (eg, VDRL, RPR, ART) (86592) Antibody screen, RBC, each serum technique (86850) Blood typing, ABO (86900) AND Blood typing, Rh (D) (86901)

80061   Lipid panel
This panel must include the following: Cholesterol, serum, total (82465) Lipoprotein, direct measurement, high density cholesterol (HDL cholesterol) (83718) Triglycerides (84478)

CIM 50-17 LABORATORY TESTS - CHRONIC RENAL DISEASE (CRD) PATIENTS

The routinely covered regimen includes the following tests:

- Per Dialysis - all hematocrit or hemoglobin and clotting time tests furnished incident to dialysis treatments
- Per Week - prothrombin time for patients on anticoagulant therapy
- Serum Creatinine
- Per Week or 13 Per Quarter
- BUN

Monthly

- Complete blood count (CBC)
- Serum calcium
- Serum potassium
- Serum chloride
- Serum bicarbonate
- Serum phosphorous
- Total protein
- Serum albumin

- Alkaline phosphatase
- Aspartate aminotransferase (AST)
- Serum glutamic oxaloacetic transaminase (SGOT)
- Lactic dehydrogenase (LDH)

Guidelines for tests other than those routinely performed include:

- Serum Aluminum - one every three months
- Serum Ferritin - one every three months

Hepatitis B surface antigen (HBsAg) and Anti-HBs are covered when patients enter a dialysis facility. Coverage of future testing depends on serologic status and the effect of immunization against hepatitis B virus. Patients in the process of receiving hepatitis B vaccines should be routinely screened as susceptible. Between one and six months after the third dose, all vaccines should be tested for anti-HBs to confirm their response to the vaccine. Laboratory tests are subject to the normal coverage requirements.

80069   Renal function panel
This panel must include the following: Albumin (82040) Calcium (82310) Carbon dioxide (bicarbonate) (82374) Chloride (82435) Creatinine (82565) Glucose (82947) Phosphorus inorganic (phosphate) (84100) Potassium (84132) Sodium (84295) Urea nitrogen (BUN) (84520)

80072   Arthritis panel
This code is deleted in 2002. See codes 84550, 85651, 86255, 86430.

80074   Acute hepatitis panel
This panel must include the following: Hepatitis A antibody (HAAb), IgM antibody (86709) Hepatitis B core antibody (HbcAb), IgM antibody (86705) Hepatitis B surface antigen (HbsAg) (87340) Hepatitis C antibody (86803)

80076   Hepatic function panel
This panel must include the following: Albumin (82040) Bilirubin, total (82247) Bilirubin, direct (82248) Phosphatase, alkaline (84075) Protein, total (84155) Transferase, alanine amino (ALT) (SGPT) (84460) Transferase, aspartate amino (AST) (SGOT) (84450)

Note that 80076 cannot be used in addition to CPT code 80053.

80090   TORCH antibody panel
This panel must include the following tests: Antibody, cytomegalovirus (CMV) (86644) Antibody, herpes simplex, non-specific type test (86694) Antibody, rubella (86762) Antibody, toxoplasma (86777)

DRUG TESTING

Consult CPT codes 82000-84999 (Chemistry) or 80150-80299 (Therapeutic drug assay) for quantitation of drugs screened.

80100   Drug screen, qualitative; multiple drug classes chromatographic method, each procedure

80101   single drug class method (eg, immunoassay, enzyme assay), each drug class

80102   Drug confirmation, each procedure

80103   Tissue preparation for drug analysis

THERAPEUTIC DRUG ASSAYS

For nonquantitative testing, consult CPT codes 80100-80103

The specimen used for analysis may be from any source.

80150   Amikacin

80152   Amitriptyline

80154   Benzodiazepines

80156	Carbamazepine; total	
80157	free	
80158	Cyclosporine	
80160	Desipramine	
80162	Digoxin	
80164	Dipropylacetic acid (valproic acid)	
80166	Doxepin	
80168	Ethosuximide	
80170	Gentamicin	
80172	Gold	
80173	Haloperidol	
80174	Imipramine	
80176	Lidocaine	
80178	Lithium	
80182	Nortriptyline	
80184	Phenobarbital	
80185	Phenytoin; total	
80186	free	
80188	Primidone	
80190	Procainamide;	
80192	with metabolites (eg, n-acetyl procainamide)	◪
80194	Quinidine	
80196	Salicylate	
80197	Tacrolimus	
80198	Theophylline	
80200	Tobramycin	
80201	Topiramate	
80202	Vancomycin	
80299	Quantitation of drug, not elsewhere specified	

EVOCATIVE/SUPPRESSION TESTING

80400 ACTH stimulation panel; for adrenal insufficiency ◪
This panel must include the following: Cortisol (82533 x 2)

80402 for 21 hydroxylase deficiency ◪
This panel must include the following: Cortisol (82533 x 2) 17 hydroxyprogesterone (83498 x 2)

80406 for 3 beta-hydroxydehydrogenase deficiency ◪
This panel must include the following: Cortisol (82533 x 2) 17 hydroxypregnenolone (84143 x 2)

80408 Aldosterone suppression evaluation panel (eg, saline infusion) ◪
This panel must include the following: Aldosterone (82088 x 2) Renin (84244 x 2)

80410 Calcitonin stimulation panel (eg, calcium, pentagastrin) ◪
This panel must include the following: Calcitonin (82308 x 3)

80412 Corticotropic releasing hormone (CRH) stimulation panel ◪
This panel must include the following: Cortisol (82533 x 6) Adrenocorticotropic hormone (ACTH) (82024 x 6)

80414 Chorionic gonadotropin stimulation panel; testosterone response ◪
This panel must include the following: Testosterone (84403 x 2 on three pooled blood samples)

80415 estradiol response ◪
This panel must include the following: Estradiol (82670 x 2 on three pooled blood samples)

80416 Renal vein renin stimulation panel (eg, captopril) ◪
This panel must include the following: Renin (84244 x 6)

80417 Peripheral vein renin stimulation panel (eg, captopril) ◪
This panel must include the following: Renin (84244 x 2)

80418 Combined rapid anterior pituitary evaluation panel ◪
This panel must include the following: Adrenocorticotropic hormone (ACTH) (82024 x 4) Luteinizing hormone (LH) (83002 x 4) Follicle stimulating hormone (FSH) (83001 x 4) Prolactin (84146 x 4) Human growth hormone (HGH) (83003 x 4) Cortisol (82533 x 4) Thyroid stimulating hormone (TSH) (84443 x 4)

80420 Dexamethasone suppression panel, 48 hour ◪
This panel must include the following: Free cortisol, urine (82530 x 2) Cortisol (82533 x 2) Volume measurement for timed collection (81050 x 2) (For single dose dexamethasone, use 82533)

If a single dose of dexamethasone is given, consult CPT code 82533.

80422 Glucagon tolerance panel; for insulinoma ◪
This panel must include the following: Glucose (82947 x 3) Insulin (83525 x 3)

80424 for pheochromocytoma ◪
This panel must include the following: Catecholamines, fractionated (82384 x 2)

80426 Gonadotropin releasing hormone stimulation panel ◪
This panel must include the following: Follicle stimulating hormone (FSH) (83001 x 4) Luteinizing hormone (LH) (83002 x 4)

CIM 45-1 L-DOPA

Whether a drug represents an allowable inpatient hospital cost during such stay depends on whether it meets the definition of a drug in §1861(t) of the Act. Levodopa (L-Dopa) has been favorably evaluated for the treatment of Parkinsonism by the American Medical Association (AMA) Drug Evaluations, First Edition 1971, and the hospital stay and related ancillary services for the administration of L-Dopa are covered if medically required for this purpose. Medicare Part A also covers:

1. Testing for optimal dosage and the control of the side effects, including a complete blood count, liver function tests such as SGOT, SGPT, and/or alkaline phosphatase, BUN or creatinine and urinalysis, blood sugar, and electrocardiogram. Lab tests in are reasonable at weekly intervals although some physicians prefer to perform the tests much less frequently.

2. Evaluative services rendered by a qualified physical therapist are payable as physical therapy, services furnished by others in connection with the carrying out of the maintenance program established by the therapist are not.

3. Initiation of L-Dopa therapy carried out in the SNF setting, applying the same guidelines used for initiation of L-Dopa therapy in the hospital, including the types of patients who should be covered for inpatient services, the role of physical therapy, and the use of laboratory tests.

Part B does not cover a self-administrable drug. However, physician services rendered in connection with L-Dopa administration and control of side effects are covered if determined to be reasonable and necessary.

80428 Growth hormone stimulation panel (eg, arginine infusion, l-dopa administration) ◪
This panel must include the following: Human growth hormone (HGH) (83003 x 4)

80430 Growth hormone suppression panel (glucose administration) ◪
This panel must include the following: Glucose (82947 x 3) Human growth hormone (HGH) (83003 x 4)

◪ CCI Comprehensive Code   50 Bilateral Procedure   + CPT Add-on Code   ⊘ Modifier -51 Exempt Code   ● New Code   ▲ Revised Code

☒ CLIA Waived Test   **M** Maternity   **N** Newborn   **P** Pediatric   **N/P** Newborn/Pediatric

80432 **Insulin-induced C-peptide suppression panel**
This panel must include the following: Insulin (83525) C-peptide (84681 x 5) Glucose (82947 x 5)

80434 **Insulin tolerance panel; for ACTH insufficiency**
This panel must include the following: Cortisol (82533 x 5) Glucose (82947 x 5)

80435 **for growth hormone deficiency**
This panel must include the following: Glucose (82947 x 5) Human growth hormone (HGH) (83003 x 5)

80436 **Metyrapone panel**
This panel must include the following: Cortisol (82533 x 2) 11 deoxycortisol (82634 x 2)

80438 **Thyrotropin releasing hormone (TRH) stimulation panel; one hour**
This panel must include the following: Thyroid stimulating hormone (TSH) (84443 x 3)

80439 **two hour**
This panel must include the following: Thyroid stimulating hormone (TSH) (84443 x 4)

80440 **for hyperprolactinemia**
This panel must include the following: Prolactin (84146 x 3)

CONSULTATIONS (CLINICAL PATHOLOGY)

80500 **Clinical pathology consultation; limited, without review of patient's history and medical records**

80502 **comprehensive, for a complex diagnostic problem, with review of patient's history and medical records**
Note that 80502 may also be used for pharmacokinetic consultations. If a patient must be examined and evaluated, consult CPT codes 99241-99275.

URINALYSIS

81000 **Urinalysis, by dip stick or tablet reagent for bilirubin, glucose, hemoglobin, ketones, leukocytes, nitrite, pH, protein, specific gravity, urobilinogen, any number of these constituents; non-automated, with microscopy**

81001 **automated, with microscopy**

81002 **non-automated, without microscopy**
Mosenthal test

81003 **automated, without microscopy**

81005 **Urinalysis; qualitative or semiquantitative, except immunoassays**
If urinalysis is performed of a non-immunoassay reagent strip, consult CPT codes 81000 and 81002. For qualitative or semiquantitative immunoassay, consult CPT code 83518.
Benedict test for dextrose

81007 **bacteriuria screen, except by culture or dipstick**
For dipstick urinalysis, consult CPT codes 81000 or 81002. For urine culture, consult CPT codes 87086-87088.

81015 **microscopic only**

81020 **two or three glass test**
Valentine's test

81025 **Urine pregnancy test, by visual color comparison methods**

81050 **Volume measurement for timed collection, each**

81099 **Unlisted urinalysis procedure**

CHEMISTRY

82000 **Acetaldehyde, blood**

82003 **Acetaminophen**

82009 **Acetone or other ketone bodies, serum; qualitative**

82010 **quantitative**

82013 **Acetylcholinesterase**
For gastric acid, free and/or total, consult CPT codes 82926 and 82928. For phosphatase, acid, consult CPT codes 84060-84066.

82016 **Acylcarnitines; qualitative, each specimen**
Report quantitative carnitine (total and free) separately, consult CPT code 82379.

82017 **quantitative, each specimen**

82024 **Adrenocorticotropic hormone (ACTH)**

82030 **Adenosine, 5'-monophosphate, cyclic (cyclic AMP)**

CIM 50-17 LABORATORY TESTS - CHRONIC RENAL DISEASE (CRD) PATIENTS
The routinely covered regimen includes the following tests:

- Per Dialysis - all hematocrit or hemoglobin and clotting time tests furnished incident to dialysis treatments
- Per Week - prothrombin time for patients on anticoagulant therapy
- Serum Creatinine
- Per Week or 13 Per Quarter
- BUN

Monthly

- Complete blood count (CBC)
- Serum calcium
- Serum potassium
- Serum chloride
- Serum bicarbonate
- Serum phosphorous
- Total protein
- Serum albumin
- Alkaline phosphatase
- Aspartate aminotransferase (AST)
- Serum glutamic oxaloacetic transaminase (SGOT)
- Lactic dehydrogenase (LDH)

Guidelines for tests other than those routinely performed include:

- Serum Aluminum - one every three months
- Serum Ferritin - one every three months

Hepatitis B surface antigen (HBsAg) and Anti-HBs are covered when patients enter a dialysis facility. Coverage of future testing depends on serologic status and the effect of immunization against hepatitis B virus. Patients in the process of receiving hepatitis B vaccines should be routinely screened as susceptible. Between one and six months after the third dose, all vaccines should be tested for anti-HBs to confirm their response to the vaccine. Laboratory tests are subject to the normal coverage requirements.

82040 **Albumin; serum**

82042 **urine or other source, quantitative, each specimen**

82043 **urine, microalbumin, quantitative**

82044 **urine, microalbumin, semiquantitative (eg, reagent strip assay)**
For prealbumin, consult CPT code 84134.

82055   **Alcohol (ethanol); any specimen except breath**   ▣
For other volatiles including isopropyl alcohol and methanol, consult CPT code 84600.

82075   **breath**

82085   **Aldolase**

82088   **Aldosterone**   ▣

82101   **Alkaloids, urine, quantitative**
For phosphatase, alkaline, consult CPT codes 84075 and 84080. For quantitative or qualitative acetone or other ketone bodies, serum, consult CPT codes 82009 and 82010. For alpha tocopherol (Vitamin E), consult CPT code 84446.

82103   **Alpha-1-antitrypsin; total**

82104   **phenotype**

82105   **Alpha-fetoprotein; serum**   ▣

82106   **amniotic fluid**   **M** ♀ ▣

82108   **Aluminum**

82120   **Amines, vaginal fluid, qualitative**   ▣
If a combined pH and amines test is performed for vaginitis, use 83986 in addition to 82120.

82127   **Amino acids; single, qualitative, each specimen**

82128   **multiple, qualitative, each specimen**   ▣

82131   **single, quantitative, each specimen**
Van Slyke method

82135   **Aminolevulinic acid, delta (ALA)**

82136   **Amino acids, 2 to 5 amino acids, quantitative, each specimen**

82139   **Amino acids, 6 or more amino acids, quantitative, each specimen**

82140   **Ammonia**

82143   **Amniotic fluid scan (spectrophotometric)**   **M** ♀
For amniotic fluid L/S ratio, consult CPT code 83611. For amobarbital, consult CPT codes 80100-80103 for qualitative analysis and 82205 for quantitative analysis.

82145   **Amphetamine or methamphetamine**
Prior to obtaining a quantitative analysis for amphetamine/methamphetamine, a qualitative drug screen (80100-80101) and drug confirmation test (80102) are normally performed.

82150   **Amylase**

82154   **Androstanediol glucuronide**

82157   **Androstenedione**

82160   **Androsterone**

82163   **Angiotensin II**

82164   **Angiotensin I - converting enzyme (ACE)**
For vasopressin (antidiuretic hormone, ADH), consult CPT code 84588. For heavy metal screening (arsenic, barium, beryllium, bismuth, antimony, mercury), consult CPT code 83015. For alpha-1-antitrypsin, consult CPT codes 82103 and 82104.

82172   **Apolipoprotein, each**

82175   **Arsenic**
For heavy metal screening (arsenic, barium, beryllium, bismuth, antimony, mercury), consult CPT code 83015.

82180   **Ascorbic acid (Vitamin C), blood**
For salicylate, consult CPT code 80196.

82190   **Atomic absorption spectroscopy, each analyte**

82205   **Barbiturates, not elsewhere specified**
Prior to obtaining a quantitative analysis for amphetamine/methamphetamine, a qualitative drug screen (80100-80101) and drug confirmation test (80102) are normally performed.

82232   **Beta-2 microglobulin**
For carbon dioxide (bicarbonate), consult CPT code 82374.

82239   **Bile acids; total**

82240   **cholylglycine**
For urine bile pigments, consult CPT codes 81000-81005.

82247   **Bilirubin; total**
Van Den Bergh test

82248   **direct**

82252   **feces, qualitative**

82261   **Biotinidase, each specimen**

▲ **82270**   **Blood, occult, by peroxidase activity (eg, guaiac), qualitative; feces, 1-3 simultaneous determinations**   ▣
Day test

▲ **82273**   **other sources**   ▣
To report fecal hemoglobin detection by immunoassay, consult CPT code 86683.

For quantitative or semiquantitative urea nitrogen, consult CPT codes 84520 and 84525.

● **82274**   **Blood, occult, by fecal hemoglobin determination by immunoassay, qualitative, feces, 1-3 simultaneous determinations**

82286   **Bradykinin**

82300   **Cadmium**

82306   **Calcifediol (25-OH Vitamin D-3)**

82307   **Calciferol (Vitamin D)**
For Dihydroxyvitamin D, 1,25-consult CPT code 82652.

82308   **Calcitonin**   ▣

82310   **Calcium; total**

82330   **ionized**

82331   **after calcium infusion test**

82340   **urine quantitative, timed specimen**

▲ **82355**   **Calculus; qualitative analysis**   ▣

82360   **quantitative analysis, chemical**   ▣

82365   **infrared spectroscopy**   ▣

82370   **x-ray diffraction**   ▣
For carbamates, see individual listings.

82373   **Carbohydrate deficient transferrin**

82374   **Carbon dioxide (bicarbonate)**
Consult also CPT code 82803.

82375   **Carbon monoxide, (carboxyhemoglobin); quantitative**

82376   **qualitative**

82378   **Carcinoembryonic antigen (CEA)**

82379   **Carnitine (total and free), quantitative, each specimen**
For acylcarnitine, qualitative, consult CPT code 82016; quantitative, consult CPT code 82017.

82380   **Carotene**

82382   **Catecholamines; total urine**

82383   **blood**

82384   **fractionated**   ▣
For metanephrine, consult CPT code 83835. For vanillylmandelic acid (VMA), consult CPT code 84585.

Pathology and Laboratory

82387 — 82666

82387	**Cathepsin-D**
82390	**Ceruloplasmin**
82397	**Chemiluminescent assay**
82415	**Chloramphenicol**
82435	**Chloride; blood**
82436	**urine**
82438	**other source**

For sweat collection by iontophoresis, consult CPT code 89360.

82441 **Chlorinated hydrocarbons, screen**

For phenothiazine, consult CPT code 84022. For calciferol (Vitamin D), consult CPT code 82307.

82465 **Cholesterol, serum or whole blood, total**

For high density lipoprotein (HDL) cholesterol, consult CPT code 83718.

82480 **Cholinesterase; serum**

82482 **RBC**

82485 **Chondroitin B sulfate, quantitative**

For quantitative or qualitative chorionic gonadotropin (hCG), consult CPT codes 84702 and 84703.

82486 **Chromatography, qualitative; column (eg, gas liquid or HPLC), analyte not elsewhere specified**

82487 **paper, 1-dimensional, analyte not elsewhere specified**

82488 **paper, 2-dimensional, analyte not elsewhere specified**

82489 **thin layer, analyte not elsewhere specified**

82491 **Chromatography, quantitative, column (eg, gas liquid or HPLC); single analyte not elsewhere specified, single stationary and mobile phase**

82492 **multiple analytes, single stationary and mobile phase**

82495 **Chromium**

82507 **Citrate**

82520 **Cocaine or metabolite**

Prior to quantification, a drug screen is normally performed and is reported separately. For drug screen, consult CPT codes 80100-80103. For quantitative urine alkaloids, consult CPT code 82101. For complement, consult CPT codes 86160-86162.

82523 **Collagen cross links, any method**

82525 **Copper**

For urine porphyrins, consult CPT codes 84119 and 84120. For hydroxycorticosteroids, 17- (17-OHCS), consult CPT code 83491.

82528 **Corticosterone**

Porter-Silber test

82530 **Cortisol; free**

82533 **total**

For C-peptide, consult CPT code 84681.

82540 **Creatine**

82541 **Column chromatography/mass spectrometry (eg, GC/MS, or HPLC/MS), analyte not elsewhere specified; qualitative, single stationary and mobile phase**

82542 **quantitative, single stationary and mobile phase**

82543 **stable isotope dilution, single analyte, quantitative, single stationary and mobile phase**

82544 **stable isotope dilution, multiple analytes, quantitative, single stationary and mobile phase**

82550 **Creatine kinase (CK), (CPK); total**

82552 **isoenzymes**

82553 **MB fraction only**

82554 **isoforms**

82565 **Creatinine; blood**

82570 **other source**

82575 **clearance**

Holten test

82585 **Cryofibrinogen**

82595 **Cryoglobulin, qualitative or semi-quantitative (eg, cryocrit)**

If quantitative cryoglobulin is performed, consult CPT codes 82784, 82785.

If crystal is identified by light microscopy with or without polarizing lens analysis, any body fluid except urine, consult CPT code 89060.

82600 **Cyanide**

82607 **Cyanocobalamin (Vitamin B-12);**

82608 **unsaturated binding capacity**

For adenosine, 5-monophosphate, cyclic (cyclic AMP), consult CPT code 82030. For guanosine monophosphate (GMP), consult CPT code 83008. For cyclosporine, consult CPT code 80158.

82615 **Cystine and homocystine, urine, qualitative**

82626 **Dehydroepiandrosterone (DHEA)**

82627 **Dehydroepiandrosterone-sulfate (DHEA-S)**

For aminolevulinic acid, delta (ALA), consult CPT code 82135.

82633 **Desoxycorticosterone, 11-**

82634 **Deoxycortisol, 11-**

For a dexamethasone suppression test, consult CPT code 80420. For amylase, consult CPT code 82150.

82638 **Dibucaine number**

For volatiles (e.g., acetic anhydride, carbon tetrachloride, dichloroethane, dichloromethane, diethylether, isopropyl alcohol, methanol), consult CPT code 84600.

82646 **Dihydrocodeinone**

A drug screen (qualitative analysis) is normally performed prior to quantitative analysis. For drug screen, consult CPT codes 80100-80103.

82649 **Dihydromorphinone**

82651 **Dihydrotestosterone (DHT)**

82652 **Dihydroxyvitamin D, 1,25-**

82654 **Dimethadione**

A drug screen (qualitative analysis) is normally performed prior to quantitative analysis. For drug screen, consult CPT codes 80100-80103. For total phenytoin, consult CPT code 80185. For dipropylacetic acid, consult CPT code 80164. For catecholamines, consult CPT codes 82382-82384. For duodenal intubation and aspiration, consult CPT code 89100. For endocrine receptor assays, consult CPT codes 84233-84235.

82657 **Enzyme activity in blood cells, cultured cells, or tissue, not elsewhere specified; nonradioactive substrate, each specimen**

82658 **radioactive substrate, each specimen**

82664 **Electrophoretic technique, not elsewhere specified**

82666 **Epiandrosterone**

For catecholamines, consult CPT codes 82382-82384.

82668	Erythropoietin	
82670	Estradiol	
82671	Estrogens; fractionated	
82672	total	

For estrogen receptor assay, consult CPT code 84233.

82677	Estriol	
82679	Estrone	

For alcohol (ethanol), consult CPT codes 82055 and 82075.

82690	Ethchlorvynol	
82693	Ethylene glycol	
82696	Etiocholanolone	

For fractionation of ketosteroids, consult CPT code 83593.

82705	Fat or lipids, feces; qualitative
82710	quantitative
82715	Fat differential, feces, quantitative
82725	Fatty acids, nonesterified
82726	Very long chain fatty acids
82728	Ferritin

For fetal hemoglobin, consult CPT codes 83030, 83033, and 85460. For fetoprotein, alpha-1, consult CPT codes 82105 and 82106.

82731	Fetal fibronectin, cervicovaginal secretions, semi-quantitative
82735	Fluoride
82742	Flurazepam

A drug screen (qualitative analysis) is normally performed prior to quantitative analysis. For drug screen, consult CPT codes 80100-80103.If a foam stability test is performed, consult CPT code 83662.

82746	Folic acid; serum
82747	RBC

For gonadotropin; follicle stimulating hormone (FSH), consult CPT code 83001.

82757	Fructose, semen

For fructosamine, consult CPT code 82985. For sugars, chromatographic, TLC or paper chromatography, consult CPT code 84375.

82759	Galactokinase, RBC
82760	Galactose
82775	Galactose-1-phosphate uridyl transferase; quantitative
82776	screen
82784	Gammaglobulin; IgA, IgD, IgG, IgM, each
	Farr test
82785	IgE

For allergen specific IgE, consult CPT code 86003 and 86005.

Farr test

82787	immunoglobulin subclasses, (IgG1, 2, 3, or 4), each

Gamma-glutamyltransferase (GGT), consult CPT code 82977.

82800	Gases, blood, pH only
82803	Gases, blood, any combination of pH, pCO2, pO2, CO2, HCO3 (including calculated O2 saturation);

Note that 82803 is to be used for two or more of the following analytes: Gases, blood, any combination of pH, Carbon Dioxide, Hydrochloric acid, including calculated oxygen saturation.

82805	with O2 saturation, by direct measurement, except pulse oximetry
82810	Gases, blood, O2 saturation only, by direct measurement, except pulse oximetry

For pulse oximetry, consult CPT code 94760.

82820	Hemoglobin-oxygen affinity (pO2 for 50% hemoglobin saturation with oxygen)
82926	Gastric acid, free and total, each specimen
82928	Gastric acid, free or total; each specimen
82938	Gastrin after secretin stimulation
82941	Gastrin

For gentamicin, consult CPT code 80170. For glutamyltransferase, gamma (GGT), consult CPT code 82977. For gas liquid or HPLA chromatography, consult CPT code 82486.

82943	Glucagon
82945	Glucose, body fluid, other than blood
82946	Glucagon tolerance test
82947	Glucose; quantitative, blood (except reagent strip)
82948	blood, reagent strip
82950	post glucose dose (includes glucose)
82951	tolerance test (GTT), three specimens (includes glucose)
82952	tolerance test, each additional beyond three specimens
82953	tolbutamide tolerance test

If an insulin tolerance test is performed, consult CPT codes 80434 and 80435. If a leucine tolerance test is performed, consult CPT code 80428. For semiquantitative urine glucose, consult CPT codes 81000, 81002, 81005, and 81099.

82955	Glucose-6-phosphate dehydrogenase (G6PD); quantitative
82960	screen

If a glucose tolerance test is performed with medication, consult CPT code 90784 in addition to 82960.

82962	Glucose, blood by glucose monitoring device(s) cleared by the FDA specifically for home use
82963	Glucosidase, beta
82965	Glutamate dehydrogenase
82975	Glutamine (glutamic acid amide)
82977	Glutamyltransferase, gamma (GGT)
82978	Glutathione
82979	Glutathione reductase, RBC
82980	Glutethimide

For glycohemoglobin, consult CPT code 83036.

82985	Glycated protein

For chorionic gonadotropin, consult CPT codes 84702 and 84703.

83001	Gonadotropin; follicle stimulating hormone (FSH)
83002	luteinizing hormone (LH)

For luteinizing releasing factor (LRH), consult CPT code 83727.

83003	Growth hormone, human (HGH) (somatotropin)

For antibody to human growth hormone, consult CPT code 86277.

83008	Guanosine monophosphate (GMP), cyclic
83010	Haptoglobin; quantitative
83012	phenotypes

▲ **83013** **Helicobacter pylori; analysis for urease activity, non-radioactive isotope**
For *H. pylori*, stool, consult CPT code 87338. For *H. pylori*, liquid scintillation counter, consult CPT codes 78267, 78268. For *H. pylori*, enzyme immunoassay, consult CPT code 87339.

83014 **drug administration and sample collection**

83015 **Heavy metal (arsenic, barium, beryllium, bismuth, antimony, mercury); screen**
Reinsch test

83018 **quantitative, each**

83020 **Hemoglobin fractionation and quantitation; electrophoresis (eg, A2, S, C, and/or F)**

83021 **chromatography (eg, A2, S, C, and/or F)**

83026 **Hemoglobin; by copper sulfate method, non-automated**

83030 **F(fetal), chemical**

83033 **F (fetal), qualitative**

83036 **glycated**
For fecal hemoglobin detection by immunoassay, consult CPT code 82274.

83045 **methemoglobin, qualitative**

83050 **methemoglobin, quantitative**

83051 **plasma**

83055 **sulfhemoglobin, qualitative**

83060 **sulfhemoglobin, quantitative**

83065 **thermolabile**

83068 **unstable, screen**

83069 **urine**

83070 **Hemosiderin; qualitative**

83071 **quantitative**
A drug screen (qualitative analysis) is normally performed prior to quantitative analysis. For drug screen, consult CPT codes 80100-80103. For hydroxyindoleacetic acid, 5-(HIAA), consult CPT code 83497. For high performance liquid chromatography HPLC, consult CPT code 82486.

83080 **b-Hexosaminidase, each assay**

83088 **Histamine**
If a hollander test is performed, consult CPT code 91052.

83090 **Homocystine**

83150 **Homovanillic acid (HVA)**
If a hydrogen breath test is performed, consult CPT code 91065.

83491 **Hydroxycorticosteroids, 17- (17-OHCS)**
For cortisol, consult CPT code 82530. For 11-deoxycortisol, consult CPT code 82634.

83497 **Hydroxyindolacetic acid, 5-(HIAA)**
If a urine qualitative test is performed, consult CPT code 81005. For 5-Hydroxytryptamine, consult CPT code 84260.

83498 **Hydroxyprogesterone, 17-d**

83499 **Hydroxyprogesterone, 20-**

83500 **Hydroxyproline; free**

83505 **total**

83516 **Immunoassay for analyte other than infectious agent antibody or infectious agent antigen, qualitative or semiquantitative; multiple step method**

83518 **single step method (eg, reagent strip)**

83519 **Immunoassay, analyte, quantitative; by radiopharmaceutical technique (eg, RIA)**

83520 **not otherwise specified**
For qualitative or semi-quantitative immunoassay excluding infectious agent antibody or infectious agent antigen, multiple step method, consult CPT code 83516; single step method, consult CPT code 83518. For quantitative immunoassay by radiopharmaceutical immunoassay or radioimmunoassay (RIA), consult CPT code 83519. For immunoassay for infectious agent antibody, qualitative or semi-quantitative, single step method (e.g., reagent strip), consult CPT code 86318. For immunoassays for infectious agent antibody, qualitative or semi-quantitative multiple step method, consult CPT codes 86602-86804. For infectious agent antigen detection by enzyme immunoassay, qualitative or semi-quantitative, consult CPT codes 87301-87899. For immunoassay for tumor antigen, consult CPT code 86316. For immunoassay for infectious agent antibody not elsewhere specified, quantitative, consult CPT code 86317.

83525 **Insulin; total**
For proinsulin, consult CPT code 84206.

83527 **free**

83528 **Intrinsic factor**
For intrinsic factor antibodies, consult CPT code 86340.

83540 **Iron**

83550 **Iron binding capacity**

83570 **Isocitric dehydrogenase (IDH)**
For isopropyl alcohol, consult CPT code 84600.

83582 **Ketogenic steroids, fractionation**
For ketone bodies for serum, consult CPT codes 82009 and 82010. For ketone bodies for urine, consult CPT codes 81000-81003.

83586 **Ketosteroids, 17- (17-KS); total**

83593 **fractionation**

83605 **Lactate (lactic acid)**

83615 **Lactate dehydrogenase (LD), (LDH);**

83625 **isoenzymes, separation and quantitation**

83632 **Lactogen, human placental (HPL) human chorionic somatomammotropin**

83633 **Lactose, urine; qualitative**

83634 **quantitative**
For tolerance, consult CPT codes 82951 and 82952. If a breath hydrogen test is performed for lactase deficiency, consult CPT code 91065.

83655 **Lead**

83661 **Fetal lung maturity assessment; lecithin sphingomyelin (L/S) ratio**

83662 **foam stability test**

83663 **fluorescence polarization**

83664 **lamellar body density**
For phosphatidylglycerol, consult CPT code 84081.

83670 **Leucine aminopeptidase (LAP)**

83690 **Lipase**

83715 **Lipoprotein, blood; electrophoretic separation and quantitation**

83716 **high resolution fractionation and quantitation of lipoprotein cholesterols (eg, electrophoresis, nuclear magnetic resonance, ultracentrifugation)**

83718	**Lipoprotein, direct measurement; high density cholesterol (HDL cholesterol)**
83719	**direct measurement VLDL cholesterol**
83721	**direct measurement LDL cholesterol**

If fractionation is performed by nuclear magnetic resonance or high-resolution electrophoresis, consult CPT code 83716.

For direct measurement, intermediate density lipoproteins (remnant lipoproteins), consult CPT Category III code 0026T.

For luteinizing hormone (LH), consult CPT code 83002.

83727 **Luteinizing releasing factor (LRH)**

If qualitative analysis is performed, consult CPT codes 80100-80103. For macroglobulins, alpha-2, consult CPT code 86329.

83735 **Magnesium**

83775 **Malate dehydrogenase**

For maltose tolerance, consult CPT codes 82951 and 82952. For mammotropin, consult CPT code 84146.

83785 **Manganese**

A drug screen (qualitative analysis) is normally performed prior to quantitative analysis. For drug screen, consult CPT codes 80100-80103.

83788 **Mass spectrometry and tandem mass spectrometry (MS, MS/MS), analyte not elsewhere specified; qualitative, each specimen**

83789 **quantitative, each specimen**

83805 **Meprobamate**

A drug screen (qualitative analysis) is normally performed prior to quantitative analysis. For drug screen, consult CPT codes 80100-80103.

83825 **Mercury, quantitative**

For mercury screen, consult CPT code 83015.

83835 **Metanephrines**

For catecholamines, consult CPT codes 82382-82384.

83840 **Methadone**

A drug screen (qualitative analysis) is normally performed prior to quantitative analysis. For drug screen, consult CPT codes 80100-80103 and 82145. For methanol, consult CPT code 84600.

83857 **Methemalbumin**

For methemoglobin, see hemoglobin CPT codes 83045 and 83050.

83858 **Methsuximide**

For methyl alcohol, consult CPT code 84600. For microalbumin, quantitative, consult CPT code 82043; semiquantitative, consult CPT code 82044. For microglobulin, beta-2, consult CPT code 82232.

83864 **Mucopolysaccharides, acid; quantitative**

83866 **screen**

83872 **Mucin, synovial fluid (Ropes test)**

83873 **Myelin basic protein, cerebrospinal fluid**

For oligoclonal bands, consult CPT code 83916.

83874 **Myoglobin**

83883 **Nephelometry, each analyte not elsewhere specified**

83885 **Nickel**

83887 **Nicotine**

83890 **Molecular diagnostics; molecular isolation or extraction**

For microbial identification, consult CPT codes 87797 and 87798.

83891 **isolation or extraction of highly purified nucleic acid**

83892 **enzymatic digestion**

83893 **dot/slot blot production**

83894 **separation by gel electrophoresis (eg, agarose, polyacrylamide)**

83896 **nucleic acid probe, each**

83897 **nucleic acid transfer (eg, Southern, Northern)**

83898 **amplification of patient nucleic acid (eg, PCR, LCR), single primer pair, each primer pair**

83901 **amplification of patient nucleic acid, multiplex, each multiplex reaction**

83902 **reverse transcription**

83903 **mutation scanning, by physical properties (eg, single strand conformational polymorphisms (SSCP), heteroduplex, denaturing gradient gel electrophoresis (DGGE), RNA'ase A), single segment, each**

83904 **mutation identification by sequencing, single segment, each segment**

83905 **mutation identification by allele specific transcription, single segment, each segment**

83906 **mutation identification by allele specific translation, single segment, each segment**

83912 **interpretation and report**

83915 **Nucleotidase 5-**

83916 **Oligoclonal immune (oligoclonal bands)**

83918 **Organic acids; total, quantitative, each specimen**

83919 **qualitative, each specimen**

83921 **Organic acid, single, quantitative**

83925 **Opiates, (eg, morphine, meperidine)**

83930 **Osmolality; blood**

83935 **urine**

83937 **Osteocalcin (bone g1a protein)**

83945 **Oxalate**

● 83950 **Oncoprotein, HER-2/neu**

To report tissues, see 88342, 88365.

83970 **Parathormone (parathyroid hormone)**

83986 **pH, body fluid, except blood**

For blood pH, consult CPT codes 82800 and 82803.

83992 **Phencyclidine (PCP)**

A drug screen (qualitative analysis) is normally performed prior to quantitative analysis. For drug screen, consult CPT codes 80100-80103. For phenobarbital, consult CPT code 80184.

84022 **Phenothiazine**

A drug screen (qualitative analysis) is normally performed prior to quantitative analysis. For drug screen, consult CPT codes 80100-80101.

84030 **Phenylalanine (PKU), blood**

For phenylalanine-tyrosine ratio, consult CPT codes 84030 and 84510.

Guthrie test

84035 **Phenylketones, qualitative**

84060 **Phosphatase, acid; total**

84061 **forensic examination**

84066 **prostatic**

84075	Phosphatase, alkaline;	
84078	heat stable (total not included)	
84080	isoenzymes	⬚
84081	Phosphatidylglycerol	

For inorganic phosphates, consult CPT code 84100. For organic phosphates, see code for specific method. For cholinesterase, consult CPT codes 82480 and 82482.

84085	Phosphogluconate, 6-, dehydrogenase, RBC	
84087	Phosphohexose isomerase	
84100	Phosphorus inorganic (phosphate);	
84105	urine	

For pituitary gonadotropins, consult CPT codes 83001-83002. For PKU, consult CPT codes 84030 and 84035.

84106	Porphobilinogen, urine; qualitative	
84110	quantitative	
84119	Porphyrins, urine; qualitative	
84120	quantitation and fractionation	
84126	Porphyrins, feces; quantitative	
84127	qualitative	

For porphyrin precursors, consult CPT codes 82135, 84106, and 84110. For protoporphyrin, RBC, consult CPT codes 84202 and 84203.

84132	Potassium; serum	
84133	urine	
84134	Prealbumin	

For microalbumin, consult CPT codes 82043 and 82044.

84135	Pregnanediol	♀
84138	Pregnanetriol	♀
84140	Pregnenolone	♀
84143	17-hydroxypregnenolone	♀
84144	Progesterone	

For progesterone receptor assay, consult CPT code 84234. For proinsulin, consult CPT code 84206.

84146	Prolactin	⬚
84150	Prostaglandin, each	
84152	Prostate specific antigen (PSA); complexed (direct measurement)	♂
84153	Prostate specific antigen (PSA); total	♂
84154	free	♂
84155	Protein; total, except refractometry	
84160	refractometric	
84165	electrophoretic fractionation and quantitation	⬚

CIM 50-52 SEROLOGIC TESTING FOR ACQUIRED IMMUNODEFICIENCY SYNDROME (AIDS)

Medicare covers serologic testing for acquired immunodeficiency syndrome (AIDS) when performed to help determine a diagnosis for symptomatic patients. They are not covered when furnished as part of a screening program for asymptomatic persons. Antibodies may be detected by a variety of immunoassay techniques, the most common is the enzyme linked immunosorbent assay (ELISA). When an assay is reactive on initial testing, it should be repeated on the same specimen. A more specific test, (Western blot, immunofluorescent assay) is usually performed following repeatedly reactive ELISA results. Two ELISA tests conducted on the same specimen must both be positive before Medicare will cover the Western blot test.

84181	Western Blot, with interpretation and report, blood or other body fluid	⬚

84182	Western Blot, with interpretation and report, blood or other body fluid, immunological probe for band identification, each	⬚

If a Western Blot tissue analysis is performed, consult CPT code 88371.

84202	Protoporphyrin, RBC; quantitative	
84203	screen	
84206	Proinsulin	

For pseudocholinesterase, consult CPT code 82480.

84207	Pyridoxal phosphate (Vitamin B-6)	
84210	Pyruvate	
84220	Pyruvate kinase	
84228	Quinine	
84233	Receptor assay; estrogen	⬚
84234	progesterone	♀ ♂
84235	endocrine, other than estrogen or progesterone (specify hormone)	⬚
84238	non-endocrine (eg, acetylcholine) (specify receptor)	⬚
84244	Renin	⬚
84252	Riboflavin (Vitamin B-2)	

For salicylates, consult CPT code 80196. If a secretin test is performed, consult CPT code 99070 and 89100 and appropriate analyses.

84255	Selenium	
84260	Serotonin	

For urine metabolites (HIAA), consult CPT code 83497.

84270	Sex hormone binding globulin (SHBG)	
84275	Sialic acid	

For sickle hemoglobin, consult CPT code 85660.

84285	Silica	
84295	Sodium; serum	
84300	urine	

For somatomammotropin, consult CPT code 83632. For somatotropin, consult CPT code 83003

84305	Somatomedin	
84307	Somatostatin	
84311	Spectrophotometry, analyte not elsewhere specified	
84315	Specific gravity (except urine)	

For specific gravity, urine, consult CPT codes 81000-81003. If stone analysis is performed, consult CPT codes 82355-82370.

84375	Sugars, chromatographic, TLC or paper chromatography	
84376	Sugars (mono-, di-, and oligosaccharides); single qualitative, each specimen	
84377	multiple qualitative, each specimen	⬚
84378	single quantitative, each specimen	⬚
84379	multiple quantitative, each specimen	⬚
84392	Sulfate, urine	

For T-3, consult CPT codes 84479-84481. For T-4, consult CPT codes 84435-84439. For sulfhemoglobin, see hemoglobin CPT codes 83055 and 83060.

84402	Testosterone; free	
84403	total	⬚
84425	Thiamine (Vitamin B-1)	
84430	Thiocyanate	

84432	**Thyroglobulin**

Thyroglobulin, antibody, see 86800. If a thyrotropin releasing hormone (TRH) test is performed, consult CPT codes 80438 and 80439.

84436 **Thyroxine; total**

84437 **requiring elution (eg, neonatal)**

84439 **free**

84442 **Thyroxine binding globulin (TBG)**

84443 **Thyroid stimulating hormone (TSH)**

▲ 84445 **Thyroid stimulating immune globulins (TSI)**

For tobramycin, consult CPT code 80200.

84446 **Tocopherol alpha (Vitamin E)**

For tolbutamide tolerance, consult CPT code 82953.

84449 **Transcortin (cortisol binding globulin)**

84450 **Transferase; aspartate amino (AST) (SGOT)**

84460 **alanine amino (ALT) (SGPT)**

84466 **Transferrin**

For iron binding capacity, consult CPT code 83550.

84478 **Triglycerides**

84479 **Thyroid hormone (T3 or T4) uptake or thyroid hormone binding ratio (THBR)**

84480 **Triiodothyronine T3; total (TT-3)**

84481 **free**

84482 **reverse**

84484 **Troponin, quantitative**

For Troponin, qualitative assay, consult CPT code 84512.

84485 **Trypsin; duodenal fluid**

84488 **feces, qualitative**

84490 **feces, quantitative, 24-hour collection**

84510 **Tyrosine**

For urate crystal identification, consult CPT code 89060.

84512 **Troponin, qualitative**

For Troponin, quantitative assay, consult CPT code 84484.

84520 **Urea nitrogen; quantitative**

84525 **semiquantitative (eg, reagent strip test)**

Patterson's test

84540 **Urea nitrogen, urine**

84545 **Urea nitrogen, clearance**

84550 **Uric acid; blood**

84560 **other source**

84577 **Urobilinogen, feces, quantitative**

84578 **Urobilinogen, urine; qualitative**

84580 **quantitative, timed specimen**

84583 **semiquantitative**

For uroporphyrins, consult CPT Code 84120. For dipropylacetic acid (valproic acid), consult CPT code 80164.

84585 **Vanillylmandelic acid (VMA), urine**

84586 **Vasoactive intestinal peptide (VIP)**

84588 **Vasopressin (antidiuretic hormone, ADH)**

84590 **Vitamin A**

For thiamine (Vitamin B-1), consult CPT code 84425. For Riboflavin (Vitamin B-2), consult CPT code 84252. For pyridoxal phosphate (Vitamin B-6), consult CPT code 84207. For cyanocobalamin (Vitamin B-12), consult CPT code 82607. If a Vitamin B-12 absorption study is performed, (e.g., Schilling test), consult CPT codes 78270 and 78271. For ascorbic acid (Vitamin C), consult CPT code 82180. For Vitamin D, consult CPT codes 82306, 82307, and 82652. For tocopherol alpha (Vitamin E), consult CPT code 84446.

84591 **Vitamin, not otherwise specified**

84597 **Vitamin K**

For vanillylmandelic acid (VMA), consult CPT code 84585.

84600 **Volatiles (eg, acetic anhydride, carbon tetrachloride, dichloroethane, dichloromethane, diethylether, isopropyl alcohol, methanol)**

For acetaldehyde, consult CPT code 8200. For plasma volume, radiopharmaceutical volume-dilution technique, consult CPT codes 78110 and 78111.

84620 **Xylose absorption test, blood and/or urine**

Administration of d-xylose is reported separately, consult CPT code 99070.

84630 **Zinc**

84681 **C-peptide**

84702 **Gonadotropin, chorionic (hCG); quantitative**

If a urine pregnancy test is conducted by visual color comparison, consult CPT code 81025.

84703 **qualitative**

84830 **Ovulation tests, by visual color comparison methods for human luteinizing hormone** ♀

84999 **Unlisted chemistry procedure**

HEMATOLOGY AND COAGULATION

85002 **Bleeding time**

For agglutinins, see the Immunology section of CPT For antiplasmin, consult CPT code 85410. For antithrombin III, consult CPT codes 85300 and 85301.

For blood banking procedures, see the Transfusion Medicine section of CPT.

85007 **Blood count; manual differential WBC count (includes RBC morphology and platelet estimation)**

For blood banking procedures, see the Transfusion Medicine section of CPT.

85008 **manual blood smear examination without differential parameters**

Consult also CPT code 85585. For other fluids (e.g., CSF), consult CPT codes 89050 and 89051.

85009 **differential WBC count, buffy coat**

For blood banking procedures, see the Transfusion Medicine section of CPT.

For eosinophils, nasal smear, consult CPT code 89190.

85013 **spun microhematocrit**

For blood banking procedures, see the Transfusion Medicine section of CPT.

85014 **other than spun hematocrit**

85018 **hemoglobin**

For other hemoglobin determination, consult CPT codes 83020-83069.

For fecal hemoglobin detection by immunoassay, consult CPT code 86683.

85021   **hemogram, automated (RBC, WBC, Hgb, Hct and indices only)**
For blood banking procedures, see the Transfusion Medicine section of CPT.

85022   **hemogram, automated, and manual differential WBC count (CBC)**

85023   **hemogram and platelet count, automated, and manual differential WBC count (CBC)**

85024   **hemogram and platelet count, automated, and automated partial differential WBC count (CBC)**

85025   **hemogram and platelet count, automated, and automated complete differential WBC count (CBC)**

85027   **hemogram and platelet count, automated**

85031   **Blood count; hemogram, manual, complete CBC (RBC, WBC, Hgb, Hct, differential and indices)**

85041   **red blood cell (RBC) only**
Consult also CPT codes 85021-85031 and 89050.

85044   **reticulocyte count, manual**
For blood banking procedures, see the Transfusion Medicine section of CPT.

85045   **reticulocyte count, flow cytometry**

85046   **reticulocytes, hemoglobin concentration**

85048   **white blood cell (WBC)**
Consult also CPT codes 85021-85031.

85060   **Blood smear, peripheral, interpretation by physician with written report**
For blood banking procedures, see the Transfusion Medicine section of CPT.

85095   ~~**Bone marrow; aspiration only**~~ This code is deleted in 2002. See code 38220.

▲ **85097**   **Bone marrow, smear interpretation**
For special stains, consult CPT codes 85540, 88312, and 88313.

85102   ~~**Bone marrow biopsy, needle or trocar**~~ This code is deleted in 2002. See code 38221.
For blood banking procedures, see the Transfusion Medicine section of CPT.

If a bone biopsy is performed, consult CPT codes 20220, 20225, 20240, 20245, 20250, and 20251.

85130   **Chromogenic substrate assay**
For blood banking procedures, see the Transfusion Medicine section of CPT.

For circulating anti-coagulant screen (mixing studies), consult CPT codes 85611 and 85732.

85170   **Clot retraction**
For blood banking procedures, see the Transfusion Medicine section of CPT.

85175   **Clot lysis time, whole blood dilution**
For clotting factor I (fibrinogen), consult CPT codes 85384 and 85385.

85210   **Clotting; factor II, prothrombin, specific**
Consult also CPT codes 85610-85613.

For blood banking procedures, see the Transfusion Medicine section of CPT.

85220   **factor V (AcG or proaccelerin), labile factor**
For blood banking procedures, see the Transfusion Medicine section of CPT.

85230   **factor VII (proconvertin, stable factor)**

85240   **factor VIII (AHG), one stage**

85244   **factor VIII related antigen**

85245   **factor VIII, VW factor, ristocetin cofactor**

85246   **factor VIII, VW factor antigen**

85247   **factor VIII, von Willebrand factor, multimetric analysis**

85250   **factor IX (PTC or Christmas)**

85260   **factor X (Stuart-Prower)**

85270   **factor XI (PTA)**

85280   **factor XII (Hageman)**

85290   **factor XIII (fibrin stabilizing)**

85291   **factor XIII (fibrin stabilizing), screen solubility**

85292   **prekallikrein assay (Fletcher factor assay)**

85293   **high molecular weight kininogen assay (Fitzgerald factor assay)**

85300   **Clotting inhibitors or anticoagulants; antithrombin III, activity**

85301   **antithrombin III, antigen assay**

85302   **protein C, antigen**

85303   **protein C, activity**

85305   **protein S, total**

85306   **protein S, free**

85307   **Activated Protein C (APC) resistance assay**

85335   **Factor inhibitor test**
For blood banking procedures, see the Transfusion Medicine section of CPT.

85337   **Thrombomodulin**
For mixing studies for inhibitors, consult CPT code 85732.

85345   **Coagulation time; Lee and White**
For blood banking procedures, see the Transfusion Medicine section of CPT.

85347   **activated**

85348   **other methods**
For a differential count, consult CPT codes 85007 et seq. For duke bleeding time, consult CPT code 85002. For eosinophils, nasal smear, consult CPT code 89190.

85360   **Euglobulin lysis**
For blood banking procedures, see the Transfusion Medicine section of CPT.

For fetal hemoglobin, consult CPT codes 83030, 83033, and 85460.

85362   **Fibrin(ogen) degradation (split) products (FDP)(FSP); agglutination slide, semiquantitative**
For blood banking procedures, see the Transfusion Medicine section of CPT.

For immunoelectrophoresis, consult CPT code 86320.

85366   **paracoagulation**
For blood banking procedures, see the Transfusion Medicine section of CPT.

85370   **quantitative**

85378	**Fibrin degradation products, D-dimer; semiquantitative**	⊡
85379	**quantitative**	⊡
85384	**Fibrinogen; activity**	⊡
85385	**antigen**	⊡
85390	**Fibrinolysins or coagulopathy screen, interpretation and report**	⊡
85400	**Fibrinolytic factors and inhibitors; plasmin**	⊡
85410	**alpha-2 antiplasmin**	⊡
85415	**plasminogen activator**	⊡
85420	**plasminogen, except antigenic assay**	⊡
85421	**plasminogen, antigenic assay**	⊡

85421 — For fragility, red blood cell, consult CPT codes 85547 and 85555-85557.

85441 Heinz bodies; direct ⊡

For blood banking procedures, see the Transfusion Medicine section of CPT.

85445 induced, acetyl phenylhydrazine ⊡

For hematocrit (PCV), consult CPT codes 85014 and 85021-85031. For hemoglobin, consult CPT codes 83020-83068 and 85018-85031.

85460 Hemoglobin or RBCs, fetal, for fetomaternal hemorrhage; differential lysis (Kleihauer-Betke) M ♀ ⊡

Consult also CPT codes 83030 and 83033. For hemogram, consult CPT codes 85021-85031. For hemolysins, consult CPT codes 86940 and 86941.

For blood banking procedures, see the Transfusion Medicine section of CPT.

85461 rosette M ♀ ⊡

85475 Hemolysin, acid ⊡

Consult also CPT codes 86940 and 86941.

Ham test

85520 Heparin assay ⊡

For blood banking procedures, see the Transfusion Medicine section of CPT.

85525 Heparin neutralization ⊡

85530 Heparin-protamine tolerance test ⊡

~~85535 Iron stain (RBC or bone marrow smears)~~ This code is deleted in 2002. See code 85536.

85536 Iron stain, peripheral blood

For iron stains on bone marrow or other tissues with physician evaluation, consult CPT code 88313.

85540 Leukocyte alkaline phosphatase with count ⊡

For blood banking procedures, see the Transfusion Medicine section of CPT.

85547 Mechanical fragility, RBC ⊡

85549 Muramidase ⊡

For nitroblue tetrazolium dye test, consult CPT code 86384.

85555 Osmotic fragility, RBC; unincubated ⊡

For blood banking procedures, see the Transfusion Medicine section of CPT.

85557 incubated ⊡

For packed cell volume, consult CPT code 85013. For partial thromboplastin time, consult CPT codes 85730 and 85732. For parasites, blood (e.g., malaria smears), consult CPT code 87207. For plasmin, consult CPT code 85400. For plasminogen, consult CPT code 85420. For plasminogen factor, consult CPT code 85415.

85576 Platelet; aggregation (in vitro), each agent ⊡

For blood banking procedures, see the Transfusion Medicine section of CPT.

85585 estimation on smear, only

Consult also CPT code 85008.

85590 manual count ⊡

For blood banking procedures, see the Transfusion Medicine section of CPT.

85595 automated count

85597 Platelet neutralization ⊡

85610 Prothrombin time; ☒ ⊡

85611 substitution, plasma fractions, each ⊡

85612 Russell viper venom time (includes venom); undiluted ⊡

85613 diluted ⊡

For red blood cell count, consult CPT codes 85021, 85031, and 85041.

85635 Reptilase test ⊡

For blood banking procedures, see the Transfusion Medicine section of CPT.

For reticulocyte count, consult CPT codes 85044 and 85045.

85651 Sedimentation rate, erythrocyte; non-automated ☒

For blood banking procedures, see the Transfusion Medicine section of CPT.

85652 automated ⊡

Westergren test

85660 Sickling of RBC, reduction ⊡

If hemoglobin electrophoresis is performed, consult CPT code 83020. For smears (e.g., for parasites, malaria), consult CPT code 87207.

85670 Thrombin time; plasma ⊡

For blood banking procedures, see the Transfusion Medicine section of CPT.

85675 titer ⊡

85705 Thromboplastin inhibition; tissue ⊡

For individual clotting factors, consult CPT codes 85245-85247.

85730 Thromboplastin time, partial (PTT); plasma or whole blood ⊡

For blood banking procedures, see the Transfusion Medicine section of CPT.

Hicks-Pitney test

85732 substitution, plasma fractions, each ⊡

85810 Viscosity

For Von Willebrand factor assay, consult CPT codes 85245-85247. For a white blood cell (WBC) count, consult CPT codes 85021-85031, 85048, and 89050.

85999 Unlisted hematology and coagulation procedure

For blood banking procedures, see the Transfusion Medicine section of CPT.

IMMUNOLOGY

Acetylcholine receptor antibody, consult CPT codes 86255, 86256.

Actinomyces to antibodies, consult CPT code 86602.

Adrenal cortex antibodies, consult CPT codes 86255, 86256.

To report tuberculosis test, cell mediated immunity measurement of gamma interferon antigen response, consult CPT Category III code 0010T.

86000 **Agglutinins, febrile (eg, Brucella, Francisella, Murine typhus, Q fever, Rocky Mountain spotted fever, scrub typhus), each antigen**

86001 **Allergen specific IgG quantitative or semiquantitative, each allergen**

For agglutinins and autohemolysins, consult CPT codes 86940 and 86941.

86003 **Allergen specific IgE; quantitative or semiquantitative, each allergen**

For total quantitative IgE, consult CPT code 82785.

86005 **qualitative, multiallergen screen (dipstick, paddle or disk)**

For total qualitative IgE, consult CPT code 83518. For alpha-1 antitrypsin, consult CPT codes 82103 and 82104. For alpha-1 feto-protein, consult CPT codes 82105 and 82106. For anti-AChR (acetylcholine receptor) antibody titer, consult CPT codes 86255 and 86256. For anticardiolipin antibody, consult CPT code 86147. For anti-DNA, consult CPT code 86225. For anti-deoxyribonuclease titer, consult CPT code 86215.

86021 **Antibody identification; leukocyte antibodies** ▣

86022 **platelet antibodies** ▣

86023 **platelet associated immunoglobulin assay** ▣

86038 **Antinuclear antibodies (ANA);** ▣

86039 **titer** ▣

For antistreptococcal antibody (e.g., anti-DNase), consult CPT code 86215. For antistreptokinase titer, consult CPT code 86590.

86060 **Antistreptolysin 0; titer** ▣

For antibodies to infectious agents, consult CPT codes 86602-86804.

86063 **screen**

For antibodies to infectious agents, consult CPT codes 86602-86804. For antibodies to Blastomyces, consult CPT code 86612.

86077 **Blood bank physician services; difficult cross match and/or evaluation of irregular antibody(s), interpretation and written report** 80

86078 **investigation of transfusion reaction including suspicion of transmissible disease, interpretation and written report** 80

86079 **authorization for deviation from standard blood banking procedures (eg, use of outdated blood, transfusion of Rh incompatible units), with written report** 80

For antibodies to candida, consult CPT code 86628. For skin testing, consult CPT code 86485. For antibodies to brucella, consult CPT code 86622.

86140 **C-reactive protein;**

For candidiasis, consult CPT code 86628.

● **86141** **high sensitivity (hsCRP)**

● **86146** **Beta 2 Glycoprotein I antibody, each**

▲ **86147** **Cardiolipin (phospholipid) antibody, each Ig class**

86148 **Anti-phosphatidylserine (phospholipid) antibody**

86155 **Chemotaxis assay, specify method**

For antibodies to coccidioides, consult CPT code 86635. For skin testing, consult CPT code 86490.

For clostridium difficile toxin, consult CPT code 87230.

86156 **Cold agglutinin; screen**

86157 **titer** ▣

86160 **Complement; antigen, each component**

86161 **functional activity, each component**

86162 **total hemolytic (CH50)**

86171 **Complement fixation tests, each antigen**

If a Coombs test is performed, consult CPT codes 86880-86886.

86185 **Counterimmunoelectrophoresis, each antigen** ▣

For antibodies to cryptococcus, consult CPT code 86641.

86215 **Deoxyribonuclease, antibody** ▣

86225 **Deoxyribonucleic acid (DNA) antibody; native or double stranded** ▣

For antibodies to echinococcus, consult the appropriate code according to the specific method used. If an HIV antibody test is performed, consult CPT codes 86701-86703.

86226 **single stranded** ▣

For fluorescent noninfectious agent antibody, consult CPT codes 86255 and 86256.

86235 **Extractable nuclear antigen, antibody to, any method (eg, nRNP, SS-A, SS-B, Sm, RNP, Sc170, J01), each antibody** ▣

86243 **Fc receptor**

For antibodies to filaria, consult the appropriate code according to the specific method used.

86255 **Fluorescent noninfectious agent antibody; screen, each antibody** ▣

86256 **titer, each antibody** ▣

For fluorescent technique for antigen identification in tissue, consult CPT code 88346; for indirect fluorescence, consult CPT code 88347. If a confirmatory test is performed for treponema pallidum, (e.g., FTA), consult CPT code 86781. For gel (agar) diffusion tests, consult CPT code 86331.

86277 **Growth hormone, human (HGH), antibody**

86280 **Hemagglutination inhibition test (HAI)**

For rubella, consult CPT code 86762. For antibodies to infectious agents, consult CPT codes 86602-86804. For hepatitis delta agent, antibody, consult CPT code 86692.

86294 **Immunoassay for tumor antigen, qualitative or semiquantitative (eg, bladder tumor antigen)** ☒

86300 **Immunoassay for tumor antigen, quantitative; CA 15-3 (27.29)**

86301 **CA 19-9**

86304 **CA 125**

For measurement of serum HER-2/neu oncoprotein, consult CPT code 83950.

86308 **Heterophile antibodies; screening** ☒

For antibodies to infectious agents, consult CPT codes 86602-86804.

86309 **titer**

86310	**titers after absorption with beef cells and guinea pig kidney**

For antibodies to histoplasma, consult CPT code 86698. For skin testing, consult CPT code 86510. For antibodies to infectious agents, consult CPT codes 86602-86804. For human growth hormone antibody, consult CPT code 86277.

86316	**Immunoassay for tumor antigen; other antigen, quantitative (eg, CA 50, 72-4, 549), each**

86317	**Immunoassay for infectious agent antibody, quantitative, not otherwise specified**

For immunoassay techniques for antigens, consult CPT codes 83516, 83518, 83519, 83520, 87301-87450, and 87810-87899. For particle agglutination procedures, consult CPT code 86403.

86318	**Immunoassay for infectious agent antibody, qualitative or semiquantitative, single step method (eg, reagent strip)**

86320	**Immunoelectrophoresis; serum**
▲ 86325	**other fluids (eg, urine, cerebrospinal fluid) with concentration**
86327	**crossed (2-dimensional assay)**
86329	**Immunodiffusion; not elsewhere specified**
86331	**gel diffusion, qualitative (Ouchterlony), each antigen or antibody**
86332	**Immune complex assay**
86334	**Immunofixation electrophoresis**
● 86336	**Inhibin A**
86337	**Insulin antibodies**
86340	**Intrinsic factor antibodies**

For antibodies to leptospira, antibodies to, consult CPT code 86720. For leukoagglutinins, consult CPT code 86021.

86341	**Islet cell antibody**
86343	**Leukocyte histamine release test (LHR)**
86344	**Leukocyte phagocytosis**
86353	**Lymphocyte transformation, mitogen (phytomitogen) or antigen induced blastogenesis**

For lymphocytes immunophenotyping, consult CPT code 88180 for cytometry and consult CPT codes 88342 and 88346 for microscopic techniques. For malaria antibodies, consult CPT code 86750.

86359	**T cells; total count**
86360	**absolute CD4 and CD8 count, including ratio**
86361	**absolute CD4 count**
86376	**Microsomal antibodies (eg, thyroid or liver-kidney), each**
86378	**Migration inhibitory factor test (MIF)**

For mitochondrial antibody, liver, consult CPT codes 86255 and 86256. For mononucleosis, consult CPT codes 86308-86310.

86382	**Neutralization test, viral**
86384	**Nitroblue tetrazolium dye test (NTD)**

For Ouchterlony diffusion, consult CPT code 86331. For platelet antibodies, consult CPT codes 86022 and 86023.

86403	**Particle agglutination; screen, each antibody**
86406	**titer, each antibody**

If a pregnancy test is conducted, consult CPT codes 84702 and 84703. If a rapid plasma reagin test (RPR) is conducted, consult CPT codes 86592 and 86593.

86430	**Rheumatoid factor; qualitative**
86431	**quantitative**

If a serologic test is performed to test for syphilis, consult CPT codes 86592 and 86593.

86485	**Skin test; candida**

For antibody, candida, consult CPT code 86628.

86490	**coccidioidomycosis**
86510	**histoplasmosis**

For histoplasma, antibody, consult CPT code 86698.

86580	**tuberculosis, intradermal**

Heaf test

86585	**tuberculosis, tine test**

To report tuberculosis test, cell mediated immunity measurement of gamma interferon antigen response, consult CPT Category III code 0010T.

If allergy tests are conducted on the skin, consult CPT codes 95010-95199. For smooth muscle antibody, consult CPT codes 86255 and 86256. For antibodies to sporothrix, consult the appropriate code according to the specific method used.

Mantoux test

86586	**unlisted antigen, each**
86590	**Streptokinase, antibody**

For antibodies to infectious agents, consult CPT codes 86602-86804. For streptolysin O antibody, see antistreptolysin O codes 86060 and 86063.

86592	**Syphilis test; qualitative (eg, VDRL, RPR, ART)**

For antibodies to infectious agents, consult CPT codes 86602-86804.

Wasserman test

86593	**quantitative**

For antibodies to infectious agents, consult CPT codes 86602-8680

86602	**Antibody; actinomyces**

For infectious agent/antigen detection, consult CPT codes 87620-87899.

86603	**adenovirus**
86606	**Aspergillus**
86609	**bacterium, not elsewhere specified**
86611	**Bartonella**
86612	**Blastomyces**

For infectious agent/antigen detection, consult CPT codes 87620-87899.

86615	**Bordetella**
86617	**Borrelia burgdorferi (Lyme disease) confirmatory test (eg, Western blot or immunoblot)**
86618	**Borrelia burgdorferi (Lyme disease)**
86619	**Borrelia (relapsing fever)**
86622	**Brucella**
86625	**Campylobacter**
86628	**Candida**

If a candida test is performed on the skin, consult CPT code 86485.

86631	**Chlamydia**

For infectious agent/antigen detection, consult CPT codes 87620-87899.

86632	**Chlamydia, IgM**

For chlamydia antigen, consult CPT codes 87270 and 87320. For fluorescent antibody technique, consult CPT codes 86255 and 86256.

86635	**Coccidioides**	

For infectious agent/antigen detection, consult CPT codes 87620-87899.

86638	**Coxiella Brunetii (Q fever)**
86641	**Cryptococcus**
86644	**cytomegalovirus (CMV)**

For TORCH panel, consult CPT code 80090.

86645	**cytomegalovirus (CMV), IgM**

For infectious agent/antigen detection, consult CPT codes 87620-87899.

86648	**Diphtheria**
86651	**encephalitis, California (La Crosse)**
86652	**encephalitis, Eastern equine**
86653	**encephalitis, St. Louis**
86654	**encephalitis, Western equine**
86658	**enterovirus (eg, coxsackie, echo, polio)**

For antibodies to trichinella, consult CPT code 86784. For antibodies to trypanosoma, consult the code appropriate for the specific method used. If skin testing is performed for tuberculosis, consult CPT code 86580. For viral antibodies, consult the code appropriate for the specific method used.

86663	**Epstein-Barr (EB) virus, early antigen (EA)**

For infectious agent/antigen detection, consult CPT codes 87620-87899.

86664	**Epstein-Barr (EB) virus, nuclear antigen (EBNA)**
86665	**Epstein-Barr (EB) virus, viral capsid (VCA)**
86666	**Ehrlichia**
86668	**Francisella Tularensis**

For infectious agent/antigen detection, consult CPT codes 87620-87899.

86671	**fungus, not elsewhere specified**
86674	**Giardia Lamblia**
86677	**Helicobacter Pylori**
86682	**helminth, not elsewhere specified**
~~86683~~	~~Antibody; hemoglobin, fecal~~ This code is deleted in 2002. See code 82274.
86684	**Hemophilus influenza**

For infectious agent/antigen detection, consult CPT codes 87620-87899.

86687	**HTLV I**
86688	**HTLV-II**

CIM 50-52 SEROLOGIC TESTING FOR ACQUIRED IMMUNODEFICIENCY SYNDROME (AIDS)

Medicare covers serologic testing for acquired immunodeficiency syndrome (AIDS) when performed to help determine a diagnosis for symptomatic patients. They are not covered when furnished as part of a screening program for asymptomatic persons. Antibodies may be detected by a variety of immunoassay techniques, the most common is the enzyme linked immunosorbent assay (ELISA). When an assay is reactive on initial testing, it should be repeated on the same specimen. A more specific test, (Western blot, immunofluorescent assay) is usually performed following repeatedly reactive ELISA results. Two ELISA tests conducted on the same specimen must both be positive before Medicare will cover the Western blot test.

86689	**HTLV or HIV antibody, confirmatory test (eg, Western Blot)**
86692	**hepatitis, delta agent**

For hepatitis delta agent, antigen, consult CPT code 87380.

86694	**herpes simplex, non-specific type test**

For infectious agent/antigen detection, consult CPT codes 87620-87899.

For TORCH panel, consult CPT code 80090.

86695	**herpes simplex, type I**

For infectious agent/antigen detection, consult CPT codes 87620-87899.

86696	**herpes simplex, type 2**
86698	**histoplasma**

For infectious agent/antigen detection, consult CPT codes 87620-87899.

86701	**HIV-1**
86702	**HIV-2**
86703	**HIV-1 and HIV-2, single assay**

For HIV-1 antigen, consult CPT code 87390. For HIV-2 antigen, consult CPT code 87391. If a confirmatory test is conducted for the HIV antibody, (e.g., Western Blot), consult CPT code 86689.

86704	**Hepatitis B core antibody (HBcAb); total**

For infectious agent/antigen detection, consult CPT codes 87620-87899.

86705	**IgM antibody**
86706	**Hepatitis B surface antibody (HBsAb)**
86707	**Hepatitis Be antibody (HBeAb)**
86708	**Hepatitis A antibody (HAAb); total**
86709	**IgM antibody**
86710	**Antibody; influenza virus**
86713	**Legionella**
86717	**Leishmania**
86720	**Leptospira**
86723	**Listeria monocytogenes**
86727	**lymphocytic choriomeningitis**
86729	**Lymphogranuloma Venereum**
86732	**mucormycosis**
86735	**mumps**
86738	**Mycoplasma**
86741	**Neisseria meningitidis**
86744	**Nocardia**
86747	**parvovirus**
86750	**Plasmodium (malaria)**
86753	**protozoa, not elsewhere specified**
86756	**respiratory syncytial virus**
86757	**Rickettsia**
86759	**rotavirus**

For infectious agent/antigen detection, consult CPT codes 87620-87899.

86762	**rubella**
86765	**rubeola**
86768	**Salmonella**
86771	**Shigella**
86774	**tetanus**
86777	**Toxoplasma**
86778	**Toxoplasma, IgM**
86781	**Treponema Pallidum, confirmatory test (eg, FTA-abs)**
86784	**trichinella**

86787		varicella-zoster
86790		virus, not elsewhere specified
86793		Yersinia
86800		**Thyroglobulin antibody**

For thyroglobulin, consult CPT code 84432.

86803		**Hepatitis C antibody;**

For infectious agent/antigen detection, consult CPT codes 87620-87899.

86804		confirmatory test (eg, immunoblot)

TISSUE TYPING

86805	**Lymphocytotoxicity assay, visual crossmatch; with titration**
86806	without titration
86807	**Serum screening for cytotoxic percent reactive antibody (PRA); standard method**
86808	quick method
86812	HLA typing; A, B, or C (eg, A10, B7, B27), single antigen
86813	A, B, or C, multiple antigens
86816	DR/DQ, single antigen
86817	DR/DQ, multiple antigens

CIM 50-45 LYMPHOCYTE MITOGEN RESPONSE ASSAYS

Medicare covers lymphocyte mitogen response assay when it is medically necessary to assess lymphocytic function in diagnosed immunodeficiency diseases and to monitor immunotherapy.

It is not covered when it is used to monitor the treatment of cancer, because its use for that purpose is experimental.

86821	lymphocyte culture, mixed (MLC)
86822	lymphocyte culture, primed (PLC)
86849	**Unlisted immunology procedure**

TRANSFUSION MEDICINE

For apheresis, consult CPT code 36520. For therapeutic phlebotomy, consult CPT code 99195.

86850	**Antibody screen, RBC, each serum technique**
86860	**Antibody elution (RBC), each elution**
86870	**Antibody identification, RBC antibodies, each panel for each serum technique**
86880	**Antihuman globulin test (Coombs test); direct, each antiserum**
86885	indirect, qualitative, each antiserum
86886	indirect, titer, each antiserum

CIM 35-30 BLOOD PLATELET TRANSFUSIONS

Blood platelet transplants, which been shown as safe and effective in correcting thrombocytopenia and other blood defects, are covered under Medicare.

86890	**Autologous blood or component, collection processing and storage; predeposited**
86891	intra- or postoperative salvage

For physician services to autologous donors, consult CPT codes 99201-99204.

86900	**Blood typing; ABO**
86901	Rh (D)
86903	antigen screening for compatible blood unit using reagent serum, per unit screened
86904	antigen screening for compatible unit using patient serum, per unit screened
86905	RBC antigens, other than ABO or Rh (D), each

86906	Rh phenotyping, complete
86910	**Blood typing, for paternity testing, per individual; ABO, Rh and MN**
86911	each additional antigen system
86915	**Bone marrow or peripheral stem cell harvest, modification or treatment to eliminate cell type(s) (eg, T-cells, metastatic carcinoma)**
86920	**Compatibility test each unit; immediate spin technique**
86921	incubation technique
86922	antiglobulin technique
86927	**Fresh frozen plasma, thawing, each unit**
86930	**Frozen blood, preparation for freezing, each unit;**
86931	with thawing
86932	with freezing and thawing
86940	**Hemolysins and agglutinins; auto, screen, each**
86941	incubated
86945	**Irradiation of blood product, each unit**

CIM 45-18 GRANULOCYTE TRANSFUSIONS

Medicare covers granulocyte transfusions to patients suffering from severe infection and granulocytopenia. Granulocytopenia is usually identified as less than 500 granulocytes/mm2 whole blood. Accepted indications for transfusions include:

- Granulocytopenia with evidence of gram negative sepsis
- Granulocytopenia in febrile patients with local progressive infections unresponsive to appropriate antibiotic therapy, thought to be due to gram negative organisms

CIM 45-27 BLOOD TRANSFUSIONS

Blood transfusions are used to restore blood volume after hemorrhage, to improve the oxygen carrying capacity of blood in severe anemia, and to combat shock in acute hemolytic anemia.

Definitions

1. Homologous blood transfusion is the infusion of blood or blood components collected from the general public.

2. An autologous blood transfusion is the collection and infusion of a patient's own blood.

3. A donor directed blood transfusion is the infusion of blood or blood components collected from a specific individual(s) other than the patient and infused into the specific patient for whom the blood is designated.

4. Perioperative blood salvage is the collection and reinfusion of blood lost during and immediately after surgery.

Medicare (Part A and Part B) generally covers medically necessary transfusion of blood, regardless of the type. The following polices apply to the preoperative collection, processing, and storage of autologous and donor-directed blood:

- Non-physician services furnished to hospital patients are covered and paid for as hospital services
- Inclusion of services provided to hospital patients by an outside supplier as part of hospital services is referred to as "bundling"
- The hospital pays the supplier when the facility obtains either autologous or donor-directed blood from an independent supplier, the supplier collects, processes, and stores the blood and, delivers it to the hospital

Under Part A payment, Medicare recognizes only a processing fee charged to the hospital by the independent blood bank. Under the prospective payment system (PPS), the diagnosis related group (DRG) payment to the hospital includes all covered blood and blood processing expenses, whether or not the blood is eventually used.

All patients share the cost of blood provided by a hospital operating its own blood collection.

Under Part B, the collection, processing, and storage of blood for later transfusion into the beneficiary is not recognized as a separate service and no blood supplier can receive direct payment under Part B for blood donation services.

When perioperative blood salvage is used in surgery on a hospital patient, payment to the hospital (under PPS or through cost reimbursement) includes payment for all related costs.

86950 **Leukocyte transfusion**
For leukapheresis, consult CPT code 36520.

86965 **Pooling of platelets or other blood products**
For apheresis, consult CPT code 36520. For therapeutic phlebotomy, consult CPT code 99195.

86970 **Pretreatment of RBC's for use in RBC antibody detection, identification, and/or compatibility testing; incubation with chemical agents or drugs, each**

86971 **incubation with enzymes, each**

86972 **by density gradient separation**

86975 **Pretreatment of serum for use in RBC antibody identification; incubation with drugs, each**

86976 **by dilution**

86977 **incubation with inhibitors, each**

86978 **by differential red cell absorption using patient RBC's or RBC's of known phenotype, each absorption**

86985 **Splitting of blood or blood products, each unit**

86999 **Unlisted transfusion medicine procedure**

MICROBIOLOGY

87001 **Animal inoculation, small animal; with observation**

87003 **with observation and dissection**

87015 **Concentration (any type), for infectious agents**
CPT code 87015 should not be reported in conjunction with CPT code 87177.

87040 **Culture, bacterial; blood, with isolation and presumptive identification of isolates (includes anaerobic culture, if appropriate)**
For definitive identification of isolates, consult CPT code 87076 or 87077. For typing of isolates, consult CPT codes 87140-87158.

87045 **feces, with isolation and preliminary examination (eg, KIA, LIA), Salmonella and Shigella species**

87046 **stool, additional pathogens, isolation and preliminary examination (eg, Campylobacter, Yersinia, Vibro, E. coli O157), each plate**

87070 **any other source except urine, blood or stool, with isolation and presumptive identification of isolates**
For urine, consult CPT codes 87086-87088.

87071 **quantitative, aerobic with isolation and presumptive identification of isolates, any source except urine, blood or stool**
For definitive identification of isolates, consult CPT code 87076 or 87077. For typing of isolates, consult CPT codes 87140-87158.

87073 **quantitative, anaerobic with isolation and presumptive identification of isolates, any source except urine, blood or stool**

87075 **any source, anaerobic with isolation and presumptive identification of isolates**

87076 **anaerobic isolate, additional methods required for definitive identification, each isolate**
For GLC (gas liquid chromatography) or HPLC (high pressure lipid chromatography consult CPT code 87143.

87077 **aerobic isolate, additional methods required for definitive identification, each isolate**

87081 **Culture, presumptive, pathogenic organisms, screening only;**

87084 **with colony estimation from density chart**

87086 **Culture, bacterial; quantitative colony count, urine**

87088 **with isolation and presumptive identification of isolates, urine**

87101 **Culture, fungi (mold or yeast) isolation, with presumptive identification of isolates; skin, hair, or nail**

87102 **other source (except blood)**

87103 **blood**

87106 **Culture, fungi, definitive identification, each organism; yeast**
Report CPT code 87106 in addition to CPT codes 87101, 87102 or 87103 when appropriate.

87107 **mold**

87109 **Culture, mycoplasma, any source**

87110 **Culture, chlamydia, any source**
For immunofluorescence staining of shell vials, consult CPT code 87140.

87116 **Culture, tubercle or other acid-fast bacilli (eg, TB, AFB, mycobacteria) any source, with isolation and presumptive identification of isolates**

87118 **Culture, mycobacterial, definitive identification, each isolate**
For nucleic acid probe identification, consult CPT code 87149. For GLC or HPLC identification consult CPT code 87143.

87140 **Culture, typing; immunofluorescent method, each antiserum**

87143 **gas liquid chromatography (GLC) or high pressure liquid chromatography (HPLC) method**

87147 **immunologic method, other than immunofluorescence (eg, agglutination grouping), per antiserum**

87149 **identification by nucleic acid probe**

87152 **identification by pulse field gel typing**

87158 **other methods**

87164 **Dark field examination, any source (eg, penile, vaginal, oral, skin); includes specimen collection**

87166 **without collection**

87168 **Macroscopic examination; arthropod**

87169 **parasite**

87172 **Pinworm exam (eg, cellophane tape prep)**

87176 **Homogenization, tissue, for culture**

87177 **Ova and parasites, direct smears, concentration and identification**
Do not report CPT code 87177 in conjunction with CPT code 87015. For coccidia or microsporidia exam, consult CPT code 87207. For trichrome, iron hematoxylin and other special stains, consult CPT code 88313. For nucleic acid probes in cytologic material, consult CPT code 88365. For molecular diagnostics, consult CPT codes 83890-83898 and 87470-87799.

87181 **Susceptibility studies, antimicrobial agent; agar dilution method, per agent (eg, antibiotic gradient strip)**

87184 **disk method, per plate (12 or fewer agents)**

87185 **enzyme detection (eg, beta lactamase), per enzyme**

87186	microdilution or agar dilution (minimum inhibitory concentration (MIC) or breakpoint), each multi-antimicrobial, per plate	
+ 87187	microdilution or agar dilution, minimum lethal concentration (MLC), each plate (List separately in addition to code for primary procedure)	

Note that 87187 is an add-on code and must be used in conjunction with CPT code 87186 or 87188.

87188	macrobroth dilution method, each agent	
87190	mycobacteria, proportion method, each agent	

To report other mycobacterial susceptibility studies, consult CPT codes 87181, 87184, 87186 87188. For fungal susceptibility studies, consult CPT codes 87181, 87184, 87187 or 87188.

87197	Serum bactericidal titer (Schlicter test)	
● 87198	Cytomegalovirus, direct fluorescent antibody (DFA)	
● 87199	Enterovirus, direct fluorescent antibody (DFA)	
87205	Smear, primary source with interpretation; Gram or Giemsa stain for bacteria, fungi, or cell types	◻
87206	fluorescent and/or acid fast stain for bacteria, fungi, parasites, viruses or cell types	◻
87207	special stain for inclusion bodies or intracellular parasites (eg, malaria, coccidia, microsporidia, cytomegalovirus, herpes viruses)	◻
	Tzank smear	
87210	wet mount for infectious agents (eg, saline, India ink, KOH preps)	◻
87220	Tissue examination by KOH slide of samples from skin, hair, or nails for fungi or ectoparasite ova or mites (eg, scabies)	◻
87230	Toxin or antitoxin assay, tissue culture (eg, Clostridium difficile toxin)	
87250	Virus isolation; inoculation of embryonated eggs, or small animal, includes observation and dissection	
87252	tissue culture inoculation, observation, and presumptive identification by cytopathic effect	
87253	tissue culture, additional studies or definitive identification (eg, hemabsorption, neutralization, immunofluorescence stain), each isolate	

For electron microscopy, consult CPT code 88348. For inclusion bodies in tissue sections, consult CPT codes 88304-88309; in smears, consult CPT codes 87207-87210; in fluids, consult CPT code 88106.

87254	shell vial, includes identification with immunofluorescence stain, each virus	

Report CPT code 87254 in addition to CPT code 87252 as appropriate.

87260	Infectious agent antigen detection by immunofluorescent technique; adenovirus	◻
87265	Bordetella pertussis/parapertussis	◻
87270	Chlamydia trachomatis	◻
87272	cryptosporidium/giardia	◻
87273	Herpes simplex virus type 2	
87274	Herpes simplex virus type 1	◻
87275	Influenza B virus	
87276	Influenza A virus	◻
87277	Legionella micdadei	
87278	Legionella pneumophila	◻
87279	Parainfluenza virus, each type	
87280	respiratory syncytial virus	◻
87281	Pneumocystis carinii	
87283	Rubeola	
87285	Treponema pallidum	◻
87290	Varicella zoster virus	◻
87299	not otherwise specified, each organism	◻
87300	Infectious agent antigen detection by immunofluorescent technique, polyvalent for multiple organisms, each polyvalent antiserum	

To report physician evaluation of infectious disease agents by immunofluoroescence, consult CPT code 88346.

87301	Infectious agent antigen detection by enzyme immunoassay technique, qualitative or semiquantitative, multiple step method; adenovirus enteric types 40/41	
87320	Chlamydia trachomatis	
87324	Clostridium difficile toxin(s)	◻
87327	Cryptococcus neoformans	

To report Cryptococcus latex agglutination, consult CPT code 86403.

87328	cryptosporidium/giardia	◻
87332	cytomegalovirus	
87335	Escherichia coli 0157	

For Giardia antigen, consult CPT code 87328.

87336	Entamoeba histolytica dispar group	
87337	Entamoeba histolytica group	
87338	Infectious agent antigen detection by enzyme immunoassay technique, qualitative or semiquantitative, multiple step method; Helicobacter pylori, stool	◻

For *H. pylori*, breath and blood by mass spectrometry, consult CPT codes 83013, 83014. For H. pylori, liquid scintillation counter, consult CPT code 78267, 78268.

87339	Helicobacter pylori	
87340	hepatitis B surface antigen (HBsAg)	◻
87341	hepatitis B surface antigen (HBsAg) neutralization	
87350	hepatitis Be antigen (HBeAg)	◻
87380	hepatitis, delta agent	
87385	Histoplasma capsulatum	
87390	HIV-1	
87391	HIV-2	
87400	Influenza, A or B, each	
87420	respiratory syncytial virus	
87425	rotavirus	◻
87427	Shiga-like toxin	
87430	Streptococcus, group A	
87449	Infectious agent antigen detection by enzyme immunoassay technique qualitative or semiquantitative; multiple step method, not otherwise specified, each organism	◻
87450	single step method, not otherwise specified, each organism	
87451	multiple step method, polyvalent for multiple organisms, each polyvalent antiserum	
87470	Infectious agent detection by nucleic acid (DNA or RNA); Bartonella henselae and Bartonella quintana, direct probe technique	◻
87471	Bartonella henselae and Bartonella quintana, amplified probe technique	◻
87472	Bartonella henselae and Bartonella quintana, quantification	◻

◻ CCI Comprehensive Code   50 Bilateral Procedure   **+** CPT Add-on Code   ⊘ Modifier -51 Exempt Code   ● New Code   ▲ Revised Code

✗ CLIA Waived Test   **M** Maternity   **N** Newborn   **P** Pediatric   **N/P** Newborn/Pediatric

Pathology and Laboratory

87475 — 87904

87475	Borrelia burgdorferi, direct probe technique	TC
87476	Borrelia burgdorferi, amplified probe technique	TC
87477	Borrelia burgdorferi, quantification	TC
87480	Candida species, direct probe technique	TC
87481	Candida species, amplified probe technique	TC
87482	Candida species, quantification	TC
87485	Chlamydia pneumoniae, direct probe technique	TC
87486	Chlamydia pneumoniae, amplified probe technique	TC
87487	Chlamydia pneumoniae, quantification	TC
87490	Chlamydia trachomatis, direct probe technique	TC
87491	Chlamydia trachomatis, amplified probe technique	TC
87492	Chlamydia trachomatis, quantification	TC
87495	cytomegalovirus, direct probe technique	TC
87496	cytomegalovirus, amplified probe technique	TC
87497	cytomegalovirus, quantification	TC
87510	Gardnerella vaginalis, direct probe technique	TC
87511	Gardnerella vaginalis, amplified probe technique	TC
87512	Gardnerella vaginalis, quantification	TC
87515	hepatitis B virus, direct probe technique	TC
87516	hepatitis B virus, amplified probe technique	TC
87517	hepatitis B virus, quantification	TC
87520	hepatitis C, direct probe technique	TC
87521	hepatitis C, amplified probe technique	TC
87522	hepatitis C, quantification	TC
87525	hepatitis G, direct probe technique	TC
87526	hepatitis G, amplified probe technique	TC
87527	hepatitis G, quantification	TC
87528	Herpes simplex virus, direct probe technique	TC
87529	Herpes simplex virus, amplified probe technique	TC
87530	Herpes simplex virus, quantification	TC
87531	Herpes virus-6, direct probe technique	TC
87532	Herpes virus-6, amplified probe technique	TC
87533	Herpes virus-6, quantification	TC
87534	HIV-1, direct probe technique	TC
87535	HIV-1, amplified probe technique	TC
87536	HIV-1, quantification	TC
87537	HIV-2, direct probe technique	TC
87538	HIV-2, amplified probe technique	TC
87539	HIV-2, quantification	TC
87540	Legionella pneumophila, direct probe technique	TC
87541	Legionella pneumophila, amplified probe technique	TC
87542	Legionella pneumophila, quantification	TC
87550	Mycobacteria species, direct probe technique	TC
87551	Mycobacteria species, amplified probe technique	TC
87552	Mycobacteria species, quantification	TC
87555	Mycobacteria tuberculosis, direct probe technique	TC
87556	Mycobacteria tuberculosis, amplified probe technique	TC
87557	Mycobacteria tuberculosis, quantification	TC
87560	Mycobacteria avium-intracellulare, direct probe technique	TC
87561	Mycobacteria avium-intracellulare, amplified probe technique	TC
87562	Mycobacteria avium-intracellulare, quantification	
87580	Mycoplasma pneumoniae, direct probe technique	TC
87581	Mycoplasma pneumoniae, amplified probe technique	TC
87582	Mycoplasma pneumoniae, quantification	TC
87590	Neisseria gonorrhoeae, direct probe technique	TC
87591	Neisseria gonorrhoeae, amplified probe technique	TC
87592	Neisseria gonorrhoeae, quantification	TC
87620	papillomavirus, human, direct probe technique	TC
87621	papillomavirus, human, amplified probe technique	TC
87622	papillomavirus, human, quantification	TC
87650	Streptococcus, group A, direct probe technique	TC
87651	Streptococcus, group A, amplified probe technique	TC
87652	Streptococcus, group A, quantification	TC

87797 Infectious agent detection by nucleic acid (DNA or RNA), not otherwise specified; direct probe technique, each organism [TC]

87798 amplified probe technique, each organism [TC]

87799 quantification, each organism [TC]

87800 Infectious agent detection by nucleic acid (DNA or RNA), multiple organisms; direct probe(s) technique

87801 amplified probe(s) technique

● 87802 Infectious agent antigen detection by immunoassay with direct optical observation; Streptococcus, group B

● 87803 Clostridium difficile toxin A

● 87804 Influenza

87810 Infectious agent detection by immunoassay with direct optical observation; Chlamydia trachomatis [TC]

87850 Neisseria gonorrhoeae [TC]

87880 Streptococcus, group A [26][TC]

87899 not otherwise specified [26][TC]

87901 Infectious agent genotype analysis by nucleic acid (DNA or RNA), HIV 1, reverse transcriptase and protease

To report infectious agent drug susceptiblity phenotype prediction for HIV-1, consult CPT Category III code 0023T.

● 87902 Hepatitis C virus

▲ 87903 Infectious agent phenotype analysis by nucleic acid (DNA or RNA) with drug resistance tissue culture analysis, HIV 1; first through 10 drugs tested

▲ + 87904 Infectious agent phenotype analysis by nucleic acid (DNA or RNA) with drug resistance tissue culture analysis, HIV 1; each additional 1 through 5 drugs tested (List separately in addition to code for primary procedure)

Note that 87904 is an add-on code and must be used in conjunction with CPT code 87903.

| 87999 | Unlisted microbiology procedure |

ANATOMIC PATHOLOGY

POSTMORTEM EXAMINATION

MCM 2070 DIAGNOSTIC X-RAY, DIAGNOSTIC LABORATORY, AND OTHER DIAGNOSTIC TESTS

Medicare covers diagnostic x-ray, diagnostic laboratory, and other diagnostic tests, including materials and the services of technicians. Medicare covers diagnostic X-ray services performed in a facility directed by a physician or group of physicians if they are performed under the direct supervision of a physician. Certain diagnostic X-ray procedures are also covered when performed by technicians without direct personal physician supervision if the technicians' general supervision and training, as well as the maintenance of the necessary equipment and supplies, are the continuing responsibility of a physician. Covered diagnostic tests include:

Histopathology

Tissue Decalcification

Bone Marrow Biopsy

Tissue Pathology

Surgical pathology

Frozen sections

Autopsy and sections

88000	**Necropsy (autopsy), gross examination only; without CNS**
88005	**with brain**
88007	**with brain and spinal cord**
88012	**infant with brain**
88014	**stillborn or newborn with brain**
88016	**macerated stillborn**
88020	**Necropsy (autopsy), gross and microscopic; without CNS**
88025	**with brain**
88027	**with brain and spinal cord**
88028	**infant with brain**
88029	**stillborn or newborn with brain**
88036	**Necropsy (autopsy), limited, gross and/or microscopic; regional**
88037	**single organ**
88040	**Necropsy (autopsy); forensic examination**
88045	**coroner's call**
88099	**Unlisted necropsy (autopsy) procedure**

CYTOPATHOLOGY

88104	**Cytopathology, fluids, washings or brushings, except cervical or vaginal; smears with interpretation**
88106	**filter method only with interpretation**
88107	**smears and filter preparation with interpretation**
88108	**Cytopathology, concentration technique, smears and interpretation (eg, Saccomanno technique)**

For gastric intubation with lavage, consult CPT codes 89130–89141 and 91055. For cervical or vaginal smears, consult CPT code 88150-88156. For x-ray localization, consult CPT code 74340.

88125	**Cytopathology, forensic (eg, sperm)**
88130	**Sex chromatin identification; Barr bodies**
88140	**peripheral blood smear, polymorphonuclear drumsticks**

For Guard stain, consult CPT code 88313.

CIM 50-20 DIAGNOSTIC PAP SMEARS

Screening Pap smears are covered when ordered and collected by a doctor of medicine or osteopathy, or other practitioner authorized under State law to perform the examination) one of the following conditions:

- Previous cancer of the cervix, uterus, or vagina that has been or is being treated
- Previous abnormal pap smear
- Any abnormal findings of the vagina, cervix, uterus, ovaries, or adnexa
- Any significant complaint by the patient referable to the female reproductive system
- Any signs or symptoms that might in the physician's judgment reasonably be related to a gynecologic disorder.

Use the following CPT codes for indicating diagnostic pap smears:

- 88150 Cytopathology, smears, cervical or vaginal (e.g., Papanicolaou), up to three smears; screening by technician under physician supervision
- 88151 Cytopathology, smears, cervical or vaginal (e.g., Papanicolaou), up to three smears; requiring interpretation by physician

When the beneficiary does not qualify for a more frequently performed screening Pap smear, the screening Pap smear is covered only after at least 23 months have passed following the month during which the beneficiary received her last covered screening Pap smear.

CIM 50-20.1 SCREENING PAP SMEARS AND PELVIC EXAMINATIONS FOR EARLY DETECTION OF CERVICAL OR VAGINAL CANCER

(For screening Pap smears, effective for services performed on or after July 1, 1990. For pelvic examinations including clinical breast examination, effective for services furnished on or after January 1, 1998.)

A screening pap smear - Use HCPCS code P3000 *Screening Papanicolaou smear, cervical or vaginal, up to three smears*; by technician under physician supervision or P3001 *Screening Papanicolaou smear, cervical or vaginal, up to three smears requiring interpretation by physician*

Use HCPCS codes:

G0123 Screening Cytopathology, cervical or vaginal (any reporting system), collected in preservative fluid, automated thin layer preparation, screening by cytotechnologist under physician supervision

or

G0124 Screening Cytopathology, cervical or vaginal (any reporting system) collected in preservative fluid, automated thin layer preparation, requiring interpretation by physician) and related medically necessary services provided to a woman for the early detection of cervical cancer (including collection of the sample of cells and a physician's interpretation of the test results) and pelvic examination (including clinical breast examination

HCPCS code G0101 cervical or vaginal cancer screening; pelvic and clinical breast examination) are covered under Medicare Part B when ordered by a physician (or authorized practitioner) under one of the following conditions:

- She has not had such a test during the preceding three years or is a woman of childbearing age
- There is evidence (on the basis of her medical history or other findings) that she is at high risk of developing cervical cancer and her physician (or authorized practitioner) recommends that she have the test performed more frequently than every three years

High risk factors for cervical and vaginal cancer are:

- Early onset of sexual activity (under 16 years of age)
- Multiple sexual partners (five or more in a lifetime)
- History of sexually transmitted disease (including HIV infection)
- Fewer than three negative or any pap smears within the previous seven years
- DES (diethylstilbestrol) - exposed daughters of women who took DES during pregnancy

NOTE: Claims for Pap smears must indicate the beneficiary's low- or high-risk status by including the appropriate ICD-9-CM on the line item (Item 24E of the HCFA-1500):

- V76.2 *special screening for malignant neoplasms of the cervix indicates low risk*
- V15.89 *other specified personal history presenting hazards to health indicates high risk*

The Common Working File will reject claims without the proper diagnostic codes.

For the purposes of Medicare reimbursement, eligibility requires that a woman of childbearing age has had a Pap smear test during any of the preceding three years that indicated the presence of cervical or vaginal cancer or other abnormality, or is at high risk of developing cervical or vaginal cancer. In addition, woman of childbearing age is one who is premenopausal and has been determined by a physician or other qualified practitioner to be of childbearing age, based upon the medical history or other findings

+ 88141   **Cytopathology, cervical or vaginal (any reporting system); requiring interpretation by physician (List separately in addition to code for technical service)** ♀
> Note that 88141 is an add-on code and must be used in conjunction with 88142-88154 and 88164-88167.

88142   **Cytopathology, cervical or vaginal (any reporting system), collected in preservative fluid, automated thin layer preparation; manual screening under physician supervision** ♀

88143   **with manual screening and rescreening under physician supervision** ♀

88144   **with manual screening and computer-assisted rescreening under physician supervision** ♀

88145   **with manual screening and computer-assisted rescreening using cell selection and review under physician supervision** ♀

88147   **Cytopathology smears, cervical or vaginal; screening by automated system under physician supervision** ♀

88148   **screening by automated system with manual rescreening under physician supervision** ♀

88150   **Cytopathology, slides, cervical or vaginal; manual screening under physician supervision** ♀

88152   **with manual screening and computer-assisted rescreening under physician supervision** ♀

88153   **with manual screening and rescreening under physician supervision** ♀

88154   **with manual screening and computer-assisted rescreening using cell selection and review under physician supervision** ♀

+ 88155   **Cytopathology, slides, cervical or vaginal, definitive hormonal evaluation (eg, maturation index, karyopyknotic index, estrogenic index) (List separately in addition to code(s) for other technical and interpretation services)** ♀
> Note that 88155 is an add-on code and must be used in conjunction with 88142-88154 and 88164-88167.

88160   **Cytopathology, smears, any other source; screening and interpretation**

88161   **preparation, screening and interpretation**

88162   **extended study involving over 5 slides and/or multiple stains**
> If specimen needs to be obtained, consult percutaneous needle biopsy under the individual organ in the Surgery section of CPT. For aerosol collection of sputum, consult CPT code 89350. For special stains, consult CPT codes 88312-88314.

88164   **Cytopathology, slides, cervical or vaginal (the Bethesda System); manual screening under physician supervision** ♀

88165   **with manual screening and rescreening under physician supervision** ♀

88166   **with manual screening and computer-assisted rescreening under physician supervision** ♀

88167   **with manual screening and computer-assisted rescreening using cell selection and review under physician supervision** ♀

~~**88170**~~   ~~**Fine needle aspiration; superficial tissue (eg, thyroid, breast, prostate)**~~ This code is deleted in 2002. See code 10021.

~~**88171**~~   ~~**Fine needle aspiration; deep tissue under radiologic guidance**~~ This code is deleted in 2002. See code 10022.

88172   **Cytopathology, evaluation of fine needle aspirate; immediate cytohistologic study to determine adequacy of specimen(s)**

88173   **interpretation and report**

88180   **Flow cytometry; each cell surface, cytoplasmic or nuclear marker**

88182   **cell cycle or DNA analysis**
> For tumor morphometry and DNA and ploidy analysis for imaging techniques, consult CPT code 88358.

88199   **Unlisted cytopathology procedure**
> For electron microscopy, consult CPT codes 88348 and 88349.

CYTOGENETIC STUDIES

For acetylcholinesterase, consult CPT code 82013. For alpha-fetoprotein, serum or amniotic fluid, consult CPT codes 82105 and 82106.

For laser microdissection of cells from tissue sample, consult CPT code 88380.

88230   **Tissue culture for non-neoplastic disorders; lymphocyte**

88233   **skin or other solid tissue biopsy**

88235   **amniotic fluid or chorionic villus cells** M ♀

88237   **Tissue culture for neoplastic disorders; bone marrow, blood cells**

88239   **solid tumor**

88240   **Cryopreservation, freezing and storage of cells, each cell line**

88241   **Thawing and expansion of frozen cells, each aliquot**

88245   **Chromosome analysis for breakage syndromes; baseline Sister Chromatid Exchange (SCE), 20-25 cells**

88248   **baseline breakage, score 50-100 cells, count 20 cells, 2 karyotypes (eg, for ataxia telangiectasia, Fanconi anemia, fragile X)**

88249   **score 100 cells, clastogen stress (eg, diepoxybutane, mitomycin C, ionizing radiation, UV radiation)**

88261   **Chromosome analysis; count 5 cells, 1 karyotype, with banding**

88262   **count 15-20 cells, 2 karyotypes, with banding**

88263   **count 45 cells for mosaicism, 2 karyotypes, with banding**

88264   **analyze 20-25 cells**

88267   **Chromosome analysis, amniotic fluid or chorionic villus, count 15 cells, 1 karyotype, with banding** M ♀

| 88269 | Chromosome analysis, in situ for amniotic fluid cells, count cells from 6-12 colonies, 1 karyotype, with banding |

| 88271 | Molecular cytogenetics; DNA probe, each (eg, FISH) |

| 88272 | chromosomal in situ hybridization, analyze 3-5 cells (eg, for derivatives and markers) |

| 88273 | chromosomal in situ hybridization, analyze 10-30 cells (eg, for microdeletions) |

| 88274 | interphase in situ hybridization, analyze 25-99 cells |

| 88275 | interphase in situ hybridization, analyze 100-300 cells |

| 88280 | Chromosome analysis; additional karyotypes, each study |

| 88283 | additional specialized banding technique (eg, NOR, C-banding) |

| 88285 | additional cells counted, each study |

| 88289 | additional high resolution study |

| 88291 | Cytogenetics and molecular cytogenetics, interpretation and report |

| 88299 | Unlisted cytogenetic study |

SURGICAL PATHOLOGY

88300 Level I - Surgical pathology, gross examination only

88302 Level II - Surgical pathology, gross and microscopic examination

Includes: Appendix, Incidental; Fallopian Tube, Sterilization; Fingers/Toes, Amputation,Traumatic; Foreskin, Newborn, Hernia Sac, Any Location; Hydrocele Sac; Nerve; Skin, Plastic Repair; Sympathetic Ganglion; Testis, Castration; Vaginal Mucosa, Incidental; Vas Deferens, Sterilization

▲ **88304** Level III - Surgical pathology, gross and microscopic examination

Includes: Abortion, Induced Abscess Aneurysm - Arterial/Ventricular Anus, Tag Appendix, Other than Incidental Artery, Atheromatous Plaque Bartholin's Gland Cyst Bone Fragment(s), Other than Pathologic Fracture Bursa/Synovial Cyst Carpal Tunnel Tissue Cartilage, Shavings Cholesteatoma Colon, Colostomy Stoma Conjunctiva - Biopsy/Pterygium Cornea Diverticulum - Esophagus/Small Intestine Dupuytren's Contracture Tissue Femoral Head, Other than Fracture Fissure/Fistula Foreskin, Other than Newborn Gallbladder Ganglion Cyst Hematoma Hemorrhoids Hydatid of Morgagni Intervertebral Disc Joint, Loose Body Meniscus Mucocele, Salivary Neuroma - Morton's/Traumatic Pilonidal Cyst/Sinus Polyps, Inflammatory - Nasal/Sinusoidal Skin - Cyst/Tag/Debridement Soft Tissue, Debridement Soft Tissue, Lipoma Spermatocele Tendon/Tendon Sheath Testicular Appendage Thrombus or Embolus Tonsil and/or Adenoids Varicocele Vas Deferens, Other than Sterilization Vein, Varicosity

▲ **88305** Level IV - Surgical pathology, gross and microscopic examination

Includes: Abortion - Spontaneous/Missed Artery, Biopsy Bone Marrow, Biopsy Bone Exostosis Brain/Meninges, Other than for Tumor Resection Breast, Biopsy, Not Requiring Microscopic Evaluation of Surgical Margins Breast, Reduction Mammoplasty Bronchus, Biopsy Cell Block, Any Source Cervix, Biopsy Colon, Biopsy Duodenum, Biopsy Endocervix, Curettings/Biopsy Endometrium, Curettings/Biopsy Esophagus, Biopsy Extremity, Amputation, Traumatic Fallopian Tube, Biopsy Fallopian Tube, Ectopic Pregnancy Femoral Head, Fracture Fingers/Toes, Amputation, Non-traumatic Gingiva/Oral Mucosa, Biopsy Heart Valve Joint, Resection Kidney, Biopsy Larynx, Biopsy Leiomyoma(s), Uterine Myomectomy - without Uterus Lip, Biopsy/Wedge Resection Lung, Transbronchial Biopsy Lymph Node, Biopsy Muscle, Biopsy Nasal Mucosa, Biopsy Nasopharynx/Oropharynx, Biopsy Nerve, Biopsy Odontogenic/Dental Cyst Omentum, Biopsy Ovary with or without Tube, Non-neoplastic Ovary, Biopsy/Wedge Resection Parathyroid Gland Peritoneum, Biopsy Pituitary Tumor Placenta, Other than Third Trimester Pleura/Pericardium - Biopsy/Tissue Polyp, Cervical/Endometrial Polyp, Colorectal Polyp, Stomach/Small Intestine Prostate, Needle Biopsy Prostate, TUR Salivary Gland, Biopsy Sinus, Paranasal Biopsy Skin, Other than Cyst/Tag/Debridement/Plastic Repair Small Intestine, Biopsy Soft Tissue, Other than Tumor/Mass/Lipoma/Debridement Spleen Stomach, Biopsy Synovium Testis, Other than Tumor/Biopsy/Castration Thyroglossal Duct/Brachial Cleft Cyst Tongue, Biopsy Tonsil, Biopsy Trachea, Biopsy Ureter, Biopsy Urethra, Biopsy Urinary Bladder, Biopsy Uterus, with or without Tubes and Ovaries, for Prolapse Vagina, Biopsy Vulva/Labia, Biopsy

▲ **88307** Level V - Surgical pathology, gross and microscopic examination

Includes: Adrenal, Resection; Bone - Biopsy/Curettings; Bone Fragment(s), Pathologic Fracture; Brain, Biopsy; Brain/Meninges, Tumor Resection; Breast, Excision of Lesion, Requiring Microscopic Evaluation of Surgical Margins; Breast, Mastectomy - Partial/Simple; Cervix, Conization; Colon, Segmental Resection, Other than for Tumor; Extremity, Amputation, Non-Traumatic; Eye, Enucleation; Kidney, Partial/Total Nephrectomy; Larynx, Partial/Total Resection; Liver, Biopsy - Needle/Wedge; Liver, Partial Resection; Lung, Wedge Biopsy; Lymph Nodes, Regional Resection; Mediastinum, Mass; Myocardium, Biopsy; Odontogenic Tumor; Ovary with or without Tube, Neoplastic; Pancreas, Biopsy; Placenta, Third Trimester; Prostate, Except Radical Resection; Salivary Gland; Sentinel Lymph Node; Small Intestine; Resection, Other than for Tumor; Soft Tissue Mass (except Lipoma) - Biopsy/Simple Excision; Stomach - Subtotal/Total Resection, Other than for Tumor; Testis, Biopsy; Thymus, Tumor; Thyroid, Total/Lobe; Ureter, Resection; Urinary Bladder, TUR; Uterus, with or without Tubes and Ovaries, Other than Neoplastic/Prolapse

---

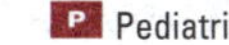

| ▣ CCI Comprehensive Code | 🔟 Bilateral Procedure | ✚ CPT Add-on Code | ⃠ Modifier -51 Exempt Code | ● New Code | ▲ Revised Code |

| ✖ CLIA Waived Test | Ⓜ Maternity | Ⓝ Newborn | Ⓟ Pediatric | N/P Newborn/Pediatric |

88309   **Level VI - Surgical pathology, gross and microscopic examination** [80]
Includes: Bone Resection; Breast, Mastectomy - with Regional Lymph Nodes; Colon, Segmental Resection for Tumor; Colon, Total Resection; Esophagus, Partial/Total Resection; Extremity, Disarticulation; Fetus, with Dissection; Larynx, Partial/Total Resection - with Regional Lymph Nodes; Lung - Total/Lobe/Segment Resection; Pancreas, Total/Subtotal Resection; Prostate, Radical Resection; Small Intestine, Resection for Tumor; Soft Tissue Tumor, Extensive Resection; Stomach - Subtotal/Total Resection for Tumor; Testis, Tumor; Tongue/Tonsil - Resection for Tumor; Urinary Bladder, Partial/Total Resection; Uterus, with or without Tubes & Ovaries, Neoplastic; Vulva, Total/Subtotal Resection
To report fine needle aspiration, consult CPT codes 10021, 10022.
To report evaluation of fine needle aspirate, consult CPT codes 88172, 88173.

+   88311   **Decalcification procedure (List separately in addition to code for surgical pathology examination)** [80]

+   88312   **Special stains (List separately in addition to code for surgical pathology examination); Group I for microorganisms (eg, Gridley, acid fast, methenamine silver), each** [80]

+   88313   **Group II, all other, (eg, iron, trichrome), except immunocytochemistry and immunoperoxidase stains, each** [80]
If immunocytochemistry and immunoperoxidase tissue studies are performed, consult CPT code 88342.

+   88314   **histochemical staining with frozen section(s)** [80]

88318   **Determinative histochemistry to identify chemical components (eg, copper, zinc)** [80]

88319   **Determinative histochemistry or cytochemistry to identify enzyme constituents, each** [80]

88321   **Consultation and report on referred slides prepared elsewhere** [80]

88323   **Consultation and report on referred material requiring preparation of slides** [80] [TC]

88325   **Consultation, comprehensive, with review of records and specimens, with report on referred material** [80] [TC]

88329   **Pathology consultation during surgery;** [80]

88331   **first tissue block, with frozen section(s), single specimen** [80] [TC]

88332   **each additional tissue block with frozen section(s)** [80] [TC]

88342   **Immunocytochemistry (including tissue immunoperoxidase), each antibody** [80]

88346   **Immunofluorescent study, each antibody; direct method** [80]

88347   **indirect method** [80]

CIM 50-18 ELECTRON MICROSCOPE

The additional expense for the electron microscope is warranted when distinguishing different types of nephritis from renal needle biopsies or when there is an uncertain diagnosis from the pathologist. When an uncertain diagnosis results from a less expensive method of exam and an electron microscope examination is necessary, both biopsy exams are covered.

88348   **Electron microscopy; diagnostic** [80] [TC]

88349   **scanning** [80]

88355   **Morphometric analysis; skeletal muscle** [80]

88356   **nerve** [80]

88358   **tumor** [80]

88362   **Nerve teasing preparations** [80]
If a physician interprets a peripheral blood smear, consult CPT code 85060.

88365   **Tissue in situ hybridization, interpretation and report** [80] [TC]

88371   **Protein analysis of tissue by Western Blot, with interpretation and report;** [TC]

88372   **immunological probe for band identification, each** [TC]

●   88380   **Microdissection (eg, mechanical, laser capture)**

88399   **Unlisted surgical pathology procedure** [80] [26]

TRANSCUTANEOUS PROCEDURES

●   88400   **Bilirubin, total, transcutaneous**

OTHER PROCEDURES

▲   89050   **Cell count, miscellaneous body fluids (eg, cerebrospinal fluid, joint fluid), except blood;** [TC]

89051   **with differential count** [TC]

89060   **Crystal identification by light microscopy with or without polarizing lens analysis, any body fluid (except urine)** [TC]

89100   **Duodenal intubation and aspiration; single specimen (eg, simple bile study or afferent loop culture) plus appropriate test procedure** [80]

89105   **collection of multiple fractional specimens with pancreatic or gallbladder stimulation, single or double lumen tube** [80] [TC]
For radiological localization, consult CPT code 74340. If chemical analyses are necessary, consult the Chemistry section of CPT. If an electrocardiogram is performed, consult CPT codes 93000-93268. If an esophagus acid perfusion test (Bernstein) is performed, consult CPT code 91030.

89125   **Fat stain, feces, urine, or respiratory secretions** [TC]

89130   **Gastric intubation and aspiration, diagnostic, each specimen, for chemical analyses or cytopathology;** [80]

89132   **after stimulation** [80]

89135   **Gastric intubation, aspiration, and fractional collections (eg, gastric secretory study); one hour** [80]

89136   **two hours** [80] [TC]

89140   **two hours including gastric stimulation (eg, histalog, pentagastrin)** [80] [TC]

89141   **three hours, including gastric stimulation** [80] [TC]
For gastric lavage, therapeutic, consult CPT code 91105. For radiologic localization of a gastric tube, consult CPT code 74340. If chemical analyses are necessary, consult CPT codes 82926 and 82928. For joint fluid chemistry, consult the Chemistry section of CPT.

89160   **Meat fibers, feces** [TC]

89190   **Nasal smear for eosinophils** [TC]
For occult blood, feces, consult CPT code 82270.
For paternity tests, consult CPT code 86910.

89250   **Culture and fertilization of oocyte(s);** ♀

89251   **with co-culture of embryos** ♀ [TC]

89252   **Assisted oocyte fertilization, microtechnique (any method)** ♀

89253   **Assisted embryo hatching, microtechniques (any method)** ♀

89254   **Oocyte identification from follicular fluid** ♀

89255	**Preparation of embryo for transfer (any method)**	♀
89256	**Preparation of cryopreserved embryos for transfer (includes thaw)**	♀ ⊡
89257	**Sperm identification from aspiration (other than seminal fluid)**	♂ ⊡

89257 — If semen is analyzed, consult CPT codes 89300-89320. If sperm is identified from testis tissue, consult CPT code 89264.

89258	**Cryopreservation; embryo**	♀
89259	**sperm**	♂
89260	**Sperm isolation; simple prep (eg, sperm wash and swim-up) for insemination or diagnosis with semen analysis**	♂ ⊡
89261	**complex prep (eg, Percoll gradient, albumin gradient) for insemination or diagnosis with semen analysis**	♂ ⊡

89261 — If semen is analyzed without sperm wash or swim-up, consult CPT code 89320.

89264	**Sperm identification from testis tissue, fresh or cryopreserved**	♂ ⊡

89264 — If the testis is biopsied, consult CPT codes 54500 and 54505. If sperm is identified from aspiration, consult CPT code 89257. If semen is analyzed, consult CPT codes 89300-89320.

89300	**Semen analysis; presence and/or motility of sperm including Huhner test (post coital)**	♂ ⊡
89310	**motility and count**	♂ ⊡
89320	**complete (volume, count, motility and differential)**	♂ ⊡

89320 — For skin tests, consult CPT codes 86485-86585 and 95010-95199.

89321	**Semen analysis, presence and/or motility of sperm**	♂
89325	**Sperm antibodies**	♂ ⊡

89325 — For medicolegal identification of sperm, consult CPT code 88125.

89329	**Sperm evaluation; hamster penetration test**	♂ ⊡
89330	**cervical mucus penetration test, with or without spinnbarkeit test**	⊡
89350	**Sputum, obtaining specimen, aerosol induced technique (separate procedure)**	TC 80
89355	**Starch granules, feces**	⊡

CIM 50-35 SWEAT TEST

Medicare covers a sweat test as a diagnostic tool in cystic fibrosis. Medicare does not cover the use of a sweat test as a predictor of efficacy of sympathectomy in peripheral vascular disease.

89360	**Sweat collection by iontophoresis**	TC 80 ⊡

89360 — For chloride and sodium analysis, consult CPT code 84295.

89365	**Water load test**	⊡
	Albarran test	
89399	**Unlisted miscellaneous pathology test**	80

MEDICINE SERVICES

CPT Expert **is not intended to replace the AMA's CPT manual. It does not include the AMA's official rules and guidelines, and Ingenix recommends you use this in conjunction with the AMA's 2002 CPT book.**

CODING INFORMATION

ORGANIZATION

The Medicine Section (90281-99199) follows the pathology and laboratory section. The diagnostic and therapeutic services include immunizations, injections, specialty-specific codes, and special services.

Subsections within the medicine section are:

Immune Globulins

Immunization Administration for Vaccines/Toxoids

Vaccines/Toxoids

Therapeutic or Diagnostic Infusions (Excludes Chemotherapy)

Therapeutic, Prophylactic or Diagnostic Injections

Psychiatry

Biofeedback

Dialysis

Gastroenterology

Ophthalmology

Special Otorhinolaryngologic Services

Cardiovascular

Non-Invasive Vascular Diagnostic Studies

Pulmonary

Allergy and Clinical Immunology

Endocrinology

Central Nervous System Assessments/Tests (eg, Neuro-Cognitive, Mental Status, Speech Testing)

Health and Behavior Assessment/Intervention

Chemotherapy Administration

Photodynamic Therapy

Special Dermatological Procedures

Physical Medicine and Rehabilitation

Medical Nutrition Therapy

Osteopathic Manipulative Treatment

Chiropractic Manipulative Treatment

Special Services, Procedures and Reports

Qualifying Circumstances for Anesthesia

Sedation With or Without Analgesia (Conscious Sedation)

Other Services and Procedures

Home Health Procedures/Services

Home Infusion Procedures

GUIDELINES

BUNDLED MEDICINE CODES

The process of coding integral services separately from a procedure or bundled service is called unbundling or fragmenting. If the component is considered part of the package or bundled service, do not code it individually. For example, 93015 is a bundled code that includes all the components of a stress test and should be reported as such when the complete procedure is performed. If the components 93016 and 93018 are reported instead of the complete test (93015), the payer will probably rebundle the two codes into 93015. However, if the procedure is performed outside the physician's office, only the services provided by the physician, e.g., interpreting the report (93018), would be reported.

SUBSECTIONS

IMMUNE GLOBULINS

Immune Globulin codes (90281-90399) report only the supply of the immune globulin product that includes broad-spectrum and anti-infective immune globulins, antitoxins, and erythrocytic isoantibodies. Administration is reported separately with codes 90780-90784.

IMMUNIZATION ADMINISTRATION FOR VACCINES/TOXOIDS

Immunization administration codes (90471-90474) are reported separately in addition to the code for the vaccine or toxoid supply (90476-90749). Significant, separately identifiable E/M services should also be reported. New to the CPT book 2002 is the addition of two codes for immunizations administered by intranasal or oral routes (90473-90474).

VACCINES/TOXOIDS

Vaccines and toxoids (90476-90749) identify only the vaccine product and should be reported with an immunization administration code (90471-90472). The exact vaccine product administered must be reported to assist in the reporting requirements of immunization registries, vaccine distribution programs, and reporting systems such as the Vaccine Adverse Event Reporting System. Note that code selection is also dependent on dosage, dose schedule, chemical formulation, and route of administration (e.g., intramuscular, subcutaneous, oral). Separate codes are available for reporting combination vaccines.

THERAPEUTIC OR DIAGNOSTIC INFUSIONS (EXCLUDES CHEMOTHERAPY)

Codes 90780 and 90781 identify therapeutic or diagnostic infusions. These infusions are prolonged intravenous injections requiring a physician's presence. The first code (90780) is for infusions up to one hour and the second (90781) is for each additional hour up to eight hours. When reporting 90781, indicate the number of hours in the unit column on the HCFA-1500 form or electronic bill. Remember that 90781 must be reported as a secondary code to 90780. Therapeutic or diagnostic injection codes (90782-90788) are for subcutaneous, intramuscular, intra-arterial, and intravenous injections of a therapeutic or diagnostic agent. Code 90788 reports the intramuscular injection of an antibiotic.

The materials injected are not included in the codes. When the drug is purchased and supplied by the physician, use 90281-90399 for immune globulin products, 99070 for supplies, including drugs, provided and not elsewhere listed, or the appropriate HCPCS Level II J-code for other drugs. Medicare bundles the administration of the medication into the E/M service. Each Medicare and Medicaid carrier has individual requirements for HCPCS Level II codes to describe the drug administered. Some carriers require the use of the CPT code for the injection and the HCPCS Level II J-code for the drug; others use only the J code and require a modifier to designate the method of administration.

PSYCHIATRY

Psychiatry codes include psychiatric diagnostic or evaluation interview procedures (90801-90802), and psychiatric therapeutic procedures (90804-90899).

Psychiatric diagnostic interview exam (90801) includes a history, mental status, and disposition, and may include communication with family or other sources and ordering/interpretation of diagnostic studies. An interactive psychiatric diagnostic interview (90802) is furnished to children and older individuals lacking expressive and receptive communication skills. These procedure codes are normally reported only on the initial visit.

The most frequently reported services are therapeutic psychiatric service codes (90804-90829) for individual psychotherapy. Individual psychotherapy services are organized first by place of service (office/outpatient, inpatient/partial hospital/residential care). Codes within these two subcategories are organized by type of psychotherapy service (insight oriented, behavior modifying, supportive, interactive), face-to-face time, and the provision of additional medical evaluation or management services.

Other psychotherapy services (90845-90857) are used to report family and group psychotherapy services. Psychiatric services and procedures (90862-

90899) are used to report medication management, electroconvulsive therapy, and hypnotherapy.

Hospital inpatient service codes (99221-99233) in the E/M section of the CPT book should be reported when the physician is involved in the medical management of an inpatient (e.g., when the attending physician reviews laboratory tests or initiates the patient's treatment plan). However, do not use hospital inpatient service codes when both psychotherapy and E/M services are provided on the same day. Combined E/M and psychotherapy services should be reported with codes designated as such in the psychiatry section (90804-90822).

BIOFEEDBACK

Biofeedback codes (90901-90911) may require prior authorization. If the payer does not cover biofeedback, enlist the help of the medical director or prior authorization (or utilization) review nurses for service coverage. Documentation may be required, such as articles or printed research material about the benefits of biofeedback.

DIALYSIS

Dialysis services (90918-90999) are divided into end stage renal disease (ESRD) services, hemodialysis, peritoneal dialysis, and miscellaneous dialysis procedures. Codes for the latter three services are selected according to whether the service includes single physician evaluations or repeated evaluations. Repeated evaluations are reported despite the lack of changes in the dialysis prescription.

Codes that report ESRD related services (90918-90921) are selected according to the age of the patient and reflect services for a full month. For less than a full month, 90922-90925 are reported for each day ESRD service is provided. Procedures for other medical problems and complications unrelated to ESRD are not included in the monthly ESRD service.

The dialysis procedure (90935-90947) includes all evaluation and management services related to the patient's ESRD rendered on a day dialysis is performed, as well as all other patient care services rendered during the dialysis procedure. Office and hospital visits are reported in addition to dialysis procedures only when they are unrelated to dialysis and cannot be rendered during a dialysis session.

GASTROENTEROLOGY

The diagnostic procedures (91000-91299) are frequently performed with consultations or other E/M services that are reported separately. Even though gastroenterology is a medicine subspecialty, the majority of procedures performed by gastroenterologists is endoscopic and listed in the surgery section.

OPHTHALMOLOGY

The medical services of ophthalmologists are described in codes 92002 through 92499. General ophthalmological services (92002-92014) are divided into new and established patient categories that are further subdivided by level of service.

INTERMEDIATE LEVEL OF SERVICE

Intermediate service codes (92002 and 92012) report the evaluation of new or existing conditions that have been complicated by a new diagnostic or management problem. This new complaint may relate to the primary diagnosis. Included in the evaluation are:

- History
- General medical observation
- External examination
- Ophthalmoscopy
- Other diagnostic procedures as indicated
  - Biomicroscopy
  - Mydriasis
  - Tonometry
- Initiation of diagnostic and treatment program

COMPREHENSIVE LEVEL OF SERVICE

Comprehensive service codes (92004 and 92014) report the evaluation of the complete visual system. This is a single service that need not be performed at one session. Included in this evaluation are:

- History
- General medical observation
- General evaluation of the complete visual system to include:
  - External examination
  - Ophthalmoscopy
  - Gross visual field
  - Basic sensorimotor examination
- Other diagnostic procedures as indicated:
  - Biomicroscopy
  - Dilation (cycloplegia)
  - Mydriasis
  - Tonometry
- Initiation of a diagnostic treatment program

SPECIAL OPHTHALMOLOGICAL SERVICES

Refractions (92015) should be reported additionally when performed at the time of a general ophthalmological service (92002-92014). Medicare allows the reporting of refractions, a noncovered service, to minimize patient confusion.

Gross visual field testing is integral to the general ophthalmic service and should not be reported separately. However, more extensive visual field examinations should be reported separately with codes 92081-92083. The CPT book recognizes three coding levels for visual field exams. The three specific visual field tests (limited, intermediate, and extended) are described as unilateral or bilateral.

Fitting and provision of contact lenses, glasses, and ocular prostheses are reported with the CPT codes 92310-92396. Use modifier -26 or 09926 with 92391 or 92396 to report the service of fitting without supply. All the codes in this section are bilateral. For prescription or fitting of one eye, append modifier -52 or 09952.

SPECIAL OTORHINOLARYNGOLOGIC SERVICES

Otorhinolaryngologic codes (92502-92599) identify the special diagnostic and treatment services not usually included in a comprehensive otorhinolaryngologic evaluation. Comprehensive ear, nose, and throat (ENT) evaluations include basic diagnostic procedures such as otoscopy and rhinoscopy. These services are an integral part of the evaluation and management service and are not itemized separately. Special services not generally included in this total evaluation are reported separately with 92502-92599, such as audiologic function tests (92551-92598). Hearing tests using calibrated electronic equipment are reportable; use of a tuning fork is not.

Hearing test codes are inherently bilateral (binaural, both ears). If only one ear is tested, the reduced service is reported with modifier -52. Codes 92590, 92592, and 92594 are the exceptions, identified in CPT as monaural (one ear). If binaural, report with 92591, 92593, or 92595.

CARDIOVASCULAR SERVICES

Cardiovascular services (92950-93799) include diagnostic and therapeutic services.

THERAPEUTIC (92950-92998)

Therapeutic services are performed for treatment of a specific condition, disorder, or disease. Some of the more frequently performed services include percutaneous placement of intracoronary stents, percutaneous transluminal coronary angioplasty (PTCA), and percutaneous transluminal coronary arthrectomy.

Percutaneous placement of coronary stents (92980-92981) includes therapeutic procedures such as PTCA and arthrectomy. Do not report stent placements for procedures 92982, 92984, 92995, and 92996.

PTCA (92982-92984) is used to treat coronary artery obstruction. A balloon catheter is placed in the affected artery and the balloon is inflated to flatten the plaque against the wall of the artery and open the obstruction.

Percutaneous transluminal coronary arthrectomy (92995-92996) may be used instead of the PTCA to treat coronary artery obstruction. Arthrectomy involves placing a catheter into the affected artery and using a rotary cutter to remove the plaque. When arthrectomy is performed with a PTCA, the PTCA is not reported separately as it is included in procedures 92995 and 92996.

CARDIOGRAPHY (93000-93278)

Cardiography services include electrocardiogram (ECG), cardiovascular stress tests, and electrocardiographic (Holter) monitoring. The Holter monitor is a diagnostic tool that creates a continuous record of the heart's electrical activity during the patient's normal activities for a 24-hour period. Cardiography codes include both a professional and a technical component. These codes have separate listings for the total component, the recording (technical component), and the review and interpretation (professional component). For example, code 93015 identifies the total service (global) for a cardiovascular stress test and includes the following components:

- Tracing (the technical component only) (93017)

- Supervision of the procedure (a portion of the professional component) (93016)

- Interpretation and report (a portion of the professional component) (93018)

ECHOCARDIOGRAPHY (93303-93350)

Echocardiography records ultrasonic waves reflected from the heart for visualizing heart size and shape, myocardial wall thickness, motion, cardiac valve structure, and function.

Echocardiography codes represent a global procedure. When the physician provides only supervision and interpretation, modifier -26 is added. In echocardiography, ultrasonic waves directed at the heart and great vessels provide a hard copy recording that serves as a diagnostic tool. To code for a follow-up echocardiogram, use 93304, 93308, and 93321, if applicable.

Transesophageal echocardiography (93312-93317) involves guiding a small ultrasonic device attached to the tip of a gastroscope into the patient's esophagus, where it rests behind the heart.

Doppler echocardiography (93320-93321) provides continuous waves but also uses a sound or frequency ultrasound to record direction of blood flow through the heart chambers. Doppler echocardiography is an add-on code and should be reported in addition to two-dimension (2-D) echocardiogram (93303-93315, 93317, 93350).

Color flow mapping (93325) converts recorded flow frequencies into different colors. These color images are superimposed on M-mode or 2-D echoes, allowing more detailed evaluation of disorders. Color flow mapping is an add-on service and should be reported in addition to echocardiography (76825-76828, 93307, 93308, 93312, 93314, 93315, 93317, 93320, 93321, and 93350).

CARDIAC CATHETERIZATION (93501-93572)

Cardiac catheterizations are invasive procedures used to visualize the heart chambers, valves, great vessels, and coronary arteries. Catheter procedures produce pressure measurements and blood volumes used to evaluate cardiac function and valve patency.

The three major components of cardiac catheterization include: introduction and positioning of the catheter (93501-93536) including repositioning, injection procedures (93539-93545) and imaging supervision, interpretation, and report (93555-93556).

Supervision and interpretation codes related to cardiac catheterization (93555 and 93556) are used with imaging performed as part of cardiac catheterization procedures. The plural presentation of the word "procedure(s)" as well as the "and/or" terminology in the descriptions of imaging services suggest the codes include imaging of one or more areas.

Aortic root aortography (93544) is the injection of a large bolus of dye into the proximal ascending aorta, just above the aortic valve. When thoracic aortography is performed without a cardiac catheterization, it should be

reported using procedure 36200 and the appropriate radiologic supervision/interpretation (75600 or 75605).

ENDOMYOCARDIAL BIOPSY (93505)

Biopsy of the inside and middle layers of the heart is a separately reportable service. It may be performed in surgery or in the cardiac cath lab with the patient under local anesthesia. The sample is usually taken from the right or left ventricle. The patient is monitored constantly with both intracardiac and external ECG leads to record cardiac response.

ELECTROPHYSIOLOGIC STUDIES (EPS) (93600-93662)

EPS evaluate the electrical conduction system of the heart. An electrode is placed and the patient is monitored constantly with both intracardiac external ECG leads to record the cardiac response. Programmed electrical stimulation is delivered through an electrode catheter to evaluate electrical conduction pathways, formation of dysrhythmia, and automaticity and refractoriness of myocardial cells. These procedures may include induction of arrhythmia to isolate the origin of the conduction problem.

NONINVASIVE VASCULAR DIAGNOSTIC STUDIES

Noninvasive vascular studies codes (93875-93990) include the patient care required to supervise the studies and interpret the results.

A Duplex scan combines both two-dimensional structure of motion with time and Doppler ultrasonic signal documentation with spectral analysis and color flow velocity mapping or imaging to produce a real-time video display of organ structure and motion.

A vascular study must produce a hard copy with data analysis for the patient's record, including bidirectional vascular flow or imaging when provided. Simple hand-held (screening) devices do not meet these requirements and are not reported separately.

PULMONARY

Pulmonary codes (94010-94799) include both diagnostic and therapeutic services. All procedures include laboratory services, interpretation, and physician services. List hospital inpatient visits, consultations, emergency department services, or office visits separately when performed on the same date as a diagnostic pulmonary service. Specify the procedures that may be performed in requesting prior authorization for pulmonary testing. If ordering tests for a patient and unsure about which test should be performed, contact the pulmonary laboratory for clarification and CPT code numbers. Include that information in documentation for prior authorization and claim review.

SPIROMETRY/BRONCHOSPASM EVALUATION

Spirometry (94010-94070) measures lung capacity. Code 94010 refers to the measurement of the lung's capacity and flow measurements using a spirometer. Expiratory flow rate is calculated generally in terms of liters per second. Maximal voluntary ventilation is included in this service. The graphic record produced by the spirometer goes into the patient's record.

Codes 94014-94016 report patient initiated spirometric recording per 30 day time period.

Bronchospasm evaluation (94060) includes spirometry before and after the use of a bronchodilator (either aerosol or parenteral). The final codes in this series report prolonged evaluation with multiple spirometric determinations.

ALLERGY AND CLINICAL IMMUNOLOGY

Allergy testing and immunology treatment (95004-95199) is performed according to the patient's history, physical findings, and clinical judgment of the provider. Specify the number of tests performed in the unit area of the claim or electronic billing form. Significant, separately identifiable E/M services should be reported in addition to allergen testing and immunotherapy.

NEUROLOGY AND NEUROMUSCULAR PROCEDURES

Neurologic services (95805-95999) are frequently performed with consultative or other evaluation and management services. The E/M services are reported separately.

MEDICINE

SLEEP TESTING

Sleep services (95805-95811) include sleep studies and polysomnography. Both types of services include continuous and simultaneous monitoring and recording of selected physiological and pathophysiological sleep parameters for a minimum of six hours. For studies of less than six hours append modifier -52. These services are global and include tracing, interpretation, and report. For interpretation only, append modifier -26. These studies are performed to diagnose a variety of sleep disorders and to evaluate a patient's response to therapies such as nasal continuous positive airway pressure (NCPAP).

Polysomnography is distinguished from sleep studies by the inclusion of sleep staging, which is defined to include:

- 1-4 lead electroencephalogram (EEG)
- Electro-oculogram (EOG)
- Submental electromyogram (EMG)

Additional parameters of sleep include:

- Electrocardiogram (ECG)
- Airflow
- Ventilation and respiratory effort
- Gas exchange by oximetry, transcutaneous monitoring, or end tidal gas analysis
- Extremity muscle activity, motor activity-movement
- Extended electroencephalogram (EEG) monitoring
- Penile tumescence
- Gastroesophageal reflux
- Continuous blood pressure monitoring
- Snoring
- Body positions

ELECTROENCEPHALOGRAM (EEG)

Electroencephalogram (EEG) codes (95812-95829, 95950-95962) include tracing, interpretation, and report. For interpretation only, append modifier -26.

NERVE CONDUCTION STUDIES

Nerve conduction study codes (95900-95967) include three new codes added to the CPT book 2002, all of which describe Magnetoencephalography (MEG) recording and analysis. Evoked response (95920-95930) describes global services and includes tracing, interpretation and report. For interpretation only, append modifier -26. Codes 95925-95927 report bilateral studies. For unilateral studies append modifier -52.

EMG/NERVE CONDUCTION STUDIES

An EMG (95860-95875) and a nerve conduction study (95900-95904, 95934-95936) are frequently performed together. Codes for EMG studies are site specific. Nerve conduction studies should be reported for each nerve studied. F-wave studies are performed on upper extremities while H-reflex studies are performed on lower extremities. Modifier -51 should not be used when reporting nerve conduction studies (95900-95904).

NEUROSTIMULATORS, ANALYSIS - PROGRAMMING

Six codes report the analysis of simple and complex implanted neurostimulators pulse generator/transmitter systems (95970-95975). These devices send electric shocks to different sites to treat symptoms of various diseases, such as Parkinson's Disease.

A simple stimulator is capable of affecting three or fewer of the following conditions, while a complex neurostimulator is capable of affecting more than three:

- Pulse amplitude
- Pulse duration
- Pulse frequency
- Eight or more electrode contacts
- Cycling

- Stimulation train duration
- Train spacing
- Number of programs
- Number of channels
- Phase angle
- Alternating electrode polarities
- Configuration of wave form
- More than one clinical feature (e.g., rigidity, dyskinesia, and tremor

Code 95970 reports analysis of implanted neurostimulator pulse generator system, simple or complex, without reprogramming. All other codes report analysis with intraoperative or subsequent programming. The analysis of simple devices requiring reprogramming is reported with a single code 95971. The analysis of complex devices requiring reprogramming is reported based on time. Report 95972 or 95974 for the first hour and 95973 or 95975 for each additional 30 minutes.

Insertion, revision, and removal of neurostimulator pulse generators are reported using codes from the Surgery Section of CPT.

MOTION ANALYSIS

A new subsection added to the CPT book 2002 should be used to report motion analysis, defined as services performed as part of a major therapeutic or diagnostic decision making process. The services are performed in laboratories dedicated to motion analysis.

CENTRAL NERVOUS SYSTEM ASSESSMENTS/TESTS

Central nervous system assessment codes (96100-96117) combine several types of testing procedures to produce information about the cognitive function of a patient. Tests include cognitive processes, visual motor responses, and abstractive abilities. When these tests are performed, material generated should be formulated into a report.

HEALTH AND BEHAVIOR ASSESSMENT/INTERVENTION

A new section in the Medicine section of CPT is health and behavior assessment/intervention (96150-96155), which are procedures used to identify the psychological, behavioral, emotional, cognitive, and social factors important to the prevention, treatment, or management of physical health problems. The codes include health and behavior assessment as well as health and behavior intervention, of which the latter is reported in 15-minute increments of direct face-to-face contact with the individual, a group, or the family of the individual.

CHEMOTHERAPY ADMINISTRATION

Chemotherapy codes (96400-96549) are reported independently of E/M services provided during the same encounter or on the same day. Most individuals receiving chemotherapy services require a separately reportable evaluation and management service at the time of chemotherapy services.

Chemotherapy codes include preparation of the chemotherapy agent. However, the supply of chemotherapy agents should be reported with HCPCS Level II J-codes or with CPT code 96545.

Administration of other medications provided in conjunction with chemotherapy should be reported separately using 90780-90788. These include antibiotics, antiemetics, narcotics, analgesics, and steroidal and biological agents. Since codes 90780-90788 report only the administration of the medications, report the medication supplied with the appropriate HCPCS Level II J-code or with CPT code 99070.

Report special filter needles, infusion sets, and other chemotherapy supplies separately with HCPCS Level II A-codes or CPT code 99070. Indicate the exact drugs and supplies for payers who do not accept HCPCS Level II codes. Include invoices to answer questions regarding cost.

Chemotherapy codes are distinguished by at least three factors. First, different codes are provided for intravenous and intra-arterial injections. Regional (isolation) chemotherapy perfusion is reported with intra-arterial infusion codes. Placement of the intra-arterial catheter should be reported using the appropriate code from the cardiovascular surgery section (36620-36640). Second, separate codes are provided for infusion and push techniques. Report the code for each technique when both techniques are used. A final factor is the element of time for infusion techniques.

PHOTODYNAMIC THERAPY

These three codes (96567-96571) report photodynamic therapy either by external application of light to destroy malignancies or by endoscopic application of light that activates photosensitive drugs to destroy abnormal tissue.

SPECIAL DERMATOLOGICAL PROCEDURES

When dermatology treatments are performed with a separately identifiable E/M service, both may be reported. Dermatologic services are typically consultative, so any of the five levels of consultation (99241-99263) may be appropriate. Similarly, E/M levels of service appropriate to dermatologic illnesses should be coded.

PHYSICAL MEDICINE AND REHABILITATION

EVALUATION SERVICES

Codes 97001-97006 report evaluation and re-evaluation services for physical, occupational, and athletic therapy. Codes 97001, 97003, and 97005 indicate the initial evaluation service. Re-evaluation services should be reported with codes 97002, 97004, and 97006.

MODALITIES

The modality range is organized into two groups. The first group (97010-97028) describes supervised procedures that do not require direct (one-on-one) patient contact. The second group (97032-97039) requires constant attendance and direct (one-on-one) patient contact.

The description for all treatment modalities specifies application of a modality to one or more areas. In other words, when hot or cold packs are applied to the arm, leg, and neck, code 97010 should be reported once. However, when different modalities are used, such as 97010 that reports the application of hot or cold pack, 97014 that reports the application of electrical stimulation, and 97022 for whirlpool therapy, each is reported separately.

Time should be reported in 15-minute increments for treatment modalities requiring constant attendance. If more than 15 minutes are required (i.e., 30 minutes) report two units on the HCFA-1500 claim form. For less than 15 minutes, append the reduced service modifier -52 and adjust the usual cost of the code based on the time actually spent.

THERAPEUTIC PROCEDURES

Therapeutic procedures describe the application of clinical skills or services to improve function. These procedures require direct (one-on-one) patient contact. Some therapeutic procedures have a time component and should be reported once for each 15 minutes of treatment. Others do not have a time component and should be reported only once per visit. For work hardening/conditioning (97545-97546), report 97545 for the initial two hours and 97546 for each additional hour. Procedure 97546 is considered an "add on" procedure. "Add on" procedures are never reduced in value and modifier -51 multiple procedures should not be appended.

ACTIVE WOUND CARE MANAGEMENT

Codes 97601 and 97602 report procedures that promote healing. Since the codes involve selective and non-selective debridement techniques, do not report codes 11040-11044 from the Surgery Section in addition to the these codes.

TESTS AND MEASUREMENTS

Use 97703 and 97750 to report tests and measurement in 15-minute increments.

MEDICAL NUTRITION THERAPY

Three codes, 97802-97804, report medical nutrition therapy face-to-face with the patient, each 15 minutes (97802) or a face-to-face re-assessment and intervention, each 15 minutes (97803). Report 97804 for therapy involving two or more patients, each 30-minute period.

OSTEOPATHIC MANIPULATIVE TREATMENT

Codes 98925-98929 report inpatient or outpatient osteopathic manipulative treatment (OMT), which is a form of manual treatment applied by a physician to eliminate or alleviate somatic dysfunction and related disorders.

The number of body regions involved in the treatment differentiate the codes (i.e., head, cervical, thoracic, lumbar, sacral, pelvic, lower extremities, upper extremities, rib cage, and abdomen and viscera). OMT includes a component of E/M service to ascertain the effectiveness of the therapy and may be identified separately when:

- A physician diagnoses the condition requiring manipulative therapy and provides the therapy during the same visit.

- The condition requiring manipulative therapy fails to respond to the therapy or the condition significantly changes or intensifies and requires E/M services beyond the usual pre- and post-service work associated with the procedure.

- The physician treats a condition unrelated to the one requiring manipulative therapy during the same visit.

CHIROPRACTIC MANIPULATIVE TREATMENT

Chiropractic manipulative treatment (CMT), reported with codes 98940-98943, is a form of manual treatment performed to influence joint and neurophysical function. CMT codes include a premanipulation patient assessment. Evaluation and management services should not be reported separately unless the patient's condition requires a separately identifiable E/M service beyond the usual pre- and post-service work normally associated with the procedure.

CMT codes are reported by region. The five spinal regions are cervical (includes atlanto-occipital joint); thoracic (includes costovertebral and costotransverse joints); lumbar, sacral; and pelvic (includes sacro-iliac joint). The five extraspinal regions are defined as follows: head (including temporomandibular joint); lower extremities; upper extremities; rib cage, and abdomen.

SPECIAL SERVICES, PROCEDURES, AND REPORTS

Special services and reports (99000-99091) allow supplemental reporting for services adjunct to the basic services provided. To justify use of these codes, identify the medical necessity of special circumstances. Document the information clearly and completely in the patient's medical record.

Code 99024 reports a postoperative follow-up visit included in the global service period. Code 99025 reports an initial (new patient) visit when a starred (*) procedure constitutes the major service at that visit. Codes 99050-99058 identify emergency office calls and services provided after hours, on Sundays, or on holidays. Other codes in this category identify medical testimony, unusual travel requirements (e.g., escorting a patient on a trip of more than 10 miles), and educational services. Codes for transportation of specimens (99000-99001) should be reported only once per visit, regardless of the number of specimens. A new code added to this subsection (99091) reports the collection and interpretation of physiologic data, with instructions to report the code only once in a 30-day period.

ANESTHESIA

Qualifying circumstances for anesthesia (99100-99140) are reported in addition to the primary anesthesia code when particularly difficult circumstances affect the regular service. Sedation with or without analgesia (conscious sedation) (99141-99142) reports a controlled state of conscious sedation while maintaining the patient's airway, reflexes, and ability to respond to stimulation or verbal commands. The codes include performance and documentation of pre- and post-sedation evaluations of the patient, administration of the sedative, and monitoring of cardiorespiratory function. The use of the codes requires an independent trained observer to assist the physician in monitoring the patient's level of consciousness and physiological status.

OTHER SERVICES AND PROCEDURES

The final series of codes (99170-99199) report services such as anogenital examinations in cases of suspected child sexual abuse, medical intervention and observation of patient following suspected cases of poisoning, and therapeutic phlebotomy.

HOME HEALTH PROCEDURES AND SERVICES

New to the CPT book 2002 is the range of codes (99500-99539) that report various home health procedures and services that are to be used by non-physician health care providers. The codes report services delivered in the patient's home, which includes a private home, an assisted living apartment, a group home, a custodial care facility, or a school.

HOME INFUSION PROCEDURES

The home infusion procedures (99551-99569) are new to the CPT book 2002 and should be used to report the home administration of a variety of drugs and medication. Each code includes a home visit by the health care provider and all solutions, equipment, and supplies (excluding the drug or medication) required for therapy in a 24-hour period. These codes do not include the patient's self-administration of the medication.

IMMUNE GLOBULINS

CPT codes 90281-90399 report the immune globulin product only. Consult CPT codes 90780-90784 for administration of immune globulin.

⊘ **90281** Immune globulin (IG), human, for intramuscular use

⊘ **90283** Immune globulin (IGIV), human, for intravenous use

⊘ **90287** Botulinum antitoxin, equine, any route

⊘ **90288** Botulism immune globulin, human, for intravenous use

⊘ **90291** Cytomegalovirus immune globulin (CMV-IGIV), human, for intravenous use

⊘ **90296** Diphtheria antitoxin, equine, any route

⊘ **90371** Hepatitis B immune globulin (HBIG), human, for intramuscular use

⊘ **90375** Rabies immune globulin (RIG), human, for intramuscular use and/or subcutaneous use

⊘ **90376** Rabies immune globulin, heat-treated (RIG-HT), human, for intramuscular and/or subcutaneous use

⊘ **90378** Respiratory syncytial virus immune globulin (RSV-IgIM), for intramuscular use, 50 mg, each

⊘ **90379** Respiratory syncytial virus immune globulin (RSV-IGIV), human, for intravenous use

⊘ **90384** Rho(D) immune globulin (RhIG), human, full-dose, for intramuscular use

⊘ **90385** Rho(D) immune globulin (RhIG), human, mini-dose, for intramuscular use

⊘ **90386** Rho(D) immune globulin (RhIGIV), human, for intravenous use

⊘ **90389** Tetanus immune globulin (TIG), human, for intramuscular use

⊘ **90393** Vaccinia immune globulin, human, for intramuscular use

⊘ **90396** Varicella-zoster immune globulin, human, for intramuscular use

⊘ **90399** Unlisted immune globulin

IMMUNIZATION ADMINISTRATION FOR VACCINES/TOXOIDS

When a significantly separately identifiable Evaluation and Management service is performed at the same visit it should be reported in addition to vaccine and toxoid administration.

▲ **90471** Immunization administration (includes percutaneous, intradermal, subcutaneous, intramuscular and jet injections); one vaccine (single or combination vaccine/toxoid)

If allergy tests are conducted, consult CPT codes 95004 et seq. For skin testing of bacterial, viral, fungal, extracts, consult CPT codes 86485-86586. If therapeutic or diagnostic injections are administered, consult CPT codes 90782-90799.

+ **90472** each additional vaccine (single or combination vaccine/toxoid) (List separately in addition to code for primary procedure)

Note that 90472 is an add-on code and must be used in conjunction with 90471. If immune globulins are administered, use CPT codes 90780-90784 and consult CPT codes 90281-90399. For intravesical administration of BCG vaccine, use CPT code 51720, and consult CPT code 90586.

● **90473** Immunization administration by intranasal or oral route; one vaccine (single or combination vaccine/toxoid)

● + **90474** each additional vaccine (single or combination vaccine/toxoid) (List separately in addition to code for primary procedure)

Note that 90474 is an add-on code and must be used in conjunction with code 90473.

VACCINES, TOXOIDS

CPT codes 90476-90748 report the vaccine or toxoid product only. Consult CPT codes 90471-90472 for administration of vaccine or toxoid.

⊘ **90476** Adenovirus vaccine, type 4, live, for oral use

⊘ **90477** Adenovirus vaccine, type 7, live, for oral use

⊘ **90581** Anthrax vaccine, for subcutaneous use

⊘ **90585** Bacillus Calmette-Guerin vaccine (BCG) for tuberculosis, live, for percutaneous use

⊘ **90586** Bacillus Calmette-Guerin vaccine (BCG) for bladder cancer, live, for intravesical use

⊘ **90632** Hepatitis A vaccine, adult dosage, for intramuscular use

⊘ **90633** Hepatitis A vaccine, pediatric/adolescent dosage-2 dose schedule, for intramuscular use

⊘ **90634** Hepatitis A vaccine, pediatric/adolescent dosage-3 dose schedule, for intramuscular use

⊘ **90636** Hepatitis A and hepatitis B vaccine (HepA-HepB), adult dosage, for intramuscular use

⊘ **90645** Hemophilus influenza b vaccine (Hib), HbOC conjugate (4 dose schedule), for intramuscular use

⊘ **90646** Hemophilus influenza b vaccine (Hib), PRP-D conjugate, for booster use only, intramuscular use

⊘ **90647** Hemophilus influenza b vaccine (Hib), PRP-OMP conjugate (3 dose schedule), for intramuscular use

⊘ **90648** Hemophilus influenza b vaccine (Hib), PRP-T conjugate (4 dose schedule), for intramuscular use

⊘ **90657** Influenza virus vaccine, split virus, 6-35 months dosage, for intramuscular or jet injection use

⊘ **90658** Influenza virus vaccine, split virus, 3 years and above dosage, for intramuscular or jet injection use

⊘ **90659** Influenza virus vaccine, whole virus, for intramuscular or jet injection use

⊘ **90660** Influenza virus vaccine, live, for intranasal use

⊘ **90665** Lyme disease vaccine, adult dosage, for intramuscular use

HCPCS code 90669 is not approved by the Food and Drug Administration (FDA). Except under specific circumstances, Medicare does not cover drugs that are not FDA approved.

90669 Pneumococcal conjugate vaccine, polyvalent, for children under five years, for intramuscular use

⊘ **90675** Rabies vaccine, for intramuscular use

⊘ **90676** Rabies vaccine, for intradermal use

⊘ **90680** Rotavirus vaccine, tetravalent, live, for oral use

⊘ **90690** Typhoid vaccine, live, oral

⊘ **90691** Typhoid vaccine, Vi capsular polysaccharide (ViCPs), for intramuscular use

⊘ **90692** Typhoid vaccine, heat- and phenol-inactivated (H-P), for subcutaneous or intradermal use

⊘ **90693** Typhoid vaccine, acetone-killed, dried (AKD), for subcutaneous or jet injection use (U.S. military)

⊘ **90700** Diphtheria, tetanus toxoids, and acellular pertussis vaccine (DTaP), for intramuscular use

⊘ **90701** Diphtheria, tetanus toxoids, and whole cell pertussis vaccine (DTP), for intramuscular use

⊘   90702   Diphtheria and tetanus toxoids (DT) adsorbed for use in individuals younger than seven years, for intramuscular use

⊘   90703   Tetanus toxoid adsorbed, for intramuscular or jet injection use

⊘   90704   Mumps virus vaccine, live, for subcutaneous or jet injection use

⊘   90705   Measles virus vaccine, live, for subcutaneous or jet injection use

⊘   90706   Rubella virus vaccine, live, for subcutaneous or jet injection use

⊘   90707   Measles, mumps and rubella virus vaccine (MMR), live, for subcutaneous or jet injection use

⊘   90708   Measles and rubella virus vaccine, live, for subcutaneous or jet injection use

⊘   90709   Rubella and mumps virus vaccine, live, for subcutaneous use

⊘   90710   Measles, mumps, rubella, and varicella vaccine (MMRV), live, for subcutaneous use

⊘   90712   Poliovirus vaccine, (any type(s)) (OPV), live, for oral use

⊘   90713   Poliovirus vaccine, inactivated, (IPV), for subcutaneous use

⊘   90716   Varicella virus vaccine, live, for subcutaneous use

⊘   90717   Yellow fever vaccine, live, for subcutaneous use

⊘   90718   Tetanus and diphtheria toxoids (Td) adsorbed for use in individuals seven years or older, for intramuscular or jet injection

⊘   90719   Diphtheria toxoid, for intramuscular use

⊘   90720   Diphtheria, tetanus toxoids, and whole cell pertussis vaccine and Hemophilus influenza B vaccine (DTP-Hib), for intramuscular use

⊘   90721   Diphtheria, tetanus toxoids, and acellular pertussis vaccine and Hemophilus influenza B vaccine (DtaP-Hib), for intramuscular use

⊘   90723   Diphtheria, tetanus toxoids, acellular pertussis vaccine, Hepatitis B, and poliovirus vaccine, inactivated (DtaP-HepB-IPV), for intramuscular use

⊘   90725   Cholera vaccine for injectable use

⊘   90727   Plague vaccine, for intramuscular or jet injection use

▲ ⊘   90732   Pneumococcal polysaccharide vaccine, 23-valent, adult or immunosuppressed patient dosage, for use in individuals 2 years or older, for subcutaneous or intramuscular use

⊘   90733   Meningococcal polysaccharide vaccine (any group(s)), for subcutaneous or jet injection use

⊘   90735   Japanese encephalitis virus vaccine, for subcutaneous use

⊘   90740   Hepatitis B vaccine, dialysis or immunosuppressed patient dosage (3 dose schedule), for intramuscular use

⊘   90743   Hepatitis B vaccine, adolescent (2 dose schedule), for intramuscular use

⊘   90744   Hepatitis B vaccine, pediatric/adolescent dosage (3 dose schedule), for intramuscular use

⊘   90746   Hepatitis B vaccine, adult dosage, for intramuscular use

⊘   90747   Hepatitis B vaccine, dialysis or immunosuppressed patient dosage (4 dose schedule), for intramuscular use

⊘   90748   Hepatitis B and Hemophilus influenza b vaccine (HepB-Hib), for intramuscular use

⊘   90749   Unlisted vaccine/toxoid

THERAPEUTIC OR DIAGNOSTIC INFUSIONS (EXCLUDES CHEMOTHERAPY)

The physician's presence is required during the infusion to report 90780-90781.

▲   90780   Intravenous infusion for therapy/diagnosis, administered by physician or under direct supervision of physician; up to one hour

+   90781   each additional hour, up to eight (8) hours (List separately in addition to code for primary procedure)

Note that 90781 is an add-on code and must be used in conjunction with 90780.

THERAPEUTIC, PROPHYLACTIC OR DIAGNOSTIC INJECTIONS

90782   Therapeutic, prophylactic or diagnostic injection (specify material injected); subcutaneous or intramuscular

For allergen immunotherapy injections see 95115-95117

If vaccines/toxoids are administered, consult CPT codes 90471-90472.

90783   intra-arterial

For allergen immunotherapy injections see 95115-95117

90784   intravenous

90788   Intramuscular injection of antibiotic (specify)

90799   Unlisted therapeutic, prophylactic or diagnostic injection

If allergy immunizations are needed, consult CPT code 95004 and subsequent codes.

PSYCHIATRY

PSYCHIATRIC DIAGNOSTIC OR EVALUATIVE INTERVIEW PROCEDURES

90801   Psychiatric diagnostic interview examination

90802   Interactive psychiatric diagnostic interview examination using play equipment, physical devices, language interpreter, or other mechanisms of communication

PSYCHIATRIC THERAPEUTIC PROCEDURES

OFFICE OR OTHER OUTPATIENT FACILITY, INSIGHT ORIENTED, BEHAVIOR MODIFYING AND/OR SUPPORTIVE PSYCHOTHERAPY

90804   Individual psychotherapy, insight oriented, behavior modifying and/or supportive, in an office or outpatient facility, approximately 20 to 30 minutes face-to-face with the patient;

90805   with medical evaluation and management services

90806   Individual psychotherapy, insight oriented, behavior modifying and/or supportive, in an office or outpatient facility, approximately 45 to 50 minutes face-to-face with the patient;

90807   with medical evaluation and management services

90808   Individual psychotherapy, insight oriented, behavior modifying and/or supportive, in an office or outpatient facility, approximately 75 to 80 minutes face-to-face with the patient;

90809   with medical evaluation and management services

⊡ CCI Comprehensive Code   🔟 Bilateral Procedure   ✚ CPT Add-on Code   ⊘ Modifier -51 Exempt Code   ● New Code   ▲ Revised Code

Ⓜ Maternity   Ⓝ Newborn   Ⓟ Pediatric   N/P Newborn/Pediatric

OFFICE OR OTHER OUTPATIENT FACILITY, INTERACTIVE PSYCHOTHERAPY

90810 Individual psychotherapy, interactive, using play equipment, physical devices, language interpreter, or other mechanisms of nonverbal communication, in an office or outpatient facility, approximately 20 to 30 minutes face-to-face with the patient; [80] [↵]

90811 with medical evaluation and management services [80] [↵]

90812 Individual psychotherapy, interactive, using play equipment, physical devices, language interpreter, or other mechanisms of nonverbal communication, in an office or outpatient facility, approximately 45 to 50 minutes face-to-face with the patient; [80] [↵]

90813 with medical evaluation and management services [80] [↵]

90814 Individual psychotherapy, interactive, using play equipment, physical devices, language interpreter, or other mechanisms of nonverbal communication, in an office or outpatient facility, approximately 75 to 80 minutes face-to-face with the patient; [80] [↵]

90815 with medical evaluation and management services [80] [↵]

INPATIENT HOSPITAL, PARTIAL HOSPITAL OR RESIDENTIAL CARE FACILITY, INSIGHT ORIENTED, BEHAVIOR MODIFYING AND/OR SUPPORTIVE PSYCHOTHERAPY

90816 Individual psychotherapy, insight oriented, behavior modifying and/or supportive, in an inpatient hospital, partial hospital or residential care setting, approximately 20 to 30 minutes face-to-face with the patient; [80] [↵]

90817 with medical evaluation and management services [80] [↵]

90818 Individual psychotherapy, insight oriented, behavior modifying and/or supportive, in an inpatient hospital, partial hospital or residential care setting, approximately 45 to 50 minutes face-to-face with the patient; [80] [↵]

90819 with medical evaluation and management services [80] [↵]

90821 Individual psychotherapy, insight oriented, behavior modifying and/or supportive, in an inpatient hospital, partial hospital or residential care setting, approximately 75 to 80 minutes face-to-face with the patient; [80] [↵]

90822 with medical evaluation and management services [80] [↵]

INPATIENT HOSPITAL, PARTIAL HOSPITAL OR RESIDENTIAL CARE FACILITY, INTERACTIVE PSYCHOTHERAPY

90823 Individual psychotherapy, interactive, using play equipment, physical devices, language interpreter, or other mechanisms of nonverbal communication, in an inpatient hospital, partial hospital or residential care setting, approximately 20 to 30 minutes face-to-face with the patient; [80] [↵]

90824 with medical evaluation and management services [80] [↵]

90826 Individual psychotherapy, interactive, using play equipment, physical devices, language interpreter, or other mechanisms of nonverbal communication, in an inpatient hospital, partial hospital or residential care setting, approximately 45 to 50 minutes face-to-face with the patient; [80] [↵]

90827 with medical evaluation and management services [80] [↵]

90828 Individual psychotherapy, interactive, using play equipment, physical devices, language interpreter, or other mechanisms of nonverbal communication, in an inpatient hospital, partial hospital or residential care setting, approximately 75 to 80 minutes face-to-face with the patient; [80] [↵]

90829 with medical evaluation and management services [80] [↵]

OTHER PSYCHOTHERAPY

90845 Psychoanalysis [80] [↵]

90846 Family psychotherapy (without the patient present) [80]

90847 Family psychotherapy (conjoint psychotherapy) (with patient present) [80] [↵]

90849 Multiple-family group psychotherapy [80] [↵]

90853 Group psychotherapy (other than of a multiple-family group) [80] [↵]

90857 Interactive group psychotherapy [80] [↵]

OTHER PSYCHIATRIC SERVICES OR PROCEDURES

90862 Pharmacologic management, including prescription, use, and review of medication with no more than minimal medical psychotherapy [80] [↵]

90865 Narcosynthesis for psychiatric diagnostic and therapeutic purposes (eg, sodium amobarbital (Amytal) interview) [80] [↵]

90870 Electroconvulsive therapy (includes necessary monitoring); single seizure [80] [↵]

90871 multiple seizures, per day [80] [↵]

90875 Individual psychophysiological therapy incorporating biofeedback training by any modality (face-to-face with the patient), with psychotherapy (eg, insight oriented, behavior modifying or supportive psychotherapy); approximately 20-30 minutes

90876 approximately 45-50 minutes

90880 Hypnotherapy [80] [↵]

90882 Environmental intervention for medical management purposes on a psychiatric patient's behalf with agencies, employers, or institutions

90885 Psychiatric evaluation of hospital records, other psychiatric reports, psychometric and/or projective tests, and other accumulated data for medical diagnostic purposes

CIM 35-14 CONSULTATIONS WITH A BENEFICIARY'S FAMILY AND ASSOCIATES

In certain types of medical conditions, including when a patient is withdrawn and uncommunicative due to a mental disorder or comatose, the physician may contact relatives and close associates to secure background information to assist in diagnosis and treatment planning. If the beneficiary is not an inpatient of a hospital, Part B reimbursement is subject to the special limitation on payments for physicians' services in connection with mental, psychoneurotic, and personality disorders. Family counseling services are covered when the primary purpose of such counseling is the treatment of the patient's condition.

MCM 2470. OUTPATIENT MENTAL HEALTH TREATMENT LIMITATION

While beneficiary is not an inpatient of a hospital at the time expenses are incurred, the Part B deductible and payment are limited to 62.5 percent of the Medicare allowed amount for those services. This limitation is called the outpatient mental health treatment limitation. Expenses for diagnostic services (e.g., psychiatric testing and evaluation to diagnose the patient's illness) are not subject to this limitation.

Do not apply the limitation to tests and evaluations performed to establish or confirm the patient's diagnosis. Diagnostic services include psychiatric or psychological tests and interpretations, diagnostic consultations, and initial evaluations. In the rare cases where a practitioner's diagnostic services take more than one visit, do not apply the limitation to the additional visits. However, when a practitioner bills for more than one visit for professional diagnostic services, request documentation to justify the reason for more than one diagnostic visit.

90887 Interpretation or explanation of results of psychiatric, other medical examinations and procedures, or other accumulated data to family or other responsible persons, or advising them how to assist patient

90889 Preparation of report of patient's psychiatric status, history, treatment, or progress (other than for legal or consultative purposes) for other physicians, agencies, or insurance carriers

90899 Unlisted psychiatric service or procedure ⬛80

BIOFEEDBACK

If psychophysiological therapy is performed incorporating biofeedback training, consult CPT codes 90875 and 90876.

90901 Biofeedback training by any modality ⬛80 ⬛

90911 Biofeedback training, perineal muscles, anorectal or urethral sphincter, including EMG and/or manometry ⬛80 ⬛

DIALYSIS

END STAGE RENAL DISEASE SERVICES

For dialysis procedures provided during an inpatient hospital stay, consult CPT codes 90945-90947. For ESRD related services during an inpatient hospital stay, consult the appropriate Evaluation and Management codes.

Report CPT codes 90918-90921 one time per month for services performed in an outpatient setting. Do not use these codes if a hospitalization occurred during the month.

These procedures do not include dialysis treatment or services provided to the patient that are non-ESRD related. Report separately any non-ERSD related Evaluation and Management services that cannot be performed during the dialysis session.

CIM 55-3 ULTRAFILTRATION MONITOR

Medicare covers ultrafiltration and ultrafiltration monitoring as a component of hemodialysis in maintaining the well-being of ESRD patients. The Ultrafiltration Monitor is covered when used to calculate fluid rates for recipients presenting difficult fluid management problems. Coverage is determined on a case-by-case basis.

MCM 15350. DIALYSIS SERVICES (CODES 90935-90999)

A. ESRD Monthly Capitation Payments.—Effective January 1, 1995, monthly capitation payments are made under the physician fee schedule. For their adult patients, physicians may bill either the monthly code (CPT code 90921) or the daily code (CPT code 90925) with units that represent the number of days in a single month, but may not bill both.

To bill for a month of services for pediatric patients, providers should bill the appropriate monthly code (CPT codes 90918, 90919, or 90920). To bill for less than a month of service, providers bill the appropriate daily code (CPT codes 90922-90925) and units that represent the number of days. Providers may bill either the monthly code or the daily code, but not both. Since billing is done at the conclusion of the month, the patient's age at the end of month is the age of the patient for billing purposes.

B. Inpatient Dialysis On Same Date As Evaluation and Management.— Payment for certain evaluation and management services (CPT codes 99231 through 99233, subsequent hospital visits, and CPT codes 99261 through 99263, follow-up inpatient consultations) is considered bundled into the payment for inpatient dialysis (CPT codes 90935 through 90947) when both are performed on the same day by the same physician for the same beneficiary. Do not pay a physician for both dialysis and a subsequent hospital visit or a follow-up inpatient consultation on the same date of service. If both are billed, pay the dialysis service and deny the evaluation and management service.

Separate payment may be made for an initial hospital visit (CPT codes 99221 through 99223), an initial inpatient consultation (CPT codes 99251 through 99255), and a hospital discharge service (CPT codes 99238 and 99239) when billed for the same date as an inpatient dialysis service. These services may be billed with a modifier -25 to indicate that they are significant and identifiable services. Payment is not allowed for more than one inpatient dialysis service per day.

90918 End stage renal disease (ESRD) related services per full month; for patients under 2 years of age to include monitoring for the adequacy of nutrition, assessment of growth and development, and counseling of parents ⬛N 80

90919 for patients between two and eleven years of age to include monitoring for the adequacy of nutrition, assessment of growth and development, and counseling of parents ⬛P 80

90920 for patients between twelve and nineteen years of age to include monitoring for the adequacy of nutrition, assessment of growth and development, and counseling of parents ⬛P 80

90921 for patients twenty years of age and over ⬛80

For dialysis procedures provided during an inpatient hospital stay, consult CPT codes 90945-90947. For ESRD related services during an inpatient hospital stay, consult the appropriate Evaluation and Management codes.

Report CPT codes 90922-90925 once per day for the days that remain in a month ESRD related services, before or after an in patient hospital stay. Report separately any non-ERSD related Evaluation and Management services that cannot be performed during the dialysis session.

90922 End stage renal disease (ESRD) related services (less than full month), per day; for patients under two years of age ⬛N 80

90923 for patients between two and eleven years of age ⬛P 80 ⬛

90924 for patients between twelve and nineteen years of age ⬛P 80

90925 for patients twenty years of age and over ⬛80 ⬛

HEMODIALYSIS

Use CPT codes 90935-90937 for inpatient ERSD and non-ESRD procedures or outpatient non-ESRD dialysis services. Use CPT codes 90935-90937 to report the hemodialysis procedure and any Evaluation and Management service that is related to the patient's renal disorder provided on the day of the hemodialysis procedure.

For an unrelated Evaluation and Management service preformed on the same day as hemodialysis, consult the appropriate Evaluation and Management code and append modifier -25 or code 09925.

For home visit hemodialysis services performed by a non-physician health care professional, use 99512.

If cannula declotting is performed, consult CPT codes 36831, 36833, 36860, and 86861. If a thrombolytic agent declots an implanted vascular access device or catheter, consult CPT code 36550. If the physician is in attendance for a prolonged period of time, consult CPT codes 99354-99360.

When collecting a blood specimen from a partially or completely implantable venous access device, consult CPT code 36540.

90935 Hemodialysis procedure with single physician evaluation ⬛80 ⬛

90937 Hemodialysis procedure requiring repeated evaluation(s) with or without substantial revision of dialysis prescription ⬛80 ⬛

● **90939** Hemodialysis access flow study to determine blood flow in grafts and arteriovenous fistulae by an indicator dilution method, hook-up; transcutaneous measurement and disconnection

---

⬛ CCI Comprehensive Code   ⬛50 Bilateral Procedure   ✚ CPT Add-on Code   ⃠ Modifier -51 Exempt Code   ● New Code   ▲ Revised Code

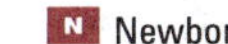 Maternity   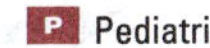 Newborn   ⬛P Pediatric   ⬛N/P Newborn/Pediatric

● **90940** **Hemodialysis access flow study to determine blood flow in grafts and arteriovenous fistulae by an indicator dilution method, hook-up; measurement and disconnection**

> Consult CPT code 93990 to report duplex scan of hemodialysis access.

MISCELLANEOUS DIALYSIS PROCEDURES

Use CPT codes 90945-90947 to report other dialysis procedures and any Evaluation and Management service that is related to the patient's renal disorder provided on the day of the dialysis procedure. For an unrelated Evaluation and Management service preformed on the same day as the dialysis procedure, consult the appropriate Evaluation and Management code and append modifier -25 or code 09925.

If the physician is in attendance for a prolonged period of time, consult CPT codes 99354-99360. If an intraperitoneal cannula or catheter is inserted, consult CPT codes 49420 and 49421.

▲ **90945** **Dialysis procedure other than hemodialysis (eg, peritoneal dialysis, hemofiltration, or other continuous renal replacement therapies), with single physician evaluation** 80 ⬏

> For home infusion of pertoneal dialysis, use 99559.

▲ **90947** **Dialysis procedure other than hemodialysis (eg, peritoneal dialysis, hemofiltration, or other continuous renal replacement therapies) requiring repeated physician evaluations, with or without substantial revision of dialysis prescription** 80 ⬏

90989 **Dialysis training, patient, including helper where applicable, any mode, completed course**

90993 **Dialysis training, patient, including helper where applicable, any mode, course not completed, per training session**

90997 **Hemoperfusion (eg, with activated charcoal or resin)**

90999 **Unlisted dialysis procedure, inpatient or outpatient** 80

GASTROENTEROLOGY

If duodenal intubation and aspiration are performed, consult CPT codes 89100-89105. If gastrointestinal radiologic procedures are performed, consult CPT codes 74210-74363. If esophagoscopy procedures are performed, consult CPT codes 43200-43228; upper GI endoscopy 43234-43259; endoscopy, small bowel and stomal 44360-44393; proctosigmoidoscopy 45300-45321; sigmoidoscopy 45330-45339; colonoscopy 45355-45385; and anoscopy 46600-46615.

91000 **Esophageal intubation and collection of washings for cytology, including preparation of specimens (separate procedure)** 80

CIM 50-25 ESOPHAGEAL MANOMETRY

Esophageal manometry is covered under Medicare where it is determined to be reasonable and necessary for the individual patient. The major use of esophageal manometry is to measure pressure within the esophagus to assist in the diagnosis of esophageal pathology including aperistalsis, spasm, achalasia, esophagitis, esophageal ulcer, esophageal congenital webs, diverticuli, scleroderma, hiatus hernia, congenital cysts, benign and malignant tumors, hypermobility, hypomobility, and extrinsic lesions.

91010 **Esophageal motility (manometric study of the esophagus and/or gastroesophageal junction) study;** 80 ⬏

91011 **with mecholyl or similar stimulant** 80 ⬏

91012 **with acid perfusion studies** 80 ⬏

91020 **Gastric motility (manometric) studies** 80 ⬏

91030 **Esophagus, acid perfusion (Bernstein) test for esophagitis** 80 ⬏

91032 **Esophagus, acid reflux test, with intraluminal pH electrode for detection of gastroesophageal reflux;** 80 ⬏

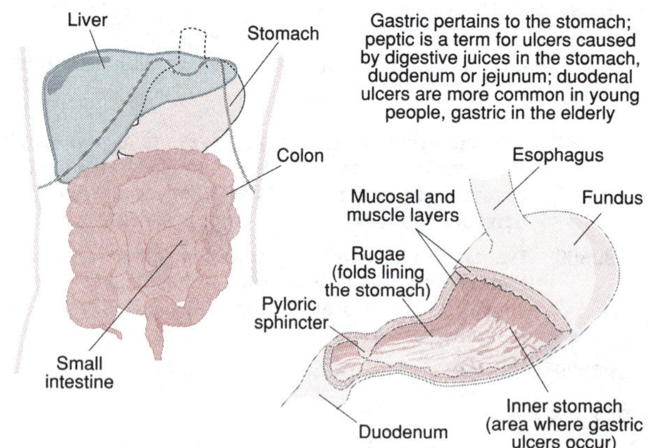

CIM 35-83 24-HOUR AMBULATORY ESOPHAGEAL PH MONITORING

Medicare covers 24-hour ambulatory pH monitoring for patients who are suspected of having gastric reflux, if the patient presents diagnostic problems associated with atypical symptoms or symptoms are suggestive of reflux, though conventional tests have not confirmed the presence of reflux.

91033 **prolonged recording** 80 ⬏

91052 **Gastric analysis test with injection of stimulant of gastric secretion (eg, histamine, insulin, pentagastrin, calcium and secretin)** 80 ⬏

> If the stomach is biopsied by capsule, peroral, or via tube, one or more specimens, consult CPT code 43600. If gastric laboratory procedures are performed, consult also CPT codes 89130-89141.

91055 **Gastric intubation, washings, and preparing slides for cytology (separate procedure)** 80 ⬏

> If therapeutic gastric lavage is performed, consult CPT code 91105.

> **Rehfuss' test**

91060 **Gastric saline load test** 80 ⬏

> If the small intestine is biopsied by capsule, peroral, or via tube (one or more specimens), consult CPT code 44100.

CIM 50-51 DIAGNOSTIC BREATH ANALYSES

Medicare covers lactose breath hydrogen to detect lactose malabsorption in gastrointestinal diseases. Medicare does not cover:

- Lactulose breath hydrogen for diagnosing small bowel bacterial overgrowth and measuring small bowel transit time
- l3CO₂ for diagnosing bile acid malabsorption
- 13CO₂ for diagnosing fat malabsorption

91065 **Breath hydrogen test (eg, for detection of lactase deficiency)** 80 ⬏

91100 **Intestinal bleeding tube, passage, positioning and monitoring** 80 ⬏

91105 **Gastric intubation, and aspiration or lavage for treatment (eg, for ingested poisons)** 80 ⬏

> If a cholangiography is performed, consult CPT codes 47500 and 74320. If abdominal paracentesis is performed, consult CPT codes 49080 and 49081; with instillation of medication, consult CPT codes 96440 and 96445. If peritoneoscopy is performed, consult CPT code 49320; with biopsy, consult CPT code 49321. If peritoneoscopy and guided transhepatic cholangiography is performed, consult CPT code 47560; with biopsy, consult CPT code 47561. If splenoportography is performed, consult CPT codes 38200 and 75810.

> If gastric intubation is performed as part of critical care services (99291-99292) do not report separately.

| | 91122 | Anorectal manometry | 80 |
| • | 91123 | Pulsed irrigation of fecal impaction | |

GASTRIC PHYSIOLOGY

•	91132	Electrogastrography, diagnostic, transcutaneous;	80
•	91133	with provocative testing	80
	91299	Unlisted diagnostic gastroenterology procedure	80

OPHTHALMOLOGY

Consult the glossary for more terms and definitions.

If surgical procedures are performed, consult Eye and Ocular Adnexa in the Surgery section of CPT (65091 and subsequent codes).

GENERAL OPHTHALMOLOGICAL SERVICES

NEW PATIENT

| 92002 | Ophthalmological services: medical examination and evaluation with initiation of diagnostic and treatment program; intermediate, new patient | 80 |
| 92004 | comprehensive, new patient, one or more visits | 80 |

ESTABLISHED PATIENT

| 92012 | Ophthalmological services: medical examination and evaluation, with initiation or continuation of diagnostic and treatment program; intermediate, established patient | 80 |
| 92014 | comprehensive, established patient, one or more visits | 80 |

SPECIAL OPHTHALMOLOGICAL SERVICES

If surgical procedures are performed, consult Eye and Ocular Adnexa in the Surgery section of CPT (65091 and subsequent codes).

OPHTHALMOSCOPY

92015	Determination of refractive state	
92018	Ophthalmological examination and evaluation, under general anesthesia, with or without manipulation of globe for passive range of motion or other manipulation to facilitate diagnostic examination; complete	80
92019	limited	80
92020	Gonioscopy (separate procedure)	80
	If gonioscopy is performed under general anesthesia, consult CPT code 92018.	
92060	Sensorimotor examination with multiple measurements of ocular deviation (eg, restrictive or paretic muscle with diplopia) with interpretation and report (separate procedure)	80

OTHER SPECIALIZED SERVICES

| 92065 | Orthoptic and/or pleoptic training, with continuing medical direction and evaluation | 80 |
| 92070 | Fitting of contact lens for treatment of disease, including supply of lens | 80 |

CIM 50-49 COMPUTER ENHANCED PERIMETRY

Medicare covers computer enhanced perimetry when used in assessing visual fields in patients with glaucoma or other neuropathologic defects.

| 92081 | Visual field examination, unilateral or bilateral, with interpretation and report; limited examination (eg, tangent screen, Autoplot, arc perimeter, or single stimulus level automated test, such as Octopus 3 or 7 equivalent) | 80 |

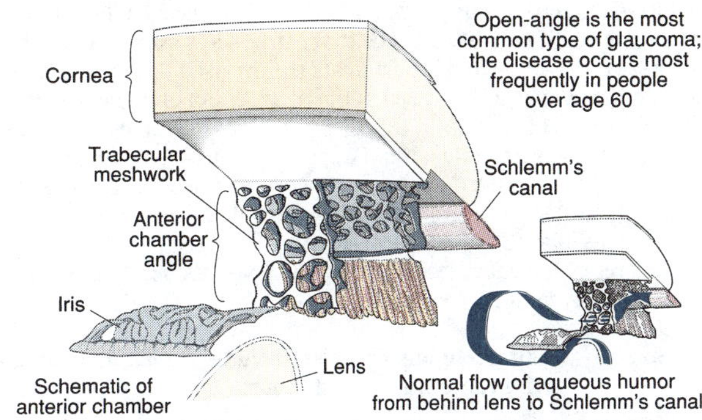

Glaucoma is caused by excessive intraocular pressure and abnormal accumulation of aqueous humor in the anterior chamber of the eye; pressure reduces blood supply to the optic nerve and causes nerve damage

| 92082 | intermediate examination (eg, at least 2 isopters on Goldmann perimeter, or semiquantitative, automated suprathreshold screening program, Humphrey suprathreshold automatic diagnostic test, Octopus program 33) | 80 |
| 92083 | extended examination (eg, Goldmann visual fields with at least 3 isopters plotted and static determination within the central 30 degrees, or quantitative, automated threshold perimetry, Octopus programs G-1, 32 or 42, Humphrey visual field analyzer full threshold programs 30-2, 24-2, or 30/60-2) | 80 |

Note that gross visual field testing (e.g., confrontation testing) is a part of general ophthalmological services and is not reported separately.

| 92100 | Serial tonometry (separate procedure) with multiple measurements of intraocular pressure over an extended time period with interpretation and report, same day (eg, diurnal curve or medical treatment of acute elevation of intraocular pressure) | 80 |

If surgical procedures are performed, consult Eye and Ocular Adnexa in the Surgery section of CPT (65091 and subsequent codes).

92120	Tonography with interpretation and report, recording indentation tonometer method or perilimbal suction method	80
92130	Tonography with water provocation	80
92135	Scanning computerized ophthalmic diagnostic imaging (eg, scanning laser) with interpretation and report, unilateral	
• 92136	Ophthalmic biometry by partial coherence interferometry with intraocular lens power calculation	
92140	Provocative tests for glaucoma, with interpretation and report, without tonography	80

OPHTHALMOSCOPY

Routine ophthalmoscopy is considered part of special or general ophthalmologic services when indicated and therefore not reported separately.

92225	Ophthalmoscopy, extended, with retinal drawing (eg, for retinal detachment, melanoma), with interpretation and report; initial	80
92226	subsequent	80
92230	Fluorescein angioscopy with interpretation and report	80

CIM 35-100 PHOTODYNAMIC THERAPY

Photodynamic therapy is a medical procedure that involves the infusion of a photosensitive (light-activated) drug with a very specific absorption peak. Once introduced to the body, the drug accumulates and is retained in diseased tissue to a greater degree than in normal tissue. Infusion is followed by the

---

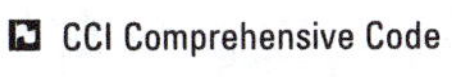 CCI Comprehensive Code   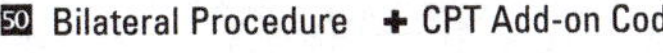 Bilateral Procedure   + CPT Add-on Code   ⊘ Modifier -51 Exempt Code   ● New Code   ▲ Revised Code

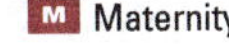 Maternity   **N** Newborn   **P** Pediatric   **N/P** Newborn/Pediatric

targeted irradiation of this tissue with a non-thermal laser, calibrated to emit light at a wavelength that corresponds to the drug's absorption peak. The drug then becomes active and locally treats the diseased tissue. Ocular photodynamic therapy (OPT) is used in the treatment of ophthalmologic diseases. Effective July 1, 2001, OPT (CPT code 67221) is only covered when used in conjunction with verteporfin. For patients with age-related macular degeneration, OPT is only covered with a diagnosis of neovascular age-related macular degeneration (ICD-9-CM 362.52) with predominately classic subfoveal choroidal neovascular (CNV) lesions (where the area of classic CNV occupies = 50% of the area of the entire lesion) at the initial visit as determined by a fluorescein angiogram (CPT code 92235).

92235   **Fluorescein angiography (includes multiframe imaging) with interpretation and report** 80

92240   **Indocyanine-green angiography (includes multiframe imaging) with interpretation and report)** 80

CIM 35-39 INTRAOCULAR PHOTOGRAPHY

Intraocular photography is covered when used by an ophthalmologist for the diagnosis of conditions such as macular degeneration, retinal neoplasms, choroid disturbances, and diabetic retinopathy, or to identify glaucoma, multiple sclerosis and other central nervous system abnormalities.

92250   **Fundus photography with interpretation and report** 80

92260   **Ophthalmodynamometry** 80
     If ophthalmoscopy is performed under general anesthesia, consult CPT code 92018.

OTHER SPECIALIZED SERVICES

92265   **Needle oculoelectromyography, one or more extraocular muscles, one or both eyes, with interpretation and report** 80

92270   **Electro-oculography with interpretation and report** 80

92275   **Electroretinography with interpretation and report** 80
     If electronystagmography is performed for vestibular function studies, consult CPT codes 92541 and subsequent codes. If ophthalmic echography is performed (diagnostic ultrasound), consult CPT codes 76511-76529.

92283   **Color vision examination, extended, eg, anomaloscope or equivalent** 80
     Note that color vision testing with pseudoisochromatic plates (such as HRR or Ishihara) is not reported separately. It is included in the appropriate general or ophthalmological service.

     Farnsworth-Munsell color test

92284   **Dark adaptation examination, with interpretation and report** 80
     If surgical procedures are performed, consult Eye and Ocular Adnexa in the Surgery section of CPT (65091 and subsequent codes).

92285   **External ocular photography with interpretation and report for documentation of medical progress (eg, close-up photography, slit lamp photography, goniophotography, stereo-photography)** 80

CIM 35-44 USE OF VISUAL TESTS PRIOR TO AND GENERAL ANESTHESIA DURING CATARACT SURGERY

When the only diagnosis is cataract(s), Medicare does not cover testing other than one comprehensive eye exam (or a combination of a brief/intermediate exam not to exceed the charge of a comprehensive exam) and an A-scan or, if medically justifiable, a B-scan. Claims for additional tests are denied unless there is an additional diagnosis and the medical need is fully documented. Because cataract surgery is an elective procedure, the patient may decide not to have the surgery until later, or to have the surgery performed by a physician other than the diagnosing physician. The use of general anesthesia in cataract surgery may be considered reasonable and necessary if, for particular medical indications, it is the accepted procedure among ophthalmologists in the local community to use general anesthesia.

CIM 50-38 ENDOTHELIAL CELL PHOTOGRAPHY

Medicare covers endothelial cell photography for patients who meet one or more of the following criteria:

- Slit lamp evidence of endothelial dystrophy (cornea guttata)
- Slit lamp evidence of corneal edema (unilateral or bilateral)
- About to undergo a secondary intraocular lens implantation or a surgical procedure associated with a higher risk to corneal endothelium
- Previous intraocular surgery and require cataract surgery
- Evidence of posterior polymorphous dystrophy of the cornea or irido-corneal- endothelium syndrome
- About to be fitted with extended wear contact lenses after intraocular surgery.

In addition, Medicare covers endothelial cell photography as part of the presurgical comprehensive eye exam or combination brief/intermediate exam prior to cataract surgery, and not in addition to it.

92286   **Special anterior segment photography with interpretation and report; with specular endothelial microscopy and cell count** 80

92287   **with fluorescein angiography** 80

CONTACT LENS SERVICES

Report the following contact lens codes separately from other ophthalmological services.

Fitting of contact lenses includes patient training and instruction as well as incidental revision of the contacts during the training period.

For therapeutic or surgical use of contact lens, consult CPT codes 68340 and 92970.

CIM 45-7 HYDROPHILIC CONTACT LENS FOR CORNEAL BANDAGE

Medicare covers a hydrophilic contact lens approved by the Food and Drug Administration (FDA) and used as a supply incident to a physician's service.

92310   **Prescription of optical and physical characteristics of and fitting of contact lens, with medical supervision of adaptation; corneal lens, both eyes, except for aphakia**
     For prescription and fitting of one eye, append modifier -52 or 09952 to 92310.

92311   **corneal lens for aphakia, one eye** 80

92312   **corneal lens for aphakia, both eyes** 80

92313   **corneoscleral lens** 80

92314   **Prescription of optical and physical characteristics of contact lens, with medical supervision of adaptation and direction of fitting by independent technician; corneal lens, both eyes, except for aphakia**
     For prescription and fitting of one eye, append modifier -52 or 09952 to 92310.

92315   **corneal lens for aphakia, one eye** 80

92316   **corneal lens for aphakia, both eyes** 80

92317   **corneoscleral lens** 80

92325   **Modification of contact lens (separate procedure), with medical supervision of adaptation** 80

92326   **Replacement of contact lens** 80

OCULAR PROSTHETICS, ARTIFICIAL EYE

If surgical procedures are performed, consult Eye and Ocular Adnexa in the Surgery section of CPT (65091 and subsequent codes).

If the supply is not included, append modifier -26 or 09926. To report supply separately, consult CPT code 92393.

92330   **Prescription, fitting, and supply of ocular prosthesis (artificial eye), with medical supervision of adaptation** 80

92335   Prescription of ocular prosthesis (artificial eye) and direction of fitting and supply by independent technician, with medical supervision of adaptation   80

SPECTACLE SERVICES (INCLUDING PROSTHESIS FOR APHAKIA)

The following codes are for the fitting and supply of spectacles only. Code the determination of prescription separately.

92340   Fitting of spectacles, except for aphakia; monofocal

92341   bifocal

92342   multifocal, other than bifocal

92352   Fitting of spectacle prosthesis for aphakia; monofocal

92353   multifocal

92354   Fitting of spectacle mounted low vision aid; single element system

92355   telescopic or other compound lens system

92358   Prosthesis service for aphakia, temporary (disposable or loan, including materials)

92370   Repair and refitting spectacles; except for aphakia

92371   spectacle prosthesis for aphakia

SUPPLY OF MATERIALS

If surgical procedures are performed, consult Eye and Ocular Adnexa in the Surgery section of CPT (65091 and subsequent codes).

92390   Supply of spectacles, except prosthesis for aphakia and low vision aids

92391   Supply of contact lenses, except prosthesis for aphakia
    If the supply of contact lenses is reported as part of the service of fitting, consult CPT codes 92310-92313. If contact lenses are replaced, consult CPT code 92326.

92392   Supply of low vision aids (A low vision aid is any lens or device used to aid or improve visual function in a person whose vision cannot be normalized by conventional spectacle correction. Includes reading additions up to 4D.)

92393   Supply of ocular prosthesis (artificial eye)
    If the supply is reported as part of the service of fitting, consult CPT code 92330.

92395   Supply of permanent prosthesis for aphakia; spectacles
    For temporary spectacle correction, see 92358.

92396   contact lenses
    If the supply is reported as part of the service of fitting, consult CPT codes 92311 and 92312. Consult CPT code 99070 for the supply of other materials, drugs, trays, etc.

OTHER PROCEDURES

92499   Unlisted ophthalmological service or procedure   80
    If surgical procedures are performed, consult Eye and Ocular Adnexa in the Surgery section of CPT (65091 and subsequent codes).

SPECIAL OTORHINOLARYNGOLOGIC SERVICES

92502   Otolaryngologic examination under general anesthesia   80
    If laryngoscopy is performed with stroboscopy, consult CPT code 31579.

92504   Binocular microscopy (separate diagnostic procedure)   80

92506   Evaluation of speech, language, voice, communication, auditory processing, and/or aural rehabilitation status   80

CIM 35-89 SPEECH PATHOLOGY SERVICES FOR THE TREATMENT OF DYSPHAGIA

Speech pathology services are covered under Medicare for the treatment of dysphagia, a swallowing disorder, regardless of a communication disability. Elements of the therapy program include thermal stimulation to heighten the sensitivity of the swallowing reflex, exercises to improve oral-motor control, training in laryngeal adduction and compensatory swallowing techniques, and positioning and dietary modifications.

MCM 2216 COVERED SPEECH PATHOLOGY

Speech pathology services are those services necessary for the diagnosis and treatment of speech and language disorders that result in communication disabilities and for the diagnosis and treatment of swallowing disorders (dysphagia), regardless of the presence of a communication disability. They must relate directly and specifically to a written treatment regimen established by the physician, after any needed consultation with the qualified speech pathologist, or by the speech pathologist providing such services.

Speech pathology services must be reasonable and necessary to the treatment of the individual's illness or injury. To be considered reasonable and necessary, the following conditions must be met:

1. Accepted standards of practice, specific and effective treatment for the patient's condition

2. Services must be of such a level of complexity and sophistication, or the patient's condition must be such that the services required can be performed only by or under the supervision of a qualified speech pathologist

3. Expectation that the patient's condition will improve significantly in a reasonable period of time based on the physician's assessment of the patient's restoration potential after any needed consultation with the qualified speech pathologist

4. Amount, frequency, and duration of the services must be reasonable under accepted standards of practice (the carrier should consult with local speech pathologists or the state chapter of the American Speech-Language-Hearing Association in the development of any utilization guidelines)

92507   Treatment of speech, language, voice, communication, and/or auditory processing disorder (includes aural rehabilitation); individual   80

92508   group, two or more individuals   80

CIM 65-14 COCHLEAR IMPLANTATION

Medicare coverage is provided only for those patients who meet all of the following guidelines:

- Diagnosis of bilateral severe-to-profound sensorineural hearing impairment with limited benefit from appropriate hearing (or vibrotactile) aids

- Cognitive ability to use auditory clues and a willingness to undergo an extended program of rehabilitation

- Freedom from middle ear infection, an accessible cochlear lumen that is structurally suited to implantation, and freedom from lesions in the auditory nerve and acoustic areas of the central nervous system

- No contraindications to surgery

- The device must be used in accordance with the FDA-approved labeling

Cochlear implants may be covered for adults (over age 18) for prelinguistically, perilinguistically, and postlinguistically deafened adults. Postlinguistically deafened adults must demonstrate test scores of 30 percent or less on sentence recognition scores from tape-recorded tests in the patient's best listening condition.

Cochlear implants may be covered for prelinguistically and postlinguistically deafened children aged 2 through 17. Bilateral profound sensorineural deafness must be demonstrated by the inability to improve on age appropriate closed-set word identification tasks with amplification.

92510   Aural rehabilitation following cochlear implant (includes evaluation of aural rehabilitation status and hearing, therapeutic services) with or without speech processor programming   80

CCI Comprehensive Code   50 Bilateral Procedure   + CPT Add-on Code   ⊘ Modifier -51 Exempt Code   ● New Code   ▲ Revised Code

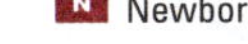 Maternity   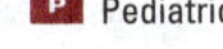 Newborn   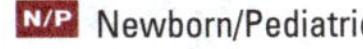 Pediatric   Newborn/Pediatric

92511 — 92599

92511	Nasopharyngoscopy with endoscope (separate procedure)	80 ▢
92512	Nasal function studies (eg, rhinomanometry)	80
92516	Facial nerve function studies (eg, electroneuronography)	80
92520	Laryngeal function studies	80
92525	Evaluation of swallowing and oral function for feeding	
92526	Treatment of swallowing dysfunction and/or oral function for feeding	80 ▢

VESTIBULAR FUNCTION TESTS

WITH OBSERVATION AND EVALUATION BY PHYSICIAN, WITHOUT ELECTRICAL RECORDING

	92531	Spontaneous nystagmus, including gaze	
▲	92532	Positional nystagmus test	
	92533	Caloric vestibular test, each irrigation (binaural, bithermal stimulation constitutes four tests) Barany caloric test	
▲	92534	Optokinetic nystagmus test	

WITH RECORDING (EG, ENG, PENG), AND MEDICAL DIAGNOSTIC EVALUATION

	92541	Spontaneous nystagmus test, including gaze and fixation nystagmus, with recording	80
	92542	Positional nystagmus test, minimum of 4 positions, with recording	80
	92543	Caloric vestibular test, each irrigation (binaural, bithermal stimulation constitutes four tests), with recording	80
	92544	Optokinetic nystagmus test, bidirectional, foveal or peripheral stimulation, with recording	80
	92545	Oscillating tracking test, with recording	80
	92546	Sinusoidal vertical axis rotational testing	80
+	92547	Use of vertical electrodes (List separately in addition to code for primary procedure) Note that 92547 is an add-on code and must be used in conjunction with 92541-92546. If vestibular tests are unlisted, consult CPT code 92599.	TC 80
	92548	Computerized dynamic posturography	80

AUDIOLOGIC FUNCTION TESTS WITH MEDICAL DIAGNOSTIC EVALUATION

The following codes describe the use of electronic equipment and differ from other otorhinolaryngologic services that include the use of tuning forks, clapping, whispering, and other stimuli. All CPT codes in this section are considered bilateral. Use modifier -52 if the test is performed on one ear only.

92551	Screening test, pure tone, air only If speech, language, and/or hearing problems are evaluated through observation and assessment of performance, consult CPT code 92506.	
92552	Pure tone audiometry (threshold); air only	TC 80
92553	air and bone	TC 80 ▢
92555	Speech audiometry threshold;	TC 80
92556	with speech recognition	TC 80 ▢
92557	Comprehensive audiometry threshold evaluation and speech recognition (92553 and 92556 combined) For hearing aid evaluation and selection, consult CPT codes 92590-92595.	TC 80 ▢
92559	Audiometric testing of groups If speech, language, and/or hearing problems are evaluated through observation and assessment of performance, consult CPT code 92506.	

92560	Bekesy audiometry; screening	
92561	diagnostic	TC 80 ▢
92562	Loudness balance test, alternate binaural or monaural	TC 80 ▢
92563	Tone decay test	TC 80 ▢
92564	Short increment sensitivity index (SISI)	TC 80 ▢
92565	Stenger test, pure tone	TC 80 ▢
92567	Tympanometry (impedance testing)	TC 80
92568	Acoustic reflex testing	TC 80
92569	Acoustic reflex decay test	TC 80 ▢
92571	Filtered speech test	TC 80 ▢
92572	Staggered spondaic word test	TC 80 ▢
92573	Lombard test	TC 80 ▢
92575	Sensorineural acuity level test	TC 80 ▢
92576	Synthetic sentence identification test	TC 80 ▢
92577	Stenger test, speech	TC 80 ▢
92579	Visual reinforcement audiometry (VRA)	TC 80 ▢
92582	Conditioning play audiometry	TC 80 ▢
92583	Select picture audiometry	TC 80 ▢
92584	Electrocochleography	TC 80 ▢

CIM 50-31 EVOKED RESPONSE TESTS
Medicare covers evoked response tests, including brain stem evoked response and visual evoked response tests.

	92585	Auditory evoked potentials for evoked response audiometry and/or testing of the central nervous system; comprehensive	80 ▢
●	92586	limited	TC 80
	92587	Evoked otoacoustic emissions; limited (single stimulus level, either transient or distortion products) If speech, language, and/or hearing problems are evaluated through observation and assessment of performance, consult CPT code 92506.	80 ▢
	92588	comprehensive or diagnostic evaluation (comparison of transient and/or distortion product otoacoustic emissions at multiple levels and frequencies)	80 ▢
	92589	Central auditory function test(s) (specify)	TC 80 ▢
	92590	Hearing aid examination and selection; monaural	
	92591	binaural	
	92592	Hearing aid check; monaural	
	92593	binaural	
	92594	Electroacoustic evaluation for hearing aid; monaural	
	92595	binaural	
	92596	Ear protector attenuation measurements	TC 80 ▢
	92597	Evaluation for use and/or fitting of voice prosthetic or augmentative/alternative communication device to supplement oral speech	
	92598	Modification of voice prosthetic or augmentative/alternative communication device to supplement oral speech	

OTHER PROCEDURES

| 92599 | Unlisted otorhinolaryngological service or procedure | 80 |

CARDIOVASCULAR

THERAPEUTIC SERVICES

For non-surgical septal reduction therapy (eg, alcohol ablation), consult CPT Category III code 0024T.

92950 **Cardiopulmonary resuscitation (eg, in cardiac arrest)** 80
> Consult also critical care services 99291 and 99292.

92953 **Temporary transcutaneous pacing** 80
> For physician direction of ambulance or rescue personnel outside the hospital, consult CPT code 99288.
>
> If temporary transcutaneous pacing is performed as part of critical care services (99291-99292) do not report separately.

92960 **Cardioversion, elective, electrical conversion of arrhythmia; external** 80

92961 **internal (separate procedure)**
> Note that 92961 cannot be reported in addition to CPT codes 93618-93624, 93631, 93640-93642, 93650-93652, and 93741-93744.

92970 **Cardioassist-method of circulatory assist; internal** 80

MCM 4277 EXTERNAL COUNTERPULSATION (ECP)

Commonly referred to as enhanced external counterpulsation, is a non-invasive outpatient treatment for coronary artery disease refractory medical and/or surgical therapy. Effective for dates of service July 1, 1999 and after, Medicare will cover ECP when its use is in patients with stable anginal pectoris, since only that use has developed sufficient evidence to demonstrate its medical effectiveness. Effective for dates of service on or after January 1, 2000, use HCPCS code G0166 (External counterpulsation, per session) to report ECP services (replaces 93799 Unlisted cardiovascular service or procedure). The codes for external cardiac assist (92971), ECG rhythm strip and report (93040 or 93041), pulse oximetry (94760 or 94761) and plethysmography (93922 or 93923) or other monitoring tests for examining the effects of this treatment are not clinically necessary with this service and should not be paid on the same day, unless they occur in a clinical setting not connected with the delivery of the ECP. Daily evaluation and management service, e.g., 99201-99205, 99211-99215, 99217-99220, 99241-99245, cannot be billed with the ECP treatments. Any evaluation and management service must be justified with adequate documentation of the medical necessity of the visit. Deductible and coinsurance apply. Professional services of a physician must be billed on Form HCFA-1500 paper or electronic equivalent.

92971 **external** 80
> If a balloon atrial-septostomy is performed, consult CPT code 92992. If catheters are placed for use in circulatory assist devices such as an intra-aortic balloon pump, consult CPT code 33970.

● + **92973** **Percutaneous transluminal coronary thrombectomy (List separately in addition to code for primary procedure)**
> Note that 92973 is an add-on code and must be used in conjunction with codes 92980, 92982.

● + **92974** **Transcatheter placement of radiation delivery device for subsequent coronary intravascular brachytherapy (List separately in addition to code for primary procedure)**
> Note that 92974 is an add-on code and must be used in conjunction with codes 92980, 92982, 93508.
>
> For intravascular radioelement application, see 77781-77784.

92975 **Thrombolysis, coronary; by intracoronary infusion, including selective coronary angiography** 80

92977 **by intravenous infusion** 80
> If thrombolysis is performed of vessels other than coronary, consult CPT codes 37201 and 75896. If cerebral thrombolysis is performed, consult CPT code 37195.

+ **92978** **Intravascular ultrasound (coronary vessel or graft) during diagnostic evaluation and/or therapeutic intervention including imaging supervision, interpretation and report; initial vessel (List separately in addition to code for primary procedure)** 80
> Note that intravascular ultrasound services include all transducer manipulations and repositioning within the specific vessel being examined, both before and after therapeutic intervention (e.g., stent placement).

+ **92979** **each additional vessel (List separately in addition to code for primary procedure)** 80
> Note that 92979 is an add-on code and must be used in conjunction with 92978.

92980 **Transcatheter placement of an intracoronary stent(s), percutaneous, with or without other therapeutic intervention, any method; single vessel** 80

+ **92981** **each additional vessel (List separately in addition to code for primary procedure)** 80
> Note that 92981 is an add-on code and must be used in conjunction with 92980. If additional vessels are treated by angioplasty or atherectomy during the same session, consult CPT codes 92984 and 92996.
>
> For transcatheter placement of radiation delivery device for coronary intravascular brachytherapy, consult CPT code 92974.
>
> For intravascular radioelement application, consult CPT codes 77781-77784.

CIM 50-32 PERCUTANEOUS TRANSLUMINAL ANGIOPLASTY (PTA)

Percutaneous transluminal angioplasty (PTA) PTA is covered to treat the following indications:

- Atherosclerotic obstructive lesions

- In the lower extremities (upper extremities do not include head or neck vessels)

- Of a single coronary artery for patients who exhibit the following characteristics:

Angina refractory to optimal medical management

Objective evidence of myocardial ischemia

Lesions amenable to angioplasty

- Of the renal arteries for patients for whom surgery is the likely alternative (i.e., PTA for this group of patients is an alternative to surgery, not simply an addition to medical management.)

- Obstructive lesions of arteriovenous dialysis fistulas and grafts when performed through either a venous or arterial approach

Effective July 1, 2001, Medicare will cover PTA of the carotid artery concurrent with carotid stent placement when furnished in accordance with the Food and Drug Administration (FDA) approved protocols governing Category B Investigational Device Exemption (IDE) clinical trials.

92982 **Percutaneous transluminal coronary balloon angioplasty; single vessel** 80

+ **92984** **each additional vessel (List separately in addition to code for primary procedure)** 80
> Note that 92984 is an add-on code and must be used in conjunction with 92980, 92982, or 92995. If a stent is placed following the completion of angioplasty or atherectomy, consult CPT codes 92980 and 92981.
>
> To report transcatheter placement of radiation delivery device for coronary intravascular brachytherapy, use 92974.
>
> For intravascular radioelement application, see 77781-77784.

92986 **Percutaneous balloon valvuloplasty; aortic valve** 80

92987 **mitral valve** 80

92990 **pulmonary valve** 80

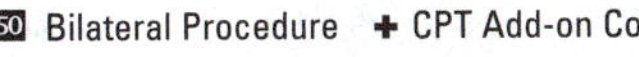
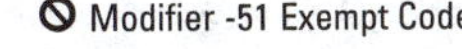
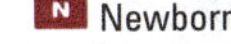
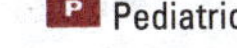

CCI Comprehensive Code   Bilateral Procedure   **+** CPT Add-on Code   Modifier -51 Exempt Code   ● New Code   ▲ Revised Code

M Maternity   **N** Newborn   **P** Pediatric   **N/P** Newborn/Pediatric

92992 Atrial septectomy or septostomy; transvenous method, balloon, (eg, Rashkind type) (includes cardiac catheterization) ⬛80 ▣

92993 blade method (Park septostomy) (includes cardiac catheterization) ⬛80 ▣

92995 Percutaneous transluminal coronary atherectomy, by mechanical or other method, with or without balloon angioplasty; single vessel ⬛80 ▣

+ 92996 each additional vessel (List separately in addition to code for primary procedure) ⬛80

Note that 92996 is an add-on code and must be used in conjunction with 92980, 92982, or 92995. If a stent is placed following the completion of angioplasty or atherectomy, consult CPT codes 92980 and 92981. If additional vessels are treated by angioplasty or atherectomy during the same session, consult CPT code 92984.

92997 Percutaneous transluminal pulmonary artery balloon angioplasty; single vessel ⬛80 ▣

+ 92998 each additional vessel (List separately in addition to code for primary procedure) ⬛80

Note that 92998 is an add-on code and must be used in conjunction with 92997.

CARDIOGRAPHY

CIM 50-15 ELECTROCARDIOGRAPHIC SERVICES

Medicare Part B covers electrocardiographic (EKG) services rendered by a physician, incident to services, or by an approved laboratory or supplier of portable X-ray services (the claim must identify the physician ordering the service and the physician making the interpretation). Practices may charge separately for an EKG interpretation by an attending or consulting physician.

In addition, Medicare covers an emergency as a laboratory service or a diagnostic service by a portable X-ray supplier only when evidence shows that a physician was in attendance at the time the service was performed or immediately thereafter. EKG services provided in the patient's home, payment is based on the reasonable charge of services supplied in the laboratory (or in the supplier's office), in the absence of documentation.

Medicare coverage of Long Term EKG Monitoring, referred to as long-term EKG recording, Holter recording, or dynamic electrocardiography depends on a complete patient evaluation prior to performance of this diagnostic study. Generally, a statement of the diagnostic impression of the referring physician with an indication of the patient's relevant signs and symptoms should be sufficient for determining medical necessity. Intermediaries or carriers may require whatever additional documentation.

Medicare covers patient-activated EKG recorders when used as an alternative to the long-term EKG for similar indications (e.g., detecting and characterizing symptomatic arrhythmias, regulation of anti-arrhythmic drug therapy). Medicare does not cover outpatient monitoring of recently discharged post-infarct patients.

Medicare covers computer interpretation of an EKG when furnished under the circumstances required for coverage of other electrocardiographic services. The certifying physician must be identified on the HCFA-1490. Where the laboratory's (or portable x-ray supplier's) reviewing physician is not identified, no professional component is involved and reimbursement is determined accordingly. If the supplying laboratory does not include professional review and certification of the hard copy, the patient's physician is reimbursed.

Medicare covers Transtelephonic Electrocardiographic Transmissions Effective as a diagnostic service for the indications described below:

- To detect, characterize, and document symptomatic transient arrhythmias

- To overcome problems in regulating antiarrhythmic drug dosage

- To carry out early post-hospital monitoring of patients discharged after myocardial infarction

The transmitting devices must meet at least the following criteria:

1. Capable of transmitting EKG Leads, I, II, or III

2. Lead transmissions must be comparable to by a conventional EKG to permit interpretation of abnormal cardiac rhythms

93000 Electrocardiogram, routine ECG with at least 12 leads; with interpretation and report ⬛80 ▣

If echocardiography is performed, consult CPT codes 93303-93350.

93005 tracing only, without interpretation and report ᵀᶜ ⬛80 ▣

93010 interpretation and report only ²⁶ ⬛80 ▣

If ECG monitoring is needed, consult CPT codes 99354-99360.

93012 Telephonic transmission of post-symptom electrocardiogram rhythm strip(s), per 30 day period of time; tracing only ᵀᶜ ⬛80 ▣

If echocardiography is performed, consult CPT codes 93303-93350.

93014 physician review with interpretation and report only ²⁶ ⬛80

CIM 35-25 CARDIAC REHABILITATION PROGRAMS

Cardiac rehabilitation programs are conducted in specialized, free-standing, cardiac rehabilitation clinics as well as in outpatient hospital departments. Exercise programs include specific types of exercise, individually prescribed for each patient.

Medicare covers cardiac rehabilitation programs for patients with a clear medical need, who are referred by their attending physician and (1) have a documented diagnosis of acute myocardial infarction within the preceding 12 months; or (2) have had coronary bypass surgery; and/or (3) have stable angina pectoris. The programs may be provided either by the outpatient department of a hospital or in a physician-directed clinic. Coverage for either program is subject to the following conditions:

1. The facility meets the definition of a hospital outpatient department or a physician- directed clinic.

2. The facility has available for immediate use all the necessary cardio-pulmonary emergency diagnostic and therapeutic life saving equipment accepted by the medical community as medically necessary.

3. The program is conducted in an area set aside for the exclusive use of the program while it is in session.

4. The program is staffed by personnel necessary to conduct the program safely and effectively, who are trained in both basic and advanced life support techniques and in exercise therapy for coronary disease.

Services of nonphysician personnel must be furnished under the direct supervision of a physician. Direct supervision means that a physician must be in the exercise program area and immediately available and accessible for an emergency at all times the exercise program is conducted. It does not require that a physician be physically present in the exercise room.

Stress testing performed to evaluate a prospective candidate may be covered for one or more of the following:

- Evaluation of chest pain, especially atypical chest pain

- Development of exercise prescriptions for patients with known cardiac disease

- Pre and postoperative evaluation of patients undergoing coronary artery by-pass procedures

A freestanding or hospital based cardiac rehabilitation clinic may provide diagnostic and therapeutic services other than stress testing and ECG monitoring, including diagnostic testing for a mental problem if the patient shows symptoms such as excessive anxiety or fear associated with the cardiac disease.

Services in connection with a cardiac rehabilitation exercise program may be provided for up to 36 sessions, usually three sessions a week in a single 12-week period. Coverage for continued participation is allowed only on a case-by-case basis with exit criteria taken into consideration. The following exit criteria guidelines apply:

- The patient has achieved a stable level of exercise tolerance without ischemia or dysrhythmia

---

- Symptoms of angina or dyspnea are stable at the patient's maximum exercise level

- Patient's resting blood pressure and heart rate are within normal limits

- The stress test is not positive during exercise

When claims are accompanied by acceptable documentation that the patient has not reached an exit level, coverage may be extended, but should not exceed 24 weeks.

MCM 2050.3 INCIDENT TO PHYSICIAN'S SERVICE IN CLINIC
A physician directed clinic is one where:

1. A physician (or a number of physicians) is present to perform medical (rather than administrative) services at all times the clinic is open

2. Each patient is under the care of a clinic physician

3. The nonphysician services are under medical supervision

In highly organized clinics, particularly those that are departmentalized, direct personal physician supervision may be the responsibility of several physicians as opposed to an individual attending physician. In this situation, medical management of all services provided in the clinic is assured. The physician ordering a particular service need not be the physician who is supervising the service. Supplies provided by the clinic during the course of treatment are also covered. When the auxiliary personnel perform services outside the clinic premises, the services are covered only if performed under the direct personal supervision of a clinic physician. If the clinic refers a patient for auxiliary services performed by personnel who are not employed by the clinic, such services are not incident to a physician's service.

93015   **Cardiovascular stress test using maximal or submaximal treadmill or bicycle exercise, continous electrocardiographic monitoring, and/or pharmacological stress; with physician supervision, with interpretation and report** 〔80〕

93016   **physician supervision only, without interpretation and report** 〔26〕〔80〕

93017   **tracing only, without interpretation and report** 〔TC〕〔80〕

93018   **interpretation and report only** 〔26〕〔80〕

93024   **Ergonovine provocation test** 〔80〕

● **93025**   **Microvolt T-wave alternans for assessment of ventricular arrhythmias**

93040   **Rhythm ECG, one to three leads; with interpretation and report** 〔80〕
     If echocardiography is performed, consult CPT codes 93303-93350.

93041   **tracing only without interpretation and report** 〔TC〕〔80〕

93042   **interpretation and report only** 〔26〕〔80〕

93224   **Electrocardiographic monitoring for 24 hours by continuous original ECG waveform recording and storage, with visual superimposition scanning; includes recording, scanning analysis with report, physician review and interpretation** 〔80〕

93225   **recording (includes hook-up, recording, and disconnection)** 〔TC〕〔80〕

93226   **scanning analysis with report** 〔TC〕〔80〕

93227   **physician review and interpretation** 〔26〕〔80〕

93230   **Electrocardiographic monitoring for 24 hours by continuous original ECG waveform recording and storage without superimposition scanning utilizing a device capable of producing a full miniaturized printout; includes recording, microprocessor-based analysis with report, physician review and interpretation** 〔80〕

93231   **recording (includes hook-up, recording, and disconnection)** 〔TC〕〔80〕

93232   **microprocessor-based analysis with report** 〔TC〕〔80〕

93233   **physician review and interpretation** 〔26〕〔80〕

93235   **Electrocardiographic monitoring for 24 hours by continuous computerized monitoring and non-continuous recording, and real-time data analysis utilizing a device capable of producing intermittent full-sized waveform tracings, possibly patient activated; includes monitoring and real time data analysis with report, physician review and interpretation** 〔80〕
     Holter monitor procedure

93236   **monitoring and real-time data analysis with report** 〔TC〕〔80〕

93237   **physician review and interpretation** 〔26〕〔80〕

93268   **Patient demand single or multiple event recording with presymptom memory loop, per 30 day period of time; includes transmission, physician review and interpretation** 〔80〕
     If postsymptom recording is needed, consult CPT codes 93012 and 93014. If implanted patient activated cardiac event recording is needed, consult CPT codes 33282 and 93727.

93270   **recording (includes hook-up, recording and disconnection)** 〔TC〕〔80〕
     If echocardiography is performed, consult CPT codes 93303-93350.

93271   **monitoring, receipt of transmissions, and analysis** 〔TC〕〔80〕
     If echocardiography is performed, consult CPT codes 93303-93350.

93272   **physician review and interpretation only** 〔26〕〔80〕
     If echocardiography is performed, consult CPT codes 93303-93350.

93278   **Signal-averaged electrocardiography (SAECG), with or without ECG** 〔80〕

ECHOCARDIOGRAPHY
This ultrasound technique of visualizing the heart and great arteries provides the physician with two-dimensional images and/or Doppler signals.

93303   **Transthoracic echocardiography for congenital cardiac anomalies; complete** 〔80〕
     If fetal echocardiography is performed, consult CPT codes 76825-76828.

93304   **follow-up or limited study** 〔80〕

93307   **Echocardiography, transthoracic, real-time with image documentation (2D) with or without M-mode recording; complete** 〔80〕

93308   **follow-up or limited study** 〔80〕

93312   **Echocardiography, transesophageal, real time with image documentation (2D) (with or without M-mode recording); including probe placement, image acquisition, interpretation and report** 〔80〕

93313   **placement of transesophageal probe only** 〔80〕

93314   **image acquisition, interpretation and report only** 〔80〕

93315   **Transesophageal echocardiography for congenital cardiac anomalies; including probe placement, image acquisisiton, interpretation and report** 〔80〕

93316   **placement of transesophageal probe only** 〔80〕

93317   **image acquisition, interpretation and report only** 〔80〕

● 93318 **Echocardiography, transesophageal (TEE) for monitoring purposes, including probe placement, real time 2-dimensional image acquisition and interpretation leading to ongoing (continuous) assessment of (dynamically changing) cardiac pumping function and to therapeutic measures on an immediate time basis** 80

+ 93320 **Doppler echocardiography, pulsed wave and/or continuous wave with spectral display (List separately in addition to codes for echocardiographic imaging); complete** 80

If fetal echocardiography is performed, consult CPT codes 76825-76828.

Note that 93320 is an add-on code and must be used in conjunction with 93303, 93304, 93307, 93308, 93312, 93314, 93315, 93317, and 93350.

+ 93321 **follow-up or limited study (List separately in addition to codes for echocardiographic imaging)** 80

If fetal echocardiography is performed, consult CPT codes 76825-76828.

Note that 93321 is an add-on code and must be used in conjunction with 93303, 93304, 93307, 93308, 93312, 93314, 93315, 93317, and 93350.

+ 93325 **Doppler echocardiography color flow velocity mapping (List separately in addition to codes for echocardiography)** 80

If fetal echocardiography is performed, consult CPT codes 76825-76828.

Note that 93325 is an add-on code and must be used in conjunction with 76825, 76826, 76827, 76828, 93303, 93304, 93307, 93308, 93312, 93314, 93315, 93317, 93320, 93321, and 93350.

93350 **Echocardiography, transthoracic, real-time with image documentation (2D, with or without M-mode recording) during rest and cardiovascular stress test using treadmill, bicycle exercise and/or pharmacologically induced stress, with interpretation and report** 80

Consult CPT codes 93015-93018 for the appropriate stress testing code that needs to be reported in addition to 93350 to capture the exercise stress portion of the study.

CARDIAC CATHETERIZATION

A number of services rely on the following cardiac catheterization codes. The procedure itself includes introduction, positioning, gauging pressure, and procuring samples.

CIM 35-45 CARDIAC CATHETERIZATION PERFORMED IN OTHER THAN A HOSPITAL

Cardiac catheterization performed in a hospital setting for either inpatients or outpatients is a covered service. The procedure may also be covered when performed in a freestanding clinic when the carrier, in consult with the appropriate Peer Review Organization (PRO), determines that the procedure can be performed safely in the particular facility. Request PRO preauthorization.

⊘ 93501 **Right heart catheterization** 80

For bundle of His recording, consult CPT code 93600.

⊘ 93503 **Insertion and placement of flow directed catheter (eg, Swan-Ganz) for monitoring purposes** 80

If subsequent monitoring is needed, consult CPT codes 99354-99360.

⊘ 93505 **Endomyocardial biopsy** 80

⊘ 93508 **Catheter placement in coronary artery(s), arterial coronary conduit(s), and/or venous coronary bypass graft(s) for coronary angiography without concomitant left heart catheterization** 80

Note that 93508 is to be used only when left heart catheterization is not performed (CPT codes 93510, 93511, 93524, and 93526). Also note that 93508 is to be used only once per procedure.

For transcatheter placement of radiation delivery device for coronary intravascular brachytherapy, consult CPT code 92974.

For intravascular radioelement application, consult CPT codes 77781-77784.

⊘ 93510 **Left heart catheterization, retrograde, from the brachial artery, axillary artery or femoral artery; percutaneous** 80

⊘ 93511 **by cutdown** 80

⊘ 93514 **Left heart catheterization by left ventricular puncture** 80

⊘ 93524 **Combined transseptal and retrograde left heart catheterization** 80

⊘ 93526 **Combined right heart catheterization and retrograde left heart catheterization** 80

⊘ 93527 **Combined right heart catheterization and transseptal left heart catheterization through intact septum (with or without retrograde left heart catheterization)** 80

⊘ 93528 **Combined right heart catheterization with left ventricular puncture (with or without retrograde left heart catheterization)** 80

⊘ 93529 **Combined right heart catheterization and left heart catheterization through existing septal opening (with or without retrograde left heart catheterization)** 80

⊘ 93530 **Right heart catheterization, for congenital cardiac anomalies** 80

⊘ 93531 **Combined right heart catheterization and retrograde left heart catheterization, for congenital cardiac anomalies** 80

⊘ 93532 **Combined right heart catheterization and transseptal left heart catheterization through intact septum with or without retrograde left heart catheterization, for congenital cardiac anomalies** 80

⊘ 93533 **Combined right heart catheterization and transseptal left heart catheterization through existing septal opening, with or without retrograde left heart catheterization, for congenital cardiac anomalies** 80

⊘ 93536 ~~Percutaneous insertion of intra-aortic balloon catheter~~ **This code is deleted in 2002. See code 33967.** 80

⊘ 93539 **Injection procedure during cardiac catheterization; for selective opacification of arterial conduits (eg, internal mammary), whether native or used for bypass** 80

When injection procedures are performed in conjunction with cardiac catheterization, these services do not include introduction of catheters but do include repositioning of catheters when necessary and use of automatic power injectors. Injection procedures represent separate identifiable services and may be coded in conjunction with one another when appropriate. The technical details of angiography, which include supervision of filming and processing and interpretation and report are not included. To report the technical details, consult CPT code 93555 and/or 93556. Note that modifier -51 should not be appended to these procedures.

⊘ 93540 **for selective opacification of aortocoronary venous bypass grafts, one or more coronary arteries** 80

⊘	93541	for pulmonary angiography	80
⊘	93542	for selective right ventricular or right atrial angiography	80
⊘	93543	for selective left ventricular or left atrial angiography	80
⊘	93544	for aortography	80
⊘	93545	for selective coronary angiography (injection of radiopaque material may be by hand)	80

⊘ **93555** Imaging supervision, interpretation and report for injection procedure(s) during cardiac catheterization; ventricular and/or atrial angiography   80

⊘ **93556** pulmonary angiography, aortography, and/or selective coronary angiography including venous bypass grafts and arterial conduits (whether native or used in bypass)   80

93561 Indicator dilution studies such as dye or thermal dilution, including arterial and/or venous catheterization; with cardiac output measurement (separate procedure)   80

If cardiac output measurements are done as part of critical care services (99291-99292), do not report separately.

Note that 93561 and 93562 are not to be used with cardiac catheterization codes. If radioisotope method is used for cardiac output, consult CPT code 78472, 78473, or 78481.

93562 subsequent measurement of cardiac output   80

If cardiac output measurements are done as part of critical care services (99291-99292), do not report separately.

Note that 93561 and 93562 are not to be used with cardiac catheterization codes. If radioisotope method is used for cardiac output, consult CPT code 78472, 78473, or 78481.

+ 93571 Intravascular doppler velocity and/or pressure derived coronary flow reserve measurement (coronary vessel or graft) during coronary angiography including pharmacologically induced stress; initial vessel (List separately in addition to code for primary procedure)   80

+ 93572 each additional vessel (List separately in addition to code for primary procedure)   80

Note that measurements of intravascular distal coronary blood flow velocity include all Doppler transducer manipulations and repositioning within the specific vessel being examined, during coronary angiography or therapeutic intervention (e.g., angioplasty). If an unlisted cardiac catheterization procedure is performed, consult CPT code 93799.

INTRACARDIAC ELECTROPHYSIOLOGICAL PROCEDURES

CIM 50-3 HIS BUNDLE STUDY

Medicare limits coverage of the His Bundle Study to patients with complex ongoing acute arrhythmias, those with intermittent or permanent heart block when pacemaker implantation is considered, and those patients who have developed heart block secondary to a myocardial infarction. When heart catheterization and the His Bundle Study are performed at the same time, the program covers only one catheterization and a small added charge for the study. When a His bundle cardiogram is part of a diagnostic endocardial electrical stimulation, no separate charge will be recognized for the His bundle study.

⊘	93600	Bundle of His recording	80
⊘	93602	Intra-atrial recording	80
⊘	93603	Right ventricular recording	80
⊘	~~93607~~	~~Left ventricular recording~~ This code is deleted in 2002. See code 93622.	80

▲ **+ 93609** Intraventricular and/or intra-atrial mapping of tachycardia site(s) with catheter manipulation to record from multiple sites to identify origin of tachycardia (List separately in addition to code for primary procedure)   80

Note that 93609 is an add-on code and must be used in conjunction with codes 93620, 93651, 93652.

⊘ **93610** Intra-atrial pacing   80

⊘ **93612** Intraventricular pacing   80

Do not report 93612 in conjunction with codes 93620, 93651, 93652.

INTRACARDIAC ELECTROPHYSIOLOGICAL PROCEDURES/STUDIES

● **+ 93613** Intracardiac electrophysiologic 3-dimensional mapping (List separately in addition to code for primary procedure)

Note that 93613 is an add-on code and must be used in conjunction with codes 93620, 93651, 93652.

INTRACARDIAC ELECTROPHYSIOLOGICAL PROCEDURES

⊘ **93615** Esophageal recording of atrial electrogram with or without ventricular electrogram(s);   80

⊘ **93616** with pacing   80

⊘ **93618** Induction of arrhythmia by electrical pacing   80

If an intracardiac phonocardiogram is performed, consult CPT code 93799.

▲ ⊘ **93619** Comprehensive electrophysiologic evaluation with right atrial pacing and recording, right ventricular pacing and recording, His bundle recording, including insertion and repositioning of multiple electrode catheters, without induction or attempted induction of arrhythmia   80

Code 993619 should not be used in conjunction with codes 93600, 93602, 93610, 93612, 93618, or 93620-93622.

▲ ⊘ **93620** Comprehensive electrophysiologic evaluation with right atrial pacing and recording, right ventricular pacing and recording, His bundle recording, including insertion and repositioning of multiple electrode catheters with induction or attempted induction of arrhythmia;   80

Code 93620 should not be used in conjunction with codes 93600, 93602, 93610, 93612, 93618, or 93619.

▲ **+ 93621** with left atrial pacing and recording from coronary sinus or left atrium (List separately in addition to code for primary procedure)   80

Note that 93621 is an add-on code and must be used in conjunction with 93620.

▲ **+ 93622** with left ventricular pacing and recording (List separately in addition to code for primary procedure)   80

Note that 93622 is an add-on code and must be used in conjunction with 93620.

+ 93623 Programmed stimulation and pacing after intravenous drug infusion (List separately in addition to code for primary procedure)   80

Note that 93623 is an add-on code and must be used in conjunction with 93619, 93620..

⊘ **93624** Electrophysiologic follow-up study with pacing and recording to test effectiveness of therapy, including induction or attempted induction of arrhythmia   80

CIM 35-75 INTRAOPERATIVE VENTRICULAR MAPPING

The intraoperative ventricular mapping procedure is covered under Medicare only for the uses and medical conditions described:

- Localize accessory pathways associated with the Wolff-Parkinson-White (WPW) and other preexcitation syndromes

- Map the sequence of atrial and ventricular activation for drug-resistant supraventricular tachycardias

---

- Delineate the anatomical course of His bundle and/or bundle branches during corrective cardiac surgery for congenital heart diseases
- Direct the surgical treatment of patients with refractory ventricular tachyarrhythmias

CIM 35-78 DIAGNOSTIC ENDOCARDIAL ELECTRICAL STIMULATION (PACING)

Diagnostic endocardial electrical stimulation (EES), also called programmed electrical stimulation of the heart, is used in the diagnosis and treatment of sustained ventricular tachycardia. However, it is also valuable in the diagnosis and management of other complex arrhythmias, conduction defects, and after cardiac arrest. Medicare covers EES when used for patients with severe cardiac arrhythmias. No separate charge is recognized for a His Bundle cardiogram.

93631   **Intra-operative epicardial and endocardial pacing and mapping to localize the site of tachycardia or zone of slow conduction for surgical correction**   80

93640   **Electrophysiologic evaluation of single or dual chamber pacing cardioverter-defibrillator leads including defibrillation threshold evaluation (induction of arrhythmia, evaluation of sensing and pacing for arrhythmia termination) at time of initial implantation or replacement;**   80

> If subsequent or periodic electronic analysis and/or reprogramming of single or dual-chamber pacing cardioverter-defibrillators is needed, consult CPT codes 93642 and 92741-93744.

93641   **with testing of single or dual chamber pacing cardioverter-defibrillator pulse generator**   80

93642   **Electrophysiologic evaluation of single or dual chamber pacing cardioverter-defibrillator (includes defibrillation threshold evaluation, induction of arrhythmia, evaluation of sensing and pacing for arrhythmia termination, and programming or reprogramming of sensing or therapeutic parameters)**   80

93650   **Intracardiac catheter ablation of atrioventricular node function, atrioventricular conduction for creation of complete heart block, with or without temporary pacemaker placement**   80

93651   **Intracardiac catheter ablation of arrhythmogenic focus; for treatment of supraventricular tachycardia by ablation of fast or slow atrioventricular pathways, accessory atrioventricular connections or other atrial foci, singly or in combination**   80

93652   **for treatment of ventricular tachycardia**   80

93660   **Evaluation of cardiovascular function with tilt table evaluation, with continuous ECG monitoring and intermittent blood pressure monitoring, with or without pharmacological intervention**   80

> If testing is performed of the autonomic nervous system function, consult CPT codes 95921-95923

+ 93662   **Intracardiac echocardiography during therapeutic/diagnostic intervention, including imaging supervision and interpretation (List separately in addition to code for primary procedure)**   80

> Note that 93662 is an add-on code and must be used in conjunction with 93621, 93622, 93651 or 93652 as appropriate.
>
> Do not report CPT code 92961 in addition to CPT code 93662.

PERIPHERAL ARTERIAL DISEASE REHABILITATION

Code 93668 identifies a service where the patient exercises under medical supervision for several sessions until symptoms of the disease abate. Each session is 45 to 60 minutes long.

93668   **Peripheral arterial disease (PAD) rehabilitation, per session**

● **93701**   **Bioimpedance, thoracic, electrical**   26

CIM 50-6 PLETHYSMOGRAPHY

Plethysmography is a noninvasive technique for diagnostic, preoperative, and postoperative evaluation of peripheral artery disease in the internal medicine or vascular surgery practice. In addition, plethysmography is used preoperative podiatric evaluation of the diabetic patient or one who has intermittent claudication or other signs or symptoms of peripheral vascular disease which bear on the patient's candidacy for foot surgery. Medicare coverage is extended to those procedures listed in Category I below when used for the accepted medical indications. The procedures in Category II are still considered experimental and are not covered.

Category I (covered)

1. Segmental Plethysmography (includes services performed with a regional plethysmograph, differential plethysmograph, recording oscillometer, and a pulse volume recorder)
2. Electrical Impedance Plethysmography
3. Ultrasonic Measurement of Blood Flow (Doppler)
4. Oculoplethysmography
5. Strain Gauge Plethysmography

Category II (not covered)

1. Inductance Plethysmography
2. Capacitance Plethysmography
3. Mechanical Oscillometry
4. Strain Gauge Plethysmography
5. Photoelectric Plethysmography

93720   **Plethysmography, total body; with interpretation and report**   80

> If arterial cannulization and recording is performed of direct arterial pressure, consult CPT code 36620. If radiographic injection procedures are performed, consult CPT codes 36000-36299. If hemodialysis is performed for vascular cannulization, consult CPT codes 36800-36821. If chemotherapy is needed for a malignant disease, consult CPT codes 96408-96549. If penile plethysmography is performed, consult CPT code 54240.

93721   **tracing only, without interpretation and report**   TC 80

93722   **interpretation and report only**   26 80

> If regional plethysmography is performed, consult CPT codes 93875-93931.

CIM 50-1 CARDIAC PACEMAKER EVALUATION SERVICES

Medicare covers a variety of services for the post-implant follow-up and evaluation of implanted cardiac pacemakers (limited to lithium battery-powered pacemakers). There are two general types of pacemakers in current use:

1. Single-chamber pacemakers sense and pace the ventricles of the heart
2. Dual-chamber pacemakers sense and pace both the atria and the ventricles

These differences require different monitoring patterns over the expected life of the units involved, which is the patient's physician responsibility. A physician's prescription is required when the monitoring is done by some entity. Where a patient is monitored both clinically and transtelephonically include frequency data on both types of monitoring.

In order for transtelephonic monitoring services to be covered, the services must consist of the following elements:

- A minimum 30-second readable strip of the pacemaker in the free-running mode
- Unless contraindicated, a minimum 30-second readable strip of the pacemaker in the magnetic mode
- A minimum 30 seconds of readable ECG strip

The following guidelines are designed to assist in claims (apply 1980 guidelines to claims for the obsolete mercury-zinc battery-powered pacemakers). The guidelines are divided into categories:

1. Guideline I applies to the majority of pacemakers in use

2. II applies only to pacemaker systems (pacemaker and leads) that meet the standards of the Inter-Society Commission for Heart Disease Resources (ICHD) for longevity and end-of-life decay

   Guideline I: Single-chamber pacemaker

   First month - every two weeks

   Second month through 36th month - every eight weeks

   37th month to failure - every four weeks

   Guideline I: Dual-chamber pacemaker

   First month - every two weeks

   Second month through 36th month - every four weeks

   37th month to failure - every four weeks

   Guideline II: Single-chamber pacemaker

   First month - every two weeks

   Second month through 48th month - every 12 weeks

   49th through 72nd month - every eight weeks

   Thereafter - every four weeks

   Guideline II: Dual-chamber pacemaker

   First month - every two weeks

   Second month through 30th month - every 12 weeks.

   31st month through 48th month every eight weeks

   Thereafter—every 4 weeks.

Pacemaker monitoring is also covered when done by pacemaker clinics. Clinic visits may be done in conjunction with transtelephonic monitoring; however, the services rendered by a pacemaker clinic are more extensive than those currently possible by telephone. They include, for example, physical examination of patients and reprogramming of pacemakers.

Frequency of clinic visits is the decision of the patient's physician, taking into account, among other things, the medical condition of the patient. The following are recommendations for monitoring guidelines on lithium-battery pacemakers:

- Single-chamber pacemakers - twice in the first six months following implant, then once every 12 months
- Dual-chamber pacemakers - twice in the first six months, then once every six months

93724 **Electronic analysis of antitachycardia pacemaker system (includes electrocardiographic recording, programming of device, induction and termination of tachycardia via implanted pacemaker, and interpretation of recordings)** 80

If arterial cannulization and recording is performed of direct arterial pressure, consult CPT code 36620. If radiographic injection procedures are performed, consult CPT codes 36000-36299. If hemodialysis is performed for vascular cannulization, consult CPT codes 36800-36821. If chemotherapy is needed for a malignant disease, consult CPT codes 96408-96549. If penile plethysmography is performed, consult CPT code 54240.

93727 **Electronic analysis of implantable loop recorder (ILR) system (includes retrieval of recorded and stored ECG data, physician review and interpretation of retrieved ECG data and reprogramming)** 26

93731 **Electronic analysis of dual-chamber pacemaker system (includes evaluation of programmable parameters at rest and during activity where applicable, using electrocardiographic recording and interpretation of recordings at rest and during exercise, analysis of event markers and device response); without reprogramming** 80

93732 with reprogramming 80

93733 **Electronic analysis of dual chamber internal pacemaker system (may include rate, pulse amplitude and duration, configuration of wave form, and/or testing of sensory function of pacemaker), telephonic analysis** 80

93734 **Electronic analysis of single chamber pacemaker system (includes evaluation of programmable parameters at rest and during activity where applicable, using electrocardiographic recording and interpretation of recordings at rest and during exercise, analysis of event markers and device response); without reprogramming** 80

93735 with reprogramming 80

93736 **Electronic analysis of single chamber internal pacemaker system (may include rate, pulse amplitude and duration, configuration of wave form, and/or testing of sensory function of pacemaker), telephonic analysis** 80

~~93737~~ ~~Electronic analysis of single or dual chamber pacing cardioverter defibrillator only (interrogation, evaluation of pulse generator status); without reprogramming~~ **This code is deleted in 2002. See codes 93741 or 93743.** 80

~~93738~~ ~~Electronic analysis of single or dual chamber pacing cardioverter defibrillator only (interrogation, evaluation of pulse generator status); with reprogramming~~ **This code is deleted in 2002. See codes 93742 or 93744.** 80

93740 **Temperature gradient studies**

93741 **Electronic analysis of pacing cardioverter-defibrillator (includes interrogation, evaluation of pulse generator status, evaluation of programmable parameters at rest and during activity where applicable, using electrocardiographic recording and interpretation of recordings at rest and during exercise, analysis of event markers and device response); single chamber, without reprogramming**

93742 single chamber, with reprogramming

93743 dual chamber, without reprogramming

93744 dual chamber, with reprogramming

CIM 50-5 THERMOGRAPHY

Thermography for any indication is excluded from Medicare coverage because the available evidence does not support this test as a useful aid in the diagnosis or treatment of illness or injury. Therefore, it is not considered effective. This exclusion was published as a CMS Final Notice in the Federal Register on November 20, 1992.

93760 **Thermogram; cephalic**

93762 **peripheral**

93770 **Determination of venous pressure**

If central venous cannulization and pressure measurements are taken, consult CPT codes 36488-36491 and 36500.

CIM 50-42 AMBULATORY BLOOD PRESSURE MONITORING WITH FULLY AND SEMI-AUTOMATIC (PATIENT-ACTIVATED) PORTABLE MONITORS - NOT COVERED

The clinical usefulness of the data obtained from these devices is not clearly established, and, accordingly, program payment may not be made for the use of such devices at this time.

93784   **Ambulatory blood pressure monitoring, utilizing a system such as magnetic tape and/or computer disk, for 24 hours or longer; including recording, scanning analysis, interpretation and report**

If arterial cannulization and recording is performed of direct arterial pressure, consult CPT code 36620. If radiographic injection procedures are performed, consult CPT codes 36000-36299. If hemodialysis is performed for vascular cannulization, consult CPT codes 36800-36821. If chemotherapy is needed for a malignant disease, consult CPT codes 96408-96549. If penile plethysmography is performed, consult CPT code 54240.

93786   **recording only**

93788   **scanning analysis with report**

93790   **physician review with interpretation and report**

OTHER PROCEDURES

CIM 35-25 CARDIAC REHABILITATION PROGRAMS

Cardiac rehabilitation programs are conducted in specialized, free-standing, cardiac rehabilitation clinics as well as in outpatient hospital departments. Exercise programs include specific types of exercise, individually prescribed for each patient.

Medicare covers cardiac rehabilitation programs for patients with a clear medical need, who are referred by their attending physician and (1) have a documented diagnosis of acute myocardial infarction within the preceding 12 months; or (2) have had coronary bypass surgery; and/or (3) have stable angina pectoris. The programs may be provided either by the outpatient department of a hospital or in a physician-directed clinic. Coverage for either program is subject to the following conditions:

1. The facility meets the definition of a hospital outpatient department or a physician- directed clinic.

2. The facility has available for immediate use all the necessary cardio-pulmonary emergency diagnostic and therapeutic life saving equipment accepted by the medical community as medically necessary.

3. The program is conducted in an area set aside for the exclusive use of the program while it is in session.

4. The program is staffed by personnel necessary to conduct the program safely and effectively, who are trained in both basic and advanced life support techniques and in exercise therapy for coronary disease.

Services of nonphysician personnel must be furnished under the direct supervision of a physician. Direct supervision means that a physician must be in the exercise program area and immediately available and accessible for an emergency at all times the exercise program is conducted. It does not require that a physician be physically present in the exercise room.

Stress testing performed to evaluate a prospective candidate may be covered for one or more of the following:

- Evaluation of chest pain, especially atypical chest pain

- Development of exercise prescriptions for patients with known cardiac disease

- Pre and postoperative evaluation of patients undergoing coronary artery by-pass procedures

A freestanding or hospital based cardiac rehabilitation clinic may provide diagnostic and therapeutic services other than stress testing and ECG monitoring, including diagnostic testing for a mental problem if the patient shows symptoms such as excessive anxiety or fear associated with the cardiac disease.

Services in connection with a cardiac rehabilitation exercise program may be provided for up to 36 sessions, usually three sessions a week in a single 12-week period. Coverage for continued participation is allowed only on a case-by-case basis with exit criteria taken into consideration. The following exit criteria guidelines apply:

- The patient has achieved a stable level of exercise tolerance without ischemia or dysrhythmia

- Symptoms of angina or dyspnea are stable at the patient's maximum exercise level

- Patient's resting blood pressure and heart rate are within normal limits

- The stress test is not positive during exercise

When claims are accompanied by acceptable documentation that the patient has not reached an exit level, coverage may be extended, but should not exceed 24 weeks.

MCM 2050.3 INCIDENT TO PHYSICIAN'S SERVICE IN CLINIC

A physician directed clinic is one where:

1. A physician (or a number of physicians) is present to perform medical (rather than administrative) services at all times the clinic is open

2. Each patient is under the care of a clinic physician

3. The nonphysician services are under medical supervision

In highly organized clinics, particularly those that are departmentalized, direct personal physician supervision may be the responsibility of several physicians as opposed to an individual attending physician. In this situation, medical management of all services provided in the clinic is assured. The physician ordering a particular service need not be the physician who is supervising the service. Supplies provided by the clinic during the course of treatment are also covered. When the auxiliary personnel perform services outside the clinic premises, the services are covered only if performed under the direct personal supervision of a clinic physician. If the clinic refers a patient for auxiliary services performed by personnel who are not employed by the clinic, such services are not incident to a physician's service.

93797   **Physician services for outpatient cardiac rehabilitation; without continuous ECG monitoring (per session)**   80 ⬚

93798   **with continuous ECG monitoring (per session)**   80 ⬚

MCM 4277. EXTERNAL COUNTERPULSATION (ECP)

Commonly referred to as enhanced external counterpulsation, is a non-invasive outpatient treatment for coronary artery disease refractory medical and/or surgical therapy. Effective for dates of service July 1, 1999 and after, Medicare will cover ECP when its use is in patients with stable anginal pectoris, since only that use has developed sufficient evidence to demonstrate its medical effectiveness. Effective for dates of service on or after January 1, 2000, use HCPCS code G0166 (External counterpulsation, per session) to report ECP services (replaces 93799 Unlisted cardiovascular service or procedure). The codes for external cardiac assist (92971), ECG rhythm strip and report (93040 or 93041), pulse oximetry (94760 or 94761) and plethysmography (93922 or 93923) or other monitoring tests for examining the effects of this treatment are not clinically necessary with this service and should not be paid on the same day, unless they occur in a clinical setting not connected with the delivery of the ECP. Daily evaluation and management service, e.g., 99201-99205, 99211-99215, 99217-99220, 99241-99245, cannot be billed with the ECP treatments. Any evaluation and management service must be justified with adequate documentation of the medical necessity of the visit. Deductible and coinsurance apply. Professional services of a physician must be billed on Form HCFA-1500 paper or electronic equivalent.

93799   **Unlisted cardiovascular service or procedure**   80

NON-INVASIVE VASCULAR DIAGNOSTIC STUDIES

CEREBROVASCULAR ARTERIAL STUDIES

CIM 50-37 NONINVASIVE TESTS OF CAROTID FUNCTION

Medicare covers the following tests, recognizing that this list is not inclusive and local medical consultants must make the determination:

DIRECT TESTS

- Carotid Phonoangiography

- Direct Bruit Analysis

- Spectral Bruit Analysis

- Doppler Flow Velocity

- Ultrasound Imaging including Real Time

- B-Scan and Doppler Devices

INDIRECT TESTS

- Periorbital Directional Doppler Ultrasonography
- Oculoplethysmography
- Ophthalmodynamometry

93875 Noninvasive physiologic studies of extracranial arteries, complete bilateral study (eg, periorbital flow direction with arterial compression, ocular pneumoplethysmography, Doppler ultrasound spectral analysis) [80]

The use of any Doppler device that produces a record that will not allow analysis of bidirectional vascular flow or that does not provide a hard copy printout is part of the physical exam of the vascular system and is not reported separately.

Consult the glossary for more terms and definitions.

93880 Duplex scan of extracranial arteries; complete bilateral study [80] [■]

93882 unilateral or limited study [80]

93886 Transcranial Doppler study of the intracranial arteries; complete study [80] [■]

93888 limited study [80]

EXTREMITY ARTERIAL STUDIES (INCLUDING DIGITS)

CIM 50-6 PLETHYSMOGRAPHY

Plethysmography is a noninvasive technique for diagnostic, preoperative, and postoperative evaluation of peripheral artery disease in the internal medicine or vascular surgery practice. In addition, plethysmography is used preoperative podiatric evaluation of the diabetic patient or one who has intermittent claudication or other signs or symptoms of peripheral vascular disease which bear on the patient's candidacy for foot surgery. Medicare coverage is extended to those procedures listed in Category I below when used for the accepted medical indications. The procedures in Category II are still considered experimental and are not covered.

Category I (covered)

1. Segmental Plethysmography (includes services performed with a regional plethysmograph, differential plethysmograph, recording oscillometer, and a pulse volume recorder)
2. Electrical Impedance Plethysmography
3. Ultrasonic Measurement of Blood Flow (Doppler)
4. Oculoplethysmography
5. Strain Gauge Plethysmography

Category II (not covered)

1. Inductance Plethysmography
2. Capacitance Plethysmography
3. Mechanical Oscillometry
4. Strain Gauge Plethysmography
5. Photoelectric Plethysmograph

MCM 4277 EXTERNAL COUNTERPULSATION (ECP)

Commonly referred to as enhanced external counterpulsation, is a non-invasive outpatient treatment for coronary artery disease refractory medical and/or surgical therapy. Effective for dates of service July 1, 1999 and after, Medicare will cover ECP when its use is in patients with stable anginal pectoris, since only that use has developed sufficient evidence to demonstrate its medical effectiveness. Effective for dates of service on or after January 1, 2000, use HCPCS code G0166 (External counterpulsation, per session) to report ECP services (replaces 93799 Unlisted cardiovascular service or procedure). The codes for external cardiac assist (92971), ECG rhythm strip and report (93040 or 93041), pulse oximetry (94760 or 94761) and plethysmography (93922 or 93923) or other monitoring tests for examining the effects of this treatment are not clinically necessary with this service and should not be paid on the same day, unless they occur in a clinical setting not connected with the delivery of the ECP. Daily evaluation and management service, e.g., 99201-99205, 99211-99215, 99217-99220, 99241-99245, cannot be billed with the ECP treatments. Any evaluation and management service must be justified with adequate documentation of the medical necessity of the visit. Deductible and coinsurance apply. Professional services of a physician must be billed on Form HCFA-1500 paper or electronic equivalent.

93922 Noninvasive physiologic studies of upper or lower extremity arteries, single level, bilateral (eg, ankle/brachial indices, Doppler waveform analysis, volume plethysmography, transcutaneous oxygen tension measurement) [80] [■]

93923 Non-invasive physiologic studies of upper or lower extremity arteries, multiple levels or with provocative functional maneuvers, complete bilateral study (eg, segmental blood pressure measurements, segmental Doppler waveform analysis, segmental volume plethysmography, segmental transcutaneous oxygen tension measurements, measurements with postural provocative tests, measurements with reactive hyperemia) [80] [■]

93924 Non-invasive physiologic studies of lower extremity arteries, at rest and following treadmill stress testing, complete bilateral study [80] [■]

93925 Duplex scan of lower extremity arteries or arterial bypass grafts; complete bilateral study [80] [■]

93926 unilateral or limited study [80] [■]

93930 Duplex scan of upper extremity arteries or arterial bypass grafts; complete bilateral study [80] [■]

93931 unilateral or limited study [80] [■]

EXTREMITY VENOUS STUDIES (INCLUDING DIGITS)

93965 Non-invasive physiologic studies of extremity veins, complete bilateral study (eg, Doppler waveform analysis with responses to compression and other maneuvers, phleborheography, impedance plethysmography) [80] [■]

93970 Duplex scan of extremity veins including responses to compression and other maneuvers; complete bilateral study [80] [■]

93971 unilateral or limited study [80] [■]

VISCERAL AND PENILE VASCULAR STUDIES

93975 Duplex scan of arterial inflow and venous outflow of abdominal, pelvic, scrotal contents and/or retroperitoneal organs; complete study [80] [■]

93976 limited study [80] [■]

93978 Duplex scan of aorta, inferior vena cava, iliac vasculature, or bypass grafts; complete study [80] [■]

93979 unilateral or limited study [80]

93980 Duplex scan of arterial inflow and venous outflow of penile vessels; complete study [80] [■]

93981 follow-up or limited study [80]

EXTREMITY ARTERIAL-VENOUS STUDIES

93990 Duplex scan of hemodialysis access (including arterial inflow, body of access and venous outflow) [80] [■]
When using indicator dilution methods for measurement of hemodialysis access flow, consult CPT code 90940.

PULMONARY

CPT codes 94010-94799 include laboratory tests and interpretation of results. Consult the appropriate Evaluation and Management CPT code and report it in addition to 94010-94799 when separate identifiable Evaluation and Management services are provided.

94010 Spirometry, including graphic record, total and timed vital capacity, expiratory flow rate measurement(s), with or without maximal voluntary ventilation [80] [■]

[■] CCI Comprehensive Code   [80] Bilateral Procedure   ✚ CPT Add-on Code   ⊘ Modifier -51 Exempt Code   ● New Code   ▲ Revised Code

[M] Maternity   [N] Newborn   [P] Pediatric   [N/P] Newborn/Pediatric

94014	Patient-initiated spirometric recording per 30-day period of time; includes reinforced education, transmission of spirometric tracing, data capture, analysis of transmitted data, periodic recalibration and physician review and interpretation	80 ⬛
94015	recording (includes hook-up, reinforced education, data transmission, data capture, trend analysis, and periodic recalibration)	TC 80 ⬛
94016	physician review and interpretation only	26 80 ⬛

| 94060 | Bronchospasm evaluation: spirometry as in 94010, before and after bronchodilator (aerosol or parenteral) | 80 ⬛ |

If a prolonged exercise test is conducted for bronchospasm with pre- and post-spirometry, consult CPT code 94620.

94070	Prolonged postexposure evaluation of bronchospasm with multiple spirometric determinations after antigen, cold air, methacholine or other chemical agent, with subsequent spirometrics	80 ⬛
94150	Vital capacity, total (separate procedure)	
94200	Maximum breathing capacity, maximal voluntary ventilation	80
94240	Functional residual capacity or residual volume: helium method, nitrogen open circuit method, or other method	80
94250	Expired gas collection, quantitative, single procedure (separate procedure)	80
94260	Thoracic gas volume	80

If plethysmography is performed, consult CPT codes 93720-93722.

94350	Determination of maldistribution of inspired gas: multiple breath nitrogen washout curve including alveolar nitrogen or helium equilibration time	80
94360	Determination of resistance to airflow, oscillatory or plethysmographic methods	80
94370	Determination of airway closing volume, single breath tests	80
94375	Respiratory flow volume loop	80

CIM 50-51 DIAGNOSTIC BREATH ANALYSES

Medicare covers lactose breath hydrogen to detect lactose malabsorption in gastrointestinal diseases. Medicare does not cover:

- Lactulose breath hydrogen for diagnosing small bowel bacterial overgrowth and measuring small bowel transit time
- l3CO$_2$ for diagnosing bile acid malabsorption
- l3CO$_2$ for diagnosing fat malabsorption

| 94400 | Breathing response to CO2 (CO2 response curve) | 80 ⬛ |
| 94450 | Breathing response to hypoxia (hypoxia response curve) | 80 ⬛ |

CIM 35-15 POSTURAL DRAINAGE PROCEDURES AND PULMONARY EXERCISES

See Medicare Carriers Manual, §2050.2.

In most cases, nursing personnel can provide postural drainage procedures and pulmonary exercises. However, in some cases patients may have acute or severe pulmonary conditions that require the skills of a physical therapist or a respiratory therapist, as determined by the attending physician as part of the plan of treatment. The physical therapy must be provided as an inpatient hospital service, extended care service, home health service, or outpatient physical therapy service. Physical therapy furnished in the outpatient department of a hospital is covered under the outpatient physical therapy benefit. If the attending physician determines that a respiratory therapist performs the services, the services are covered when provided as an inpatient hospital service, outpatient hospital service, or extended care service, assuming that services are furnished to the skilled nursing facility by a hospital with a transfer agreement. Since the services of a respiratory therapist are not covered under the home health benefit, payment may not be made under the home health benefit for visits by a respiratory therapist to a patient's home. In addition, postural drainage procedures and pulmonary exercises are covered when furnished by a physical or a respiratory therapist as incident to a physician's professional service.

MCM 2050.2 SERVICES OF NONPHYSICIAN PERSONNEL FURNISHED INCIDENT TO PHYSICIAN'S SERVICES

In addition to coverage for the services of nonphysician personnel as nurses, technicians, and therapists when furnished incident to the professional services of a physician, a physician may also have the services of certain nonphysician practitioners covered as incident to a physician's professional services. These nonphysician practitioners, include, for example, certified nurse midwives, certified registered nurse anesthetists, clinical psychologists, clinical social workers, physician assistants, nurse practitioners, and clinical nurse specialists. The nonphysician practitioner may provide services ordinarily provided in the office (e.g., medical services such as taking blood pressures and temperatures, giving injections, and changing dressings) and services, and other activities that involve evaluation or treatment of a patient's condition.

| 94620 | Pulmonary stress testing; simple (eg, prolonged exercise test for bronchospasm with pre- and post-spirometry) | 80 ⬛ |

CIM 50-15 ELECTROCARDIOGRAPHIC SERVICES

Medicare Part B covers electrocardiographic (EKG) services rendered by a physician, incident to services, or by an approved laboratory or supplier of portable X-ray services (the claim must identify the physician ordering the service and the physician making the interpretation). Practices may charge separately for an EKG interpretation by an attending or consulting physician.

In addition, Medicare covers an emergency as a laboratory service or a diagnostic service by a portable X-ray supplier only when evidence shows that a physician was in attendance at the time the service was performed or immediately thereafter. EKG services provided in the patient's home, payment is based on the reasonable charge of services supplied in the laboratory (or in the supplier's office), in the absence of documentation.

Medicare coverage of Long Term EKG Monitoring, referred to as long-term EKG recording, Holter recording, or dynamic electrocardiography depends on a complete patient evaluation prior to performance of this diagnostic study. Generally, a statement of the diagnostic impression of the referring physician with an indication of the patient's relevant signs and symptoms should be sufficient for determining medical necessity. Intermediaries or carriers may require whatever additional documentation.

Medicare covers patient-activated EKG recorders when used as an alternative to the long-term EKG for similar indications (e.g., detecting and characterizing symptomatic arrhythmias, regulation of anti-arrhythmic drug therapy). Medicare does not cover outpatient monitoring of recently discharged post-infarct patients.

Medicare covers computer interpretation of an EKG when furnished under the circumstances required for coverage of other electrocardiographic services. The certifying physician must be identified on the HCFA-1490. Where the laboratory's (or portable x-ray supplier's) reviewing physician is not identified, no professional component is involved and reimbursement is determined accordingly. If the supplying laboratory does not include professional review and certification of the hard copy, the patient's physician is reimbursed.

Medicare covers Transtelephonic Electrocardiographic Transmissions Effective as a diagnostic service for the indications described below:

- To detect, characterize, and document symptomatic transient arrhythmias
- To overcome problems in regulating antiarrhythmic drug dosage
- To carry out early post-hospital monitoring of patients discharged after myocardial infarction

The transmitting devices must meet at least the following criteria:

1. Capable of transmitting EKG Leads, I, II, or III
2. Lead transmissions must be comparable to by a conventional EKG to permit interpretation of abnormal cardiac rhythms

| 94621 | complex (including measurements of CO2 production, O2 uptake, and electrocardiographic recordings) | 80 ⬜ |

94640 Nonpressurized inhalation treatment for acute airway obstruction 80 ⬜

94642 Aerosol inhalation of pentamidine for pneumocystis carinii pneumonia treatment or prophylaxis 80

94650 Intermittent positive pressure breathing (IPPB) treatment, air or oxygen, with or without nebulized medication; initial demonstration and/or evaluation 80 ⬜

94651 subsequent 80

94652 newborn infants N 80

94656 Ventilation assist and management, initiation of pressure or volume preset ventilators for assisted or controlled breathing; first day 80

If ventilation assist and management is performed as part of critical care services (99291-99292), do not report separately.

94657 subsequent days 80

94660 Continuous positive airway pressure ventilation (CPAP), initiation and management 80

If CPAP is performed as part of critical care services (99291-99292), do not report separately.

94662 Continuous negative pressure ventilation (CNP), initiation and management 80

If CNP is performed as part of critical care services 99291-99292), do not report separately.

94664 Aerosol or vapor inhalations for sputum mobilization, bronchodilation, or sputum induction for diagnostic purposes; initial demonstration and/or evaluation 80

94665 subsequent 80

CIM 35-2 MANIPULATION

Manual manipulation of the rib cage contributes to the treatment of respiratory conditions such as bronchitis, emphysema, and asthma as part of a regimen that includes other elements of therapy. It is covered only under such circumstances. Manipulation of the occipitocervical or temporomandibular regions of the head when indicated for conditions affecting those portions of the head and neck is a covered service.

94667 Manipulation chest wall, such as cupping, percussing, and vibration to facilitate lung function; initial demonstration and/or evaluation 80

94668 subsequent 80

CIM 35-15 POSTURAL DRAINAGE PROCEDURES AND PULMONARY EXERCISES

See Medicare Carriers Manual, §2050.2.

In most cases, nursing personnel can provide postural drainage procedures and pulmonary exercises. However, in some cases patients may have acute or severe pulmonary conditions that require the skills of a physical therapist or a respiratory therapist, as determined by the attending physician as part of the plan of treatment. The physical therapy must be provided as an inpatient hospital service, extended care service, home health service, or outpatient physical therapy service. Physical therapy furnished in the outpatient department of a hospital is covered under the outpatient physical therapy benefit. If the attending physician determines that a respiratory therapist performs the services, the services are covered when provided as an inpatient hospital service, outpatient hospital service, or extended care service, assuming that services are furnished to the skilled nursing facility by a hospital with a transfer agreement. Since the services of a respiratory therapist are not covered under the home health benefit, payment may not be made under the home health benefit for visits by a respiratory therapist to a patient's home. In addition, postural drainage procedures and pulmonary exercises are covered when furnished by a physical or a respiratory therapist as incident to a physician's professional service.

MCM 2050.2 SERVICES OF NONPHYSICIAN PERSONNEL FURNISHED INCIDENT TO PHYSICIAN'S SERVICES

In addition to coverage for the services of nonphysician personnel as nurses, technicians, and therapists when furnished incident to the professional services of a physician, a physician may also have the services of certain nonphysician practitioners covered as incident to a physician's professional services. These nonphysician practitioners, include, for example, certified nurse midwives, certified registered nurse anesthetists, clinical psychologists, clinical social workers, physician assistants, nurse practitioners, and clinical nurse specialists. The nonphysician practitioner may provide services ordinarily provided in the office (e.g., medical services such as taking blood pressures and temperatures, giving injections, and changing dressings) and services, and other activities that involve evaluation or treatment of a patient's condition.

94680 Oxygen uptake, expired gas analysis; rest and exercise, direct, simple 80 ⬜

For analysis of arterial blood gas results, see appropriate Evaluation and Mangement code. For testing consult CPT codes 82800-82810.

94681 including CO2 output, percentage oxygen extracted 80 ⬜

94690 rest, indirect (separate procedure) 80

If a single arterial procedure is performed, consult CPT code 36600.

▲ **94720** Carbon monoxide diffusing capacity (eg, single breath, steady state) 80

94725 Membrane diffusion capacity 80

▲ **94750** Pulmonary compliance study (eg, plethysmography, volume and pressure measurements) 80

MCM 4277. EXTERNAL COUNTERPULSATION (ECP)

Commonly referred to as enhanced external counterpulsation, is a non-invasive outpatient treatment for coronary artery disease refractory medical and/or surgical therapy. Effective for dates of service July 1, 1999 and after, Medicare will cover ECP when its use is in patients with stable anginal pectoris, since only that use has developed sufficient evidence to demonstrate its medical effectiveness. Effective for dates of service on or after January 1, 2000, use HCPCS code G0166 (External counterpulsation, per session) to report ECP services (replaces 93799 Unlisted cardiovascular service or procedure). The codes for external cardiac assist (92971), ECG rhythm strip and report (93040 or 93041), pulse oximetry (94760 or 94761) and plethysmography (93922 or 93923) or other monitoring tests for examining the effects of this treatment are not clinically necessary with this service and should not be paid on the same day, unless they occur in a clinical setting not connected with the delivery of the ECP. Daily evaluation and management service, e.g., 99201-99205, 99211-99215, 99217-99220, 99241-99245, cannot be billed with the ECP treatments. Any evaluation and management service must be justified with adequate documentation of the medical necessity of the visit. Deductible and coinsurance apply. Professional services of a physician must be billed on Form HCFA-1500 paper or electronic equivalent.

94760 Noninvasive ear or pulse oximetry for oxygen saturation; single determination TC 80 ⬜

For blood gases, consult CPT codes 82803-82810.

94761 multiple determinations (eg, during exercise) TC 80 ⬜

94762 by continuous overnight monitoring (separate procedure) TC 80

94770	Carbon dioxide, expired gas determination by infrared analyzer [80]

If bronchoscopy is performed, consult CPT codes 31622-31659. If a flow directed catheter is placed, consult CPT code 93503. If venipuncture is performed, consult CPT code 36410. If a central venous catheter is placed, consult CPT codes 36488-36491. If an arterial puncture is performed, consult CPT code 36600. If arterial catheterization is performed, consult CPT code 36620. If thoracentesis is performed, consult CPT code 32000. If a therapeutic phlebotomy is performed, consult CPT code 99195. If a needle biopsy is performed on the lung, consult CPT code 32405.If orotracheal or nasotracheal intubation is necessary, consult CPT code 31500.

94772 Circadian respiratory pattern recording (pediatric pneumogram), 12 to 24 hour continuous recording, infant [N] [80]

Separate procedure codes for electromyograms, EEG, ECG, and recordings of respiration cannot be reported with this procedural code.

94799 Unlisted pulmonary service or procedure [80]

ALLERGY AND CLINICAL IMMUNOLOGY

ALLERGY TESTING

MCM 15050. ALLERGY TESTING AND IMMUNOTHERAPY

A. Allergy Testing.—Allergy testing services billed under codes 95004-95078 are paid under the Medicare fee schedule for physician services using the national RVUs included in the data base. The RVUs shown for each code are per test. Therefore, instruct physicians to show the quantity of tests provided when billing. Multiply the payment for one test by the quantity for the code.

EXAMPLE: If a physician performs 25 percutaneous tests (scratch, puncture, or prick) with allergenic extract, the physician must bill code 95004 and specify 25 in the units field of Form HCFA-1500 (paper claims or electronic format). To compute payment, the Medicare carrier multiplies the payment for one test (i.e., the payment listed in the fee schedule) by the quantity listed in the units field.

95004 Percutaneous tests (scratch, puncture, prick) with allergenic extracts, immediate type reaction, specify number of tests [80]

95010 Percutaneous tests (scratch, puncture, prick) sequential and incremental, with drugs, biologicals or venoms, immediate type reaction, specify number of tests [80]

95015 Intracutaneous (intradermal) tests, sequential and incremental, with drugs, biologicals, or venoms, immediate type reaction, specify number of tests [80]

95024 Intracutaneous (intradermal) tests with allergenic extracts, immediate type reaction, specify number of tests [80]

95027 Skin end point titration [TC] [80]

95028 Intracutaneous (intradermal) tests with allergenic extracts, delayed type reaction, including reading, specify number of tests [TC] [80]

95044 Patch or application test(s) (specify number of tests) [80]

95052 Photo patch test(s) (specify number of tests) [80]

95056 Photo tests [80]

95060 Ophthalmic mucous membrane tests [TC] [80]

95065 Direct nasal mucous membrane test [TC] [80]

CIM 50-22 CHALLENGE INGESTION FOOD TESTING

Challenge ingestion food testing is a safe and effective technique in the diagnosis of food allergies. This procedure is covered when it is used on an outpatient basis if it is reasonable and necessary for the individual patient. Challenge ingestion food testing has not been proven to be effective in the diagnosis of rheumatoid arthritis, depression, or respiratory disorders, and no program payment is made for this procedure when it is so used.

95070 Inhalation bronchial challenge testing (not including necessary pulmonary function tests); with histamine, methacholine, or similar compounds [TC] [80] [CL]

95071 with antigens or gases, specify [TC] [80] [CL]

If pulmonary function tests are performed, consult CPT codes 94060 and 94070.

95075 Ingestion challenge test (sequential and incremental ingestion of test items, eg, food, drug or other substance such as metabisulfite) [80]

95078 Provocative testing (eg, Rinkel test) [TC] [80]

If allergy laboratory tests are conducted, consult CPT codes 86000-86999. If intravenous therapy is needed for severe or intractable allergic disease, consult CPT codes 90780, 90781, and 90784.

ALLERGEN IMMUNOTHERAPY

95115 Professional services for allergen immunotherapy not including provision of allergenic extracts; single injection [80]

95117 two or more injections [80] [CL]

95120 Professional services for allergen immunotherapy in prescribing physician's office or institution, including provision of allergenic extract; single injection

95125 two or more injections

95130 single stinging insect venom

95131 two stinging insect venoms

95132 three stinging insect venoms

95133 four stinging insect venoms

95134 five stinging insect venoms

CIM 45-28 ANTIGENS PREPARED FOR SUBLINGUAL ADMINISTRATION

Medicare does not cover antigens administered sublingually (i.e., by placing drops under the patient's tongue). Antigens are covered only if they are administered by injection.

▲ **95144** Professional services for the supervision of preparation and provision of antigens for allergen immunotherapy; single dose vial(s) (specify number of vials) [80]

A single dose vial is defined as a single dose of antigen administered in one injection.

▲ **95145** Professional services for the supervision of preparation and provision of antigens for allergen immunotherapy (specify number of doses); single stinging insect venom [80]

95146 two single stinging insect venoms [80] [CL]

95147 three single stinging insect venoms [80] [CL]

95148 four single stinging insect venoms [80] [CL]

95149 five single stinging insect venoms [80] [CL]

▲ **95165** Professional services for the supervision of preparation and provision of antigens for allergen immunotherapy; single or multiple antigens (specify number of doses) [80]

95170 whole body extract of biting insect or other arthropod (specify number of doses) [80]

When reporting allergy immunotherapy, a dose is the amount of antigen(s) administered in a single injection from a multiple dose vial.

▲ **95180** Rapid desensitization procedure, each hour (eg, insulin, penicillin, equine serum) [80]

95199 Unlisted allergy/clinical immunologic service or procedure [80]

If skin testing for bacterial, viral, and fungal extracts is performed, consult CPT codes 86485-86586 and 95028. If special reports are filed for an allergy patient, consult CPT code 99080. If testing procedures such as allergosorbent testing (RAST), rat mast cell technique (RMCT), mast cell degranulation test (MCDT), lymphocytic transformation test (LTT), leukocyte histamine release (LHR), migration inhibitory factor test (MIF), transfer factor test (TFT), nitroblue tetrazolium dye test (NTD) are performed, consult the Immunology section in Pathology or use 95199.

ENDOCRINOLOGY

● **95250** Glucose monitoring for up to 72 hours by continuous recording and storage of glucose values from interstitial tissue fluid via a subcutaneous sensor (includes hook-up, calibration, patient initiation and training, recording, disconnection, downloading with printout of data)

Code 95250 should not be used in conjunction with 99091.

For physician review, interpretation and written report associated with code 95250, see Evaluation and Management services section.

NEUROLOGY AND NEUROMUSCULAR PROCEDURES

SLEEP TESTING

In these codes, a patient's physiology is monitored while asleep to determine the cause or type of complaint or institute a therapy. CPT specifies that the patient sleep six or more hours with physician review, interpretation, and report.

95805 Multiple sleep latency or maintenance of wakefulness testing, recording, analysis and interpretation of physiological measurements of sleep during multiple trials to assess sleepiness [80]

If less than six hours of recording takes place of if there are other reduced services, append modifier -52.

95806 Sleep study, simultaneous recording of ventilation, respiratory effort, ECG or heart rate, and oxygen saturation, unattended by a technologist [80]

95807 Sleep study, simultaneous recording of ventilation, respiratory effort, ECG or heart rate, and oxygen saturation, attended by a technologist [80]

95808 Polysomnography; sleep staging with 1-3 additional parameters of sleep, attended by a technologist [80]

95810 sleep staging with 4 or more additional parameters of sleep, attended by a technologist [80]

95811 sleep staging with 4 or more additional parameters of sleep, with initiation of continuous positive airway pressure therapy or bilevel ventilation, attended by a technologist [80]

CIM 50-39 TELEPHONE TRANSMISSION OF ELECTROENCEPHALOGRAMS

Medicare covers telephone transmission of electroencephalograms (EEGs) in the following situations:

- Altered consciousness such as stuporous, semicomatose, or comatose states

- Atypical seizure variants in patients experiencing bizarre, distressing symptoms as seen with "spike and wave stupor" or other forms of seizure disorders

- Diagnosis of a suspected intracranial tumor

- Head injury, where a subdural hematoma may be identified

- Headaches during the acute phase where, for instance, in migraine syndrome, abnormal responses may be seen

95812 Electroencephalogram (EEG) extended monitoring; up to one hour [80]

95813 greater than one hour [80]

95816 Electroencephalogram (EEG) including recording awake and drowsy (including hyperventilation and/or photic stimulation when appropriate) [80]

If EEG monitoring is extended, consult CPT codes 95812 and 95813.

95819 Electroencephalogram (EEG) including recording awake and asleep (including hyperventilation and/or photic stimulation when appropriate) [80]

If EEG monitoring is extended, consult CPT codes 95812 and 95813. If the EEG is analyzed digitally, consult CPT code 95957.

95822 Electroencephalogram (EEG); sleep only [80]

If EEG monitoring is extended, consult CPT codes 95812 and 95813.

95824 cerebral death evaluation only [26] [80]

95827 all night sleep only [80]

If ambulatory 24-hour EEG monitoring is needed, consult CPT code 95950. If an EEG is performed during nonintracranial surgery, consult CPT code 95955. If a Wada activation test is performed, consult CPT code 95958. If circadian respiratory patterns of infants are recorded, consult CPT code 94772.

95829 Electrocorticogram at surgery (separate procedure) [80]

95830 Insertion by physician of sphenoidal electrodes for electroencephalographic (EEG) recording [80]

95831 Muscle testing, manual (separate procedure) with report; extremity (excluding hand) or trunk [80]

95832 hand, with or without comparison with normal side [80]

95833 total evaluation of body, excluding hands [80]

95834 total evaluation of body, including hands [80]

95851 Range of motion measurements and report (separate procedure); each extremity (excluding hand) or each trunk section (spine) [80]

95852 hand, with or without comparison with normal side [80]

95857 Tensilon test for myasthenia gravis; [80]

95858 with electromyographic recording [80]

95860 Needle electromyography, one extremity with or without related paraspinal areas [80]

95861 Needle electromyography, two extremities with or without related paraspinal areas [80]

To report dynamic electromyography performed during motion analysis studies, consult CPT codes 96002-96003.

95863 Needle electromyography, three extremities with or without related paraspinal areas [80]

95864 Needle electromyography, four extremities with or without related paraspinal areas [80]

95867 Needle electromyography, cranial nerve supplied muscles, unilateral [80]

95868 Needle electromyography, cranial nerve supplied muscles, bilateral [80]

□ CCI Comprehensive Code   [50] Bilateral Procedure   ✚ CPT Add-on Code   ⊘ Modifier -51 Exempt Code   ● New Code   ▲ Revised Code

[M] Maternity   [N] Newborn   [P] Pediatric   [N/P] Newborn/Pediatric

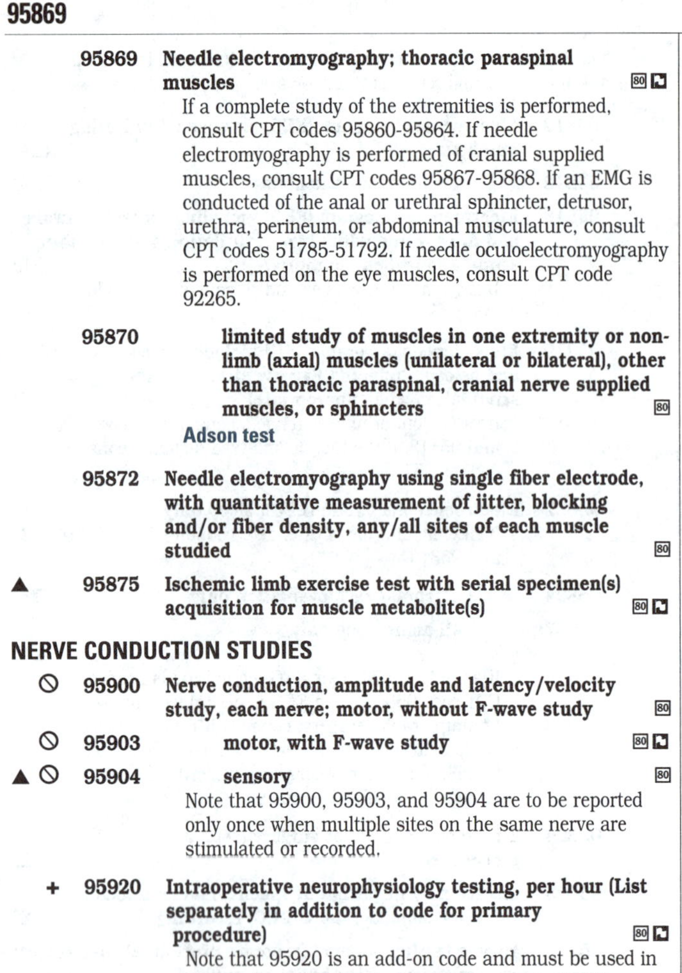

95869 Needle electromyography; thoracic paraspinal muscles [80] [▣]

If a complete study of the extremities is performed, consult CPT codes 95860-95864. If needle electromyography is performed of cranial supplied muscles, consult CPT codes 95867-95868. If an EMG is conducted of the anal or urethral sphincter, detrusor, urethra, perineum, or abdominal musculature, consult CPT codes 51785-51792. If needle oculoelectromyography is performed on the eye muscles, consult CPT code 92265.

95870 limited study of muscles in one extremity or non-limb (axial) muscles (unilateral or bilateral), other than thoracic paraspinal, cranial nerve supplied muscles, or sphincters [80]

Adson test

95872 Needle electromyography using single fiber electrode, with quantitative measurement of jitter, blocking and/or fiber density, any/all sites of each muscle studied [80]

▲ **95875** Ischemic limb exercise test with serial specimen(s) acquisition for muscle metabolite(s) [80] [▣]

NERVE CONDUCTION STUDIES

⊘ **95900** Nerve conduction, amplitude and latency/velocity study, each nerve; motor, without F-wave study [80]

⊘ **95903** motor, with F-wave study [80] [▣]

▲ ⊘ **95904** sensory [80]

Note that 95900, 95903, and 95904 are to be reported only once when multiple sites on the same nerve are stimulated or recorded.

+ **95920** Intraoperative neurophysiology testing, per hour (List separately in addition to code for primary procedure) [80] [▣]

Note that 95920 is an add-on code and must be used in conjunction with the study performed (e.g., 92585, 95822, 95860, 95861, 95867, 95868, 95900, 95904, 95925, 95926, 95927, 95930, 95933, 95934, 95936, 95937).

Code 95920 describes ongoing electrophysiologic testing and monitoring performed during surgical procedures. Code 95920 is reported per hour of service, and includes only the ongoing electrophysiologic monitoring time distinct from performance of specific type(s) of baseline electrophysiologic study(ies) (95860, 95861, 95867, 95868, 95900, 95904, 95933, 95934, 95936, 95937) or interpretation of specific type(s) of baseline electrophysiologic study(ies) (92585, 95822, 95925, 95926, 95927, 95930). The time spent performing or interpreting the baseline electrophysiologic study(ies) should not be counted as intraoperative monitoring, but represents separately reportable procedures. Code 95920 should beused once per hour even if multiple electrophysiologic studies are performed. The baseline electrophysiologic study(ies) should be used once per operative session.

95921 Testing of autonomic nervous system function; cardiovagal innervation (parasympathetic function), including two or more of the following; heart rate response to deep breathing with recorded R-R interval, Valsalva ratio, and 30:15 ratio [80] [▣]

95922 vasomotor adrenergic innervation (sympathetic adrenergic function), including beat-to-beat blood pressure and R-R interval changes during Valsalva maneuver and at least five minutes of passive tilt [80] [▣]

95923 sudomotor, including one or more of the following: quantitative sudomotor axon reflex test (QSART), silastic sweat imprint, thermoregulatory sweat test, and changes in sympathetic skin potential [80] [▣]

95925 Short-latency somatosensory evoked potential study, stimulation of any/all peripheral nerves or skin sites, recording from the central nervous system; in upper limbs [80]

95926 in lower limbs [80]

95927 in the trunk or head [80]

If this procedure is performed unilaterally, append modifier -52 to the procedural code. If visual evoked potential testing is performed on the central nervous system, consult CPT code 95930. If brainstem evoked response recording takes place, consult CPT code 92585. If auditory evoked potentials testing is conducted on the central nervous system, consult CPT code 92585.

CIM 50-31 EVOKED RESPONSE TESTS

Medicare covers evoked response tests, including brain stem evoked response and visual evoked response tests.

95930 Visual evoked potential (VEP) testing central nervous system, checkerboard or flash [80]

95933 Orbicularis oculi (blink) reflex, by electrodiagnostic testing [80]

95934 H-reflex, amplitude and latency study; record gastrocnemius/soleus muscle [80] [50]

95936 record muscle other than gastrocnemius/soleus muscle [80] [50]

95937 Neuromuscular junction testing (repetitive stimulation, paired stimuli), each nerve, any one method [80] [▣]

CIM 50-39.1 AMBULATORY ELECTROENCEPHALOGRAPHIC (EEG) MONITORING

Ambulatory electroencephalographic (EEG) monitoring is a diagnostic procedure when seizure diathesis is suspected but not defined by history, physical, or resting EEG. Ambulatory EEG can be utilized in the differential diagnosis of syncope and transient ischemic attacks if not elucidated by conventional studies. A resting EEG precedes an ambulatory EEG. Ambulatory EEG monitoring is considered an established technique and covered under Medicare for the above purposes.

95950 Monitoring for identification and lateralization of cerebral seizure focus, electroencephalographic (eg, 8 channel EEG) recording and interpretation, each 24 hours [80] [▣]

95951 Monitoring for localization of cerebral seizure focus by cable or radio, 16 or more channel telemetry, combined electroencephalographic (EEG) and video recording and interpretation (eg, for presurgical localization), each 24 hours [80] [▣]

95953 Monitoring for localization of cerebral seizure focus by computerized portable 16 or more channel EEG; electroencephalographic (EEG) recording and interpretation, each 24 hours [80] [▣]

95954 Pharmacological or physical activation requiring physician attendance during EEG recording of activation phase (eg, thiopental activation test) [80]

If an EEG is analyzed digitally, consult CPT code 95957.

95955 Electroencephalogram (EEG) during nonintracranial surgery (eg, carotid surgery) [80]

95956 Monitoring for localization of cerebral seizure focus by cable or radio, 16 or more channel telemetry, electroencephalographic (EEG) recording and interpretation, each 24 hours [80] [▣]

95957	**Digital analysis of electroencephalogram (EEG) (eg, for epileptic spike analysis)** [80]
95958	**Wada activation test for hemispheric function, including electroencephalographic (EEG) monitoring** [80]

CIM 35-20 TREATMENT OF MOTOR FUNCTION DISORDERS WITH ELECTRIC NERVE STIMULATION - NOT COVERED

No reimbursement may be made for electric nerve stimulation or for the services related to its implantation since this treatment cannot be considered reasonable and necessary. However, Medicare covers deep brain stimulation by implanting a stimulator device at the carrier's discretion.

CIM 65-8 ELECTRICAL NERVE STIMULATORS

Two general classifications of electrical nerve stimulators are employed to treat chronic intractable pain: peripheral nerve stimulators and central nervous system stimulators.

There are two types of implantations covered by this instruction:

- Dorsal column (spinal cord) neurostimulation.
- Depth brain neurostimulation

No payment may be made unless all of the conditions listed below have been met:

a. The implantation of the stimulator is used only as a late resort (if not a last resort) for patients with chronic intractable pain

b. Other treatment modalities (pharmacological, surgical, physical, or psychological therapies) have been tried and did not prove satisfactory, or are judged to be unsuitable or contraindicated for the given patient

c. Patients have undergone careful screening, evaluation and diagnosis by a multidisciplinary team prior to implantation. (psychological and physical evaluation)

d. All the facilities, equipment, and professional and support personnel required for the proper diagnosis, treatment training, and follow-up of the patient must be available

e. Demonstration of pain relief with a temporarily implanted electrode precedes permanent implantation

95961	**Functional cortical and subcortical mapping by stimulation and/or recording of electrodes on brain surface, or of depth electrodes, to provoke seizures or identify vital brain structures; initial hour of physician attendance** [80]
+ 95962	**each additional hour of physician attendance (List separately in addition to code for primary procedure)** [80]

Note that 95962 is an add-on code and must be used in conjunction with 95961.

● **95965**	**Magnetoencephalography (MEG), recording and analysis; for spontaneous brain magnetic activity (eg, epileptic cerebral cortex localization)** [26]
● **95966**	**for evoked magnetic fields, single modality (eg, sensory, motor, language, or visual cortex localization)** [26]
● + **95967**	**for evoked magnetic fields, each additional modality (eg, sensory, motor, language, or visual cortex localization) (List separately in addition to code for primary procedure)** [26]

Note that 95967 is an add-on code and must be used in conjunction with code 95966.

To report electroencephalography performed in addition to magnetoencephalography, consult CPT codes 95812-95827.

For somatosensory evoked potentials, auditory evoked potentials, and visual evoked potentials performed in addition to magnetic evoked field responses, see 92585, 95925, 95926, and/or 95930.

For computerized tomography performed in addition to magnetoencephalography, see 70450-70470, 70496.

For magnetic resonance imaging performed in addition to magnetoencephalography, see 70551-70553.

NEUROSTIMULATORS, ANALYSIS-PROGRAMMING

The following codes discuss the analysis and programming of neurostimulators. Neurostimulator pulse generators and transmitters affect pulse amplitude, duration, and frequency; more than eight electrode contacts; cycling; stimulation duration and spacing; number of programs and channels; phase angle; alternating polarities; configuration of wave form; and more than one clinical symptom.

CPT defines a simple neurostimulator as affecting up to three of these and a complex neurostimulator as affecting three or more.

CIM 45-25 SUPPLIES USED IN THE DELIVERY OF TRANSCUTANEOUS ELECTRICAL NERVE STIMULATION (TENS) AND NEUROMUSCULAR ELECTRICAL STIMULATION (NMES)

There are times patients receiving Transcutaneous Electrical Nerve Stimulation (TENS) and/or Neuromuscular Electrical Stimulation (NMES) treatment may need to use adhesive tapes and lead wires, a form-fitting conductive garment. A form-fitting conductive garment (and medically necessary related supplies) may be covered under the program when:

1. It has received permission or approval for marketing by the Food and Drug Administration (FDA)

2. It has been prescribed by a physician for use in delivering covered TENS or NMES treatment

3. One of the medical indications outlined below is met:

- Patient cannot manage without the conductive garment due to the large area or number of areas requiring stimulation

- Patient cannot manage without the conductive garment because the areas or sites to be stimulated are inaccessible with the use of conventional methods

- Patient has a documented medical condition such as skin problems that preclude the application of conventional devices

- Patient requires electrical stimulation beneath a cast either to treat disuse atrophy or to treat chronic intractable pain

- Patient has a medical need for rehabilitation strengthening (pursuant to a written plan of rehabilitation) following an injury

A conductive garment is covered for use with a TENS device during the trial period when:

1. Patient has a documented skin problem prior to the start of the trial period

2. Carrier's medical consultants are satisfied that use is medically necessary

---

95970   Electronic analysis of implanted neurostimulator pulse generator system (eg, rate, pulse amplitude and duration, configuration of wave form, battery status, electrode selectability, output modulation, cycling, impedance and patient compliance measurements); simple or complex brain, spinal cord, or peripheral (ie, cranial nerve, peripheral nerve, autonomic nerve, neuromuscular) neurostimulator pulse generator/transmitter, without reprogramming ⟨80⟩

> If a neurostimulator pulse generator is inserted, consult CPT codes 61885, 63685, 63688, and 64590. If a neurostimulator pulse generator or receiver is revised or removed, consult CPT codes 61888, 63688, and 64595. If neurostimulator electrodes are implanted, consult CPT codes 61850-61875, 63650-63655, and 64553-64580. If neurostimulator electrodes are revised or removed, consult CPT codes 61880, 63660, and 64585.

95971   simple brain, spinal cord, or peripheral (ie, peripheral nerve, autonomic nerve, neuromuscular) neurostimulator pulse generator/transmitter, with intraoperative or subsequent programming ⟨80⟩

95972   complex brain, spinal cord, or peripheral (except cranial nerve) neurostimulator pulse generator/transmitter, with intraoperative or subsequent programming, first hour ⟨80⟩

+ 95973   complex brain, spinal cord, or peripheral (except cranial nerve) neurostimulator pulse generator/transmitter, with intraoperative or subsequent programming, each additional 30 minutes after first hour (List separately in addition to code for primary procedure) ⟨80⟩

> Note that 95973 is an add-on code and must be used in conjunction with 95972.

95974   complex cranial nerve neurostimulator pulse generator/transmitter, with intraoperative or subsequent programming, with or without nerve interface testing, first hour ⟨80⟩

+ 95975   complex cranial nerve neurostimulator pulse generator/transmitter, with intraoperative or subsequent programming, each additional 30 minutes after first hour (List separately in addition to code for primary procedure) ⟨80⟩

> Note that 95975 is an add-on code and must be used in conjunction with 95974.

OTHER PROCEDURES

95999   Unlisted neurological or neuromuscular diagnostic procedure ⟨80⟩

MOTION ANALYSIS

For performance of needle electromyography procedures, consult CPT codes 95860-95875.

To report gait training, consult CPT code 97116.

●   **96000**   Comprehensive computer-based motion analysis by video-taping and 3-D kinematics;

●   **96001**   with dynamic plantar pressure measurements during walking

●   **96002**   Dynamic surface electromyography, during walking or other functional activities, 1-12 muscles

●   **96003**   Dynamic fine wire electromyography, during walking or other functional activities, 1 muscle

> Codes 95860-95875 should not be used in addition to 96002, 96003.

●   **96004**   Physician review and interpretation of comprehensive computer based motion analysis, dynamic plantar pressure measurements, dynamic surface electromyography during walking or other functional activities, and dynamic fine wire electromyography, with written report

CENTRAL NERVOUS SYSTEM ASSESSMENTS/TESTS (EG, NEURO-COGNITIVE, MENTAL STATUS, SPEECH TESTING)

The reports resulting from the following tests address the cognitive function of the patient.

96100   Psychological testing (includes psychodiagnostic assessment of personality, psychopathology, emotionality, intellectual abilities, eg, WAIS-R, Rorschach, MMPI) with interpretation and report, per hour ⟨80⟩

> If cognitive skills are developed to improve attention, memory, and problem solving, consult CPT code 97770.

Bender-Gestalt test

96105   Assessment of aphasia (includes assessment of expressive and receptive speech and language function, language comprehension, speech production ability, reading, spelling, writing, eg, by Boston Diagnostic Aphasia Examination) with interpretation and report, per hour ⟨80⟩

96110   Developmental testing; limited (eg, Developmental Screening Test II, Early Language Milestone Screen), with interpretation and report ⟨80⟩

96111   extended (includes assessment of motor, language, social, adaptive and/or cognitive functioning by standardized developmental instruments, eg, Bayley Scales of Infant Development) with interpretation and report, per hour ⟨80⟩

96115   Neurobehavorial status exam (clinical assessment of thinking, reasoning and judgment, eg, acquired knowledge, attention, memory, visual spatial abilities, language functions, planning) with interpretation and report, per hour ⟨80⟩

> To report mini-mental status examination performed by a physician, consult Evaluation and Management services codes.

96117   Neuropsychological testing battery (eg, Halstead-Reitan, Luria, WAIS-R) with interpretation and report, per hour ⟨80⟩

> If cognitive skills are developed to improve attention, memory, and problem solving, consult CPT codes 97532, 97533.

HEALTH AND BEHAVIOR ASSESSMENT/INTERVENTION

●   **96150**   Health and behavior assessment (eg, health-focused clinical interview, behavioral observations, psychophysicological monitoring, health-oriented questionnaires), each 15 minutes face-to-face with the patient; initial assessment

●   **96151**   re-assessment

●   **96152**   Health and behavior intervention, each 15 minutes, face-to-face; individual

●   **96153**   group (2 or more patients)

●   **96154**   family (with the patient present)

●   **96155**   family (without the patient present)

> For health and behavior assessment and/or intervention performed by a physician, see Evaluation and Management or Preventive Medicine services codes.

CHEMOTHERAPY ADMINISTRATION

CIM 45-21 SCALP HYPOTHERMIA DURING CHEMOTHERAPY, TO PREVENT HAIR LOSS
Cooling may be done by packing the scalp with ice-filled bags or bandages, or by cold-producing chemicals activated during chemotherapy. While the devices used for scalp hypothermia during chemotherapy may be covered as supplies of the kind commonly furnished without a separate charge, no separate charge for them would be recognized.

MCM 15400 CHEMOTHERAPY ADMINISTRATION (CODES 96400-96549)
Chemotherapy administration codes, 96400 through 96450, 96542, 96545, and 96549, are only to be used when reporting chemotherapy administration when the drug being used is an antineoplastic and the diagnosis is cancer. The administration of other drugs, such as growth factors, saline, and diuretics, to patients with cancer, or the administration of antineoplastics to patients with a diagnosis other than cancer, are reported with codes 90780 through 90784 as appropriate.

96400 **Chemotherapy administration, subcutaneous or intramuscular, with or without local anesthesia**

96405 **Chemotherapy administration, intralesional; up to and including 7 lesions**

96406 **more than 7 lesions**

96408 **Chemotherapy administration, intravenous; push technique**

96410 **infusion technique, up to one hour**

+ **96412** **infusion technique, one to 8 hours, each additional hour (List separately in addition to code for primary procedure)**
Note that 96412 is an add-on code and must be used in conjunction with 96410.

96414 **infusion technique, initiation of prolonged infusion (more than 8 hours), requiring the use of a portable or implantable pump**
If the pump or reservoir is refilled, consult CPT codes 96520 and 96530.

96420 **Chemotherapy administration, intra-arterial; push technique**

96422 **infusion technique, up to one hour**
If regional chemotherapy perfusion to an extremity is performed, consult CPT code 36823.

+ **96423** **infusion technique, one to 8 hours, each additional hour (List separately in addition to code for primary procedure)**
Note that 96423 is an add-on code and must be used in conjunction with 96422.
For regional chemotherapy perfusion via membrane oxygenator perfusion pump to an extremity, use 36823.

96425 **infusion technique, initiation of prolonged infusion (more than 8 hours), requiring the use of a portable or implantable pump**
If an implanted pump or reservoir is refilled, consult CPT codes 96520 and 96530.

96440 **Chemotherapy administration into pleural cavity, requiring and including thoracentesis**

96445 **Chemotherapy administration into peritoneal cavity, requiring and including peritoneocentesis**

▲ **96450** **Chemotherapy administration, into CNS (eg, intra-thecal), requiring and including spinal puncture**
If intravesical (bladder) chemotherapy is administered, consult CPT code 51720. If a subarachnoid catheter and reservoir is inserted for drug infusion, consult CPT codes 62350, 62351, and 62360-62362. If an intraventricular catheter and reservoir is inserted, consult CPT codes 61210 and 61215.

96520 **Refilling and maintenance of portable pump**

96530 **Refilling and maintenance of implantable pump or reservoir**
Note that access of pump port is included in filling of implantable pump.

96542 **Chemotherapy injection, subarachnoid or intraventricular via subcutaneous reservoir, single or multiple agents**

96545 **Provision of chemotherapy agent**
If radioactive isotope therapy is given, consult CPT codes 79000-79999.

96549 **Unlisted chemotherapy procedure**

PHOTODYNAMIC THERAPY

● **96567** **Photodynamic therapy by external application of light to destroy premalignant and/or malignant lesions of the skin and adjacent mucosa (eg, lip) by activation of photosensitive drug(s), each phototherapy exposure session**

CIM 35-59 ENDOSCOPY
Although endoscopy is primarily a diagnostic tool, it includes certain therapeutic procedures such as removal of polyps, and endoscopic papillotomy, by which stones are removed from the bile duct. Endoscopic procedures are covered when reasonable and necessary for the individual patient.

+ **96570** **Photodynamic therapy by endoscopic application of light to ablate abnormal tissue via activation of photosensitive drug(s); first 30 minutes (List separately in addition to code for endoscopy or bronchoscopy procedures of lung and esophagus)**
Note that 96570 and 96571 are to be used in addition to bronchoscopy, endoscopy codes. Note that 96570-96571 are add-on codes and must be used in conjunction with 31641 or 43228 as appropriate.
For reporting ocular photodynamic therapy consult CPT code 67221.

+ **96571** **each additional 15 minutes (List separately in addition to code for endoscopy or bronchoscopy procedures of lung and esophagus)**
Note that 96570 and 96571 are to be used in addition to bronchoscopy, endoscopy codes. Note that 96570-96571 are add-on codes and must be used in conjunction with 31641 or 43228 as appropriate.
For reporting ocular photodynamic therapy, consult CPT code 67221.

SPECIAL DERMATOLOGICAL PROCEDURES

96900 **Actinotherapy (ultraviolet light)**
If intralesional injections are administered, consult CPT codes 11900 and 11901. If a Tzanck smear is performed, consult CPT code 87207.

CIM 50-24 HAIR ANALYSIS - NOT COVERED
Hair analysis to detect mineral traces as an aid in diagnosing human disease is not a covered service under Medicare.

96902 **Microscopic examination of hairs plucked or clipped by the examiner (excluding hair collected by the patient) to determine telogen and anagen counts, or structural hair shaft abnormality**

CIM 35-66 TREATMENT OF PSORIASIS
Psoriasis treatment uses a psoralen derivative drug in combination with ultraviolet A light, known as PUVA. PUVA therapy is covered for treatment of intractable, disabling psoriasis, but only after the psoriasis has not responded to more conventional treatment. The contractor should document this before paying for PUVA therapy and limit reimbursement to amounts paid for other types of photochemotherapy. Payment should not extend over 30 days of treatment, unless improvement is documented.

□ CCI Comprehensive Code   50 Bilateral Procedure   + CPT Add-on Code   ◊ Modifier -51 Exempt Code   ● New Code   ▲ Revised Code

M Maternity   **N** Newborn   **P** Pediatric   **N/P** Newborn/Pediatric

| 96910 | Photochemotherapy; tar and ultraviolet B (Goeckerman treatment) or petrolatum and ultraviolet B | 80 |

CIM 35-66 TREATMENT OF PSORIASIS

Psoriasis treatment uses a psoralen derivative drug in combination with ultraviolet A light, known as PUVA. PUVA therapy is covered for treatment of intractable, disabling psoriasis, but only after the psoriasis has not responded to more conventional treatment. The contractor should document this before paying for PUVA therapy and limit reimbursement to amounts paid for other types of photochemotherapy. Payment should not extend over 30 days of treatment, unless improvement is documented.

96912	psoralens and ultraviolet A (PUVA)	80
96913	Photochemotherapy (Goeckerman and/or PUVA) for severe photoresponsive dermatoses requiring at least four to eight hours of care under direct supervision of the physician (includes application of medication and dressings)	80
96999	Unlisted special dermatological service or procedure	80

PHYSICAL MEDICINE AND REHABILITATION

MCM 2050.3 INCIDENT TO PHYSICIAN'S SERVICE IN CLINIC

A physician directed clinic is one where:

1. A physician (or a number of physicians) is present to perform medical (rather than administrative) services at all times the clinic is open

2. Each patient is under the care of a clinic physician

3. The nonphysician services are under medical supervision

In highly organized clinics, particularly those that are departmentalized, direct personal physician supervision may be the responsibility of several physicians as opposed to an individual attending physician. In this situation, medical management of all services provided in the clinic is assured. The physician ordering a particular service need not be the physician who is supervising the service. Supplies provided by the clinic during the course of treatment are also covered. When the auxiliary personnel perform services outside the clinic premises, the services are covered only if performed under the direct personal supervision of a clinic physician. If the clinic refers a patient for auxiliary services performed by personnel who are not employed by the clinic, such services are not incident to a physician's service.

| 97001 | Physical therapy evaluation | 80 |

If muscles are tested for range of joint motion, electromyography, consult CPT codes 95831 et seq. For biofeedback training by EMG, consult CPT code 90901. For transcutaneous nerve stimulation (TNS), consult CPT code 64550.

97002	Physical therapy re-evaluation	80
97003	Occupational therapy evaluation	80
97004	Occupational therapy re-evaluation	80
● 97005	Athletic training evaluation	
● 97006	Athletic training re-evaluation	

MODALITIES

SUPERVISED

97010	Application of a modality to one or more areas; hot or cold packs	
97012	traction, mechanical	80
97014	electrical stimulation (unattended)	80

If acupuncture is performed with electrical stimulation, consult CPT code 97781.

97016	vasopneumatic devices	80
97018	paraffin bath	80
97020	microwave	80
97022	whirlpool	80

CIM 35-3 HEAT TREATMENT, INCLUDING THE USE OF DIATHERMY AND ULTRA- SOUND FOR PULMONARY CONDITIONS - NOT COVERED

There is no physiological rationale or valid scientific documentation that diathermy or ultrasound heat treatments for asthma, bronchitis, or any other pulmonary condition is effective and, thus, cannot be considered reasonable and necessary.

CIM 35-41 DIATHERMY TREATMENT

High energy pulsed wave diathermy machines, which produce therapeutic benefit for essentially the same conditions as standard diathermy is considered a covered service, but only for those conditions for which standard diathermy is medically indicated and only when rendered by a physician or incident to a physician's professional services. Payment for high-energy diathermy treatment is based on the reasonable charge for standard diathermy (CPT-4 code 97024, ICD-9-CM code 93.34).

97024	diathermy	80
97026	infrared	80
97028	ultraviolet	80

CONSTANT ATTENDANCE

CIM 35-72 ELECTROTHERAPY FOR TREATMENT OF FACIAL NERVE PARALYSIS (BELL'S PALSY) - NOT COVERED

Electrotherapy for the treatment of facial nerve paralysis, commonly known as Bell's Palsy, is not covered under Medicare because its clinical effectiveness has not been established.

97032	Application of a modality to one or more areas; electrical stimulation (manual), each 15 minutes	80
97033	iontophoresis, each 15 minutes	80
97034	contrast baths, each 15 minutes	80

CIM 35-3 HEAT TREATMENT, INCLUDING THE USE OF DIATHERMY AND ULTRA- SOUND FOR PULMONARY CONDITIONS - NOT COVERED

There is no physiological rationale or valid scientific documentation that diathermy or ultrasound heat treatments for asthma, bronchitis, or any other pulmonary condition is effective and, thus, cannot be considered reasonable and necessary.

97035	ultrasound, each 15 minutes	80
97036	Hubbard tank, each 15 minutes	80
97039	Unlisted modality (specify type and time if constant attendance)	80

THERAPEUTIC PROCEDURES

97110	Therapeutic procedure, one or more areas, each 15 minutes; therapeutic exercises to develop strength and endurance, range of motion and flexibility	80
▲ 97112	neuromuscular reeducation of movement, balance, coordination, kinesthetic sense, posture, and/or proprioception for sitting and/or standing activities	80
97113	aquatic therapy with therapeutic exercises	80
97116	gait training (includes stair climbing)	80

To report comprehensive gait and motion analysis procedures, consult CPT codes 96000-96003.

| 97124 | massage, including effleurage, petrissage and/or tapotement (stroking, compression, percussion) | 80 |

For myofascial release, consult CPT code 97140.

| 97139 | unlisted therapeutic procedure (specify) | 80 |
| 97140 | Manual therapy techniques (eg, mobilization/manipulation, manual lymphatic drainage, manual traction), one or more regions, each 15 minutes | 80 |

97150	**Therapeutic procedure(s), group (2 or more individuals)**	80 ⬚

Note that 97150 is reported for each member of the group. Group therapy procedures involve constant attendance of the physician or therapist, but by definition do not require one-on-one patient contact by the physician or therapist. If manipulation under general anesthesia is performed, consult the appropriate anatomic section in Musculoskeletal System. If osteopathic manipulative treatment (OMT) is given, consult CPT codes 98925-98929.

▲ 97504 **Orthotic(s) fitting and training, upper extremity(ies), lower extremity(ies), and/or trunk, each 15 minutes** 80 ⬚

Note that 97504 cannot be reported with 97116. If casting and strapping is needed for a fracture, injury, or dislocation, consult CPT codes 29000 and 29590.

97520 **Prosthetic training, upper and/or lower extremities, each 15 minutes** 80 ⬚

97530 **Therapeutic activities, direct (one on one) patient contact by the provider (use of dynamic activities to improve functional performance), each 15 minutes** 80 ⬚

97532 **Development of cognitive skills to improve attention, memory, problem solving, (includes compensatory training), direct (one-on-one) patient contact by the provider, each 15 minutes** 80

97533 **Sensory integrative techniques to enhance sensory processing and promote adaptive responses to environmental demands, direct (one-on-one) patient contact by the provider, each 15 minutes** 80

▲ 97535 **Self-care/home management training (eg, activities of daily living (ADL) and compensatory training, meal preparation, safety procedures, and instructions in use of assistive technology devices/adaptive equipment) direct one-on-one contact by provider, each 15 minutes** 80 ⬚

97537 **Community/work reintegration training (eg, shopping, transportation, money management, avocational activities and/or work environment/modification analysis, work task analysis), direct one on one contact by provider, each 15 minutes** 80 ⬚

If wheelchair management/propulsion training is conducted, consult CPT code 97542.

97542 **Wheelchair management/propulsion training, each 15 minutes** 80 ⬚

97545 **Work hardening/conditioning; initial 2 hours** 80 ⬚

+ 97546 **each additional hour (List separately in addition to code for primary procedure)** 80

Note that 97546 is an add-on code and must be used in conjunction with 97545.

ACTIVE WOUND CARE MANAGEMENT

▲ 97601 **Removal of devitalized tissue from wound(s); selective debridement, without anesthesia (eg, high pressure waterjet, sharp selective debridement with scissors, scalpel and tweezers), including topical application(s), wound assessment, and instruction(s) for ongoing care, per session** ⬚

97602 **non-selective debridement, without anesthesia (eg, wet-to-moist dressings, enzymatic, abrasion), including topical application(s), wound assessment, and instruction(s) for ongoing care, per session**

Do not report CPT codes 97601, 97602 when reporting CPT codes 11040-11044.

TESTS AND MEASUREMENTS

97703 **Checkout for orthotic/prosthetic use, established patient, each 15 minutes** 80

97750 **Physical performance test or measurement (eg, musculoskeletal, functional capacity), with written report, each 15 minutes** 80 ⬚

OTHER PROCEDURES

For extracorporeal shock wave musculoskeletal therapy, consult CPT Category III code 0019T.

CIM 35-8 ACUPUNCTURE - NOT COVERED

Three units of the National Institutes of Health - National Institute of General Medical Sciences, National Institute of Neurological Diseases and Stroke, and Fogarty International Center - have been designed to assess and identify specific opportunities for the use of acupuncture for surgical anesthesia and relief of chronic pain. Until the pending scientific assessment of the technique has been completed and its efficacy has been established, Medicare reimbursement may not be made as an anesthetic or as an analgesic or for other therapeutic purposes.

CIM 35-21.1 OUTPATIENT HOSPITAL PAIN REHABILITATION PROGRAMS

Generally, hospital pain rehabilitation programs for outpatients are provided in group settings. Coverage is available if the patient's pain is attributed to a physical cause, the usual methods of treatment are unsuccessful, and the patient has a significant loss in the ability to function independently. Noncovered services (e.g., vocational counseling, meals for outpatients, or acupuncture) are excluded from coverage and intermediaries may find that the pain rehabilitation program is not reasonable and necessary for the treatment of their conditions.

97780 **Acupuncture, one or more needles; without electrical stimulation**

97781 **with electrical stimulation**

97799 **Unlisted physical medicine/rehabilitation service or procedure** 80

MEDICAL NUTRITION THERAPY

CIM 35-26.1 SUPPLEMENTED FASTING

Serious questions exist about the safety of prolonged adherence to low calorie weight reduction, therefore supplemented fasting is not covered as a general treatment for obesity. However, Medicare may cover supplemental fasting for a patient who must lose weight before surgery to ameliorate complications posed by obesity when it coexists with pathological conditions such as cardiac and respiratory diseases, diabetes or hypertension. The risks associated with the achievement of rapid weight loss must be carefully balanced against the risk posed by the condition requiring surgical treatment.

97802 **Medical nutrition therapy; initial assessment and intervention, individual, face-to-face with the patient, each 15 minutes**

Consult Evaluation and Management or Preventive Medicine service codes for medical nutrition therapy assessment and/or intervention performed by physician.

97803 **re-assessment and intervention, individual, face-to-face with the patient, each 15 minutes**

97804 **group (2 or more individual(s)), each 30 minutes**

OSTEOPATHIC MANIPULATIVE TREATMENT

Consult the appropriate Evaluation and Management CPT code and append modifier -25 or code 09925 in addition to OMT when separately identifiable Evaluation and Management services, above and beyond any pre or post service work associated with OMT, are provided.

Consult the glossary for more terms and definitions.

CIM 35-2 MANIPULATION

Manual manipulation of the rib cage contributes to the treatment of respiratory conditions such as bronchitis, emphysema, and asthma as part of a regimen that includes other elements of therapy. It is covered only under such circumstances. Manipulation of the occipitocervical or temporomandibular regions of the head when indicated for conditions affecting those portions of the head and neck is a covered service.

98925	Osteopathic manipulative treatment (OMT); one to two body regions involved	80 ▣
98926	three to four body regions involved	80 ▣
98927	five to six body regions involved	80 ▣
98928	seven to eight body regions involved	80 ▣
98929	nine to ten body regions involved	80 ▣

CHIROPRACTIC MANIPULATIVE TREATMENT

Consult the appropriate Evaluation and Management CPT code and append modifier -25 or code 09925 in addition to CMT when separately identifiable Evaluation and Management services, above and beyond any pre or post service work associated with CMT, are provided.

Consult the glossary for more terms and definitions.

98940	Chiropractic manipulative treatment (CMT); spinal, one to two regions	80 ▣
98941	spinal, three to four regions	80 ▣
98942	spinal, five regions	80 ▣
98943	extraspinal, one or more regions	

SPECIAL SERVICES, PROCEDURES AND REPORTS

MISCELLANEOUS SERVICES

The following codes are for use when services adjunct to the service performed must be reported.

99000 **Handling and/or conveyance of specimen for transfer from the physician's office to a laboratory**

99001 **Handling and/or conveyance of specimen for transfer from the patient in other than a physician's office to a laboratory (distance may be indicated)**

99002 **Handling, conveyance, and/or any other service in connection with the implementation of an order involving devices (eg, designing, fitting, packaging, handling, delivery or mailing) when devices such as orthotics, protectives, prosthetics are fabricated by an outside laboratory or shop but which items have been designed, and are to be fitted and adjusted by the attending physician**
   For a routine collection of venous blood, consult CPT code 36415.

99024 **Postoperative follow-up visit, included in global service**
   Note that 99024 is a component of a surgical "package." Consult surgery guidelines.

99025 **Initial (new patient) visit when starred (*) surgical procedure constitutes major service at that visit**

99050 **Services requested after office hours in addition to basic service**

99052 **Services requested between 10:00 PM and 8:00 AM in addition to basic service**

99054 **Services requested on Sundays and holidays in addition to basic service**

99056 **Services provided at request of patient in a location other than physician's office which are normally provided in the office**

99058 **Office services provided on an emergency basis**

99070 **Supplies and materials (except spectacles), provided by the physician over and above those usually included with the office visit or other services rendered (list drugs, trays, supplies, or materials provided)**
   For a supply of spectacles, consult CPT codes 92390-92395.

99071 **Educational supplies, such as books, tapes, and pamphlets, provided by the physician for the patient's education at cost to physician**

99075 **Medical testimony**

MCM 2050.3 INCIDENT TO PHYSICIAN'S SERVICE IN CLINIC

A physician directed clinic is one where:

1. A physician (or a number of physicians) is present to perform medical (rather than administrative) services at all times the clinic is open

2. Each patient is under the care of a clinic physician

3. The nonphysician services are under medical supervision

In highly organized clinics, particularly those that are departmentalized, direct personal physician supervision may be the responsibility of several physicians as opposed to an individual attending physician. In this situation, medical management of all services provided in the clinic is assured. The physician ordering a particular service need not be the physician who is supervising the service. Supplies provided by the clinic during the course of treatment are also covered. When the auxiliary personnel perform services outside the clinic premises, the services are covered only if performed under the direct personal supervision of a clinic physician. If the clinic refers a patient for auxiliary services performed by personnel who are not employed by the clinic, such services are not incident to a physician's service.

CIM 80-2 OUTPATIENT DIABETIC EDUCATION PROGRAMS

Medicare covers outpatient hospital diabetic education programs provided the services are furnished under a physician's order by the provider's personnel and under medical staff supervision to individuals who are registered patients of that provider. The services must be closely related to the care and treatment of the individual patient and must provide the patient with essential knowledge that aids in the patient's active participation in his or her own treatment and the skills that enable self-management. Not all diabetic patients are eligible to participate in these programs. In general, the kinds of patients that are likely to be suitable candidates for outpatient education programs are newly diagnosed diabetics and/or unstable diabetics (e.g., a long-term diabetic with current management problems).

99078 **Physician educational services rendered to patients in a group setting (eg, prenatal, obesity, or diabetic instructions)**

99080 **Special reports such as insurance forms, more than the information conveyed in the usual medical communications or standard reporting form**

MCM 15026 UNUSUAL TRAVEL (CPT CODE 99082)

In general, travel has been incorporated in the practice expense RVUs and is thus not separately payable. Pay separately for unusual travel (CPT code 99082) only when the physician submits documentation to demonstrate that the travel was very unusual.

99082 **Unusual travel (eg, transportation and escort of patient)** 80

▲ 99090 **Analysis of clinical data stored in computers (eg, ECGs, blood pressures, hematologic data)**
   For physician/health care professional collection and interpretation of physiologic data stored/transmitted by patient/caregiver, see 99091.

   Do not report 99090 if other more specific CPT codes exist, eg, 93014, 93227, 93233, 93272 for cardiographic services; 95250 for continuous glucose monitoring, 97750 for musculoskeletal function testing.

- **99091** **Collection and interpretation of physiologic data (eg, ECG, blood pressure, glucose monitoring) digitally stored and/or transmitted by the patient and/or caregiver to the physician or other qualified health care professional, requiring a minimum of 30 minutes of time**

QUALIFYING CIRCUMSTANCES FOR ANESTHESIA

+ **99100** **Anesthesia for patient of extreme age, under one year and over seventy (List separately in addition to code for primary anesthesia procedure)**
  If an explanation is needed for these services, consult the Anesthesia guidelines.

+ **99116** **Anesthesia complicated by utilization of total body hypothermia (List separately in addition to code for primary anesthesia procedure)**

+ **99135** **Anesthesia complicated by utilization of controlled hypotension (List separately in addition to code for primary anesthesia procedure)**

+ **99140** **Anesthesia complicated by emergency conditions (specify) (List separately in addition to code for primary anesthesia procedure)**
  An emergency is defined as existing when delay in treatment of the patient would lead to a significant increase in the threat to life or body part.

SEDATION WITH OR WITHOUT ANALGESIA (CONSCIOUS SEDATION)

99141 **Sedation with or without analgesia (conscious sedation); intravenous, intramuscular or inhalation**
  If sedation with or without analgesia (conscious sedation) is administered in support of a procedure provided by another physician, see Anesthesia section. Note that 94760-94762 cannot be reported in addition to 99141-99142.

99142 **oral, rectal and/or intranasal**

OTHER SERVICES AND PROCEDURES

99170 **Anogenital examination with colposcopic magnification in childhood for suspected trauma**
  If conscious sedation is used, consult CPT codes 99141 and 99142

- **99172** **Visual function screening, automated or semi-automated bilateral quantitative determination of visual acuity, ocular alignment, color vision by pseudoisochromatic plates, and field of vision (may include all or some screening of the determination(s) for contrast sensitivity, vision under glare)**
  This service MUST consist of graduated visual acuity stimuli that allow a quantitative determination of visual acuity (eg, Snellen chart).
  This service may not be used in addition to a general opthalmological service or an E/M service.
  Do not report CPT code 99172 in conjunction with CPT code 99173.

99173 **Screening test of visual acuity, quantitative, bilateral**
  Do not report CPT code 99173 in conjunction with CPT code 99172.

99175 **Ipecac or similar administration for individual emesis and continued observation until stomach adequately emptied of poison**
  If diagnostic intubation is needed, consult CPT codes 82926-82928 and 89130-98141. If gastric lavage is used for diagnostic purposes, consult CPT code 91055.

CIM 35-10 HYPERBARIC OXYGEN THERAPY

Hyperbaric oxygen (HBO) therapy is a modality exposing the entire body to oxygen under increased atmospheric pressure. HBO therapy should not be a replacement for other standard therapeutic measures and reimbursement depends upon the constant attendance of a physician who holds credentials in hyperbaric medicine and the management of acute cardiopulmonary emergencies, including placement of chest tube. This requirement applies in all settings: no payment will be made under Part A or Part B, unless the physician holds credentials and is in constant attendance during the HBO therapy procedure.

Depending on the response of the individual patient and the severity of the original problem, treatment may range from less than one week to several months, the average being two to four weeks. Further reimbursement is based on a review and documentation of medical necessity for more than two months, regardless of the condition of the patient. Program reimbursement for HBO therapy requires administration in a chamber (including a single unit) and is limited to the following conditions:

1. Acute carbon monoxide intoxication, (ICD-9-CM diagnosis 986).

2. Decompression illness, (ICD-9-CM diagnosis 993.2, 993.3).

3. Gas embolism, (ICD-9-CM diagnosis 958.0, 999.1).

4. Gas gangrene, (ICD-9-CM diagnosis 0400).

5. Acute traumatic peripheral ischemia. HBO therapy is n aadjunctive treatment used in combination with accepted standard therapeutic measures when loss of function, limb, or life is threatened. (ICD-9-CM diagnosis 902.53, 903.01, 903.1, 904.0, 904.41.)

6. Crush injuries and suturing of severed limbs. As in the previous conditions, HBO therapy would be an adjunctive treatment when loss of function, limb, or life is threatened. (ICD-9-CM diagnosis 927.00-927.03, 927.09-927.11, 927.20-927.21, 927.8-927.9, 928.00-928.01, 928.10-928.11, 928.20-928.21, 928.3, 928.8-928.9, 929.0, 929.9, 996.90-996.99.)

7. Progressive necrotizing infections (necrotizing fasciitis), (ICD-9-CM diagnosis 728.86).

8. Acute peripheral arterial insufficiency (ICD-9-CM diagnosis 444.21, 444.22, 444.81).

9. Treatment of compromised skin grafts (ICD-9-CM diagnosis 996.52; excludes artificial skin graft).

10. Chronic refractory osteomyelitis, unresponsive to conventional medical and surgical management (ICD-9-CM diagnosis 730.10-730.19).

11. Osteoradionecrosis as an adjunct to conventional treatment (ICD-9-CM diagnosis 526.89).

12. Soft tissue radionecrosis as an adjunct to conventional treatment (ICD-9-CM diagnosis 990).

13. Cyanide poisoning (ICD-9-CM diagnosis 987.7, 989.0).

14. Actinomycosis, only as an adjunct to conventional therapy when the disease process is refractory to antibiotics and surgical treatment, (ICD-9-CM diagnosis 039.0-039.4, 039.8, 039.9).

No program payment may be made for any conditions other than those listed. In addition, Medicare does not cover the topical application of oxygen due to the lack of clinical efficacy.

99183 **Physician attendance and supervision of hyperbaric oxygen therapy, per session**
  Note that Evaluation and Management services and/or procedures (e.g., wound debridement) provided in a hyperbaric oxygen treatment facility in conjunction with a hyperbaric oxygen therapy session should be reported separately.

99185 **Hypothermia; regional**

99186 **total body**

99190 **Assembly and operation of pump with oxygenator or heat exchanger (with or without ECG and/or pressure monitoring); each hour**

99191 **3/4 hour**

99192 **1/2 hour**

99195 **Phlebotomy, therapeutic (separate procedure)**

99199 **Unlisted special service, procedure or report**

HOME HEALTH PROCEDURES/SERVICES

- **99500** Home visit for prenatal monitoring and assessment to include fetal heart rate, non-stress test, uterine monitoring, and gestational diabetes monitoring
- **99501** Home visit for postnatal assessment and follow-up care
- **99502** Home visit for newborn care and assessment
- **99503** Home visit for respiratory therapy care (eg, bronchodilator, oxygen therapy, respiratory assessment, apnea evaluation)
- **99504** Home visit for patients receiving mechanical ventilation
- **99505** Home visit for stoma care and maintenance including colostomy and cystostomy
- **99506** Home visit for intramuscular injections
- **99507** Home visit for care and maintenance of catheter(s) (eg, urinary, drainage, and enteral)
- **99508** Home visit for polysomnography and sleep studies
- **99509** Home visit for assistance with activities of daily living and personal care

  To report self-care/home management training, see 97535.

  To report home medical nutrition assessment and intervention services, see 97802-97804.

  To report home speech therapy services, see 92507-92508.

- **99510** Home visit for individual, family, or marriage counseling
- **99511** Home visit for fecal impaction management and enema administration
- **99512** Home visit for hemodialysis, per diem

  For home infusion of peritoneal dialysis, use 99559.

- **99539** Unlisted home visit service or procedure

HOME INFUSION PROCEDURES

- **99551** Home infusion for pain management (intravenous or subcutaneous), per diem
- **99552** Home infusion for pain management (epidural or intrathecal), per diem
- **99553** Home infusion for tocolytic therapy, per diem
- **99554** Home infusion for hematopoietic hormones (eg, erythropoietin, G-CSF, CM-CSF) or platelets, per diem
- **99555** Home infusion for chemotherapy, per diem
- **99556** Home infusion for antibiotics/antifungals/antivirals, per diem
- **99557** Home infusion of continuous anticoagulant therapy (eg, heparin), per diem
- **99558** Home infusion of immunotherapy, per diem
- **99559** Home infusion of peritoneal dialysis, per diem

  For home visit for hemodialysis, use 999512.

- **99560** Home infusion of enteral nutrition, per diem
- **99561** Home infusion of hydration therapy, per diem
- **99562** Home infusion of total parenteral nutrition, per diem
- **99563** Home administration of aerosolized pentamidine, per diem
- **99564** Home infusion for anti-hemophilic agents (eg, Factor VIII), per diem
- **99565** Home infusion of alpha-1-proteinase inhibitor (eg, Prolastin), per diem
- **99566** Home infusion for uninterrupted, long-term intravenous treatment (eg, epoprostenol), per diem
- **99567** Home infusion of sympathomimetic agents (eg, dobutamine), per diem
- **99568** Home infusion of miscellaneous drugs, per diem
- **+** **99569** Home infusion, each additional therapy given on same day (List separately in addition to code for primary visit)

CATEGORY III CODES

The following is taken from information provided by the American Medical Association (AMA).

New to the CPT code set are Category III codes, alphanumeric codes intended to allow data collection for the services and procedures below. This is an activity that is critically important in the evaluation of health care delivery and the formation of public and private policy. The use of the codes in this section will allow physicians and other qualified health care professionals, payers, health services researchers, and health policy experts to identify emerging technology, services, and procedures for clinical efficacy, utilization and outcomes.

Category I codes are the long-used, 5-digit codes that make up the rest of the book. **If a Category III code is available for a given service or procedure, use the Category III code instead of a Category I Unlisted code.**

The inclusion of a service or procedure in this section neither implies nor endorses clinical efficacy, safety or the applicability to clinical practice. The codes in this section do not conform to the usual requirements for CPT Category I codes. For Category I codes, the AMA requires that the service or procedure be performed by many health care professionals in clinical practice in multiple locations and that necessary FDA approval has already been received. The nature of emerging technology, services, and procedures is that these requirements may not be met. New temporary codes for emerging technology, services, and procedures have been placed in a separate section of the CPT book and the codes are differentiated from Category I CPT codes by the use of alphanumeric characters.

Since these are temporary codes, they may or may not receive placement in the CPT book; and, those not adopted as permanent codes will be archived by the AMA after five years unless it is believed the temporary code is still needed. If made a permanent code in the CPT book, the existing numbers do not imply where they will be placed.

CATEGORY III CODES

● **0001T** Endovascular repair of infrarenal abdominal aortic aneurysm or dissection; modular bifurcated prosthesis (two docking limbs)

● **0002T** aorto-uni-iliac or aorto-unifemoral prosthesis
For radiological supervision and interpretation, use 75952 in conjunction with 0001T–0002T.

● **0003T** Cervicography

● **0005T** Transcatheter placement of extracranial cerebrovascular artery stent(s), percutaneous; initial vessel

● + **0006T** each additional vessel (List separately in addition to code for primary procedure
Use 0006T in conjunction with code 0005T.

For radiological supervision and interpretation, use 0007T.

● **0007T** Transcatheter placement of extracranial cerebrovascular artery stent(s), percutaneous, radiological supervision and interpretation, each vessel
For procedure, see 0005T, 0006T.

● **0008T** Upper gastrointestinal endoscopy including esophagus, stomach, and either the duodenum and/or jejunum as appropriate; with suturing of the esophagogastric junction

● **0009T** Endometrial cryoablation with ultrasonic guidance

● **0010T** Tuberculosis test, cell mediated immunity measurement of gamma interferon antigen response

● **0012T** Arthroscopy, knee, surgical, implantation of osteochondral graft(s) for treatment of articular surface defect; autografts

● **0013T** allografts

● **0014T** Meniscal transplantation, medial or lateral, knee (any method)

● **0016T** Destruction of localized lesion of choroid (eg, choroidal neovascularization), transpupillary thermotherapy

● **0017T** Destruction of macular drusen, photocoagulation

● **0018T** Delivery of high power, focal magnetic pulses for direct stimulation to cortical neurons

● **0019T** Extracorporeal shock wave therapy; involving musculoskeletal system

● **0020T** involving plantar fascia

● **0021T** Insertion of transcervical or transvaginal fetal oximetry sensor

● **0023T** Infectious agent drug susceptibility phenotype prediction using genotypic comparison to known genotypic/phenotypic database, HIV 1

● **0024T** Non-surgical septal reduction therapy (eg, alcohol ablation), for hypertrophic obstructive cardiomyopathy; with coronary arteriograms, with or without temporary pacemaker

● **0025T** Determination of corneal thickness (eg, pachymetry) with interpretation and report, bilateral

● **0026T** Lipoprotein, direct measurement, intermediate density lipoproteins (IDL) (remnant

---

● CCI Comprehensive Code   50 Bilateral Procedure   + CPT Add-on Code   ⊘ Modifier -51 Exempt Code   ● New Code   ▲ Revised Code

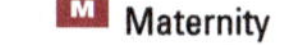 Maternity   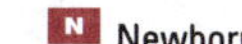 Newborn   P Pediatric   N/P Newborn/Pediatric

APPENDIX A—MODIFIERS

CPT MODIFIERS

This list includes all of the modifiers applicable to CPT codes.

-21 **Prolonged Evaluation and Management Services:** When the face-to-face or floor/unit service(s) provided is prolonged or otherwise greater than that usually required for the highest level of evaluation and management service within a given category, it may be identified by adding modifier '-21' to the evaluation and management code number or by use of the separate five digit modifier code 09921. A report may also be appropriate.

-22 **Unusual Procedural Services:** When the service(s) provided is greater than that usually required for the listed procedure, it may be identified by adding modifier '-22' to the usual procedure number or by use of the separate five digit modifier code 09922. A report may also be appropriate.

-23 **Unusual Anesthesia:** Occasionally, a procedure, which usually requires either no anesthesia or local anesthesia, because of unusual circumstances must be done under general anesthesia. This circumstance may be reported by adding modifier '-23' to the procedure code of the basic service or by use of the separate five digit modifier code 09923.

-24 **Unrelated Evaluation and Management Service by the Same Physician During a Postoperative Period:** The physician may need to indicate that an evaluation and management service was performed during a postoperative period for a reason(s) unrelated to the original procedure. This circumstance may be reported by adding modifier '-24' to the appropriate level of E/M service, or the separate five digit modifier 09924 may be used.

-25 **Significant, Separately Identifiable Evaluation and Management Service by the Same Physician on the Same Day of the Procedure or Other Service:** The physician may need to indicate that on the day a procedure or service identified by a CPT code was performed, the patient's condition required a significant, separately identifiable E/M service above and beyond the other service provided or beyond the usual preoperative and postoperative care associated with the procedure that was performed. The E/M service may be prompted by the symptom or condition for which the procedure and/or service was provided. As such, different diagnoses are not required for reporting of the E/M services on the same date. This circumstance may be reported by adding modifier '-25' to the appropriate level of E/M service, or the separate five digit modifier 09925 may be used. Note: This modifier is not used to report an E/M service that resulted in a decision to perform surgery. See modifier '-57.'

-26 **Professional Component:** Certain procedures are a combination of a physician component and a technical component. When the physician component is reported separately, the service may be identified by adding modifier '-26' to the usual procedure number or the service may be reported by use of the five digit modifier code 09926.

-32 **Mandated Services:** Services related to mandated consultation and/or related services (eg, PRO, third party payer, governmental, legislative, or regulatory requirement) may be identified by adding modifier '-32' to the basic procedure or the service may be reported by use of the five digit modifier 09932.

-47 **Anesthesia by Surgeon:** Regional or general anesthesia provided by the surgeon may be reported by adding modifier '-47' to the basic service or by use of the separate five digit modifier code 09947. (This does not include local anesthesia.) Note: Modifier '-47' or 09947 would not be used as a modifier for the anesthesia procedures 00100-01999.

-50 **Bilateral Procedure:** Unless otherwise identified in the listings, bilateral procedures that are performed at the same operative session should be identified by adding modifier '-50' to the appropriate five digit code or by use of the separate five digit modifier code 09950.

-51 **Multiple Procedures:** When multiple procedures, other than Evaluation and Management Services, are performed at the same session by the same provider, the primary procedure or service may be reported as listed. The additional procedure(s) or service(s) may be identified by appending modifier '-51' to the additional procedure or service code(s) or by the use of the separate five digit modifier code

09951. Note: This modifier should not be appended to designated "add-on" codes.

-52 **Reduced Services:** Under certain circumstances a service or procedure is partially reduced or eliminated at the physician's discretion. Under these circumstances the service provided can be identified by its usual procedure number and the addition of modifier '-52', signifying that the service is reduced. This provides a means of reporting reduced services without disturbing the identification of the basic service. Modifier code 09952 may be used as an alternative to modifier '-52.' Note: For hospital outpatient reporting of a previously scheduled procedure/service that is partially reduced or cancelled as a result of extenuating circumstances or those that threaten the well-being of the patient prior to or after administration of anesthesia, see modifiers '-73' and '-74' (see modifiers approved for ASC hospital outpatient use).

-53 **Discontinued Procedure:** Under certain circumstances, the physician may elect to terminate a surgical or diagnostic procedure. Due to extenuating circumstances or those that threaten the well being of the patient, it may be necessary to indicate that a surgical or diagnostic procedure was started but discontinued. This circumstance may be reported by adding modifier '-53' to the code reported by the physician for the discontinued procedure or by use of the separate five digit modifier code 09953. Note: This modifier is not used to report the elective cancellation of a procedure prior to the patient's anesthesia induction and/or surgical preparation in the operating suite. For outpatient hospital/ambulatory surgery center (ASC) reporting of a previously scheduled procedure/service that is partially reduced or cancelled as a result of extenuating circumstances or those that threaten the well being of the patient prior to or after administration of anesthesia, see modifiers '-73' and '-74' (see modifiers approved for ASC hospital outpatient use).

-54 **Surgical Care Only:** When one physician performs a surgical procedure and another provides preoperative and/or postoperative management, surgical services may be identified by adding modifier '-54' to the usual procedure number or by use of the separate five digit modifier code 09954.

-55 **Postoperative Management Only:** When one physician performs the postoperative management and another physician has performed the surgical procedure, the postoperative component may be identified by adding modifier '-55' to the usual procedure number or by use of the separate five digit modifier code 09955.

-56 **Preoperative Management Only:** When one physician performs the preoperative care and evaluation and another physician performs the surgical procedure, the preoperative component may be identified by adding modifier '-56' to the usual procedure number or by use of the separate five digit modifier code 09956.

-57 **Decision for Surgery:** An evaluation and management service that resulted in the initial decision to perform the surgery may be identified by adding modifier '-57' to the appropriate level of E/M service, or the separate five digit modifier 09957 may be used.

-58 **Staged or Related Procedure or Service by the Same Physician During the Postoperative Period:** The physician may need to indicate that the performance of a procedure or service during the postoperative period was: a) planned prospectively at the time of the original procedure (staged); b) more extensive than the original procedure; or c) for therapy following a diagnostic surgical procedure. This circumstance may be reported by adding modifier '-58' to the staged or related procedure, or the separate five digit modifier 09958 may be used. Note: This modifier is not used to report the treatment of a problem that requires a return to the operating room. See modifier '-78.'

-59 **Distinct Procedural Service:** Under certain circumstances, the physician may need to indicate that a procedure or service was distinct or independent from other services performed on the same day. Modifier '-59' is used to identify procedures/services that are not normally reported together, but are appropriate under the circumstances. This may represent a different session or patient encounter, different procedure or surgery, different site or organ system, separate incision/excision, separate lesion, or separate injury (or area of injury in extensive injuries) not ordinarily encountered or performed on the same day by the same physician. However, when another already established modifier is appropriate it should be used rather than modifier '-59.' Only if no more descriptive modifier is available, and the use of modifier '-59' best explains the circumstances, should modifier '-59' be used. Modifier code 09959 may be used as an alternative to modifier '-59.'

-62 **Two Surgeons:** When two surgeons work together as primary surgeons performing distinct part(s) of a procedure, each surgeon should report his/her distinct operative work by adding modifier '-62' to the procedure code and any associated add-on code(s) for that procedure as long as both surgeons continue to work together as primary surgeons. Each surgeon should report the co-surgery once using the same procedure code. If an additional procedure(s) (including an add-on procedure(s)) is performed during the same surgical session, a separate code(s) may be reported with the modifier '-62' added. Modifier code 09962 may be used as an alternative to modifier '-62'. Note: If a co-surgeon acts as an assistant in the performance of an additional procedure(s) during the same surgical session, the service(s) may be reported using a separate procedure code(s) with modifier '-80' or modifier '-82' added, as appropriate.

-66 **Surgical Team:** Under some circumstances, highly complex procedures (requiring the concomitant services of several physicians, often of different specialties, plus other highly skilled, specially trained personnel, various types of complex equipment) are carried out under the "surgical team" concept. Such circumstances may be identified by each participating physician with the addition of modifier '-66' to the basic procedure number used for reporting services. Modifier code 09966 may be used as an alternative to modifier '-66.'

-76 **Repeat Procedure by Same Physician:** The physician may need to indicate that a procedure or service was repeated subsequent to the original procedure or service. This circumstance may be reported by adding modifier '-76' to the repeated procedure/service or the separate five digit modifier code 09976 may be used.

-77 **Repeat Procedure by Another Physician:** The physician may need to indicate that a basic procedure or service performed by another physician had to be repeated. This situation may be reported by adding modifier '-77' to the repeated procedure/service or the separate five digit modifier code 09977 may be used.

-78 **Return to the Operating Room for a Related Procedure During the Postoperative Period:** The physician may need to indicate that another procedure was performed during the postoperative period of the initial procedure. When this subsequent procedure is related to the first, and requires the use of the operating room, it may be reported by adding modifier '-78' to the related procedure, or by using the separate five digit modifier 09978. (For repeat procedures on the same day, see modifier '-76'.)

-79 **Unrelated Procedure or Service by the Same Physician During the Postoperative Period:** The physician may need to indicate that the performance of a procedure or service during the postoperative period was unrelated to the original procedure. This circumstance may be reported by using modifier '-79' or by using the separate five digit modifier code 09979. (For repeat procedures on the same day, see modifier '-76'.)

-80 **Assistant Surgeon:** Surgical assistant services may be identified by adding modifier '-80' to the usual procedure number(s) or by use of the separate five digit modifier code 09980.

-81 **Minimum Assistant Surgeon:** Minimum surgical assistant services are identified by adding modifier '-81' to the usual procedure number or by use of the separate five digit modifier code 09981.

-82 **Assistant Surgeon (when qualified resident surgeon not available):** The unavailability of a qualified resident surgeon is a prerequisite for use of modifier '-82' appended to the usual procedure code number(s) or by use of the separate five digit modifier code 09982.

-90 **Reference (Outside) Laboratory:** When laboratory procedures are performed by a party other than the treating or reporting physician, the procedure may be identified by adding modifier '-90' to the usual procedure number or by use of the separate five digit modifier code 09990.

-91 **Repeat Clinical Diagnostic Laboratory Test:** In the course of treatment of the patient, it may be necessary to repeat the same laboratory test on the same day to obtain subsequent (multiple) test results. Under these circumstances, the laboratory test performed can be identified by its usual procedure number and the addition of modifier '-91'. Note: This modifier may not be used when tests are rerun to confirm initial results; due to testing problems with specimens or equipment; or for any other reason when a normal, one-time, reportable result is all that is required. This modifier may not

be used when another code(s) describes a series of test results (eg, glucose tolerance tests, evocative/suppression testing). This modifier may only be used for a laboratory test(s) performed more than once on the same day on the same patient.

-99 Multiple Modifiers: Under certain circumstances two or more modifiers may be necessary to completely delineate a service. In such situations, modifier '-99' should be added to the basic procedure and other applicable modifiers may be listed as part of the description of the service. Modifier code 09999 may be used as an alternative to modifier '-99.'

ANESTHESIA PHYSICAL STATUS MODIFIERS

All anesthesia services are reported by use of the five-digit anesthesia procedure code with the appropriate physical status modifier appended.

-P1 A normal healthy patient

-P2 A patient with mild systemic disease

-P3 A patient with severe systemic disease

-P4 A patient with severe systemic disease that is a constant threat to life

-P5 A moribund patient who is not expected to survive without the operation

-P6 A declared brain-dead patient whose organs are being removed for donor purposes

MODIFIERS APPROVED FOR AMBULATORY SURGERY CENTER (ASC) HOSPITAL OUTPATIENT USE

CPT LEVEL I MODIFIERS

-25 **Significant, Separately Identifiable Evaluation and Management Service by the Same Physician on the Same Day of the Procedure or Other Service:** The physician may need to indicate that on the day a procedure or service identified by a CPT code was performed, the patient's condition required a significant, separately identifiable E/M service above and beyond the other service provided or beyond the usual preoperative and postoperative care associated with the procedure that was performed. The E/M service may be prompted by the symptom or condition for which the procedure and/or service was provided. As such, different diagnoses are not required for reporting of the E/M services on the same date. This circumstance may be reported by adding modifier '-25' to the appropriate level of E/M service, or the separate five digit modifier 09925 may be used. Note: This modifier is not used to report an E/M service that resulted in a decision to perform surgery. See modifier '-57.'

-27 **Multiple Outpatient Hospital E/M Encounters on the Same Date:** For hospital outpatient reporting purposes, utilization of hospital resources related to separate and distinct E/M encounters performed in multiple outpatient hospital settings on the same date may be reported by adding modifier '-27' to each appropriate level outpatient and/or emergency department E/M code(s). This modifier provides a means of reporting circumstances involving evaluation and management services provided by a physician(s) in more than one (multiple) outpatient hospital setting(s) (eg, hospital emergency department, clinic). Note: This modifier is not to be used for physician reporting of multiple E/M services performed by the same physician on the same date. For physician reporting of all outpatient evaluation and management services provided by the same physician on the same date and performed in multiple outpatient settings (eg, hospital emergency department, clinic), see Evaluation and Management, Emergency Department, or Preventive Medicine Services codes.

-50 **Bilateral Procedure:** Unless otherwise identified in the listings, bilateral procedures that are performed at the same operative session should be identified by adding modifier '-50' to the appropriate five digit code or by use of the separate five digit modifier code 09950.

-52 **Reduced Services:** Under certain circumstances a service or procedure is partially reduced or eliminated at the physician's discretion. Under these circumstances the service provided can be identified by its usual procedure number and the addition of modifier '-52', signifying that the service is reduced. This provides a means of reporting reduced services without disturbing the identification of the basic service. Modifier code 09952 may be used as an alternative to modifier '-52.' Note: For hospital outpatient reporting of a previously scheduled procedure/service that is partially reduced or cancelled as a result of extenuating circumstances or those that threaten the well-being of the patient prior to or after administration of anesthesia, see modifiers '-73' and '-74' (see modifiers approved for ASC hospital outpatient use).

-58 **Staged or Related Procedure or Service by the Same Physician During the Postoperative Period:** The physician may need to indicate that the performance of a procedure or service during the postoperative period was: a) planned prospectively at the time of the original procedure (staged); b) more extensive than the original procedure; or c) for therapy following a diagnostic surgical procedure. This circumstance may be reported by adding modifier '-58' to the staged or related procedure, or the separate five digit modifier 09958 may be used. Note: This modifier is not used to report the treatment of a problem that requires a return to the operating room. See modifier '-78.'

-59 **Distinct Procedural Service:** Under certain circumstances, the physician may need to indicate that a procedure or service was distinct or independent from other services performed on the same day. Modifier '-59' is used to identify procedures/services that are not normally reported together, but are appropriate under the circumstances. This may represent a different session or patient encounter, different procedure or surgery, different site or organ system, separate incision/excision, separate lesion, or separate injury (or area of injury in extensive injuries) not ordinarily encountered or performed on the same day by the same physician. However, when another already established modifier is appropriate it should be used rather than modifier '-59.' Only if no more descriptive modifier is available, and the use of modifier '-59' best explains the circumstances, should modifier '-59' be used. Modifier code 09959 may be used as an alternative to modifier '-59.'

-73 **Discontinued Out-Patient Hospital/Ambulatory Surgery Center (ASC) Procedure Prior to the Administration of Anesthesia:** Due to extenuating circumstances or those that threaten the well being of the patient, the physician may cancel a surgical or diagnostic procedure subsequent to the patient's surgical preparation (including sedation when provided, and being taken to the room where the procedure is to be performed), but prior to the administration of anesthesia (local, regional block(s), or general). Under these circumstances, the intended service that is prepared for but cancelled can be reported by its usual procedure number and the addition of modifier '-73' or by use of the separate five digit modifier code 09973. Note: The elective cancellation of a service prior to the administration of anesthesia and/or surgical preparation of the patient should not be reported. For physician reporting of a discontinued procedure, see modifier '-53.'

-74 **Discontinued Out-Patient Hospital/Ambulatory Surgery Center (ASC) Procedure After Administration of Anesthesia:** Due to extenuating circumstances or those that threaten the well being of the patient, the physician may terminate a surgical or diagnostic procedure after the administration of anesthesia (local, regional block(s), general) or after the procedure was started (incision made, intubation started, scope inserted, etc.). Under these circumstances, the procedure started but terminated can be reported by its usual procedure number and the addition of modifier '-74' or by use of the separate five digit modifier code 09974. Note: The elective cancellation of a service prior to the administration of anesthesia and/or surgical preparation of the patient should not be reported. For physician reporting of a discontinued procedure, see modifier '-53.'

-76 **Repeat Procedure by Same Physician:** The physician may need to indicate that a procedure or service was repeated subsequent to the original procedure or service. This circumstance may be reported by adding modifier '-76' to the repeated procedure/service or the separate five digit modifier code 09976 may be used.

-77 **Repeat Procedure by Another Physician:** The physician may need to indicate that a basic procedure or service performed by another physician had to be repeated. This situation may be reported by adding modifier '-77' to the repeated procedure/service or the separate five digit modifier code 09977 may be used.

-78 **Return to the Operating Room for a Related Procedure During the Postoperative Period:** The physician may need to indicate that another procedure was performed during the postoperative period of the initial procedure. When this subsequent procedure is related to the first, and requires the use of the operating room, it may be reported by adding modifier '-78' to the related procedure, or by using the separate five digit modifier 09978. (For repeat procedures on the same day, see modifier '-76'.)

-79 **Unrelated Procedure or Service by the Same Physician During the Postoperative Period:** The physician may need to indicate that the performance of a procedure or service during the postoperative period was unrelated to the original procedure. This circumstance may be reported by using modifier '-79' or by using the separate five digit modifier code 09979. (For repeat procedures on the same day, see modifier '-76'.)

-91 **Repeat Clinical Diagnostic Laboratory Test:** In the course of treatment of the patient, it may be necessary to repeat the same laboratory test on the same day to obtain subsequent (multiple) test results. Under these circumstances, the laboratory test performed can be identified by its usual procedure number and the addition of modifier '-91'. Note: This modifier may not be used when tests are rerun to confirm initial results; due to testing problems with specimens or equipment; or for any other reason when a normal, one-time, reportable result is all that is required. This modifier may not be used when another code(s) describe a series of test results (eg, glucose tolerance tests, evocative/suppression testing). This modifier may only be used for a laboratory test(s) performed more than once on the same day on the same patient.

LEVEL II (HCPCS/NATIONAL) MODIFIERS

ANATOMICAL MODIFIERS

-E1	Upper left, eyelid
-E2	Lower left, eyelid
-E3	Upper right, eyelid
-E4	Lower right, eyelid
-F1	Left hand, second digit
-F2	Left hand, third digit
-F3	Left hand, fourth digit
-F4	Left hand, fifth digit
-F5	Right hand, thumb
-F6	Right hand, second digit
-F7	Right hand, third digit
-F8	Right hand, fourth digit
-F9	Right hand, fifth digit
-FA	Left hand, thumb
-LT	Left side (used to identify procedures performed on the left side of the body)
-RT	Right side (used to identify procedures performed on the right side of the body)
-T1	Left foot, second digit
-T2	Left foot, third digit
-T3	Left foot, fourth digit
-T4	Left foot, fifth digit
-T5	Right foot, great toe
-T6	Right foot, second digit
-T7	Right foot, third digit
-T8	Right foot, fourth digit
-T9	Right foot, fifth digit
-TA	Left foot, great toe

AMBULANCE MODIFIERS

-GM	Multiple patients on one ambulance trip
-QM	Ambulance service provided under arrangement by a provider of services
-QN	Ambulance service furnished directly by a provider of services
-QL	Patient pronounced dead after ambulance called

ANESTHESIA MODIFIERS

-AA Anesthesia services performed personally by anesthesiologist

-AD Medical supervision by a physician: more than four concurrent anesthesia procedures

-G8 Monitored anesthesia care (MAC) for deep complex, complicated, or markedly invasive surgical procedure

-G9 Monitored anesthesia care for patient who has history of severe cardio-pulmonary condition

-QK Medical direction of two, three, or four concurrent anesthesia procedures involving qualified individuals

-QS Monitored anesthesia care service

-QY Medical direction of one certified registered nurse anesthetist (CRNA) by an anesthesiologist

-QZ CRNA service: without medical direction by a physician

CORONARY ARTERY MODIFIERS

-LC Left circumflex coronary artery (Hospitals use with codes 92980-92984, 92995, 92996)

-LD Left anterior descending coronary artery (Hospitals use with codes 92980-92984, 92995, 92996)

-RC Right coronary artery (Hospitals use with codes 92980-92984, 92995, 92996)

OPHTHALMOLOGY MODIFIERS

-AP Determination of refractive state was not performed in the course of diagnostic ophthalmological examination

-LS FDA-monitored intraocular lens implant

-PL Progressive addition lenses

-VP Aphakic patient

PROFESSIONAL SERVICES

-AH Clinical psychologist

-AJ Clinical social worker

-AM Physician, team member service

-AS Physician assistant, nurse practitioner, or clinical nurse specialist services for assistant at surgery

-AT Acute treatment (this modifier should be used when reporting service 98940, 98941, 98942)

-CC Procedure code change (use 'CC' when the procedure code submitted was changed either for administrative reasons or because an incorrect code was filed)

-EP Service provided as part of medicaid early periodic screening diagnosis and treatment (EPSDT) program

-ET Emergency services

-G7 Pregnancy resulted from rape or incest or pregnancy certified by physician as life threatening

-GA Waiver of liability statement on file

-GB Claim being resubmitted for payment because it is no longer covered under a global payment demonstration

-GC This service has been performed in part by a resident under the direction of a teaching physician

-GE This service has been performed by a resident without the presence of a teaching physician under the primary care exception

-GG Performance and payment of a screening mammogram and diagnostic mammogram on the same patient, same day

-GH Diagnostic mammogram converted from screening mammogram on same day

-GJ "OPT OUT" physician or practitioner emergency or urgent service

-GK Actual item/service ordered byphysician, item associated with –GA or –GZ modifier

-GL Medically unnecessary upgrade provided instead of standard item, no charge, no advance beneficiary notice (ABN)

-GN Service delivered personally by a speech-language pathologist or under an outpatient speech-language pathology plan of care

-GO Service delivered personally by an occupational therapist or under an outpatient occupational therapy plan of care

-GP Service delivered personally by a physical therapist or under an outpatient physical therapy plan of care

-GQ Via asynchronous telecommunications system

-GT Via interactive audio and video telecommunication systems

-GV Attending physician not employed or paid under arrangement by the patient's hospice provider

-GW Service not related to the hospice patient's terminal condition

-GY Item or service statutorily excluded or does not meet the definition of any medicare benefit

-GZ Item or service expected to be denied as not reasonable and necessary

-Q4 Service for ordering/referring physician qualifies as a service exemption

-Q5 Service furnished by a substitute physician under a reciprocal billing arrangement

-Q6 Service furnished by a locum tenens physician

-QB Physician providing service in a rural HPSA

-QP Documentation is on file showing that the laboratory test(s) was ordered individually or ordered as a CPT-recognized panel other than automated profile codes 80002-80019, G0058, G0059, and G0060

-QQ Claim submitted with a written statement of intent

-QR Repeat laboratory test performed on the same day

-QS Monitored anesthesia care service

-QV Item or service provided as routine care in a Medicare qualifying clinical trial

-QW CLIA waived test

-QX CRNA service: with medical direction by a physician

-QY Medical direction of one certified registered nurse anesthetist (CRNA) by an anesthesiologist

-QZ CRNA service: without medical direction by a physician

-SA Nurse practitioner rendering service in collaboration with a physician

-SB Nurse Midwife

-SC Medically necessary service or supply

-SD Services provided by registered nurse with specialized, highly technical home infusion training

-SE State and/or federally funded programs/services

-SG Ambulatory surgical center (ASC) facility service

-SH Second concurrently administered infusion therapy

-SJ Third or more concurrently administered infusion therapy

-TC Technical component. Under certain circumstances, a charge may be made for the technical component alone. Under those circumstances the technical component charge is identified by adding modifier 'TC' to the usual procedure number. Technical component charges are institutional charges and not billed separately by physicians. However, portable x-ray suppliers only bill for technical component and should utilize modifier TC. The charge data from portable x-ray suppliers will then be used to build customary and prevailing profiles.

-TD RN

-TE LPN/LVN

-TF Intermediate level of care

-TG Complex/high level of care

-TH Obstetrical treatment/services, prenatal or postpartum

-TJ Program group, child and/or adolescent

ESRD MODIFIERS

-EJ Subsequent claims for a defined course of therapy, e.g., EPO, sodium hyaluronate, infliximab

-EM Emergency reserve supply (for ESRD benefit only)

-G1 Most recent urea reduction ratio (URR) reading of less than 60

-G2 Most recent urea reduction ration (URR) reading of 60 to 64.9

-G3 Most recent urea reduction ratio (URR) reading of 65 to 69.9

-G4 Most recent urea reduction ratio (URR) reading of 70 to 74.9

APPENDIX A—MODIFIERS

-G5   Most recent urea reduction ratio (URR) reading of 75 or greater

-G6   ESRD patient for whom less than six dialysis sessions have been provided in a month

-Q3   Live kidney donor: services associated with postoperative medical complications directly related to the donation

DENTAL MODIFIERS

-ET   Emergency services (dental procedures performed in emergency situations should show the modifier 'ET')

APPENDIX B—SUMMARY OF ADDITIONS, DELETIONS, AND REVISIONS

NEW CODES

0001T Endovascular repair of infrarenal abdominal aortic aneurysm or dissection; modular bifurcated prosthesis (two docking limbs)

0002T Endovascular repair of infrarenal abdominal aortic aneurysm or dissection; aorto-uni-iliac or aorto-unifemoral prosthesis

0003T Cervicography

0005T Transcatheter placement of extracranial cerebrovascular artery stent(s), percutaneous; initial vessel

0006T Transcatheter placement of extracranial cerebrovascular artery stent(s), percutaneous; each additional vessel (List separately in addition to code for primary procedure

0007T Transcatheter placement of extracranial cerebrovascular artery stent(s), percutaneous, radiological supervision and interpretation, each vessel

0008T Upper gastrointestinal endoscopy including esophagus, stomach, and either the duodenum and/or jejunum as appropriate; with suturing of the esophagogastric junction

0009T Endometrial cryoablation with ultrasonic guidance

0010T Tuberculosis test, cell mediated immunity measurement of gamma interferon antigen response

0012T Arthroscopy, knee, surgical, implantation of osteochondral graft(s) for treatment of articular surface defect; autografts

0013T Arthroscopy, knee, surgical, implantation of osteochondral graft(s) for treatment of articular surface defect; allografts

0014T Meniscal transplantation, medial or lateral, knee (any method)

0016T Destruction of localized lesion of choroid (eg, choroidal neovascularization), transpupillary thermotherapy

0017T Destruction of macular drusen, photocoagulation

0018T Delivery of high power, focal magnetic pulses for direct stimulation to cortical neurons

0019T Extracorporeal shock wave therapy; involving musculoskeletal system

0020T Extracorporeal shock wave therapy; involving plantar fascia

0021T Insertion of transcervical or transvaginal fetal oximetry sensor

0023T Infectious agent drug susceptibility phenotype prediction using genotypic comparison to known genotypic/phenotypic database, HIV 1

0024T Non-surgical septal reduction therapy (eg, alcohol ablation), for hypertrophic obstructive cardiomyopathy; with coronary arteriograms, with or without temporary pacemaker

0025T Determination of corneal thickness (eg, pachymetry) with interpretation and report, bilateral

0026T Lipoprotein, direct measurement, intermediate density lipoproteins (IDL) (remnant lipoproteins)

00797 Anesthesia for intraperitoneal procedures in upper abdomen including laparoscopy; gastric restrictive procedure for morbid obesity

00851 Anesthesia for intraperitoneal procedures in lower abdomen including laparoscopy; tubal ligation/transection

00869 Anesthesia for extraperitoneal procedures in lower abdomen, including urinary tract; vasectomy, unilateral/bilateral

01905 Anesthesia for myelography, diskography, vertebroplasty

01924 Anesthesia for therapeutic interventional radiologic procedures involving the arterial system; not otherwise specified

01925 Anesthesia for therapeutic interventional radiologic procedures involving the arterial system; carotid or coronary

01926 Anesthesia for therapeutic interventional radiologic procedures involving the arterial system; intracranial, intracardiac, or aortic

01930 Anesthesia for therapeutic interventional radiologic procedures involving the venous/lymphatic system (not to include access to the central circulation); not otherwise specified

01931 Anesthesia for therapeutic interventional radiologic procedures involving the venous/lymphatic system (not to include access to the central circulation); intrahepatic or portal circulation (eg, transcutaneous porto-caval shunt (TIPS))

01932 Anesthesia for therapeutic interventional radiologic procedures involving the venous/lymphatic system (not to include access to the central circulation); intrathoracic or jugular

01933 Anesthesia for therapeutic interventional radiologic procedures involving the venous/lymphatic system (not to include access to the central circulation); intracranial

01960 Anesthesia for; vaginal delivery only

01961 Anesthesia for; cesarean delivery only

01962 Anesthesia for; urgent hysterectomy following delivery

01963 Anesthesia for; cesarean hysterectomy without any labor analgesia/anesthesia care

01964 Anesthesia for; abortion procedures

01967 Neuraxial labor analgesia/anesthesia for planned vaginal delivery (this includes any repeat subarachnoid needle placement and drug injection and/or any necessary replacement of an epidural catheter during labor)

01968 Cesarean delivery following neuraxial labor analgesia/anesthesia (List separately in addition to code for primary procedure)

01969 Cesarean hysterectomy following neuraxial labor analgesia/anesthesia (List separately in addition to code for primary procedure)

10021 Fine needle aspiration; without imaging guidance

10022 Fine needle aspiration; with imaging guidance

11981 Insertion, non-biodegradable drug delivery implant

11982 Removal, non-biodegradable drug delivery implant

11983 Removal with reinsertion, non-biodegradable drug delivery implant

20526 Injection, therapeutic (eg, local anesthetic, corticosteroid), carpal tunnel

20551 Injection; tendon origin/insertion

20552 Injection; single or multiple trigger point(s), one or two muscle group(s)

20553 Injection; single or multiple trigger point(s), three or more muscle groups

24300 Manipulation, elbow, under anesthesia

24332 Tenolysis, triceps

24343 Repair lateral collateral ligament, elbow, with local tissue

24344 Reconstruction lateral collateral ligament, elbow, with tendon graft (includes harvesting of graft)

24345 Repair medial collateral ligament, elbow, with local tissue

24346 Reconstruction medial collateral ligament, elbow, with tendon graft (includes harvesting of graft)

25001 Incision, flexor tendon sheath, wrist (eg, flexor carpi radialis)

25024 Decompression fasciotomy, forearm and/or wrist, flexor AND extensor compartment; without debridement of nonviable muscle and/or nerve

25025 Decompression fasciotomy, forearm and/or wrist, flexor AND extensor compartment; with debridement of nonviable muscle and/or nerve

25259 Manipulation, wrist, under anesthesia

25275 Repair, tendon sheath, extensor, forearm and/or wrist, with free graft (includes obtaining graft) (eg, for extensor carpi ulnaris subluxation)

25394 Osteoplasty, carpal bone, shortening

25430 Insertion of vascular pedicle into carpal bone (eg, Harii procedure)

25431 Repair of nonunion of carpal bone (excluding carpal scaphoid (navicular)) (includes obtaining graft and necessary fixation), each bone

25651 Percutaneous skeletal fixation of ulnar styloid fracture

25652 Open treatment of ulnar styloid fracture

25671 Percutaneous skeletal fixation of distal radioulnar dislocation

26340 Manipulation, finger joint, under anesthesia, each joint

29086 Application, cast; finger (eg, contracture)

29805 Arthroscopy, shoulder, diagnostic, with or without synovial biopsy (separate procedure)

29806   Arthroscopy, shoulder, surgical; capsulorrhaphy

29807   Arthroscopy, shoulder, surgical; repair of slap lesion

29824   Arthroscopy, shoulder, surgical; distal claviculectomy including distal articular surface (Mumford procedure)

29900   Arthroscopy, metacarpophalangeal joint, diagnostic, includes synovial biopsy

29901   Arthroscopy, metacarpophalangeal joint, surgical; with debridement

29902   Arthroscopy, metacarpophalangeal joint, surgical; with reduction of displaced ulnar collateral ligament (eg, Stenar lesion)

29999   Unlisted procedure, arthroscopy

33967   Insertion of intra-aortic balloon assist device, percutaneous

33979   Insertion of ventricular assist device, implantable intracorporeal, single ventricle

33980   Removal of ventricular assist device, implantable intracorporeal, single ventricle

35647   Bypass graft, with other than vein; aortofemoral

35685   Placement of vein patch or cuff at distal anastomosis of bypass graft, synthetic conduit (List separately in addition to code for primary procedure)

35686   Creation of distal arteriovenous fistula during lower extremity bypass surgery (non-hemodialysis) (List separately in addition to code for primary procedure)

36002   Injection procedures (eg, thrombin) for percutaneous treatment of extremity pseudoaneurysm

36820   Arteriovenous anastomosis, open; by forearm vein transposition

38220   Bone marrow aspiration

38221   Bone marrow biopsy, needle or trocar

43313   Esophagoplasty for congenital defect, (plastic repair or reconstruction), thoracic approach; without repair of congenital tracheoesophageal fistula

43314   Esophagoplasty for congenital defect, (plastic repair or reconstruction), thoracic approach; with repair of congenital tracheoesophageal fistula

44126   Enterectomy, resection of small intestine for congenital atresia, single resection and anastomosis of proximal segment of intestine; without tapering

44127   Enterectomy, resection of small intestine for congenital atresia, single resection and anastomosis of proximal segment of intestine; with tapering

44128   Enterectomy, resection of small intestine for congenital atresia, single resection and anastomosis of proximal segment of intestine; each additional resection and anastomosis (List separately in addition to code for primary procedure)

44203   Laparoscopy, surgical; each additional small intestine resection and anastomosis (List separately in addition to code for primary procedure)

44204   Laparoscopy, surgical; colectomy, partial, with anastomosis

44205   Laparoscopy, surgical; colectomy, partial, with removal of terminal ileum with ileocolostomy

45136   Excision of ileoanal reservoir with ileostomy

46020   Placement of seton

47370   Laparoscopy, surgical, ablation of one or more liver tumor(s); radiofrequency

47371   Laparoscopy, surgical, ablation of one or more liver tumor(s); cryosurgical

47380   Ablation, open, of one or more liver tumor(s); radiofrequency

47381   Ablation, open, of one or more liver tumor(s); cryosurgical

47382   Ablation, one or more liver tumor(s), percutaneous, radiofrequency

49491   Repair, initial inguinal hernia, preterm infant (less than 37 weeks gestation at birth), performed from birth up to 50 weeks post-conceptual age, with or without hydrocelectomy; reducible

49492   Repair, initial inguinal hernia, preterm infant (less than 37 weeks gestation at birth), performed from birth up to 50 weeks post-conceptual age, with or without hydrocelectomy; incarcerated or strangulated

52001   Cystourethroscopy with irrigation and evacuation of clots

52347   Cystourethroscopy with transurethral resection or incision of ejaculatory ducts

53431   Urethroplasty with tubularization of posterior urethra and/or lower bladder for incontinence (eg, Tenago, Leadbetter procedure)

53444   Insertion of tandem cuff (dual cuff)

53446   Removal of inflatable urethral/bladder neck sphincter, including pump, reservoir, and cuff

53448   Removal and replacement of inflatable urethral/bladder neck sphincter including pump, reservoir, and cuff through an infected field at the same operative session including irrigation and debridement of infected tissue

53853   Transurethral destruction of prostate tissue; by water-induced thermotherapy

54162   Lysis or excision of penile post-circumcision adhesions

54163   Repair incomplete circumcision

54164   Frenulotomy of penis

54406   Removal of all components of a multi-component, inflatable penile prosthesis without replacement of prosthesis

54408   Repair of component(s) of a multi-component, inflatable penile prosthesis

54410   Removal and replacement of all component(s) of a multi-component, inflatable penile prosthesis at the same operative session

54411   Removal and replacement of all components of a multi-component inflatable penile prosthesis through an infected field at the same operative session, including irrigation and debridement of infected tissue

54415   Removal of non-inflatable (semi-rigid) or inflatable (self-contained) penile prosthesis, without replacement of prosthesis

54416   Removal and replacement of non-inflatable (semi-rigid) or inflatable (self-contained) penile prosthesis at the same operative session

54417   Removal and replacement of non-inflatable (semi-rigid) or inflatable (self-contained) penile prosthesis through an infected field at the same operative session, including irrigation and debridement of infected tissue

57155   Insertion of uterine tandems and/or vaginal ovoids for clinical brachytherapy

58346   Insertion of Heyman capsules for clinical brachytherapy

58953   Bilateral salpingo-oophorectomy with omentectomy, total abdominal hysterectomy and radical dissection for debulking;

58954   Bilateral salpingo-oophorectomy with omentectomy, total abdominal hysterectomy and radical dissection for debulking; with pelvic lymphadenectomy and limited para-aortic lymphadenectomy

59001   Amniocentesis; therapeutic amniotic fluid reduction (includes ultrasound guidance)

64561   Percutaneous implantation of neurostimulator electrodes; sacral nerve (transforaminal placement)

64581   Incision for implantation of neurostimulator electrodes; sacral nerve (transforaminal placement)

64821   Sympathectomy; radial artery

64822   Sympathectomy; ulnar artery

64823   Sympathectomy; superficial palmar arch

67225   Destruction of localized lesion of choroid (eg, choroidal neovascularization); photodynamic therapy, second eye, at single session (List separately in addition to code for primary eye treatment)

76085   Digitization of film radiographic images with computer analysis for lesion detection and further physician review for interpretation, screening mammography (List separately in addition to code for primary procedure)

76362   Computerized axial tomographic guidance for, and monitoring of, tissue ablation

76394   Magnetic resonance guidance for, and monitoring of, tissue ablation

76490   Ultrasound guidance for, and monitoring of, tissue ablation

77301   Intensity modulated radiotherapy plan, including dose-volume histograms for target and critical structure partial tolerance specifications

Appendixes

77418	Intensity modulated treatment delivery, single or multiple fields/arcs, via narrow spatially and temporally modulated beams (eg, binary, dynamic MLC), per treatment session
82274	Blood, occult, by fecal hemoglobin determination by immunoassay, qualitative, feces, 1-3 simultaneous determinations
83950	Oncoprotein, HER-2/neu
86141	C-reactive protein; high sensitivity (hsCRP)
86336	Inhibin A
87198	Cytomegalovirus, direct fluorescent antibody (DFA)
87199	Enterovirus, direct fluorescent antibody (DFA)
87802	Infectious agent antigen detection by immunoassay with direct optical observation; Streptococcus, group B
87803	Infectious agent antigen detection by immunoassay with direct optical observation; Clostridium difficile toxin A
87804	Infectious agent antigen detection by immunoassay with direct optical observation; Influenza
87902	Infectious agent genotype analysis by nucleic acid (DNA or RNA); Hepatitis C virus
88380	Microdissection (eg, mechanical, laser capture)
90473	Immunization administration by intranasal or oral route; one vaccine (single or combination vaccine/toxoid)
90474	Immunization administration by intranasal or oral route; each additional vaccine (single or combination vaccine/toxoid) (List separately in addition to code for primary procedure)
90939	Hemodialysis access flow study to determine blood flow in grafts and arteriovenous fistulae by an indicator dilution method, hook-up; transcutaneous measurement and disconnection
91123	Pulsed irrigation of fecal impaction
92136	Ophthalmic biometry by partial coherence interferometry with intraocular lens power calculation
92973	Percutaneous transluminal coronary thrombectomy (List separately in addition to code for primary procedure)
92974	Transcatheter placement of radiation delivery device for subsequent coronary intravascular brachytherapy (List separately in addition to code for primary procedure)
93025	Microvolt T-wave alternans for assessment of ventricular arrhythmias
93613	Intracardiac electrophysiologic 3-dimensional mapping (List separately in addition to code for primary procedure)
93701	Bioimpedance, thoracic, electrical
95250	Glucose monitoring for up to 72 hours by continuous recording and storage of glucose values from interstitial tissue fluid via a subcutaneous sensor (includes hook-up, calibration, patient initiation and training, recording, disconnection, downloading with printout of data)
95965	Magnetoencephalography (MEG), recording and analysis; for spontaneous brain magnetic activity (eg, epileptic cerebral cortex localization)
95966	Magnetoencephalography (MEG), recording and analysis; for evoked magnetic fields, single modality (eg, sensory, motor, language, or visual cortex localization)
95967	Magnetoencephalography (MEG), recording and analysis; for evoked magnetic fields, each additional modality (eg, sensory, motor, language, or visual cortex localization) (List separately in addition to code for primary procedure)
96000	Comprehensive computer-based motion analysis by video-taping and 3-D kinematics;
96001	Comprehensive computer-based motion analysis by video-taping and 3-D kinematics; with dynamic plantar pressure measurements during walking
96002	Dynamic surface electromyography, during walking or other functional activities, 1-12 muscles
96003	Dynamic fine wire electromyography, during walking or other functional activities, 1 muscle
96004	Physician review and interpretation of comprehensive computer based motion analysis, dynamic plantar pressure measurements, dynamic surface electromyography during walking or other functional
	activities, and dynamic fine wire electromyography, with written report
96150	Health and behavior assessment (eg, health-focused clinical interview, behavioral observations, psychophysicological monitoring, health-oriented questionnaires), each 15 minutes face-to-face with the patient; initial assessment
96151	Health and behavior assessment (eg, health-focused clinical interview, behavioral observations, psychophysicological monitoring, health-oriented questionnaires), each 15 minutes face-to-face with the patient; re-assessment
96152	Health and behavior intervention, each 15 minutes, face-to-face; individual
96153	Health and behavior intervention, each 15 minutes, face-to-face; group (2 or more patients)
96154	Health and behavior intervention, each 15 minutes, face-to-face; family (with the patient present)
96155	Health and behavior intervention, each 15 minutes, face-to-face; family (without the patient present)
96567	Photodynamic therapy by external application of light to destroy premalignant and/or malignant lesions of the skin and adjacent mucosa (eg, lip) by activation of photosensitive drug(s), each phototherapy exposure session
97005	Athletic training evaluation
97006	Athletic training re-evaluation
99091	Collection and interpretation of physiologic data (eg, ECG, blood pressure, glucose monitoring) digitally stored and/or transmitted by the patient and/or caregiver to the physician or other qualified health care professional, requiring a minimum of 30 minutes of time
99289	Physician constant attention of the critically ill or injured patient during an interfacility transport; first 30-74 minutes
99290	Physician constant attention of the critically ill or injured patient during an interfacility transport; each additional 30 minutes (List separately in addition to code for primary service)
99500	Home visit for prenatal monitoring and assessment to include fetal heart rate, non-stress test, uterine monitoring, and gestational diabetes monitoring
99501	Home visit for postnatal assessment and follow-up care
99502	Home visit for newborn care and assessment
99503	Home visit for respiratory therapy care (eg, bronchodilator, oxygen therapy, respiratory assessment, apnea evaluation)
99504	Home visit for patients receiving mechanical ventilation
99505	Home visit for stoma care and maintenance including colostomy and cystostomy
99506	Home visit for intramuscular injections
99507	Home visit for care and maintenance of catheter(s) (eg, urinary, drainage, and enteral)
99508	Home visit for polysomnography and sleep studies
99509	Home visit for assistance with activities of daily living and personal care
99510	Home visit for individual, family, or marriage counseling
99511	Home visit for fecal impaction management and enema administration
99512	Home visit for hemodialysis, per diem
99539	Unlisted home visit service or procedure
99551	Home infusion for pain management (intravenous or subcutaneous), per diem
99552	Home infusion for pain management (epidural or intrathecal), per diem
99553	Home infusion for tocolytic therapy, per diem
99554	Home infusion for hematopoietic hormones (eg, erythropoietin, G-CSF, CM-CSF) or platelets, per diem
99555	Home infusion for chemotherapy, per diem
99556	Home infusion for antibiotics/antifungals/antivirals, per diem
99557	Home infusion of continuous anticoagulant therapy (eg, heparin), per diem

99558	Home infusion of immunotherapy, per diem
99559	Home infusion of peritoneal dialysis, per diem
99560	Home infusion of enteral nutrition, per diem
99561	Home infusion of hydration therapy, per diem
99562	Home infusion of total parenteral nutrition, per diem
99563	Home administration of aerosolized pentamidine, per diem
99564	Home infusion for anti-hemophilic agents (eg, Factor VIII), per diem
99565	Home infusion of alpha-1-proteinase inhibitor (eg, Prolastin), per diem
99566	Home infusion for uninterrupted, long-term intravenous treatment (eg, epoprostenol), per diem
99567	Home infusion of sympathomimetic agents (eg, dobutamine), per diem
99568	Home infusion of miscellaneous drugs, per diem
99569	Home infusion, each additional therapy given on same day (List separately in addition to code for primary visit)

CHANGED CODES

00220	Anesthesia for intracranial procedures; cerebrospinal fluid shunting procedures
00560	Anesthesia for procedures on heart, pericardial sac, and great vessels of chest; without pump oxygenator
00942	Anesthesia for vaginal procedures (including biopsy of labia, vagina, cervix or endometrium); colpotomy, vaginectomy, colporrhaphy, and open urethral procedures
01214	Anesthesia for open procedures involving hip joint; total hip arthroplasty
01402	Anesthesia for open procedures on knee joint; total knee arthroplasty
01916	Anesthesia for diagnostic arteriography/venography
01920	Anesthesia for cardiac catheterization including coronary angiography and ventriculography (not to include Swan-Ganz catheter)
01951	Anesthesia for second and third degree burn excision or debridement with or without skin grafting, any site, for total body surface area (TBSA) treated during anesthesia and surgery; less than four percent total body surface area
01952	Anesthesia for second and third degree burn excision or debridement with or without skin grafting, any site, for total body surface area (TBSA) treated during anesthesia and surgery; between four and nine percent of total body surface area
01995	Regional intravenous administration of local anesthetic agent or other medication (upper or lower extremity)
11755	Biopsy of nail unit (eg, plate, bed, matrix, hyponychium, proximal and lateral nail folds) (separate procedure)
15732	Muscle, myocutaneous, or fasciocutaneous flap; head and neck (eg, temporalis, masseter muscle, sternocleidomastoid, levator scapulae)
15860	Intravenous injection of agent (eg, fluorescein) to test vascular flow in flap or graft
17000	Destruction (eg, laser surgery, electrosurgery, cryosurgery, chemosurgery, surgical curettement), all benign or premalignant lesions (eg, actinic keratoses) other than skin tags or cutaneous vascular proliferative lesions; first lesion
17004	Destruction (eg, laser surgery, electrosurgery, cryosurgery, chemosurgery, surgical curettement), all benign or premalignant lesions (eg, actinic keratoses) other than skin tags or cutaneous vascular proliferative lesions; 15 or more lesions
17110	Destruction (eg, laser surgery, electrosurgery, cryosurgery, chemosurgery, surgical curettement), of flat warts, molluscum contagiosum, or milia; up to 14 lesions
17260	Destruction, malignant lesion (eg, laser surgery, electrosurgery, cryosurgery, chemosurgery, surgical curettement), trunk, arms or legs; lesion diameter 0.5 cm or less
17270	Destruction, malignant lesion (eg, laser surgery, electrosurgery, cryosurgery, chemosurgery, surgical curettement), scalp, neck, hands, feet, genitalia; lesion diameter 0.5 cm or less
17280	Destruction, malignant lesion (eg, laser surgery, electrosurgery, cryosurgery, chemosurgery, surgical curettement), face, ears, eyelids, nose, lips, mucous membrane; lesion diameter 0.5 cm or less
20225	Biopsy, bone, trocar, or needle; deep (eg, vertebral body, femur)

20550	Injection; tendon sheath, ligament, ganglion cyst
21182	Reconstruction of orbital walls, rims, forehead, nasoethmoid complex following intra- and extracranial excision of benign tumor of cranial bone (eg, fibrous dysplasia), with multiple autografts (includes obtaining grafts); total area of bone grafting less than 40 sq cm
21183	Reconstruction of orbital walls, rims, forehead, nasoethmoid complex following intra- and extracranial excision of benign tumor of cranial bone (eg, fibrous dysplasia), with multiple autografts (includes obtaining grafts); total area of bone grafting greater than 40 sq cm but less than 80 sq cm
21184	Reconstruction of orbital walls, rims, forehead, nasoethmoid complex following intra- and extracranial excision of benign tumor of cranial bone (eg, fibrous dysplasia), with multiple autografts (includes obtaining grafts); total area of bone grafting greater than 80 sq cm
21750	Closure of median sternotomy separation with or without debridement (separate procedure)
23000	Removal of subdeltoid calcareous deposits, open
23350	Injection procedure for shoulder arthrography or enhanced CT/MRI shoulder arthrography
24075	Excision, tumor, soft tissue of upper arm or elbow area; subcutaneous
25020	Decompression fasciotomy, forearm and/or wrist, flexor OR extensor compartment; without debridement of nonviable muscle and/or nerve
25075	Excision, tumor, soft tissue of forearm and/or wrist area; subcutaneous
25274	Repair, tendon or muscle, extensor, forearm and/or wrist; secondary, with free graft (includes obtaining graft), each tendon or muscle
25405	Repair of nonunion or malunion, radius OR ulna; with autograft (includes obtaining graft)
25420	Repair of nonunion or malunion, radius AND ulna; with autograft (includes obtaining graft)
25440	Repair of nonunion, scaphoid carpal (navicular) bone, with or without radial styloidectomy (includes obtaining graft and necessary fixation)
25443	Arthroplasty with prosthetic replacement; scaphoid carpal (navicular)
25520	Closed treatment of radial shaft fracture and closed treatment of dislocation of distal radioulnar joint (Galeazzi fracture/dislocation)
25526	Open treatment of radial shaft fracture, with internal and/or external fixation and open treatment, with or without internal or external fixation of distal radioulnar joint (Galeazzi fracture/dislocation), includes repair of triangular fibrocartilage complex
25645	Open treatment of carpal bone fracture (other than carpal scaphoid (navicular)), each bone
26115	Excision, tumor or vascular malformation, soft tissue of hand or finger; subcutaneous
26116	Excision, tumor or vascular malformation, soft tissue of hand or finger; deep (subfascial or intramuscular)
26160	Excision of lesion of tendon sheath or joint capsule (eg, cyst, mucous cyst, or ganglion), hand or finger
26350	Repair or advancement, flexor tendon, not in zone 2 digital flexor tendon sheath (eg, no man's land); primary or secondary without free graft, each tendon
26356	Repair or advancement, flexor tendon, in zone 2 digital flexor tendon sheath (eg, no man's land); primary or secondary without free graft, each tendon
26390	Excision flexor tendon, with implantation of synthetic rod for delayed tendon graft, hand or finger, each rod
26392	Removal of synthetic rod and insertion of flexor tendon graft, hand or finger (includes obtaining graft), each rod
26415	Excision of extensor tendon, with implantation of synthetic rod for delayed tendon graft, hand or finger, each rod
26416	Removal of synthetic rod and insertion of extensor tendon graft (includes obtaining graft), hand or finger, each rod
26426	Repair of extensor tendon, central slip, secondary (eg, boutonniere deformity); using local tissue(s), including lateral band(s), each finger
26428	Repair of extensor tendon, central slip, secondary (eg, boutonniere deformity); with free graft (includes obtaining graft), each finger
26445	Tenolysis, extensor tendon, hand OR finger; each tendon

26510   Cross intrinsic transfer, each tendon

26587   Reconstruction of polydactylous digit, soft tissue and bone

26590   Repair macrodactylia, each digit

26607   Closed treatment of metacarpal fracture, with manipulation, with external fixation, each bone

26670   Closed treatment of carpometacarpal dislocation, other than thumb, with manipulation, each joint; without anesthesia

26676   Percutaneous skeletal fixation of carpometacarpal dislocation, other than thumb, with manipulation, each joint

26685   Open treatment of carpometacarpal dislocation, other than thumb; with or without internal or external fixation, each joint

26843   Arthrodesis, carpometacarpal joint, digit, other than thumb, each;

27110   Transfer iliopsoas; to greater trochanter of femur

27130   Arthroplasty, acetabular and proximal femoral prosthetic replacement (total hip arthroplasty), with or without autograft or allograft

27132   Conversion of previous hip surgery to total hip arthroplasty, with or without autograft or allograft

27140   Osteotomy and transfer of greater trochanter of femur (separate procedure)

27185   Epiphyseal arrest by epiphysiodesis or stapling, greater trochanter of femur

27447   Arthroplasty, knee, condyle and plateau; medial AND lateral compartments with or without patella resurfacing (total knee arthroplasty)

28104   Excision or curettage of bone cyst or benign tumor, tarsal or metatarsal, except talus or calcaneus;

28238   Reconstruction (advancement), posterior tibial tendon with excision of accessory tarsal navicular bone (eg, Kidner type procedure)

28299   Correction, hallux valgus (bunion), with or without sesamoidectomy; by double osteotomy

28737   Arthrodesis, with tendon lengthening and advancement, midtarsal, tarsal navicular-cuneiform (eg, Miller type procedure)

29049   Application, cast; figure-of-eight

30117   Excision or destruction (eg, laser), intranasal lesion; internal approach

30801   Cautery and/or ablation, mucosa of turbinates, unilateral or bilateral, any method, (separate procedure); superficial

30905   Control nasal hemorrhage, posterior, with posterior nasal packs and/or cautery, any method; initial

31238   Nasal/sinus endoscopy, surgical; with control of nasal hemorrhage

31528   Laryngoscopy direct, with or without tracheoscopy; with dilation, initial

31529   Laryngoscopy direct, with or without tracheoscopy; with dilation, subsequent

31641   Bronchoscopy, (rigid or flexible); with destruction of tumor or relief of stenosis by any method other than excision (eg, laser therapy, cryotherapy)

32420   Pneumocentesis, puncture of lung for aspiration

32650   Thoracoscopy, surgical; with pleurodesis (eg, mechanical or chemical)

33250   Operative ablation of supraventricular arrhythmogenic focus or pathway (eg, Wolff-Parkinson-White, atrioventricular node re-entry), tract(s) and/or focus (foci); without cardiopulmonary bypass

33406   Replacement, aortic valve, with cardiopulmonary bypass; with allograft valve (freehand)

33413   Replacement, aortic valve; by translocation of autologous pulmonary valve with allograft replacement of pulmonary valve (Ross procedure)

33610   Repair of complex cardiac anomalies (eg, single ventricle with subaortic obstruction) by surgical enlargement of ventricular septal defect

33975   Insertion of ventricular assist device; extracorporeal, single ventricle

33976   Insertion of ventricular assist device; extracorporeal, biventricular

33977   Removal of ventricular assist device; extracorporeal, single ventricle

33978   Removal of ventricular assist device; extracorporeal, biventricular

35001   Direct repair of aneurysm, pseudoaneurysm, or excision (partial or total) and graft insertion, with or without patch graft; for aneurysm and associated occlusive disease, carotid, subclavian artery, by neck incision

35005   Direct repair of aneurysm, pseudoaneurysm, or excision (partial or total) and graft insertion, with or without patch graft; for aneurysm, pseudoaneurysm, and associated occlusive disease, vertebral artery

35021   Direct repair of aneurysm, pseudoaneurysm, or excision (partial or total) and graft insertion, with or without patch graft; for aneurysm, pseudoaneurysm, and associated occlusive disease, innominate, subclavian artery, by thoracic incision

35045   Direct repair of aneurysm, pseudoaneurysm, or excision (partial or total) and graft insertion, with or without patch graft; for aneurysm, pseudoaneurysm, and associated occlusive disease, radial or ulnar artery

35081   Direct repair of aneurysm, pseudoaneurysm, or excision (partial or total) and graft insertion, with or without patch graft; for aneurysm, pseudoaneurysm, and associated occlusive disease, abdominal aorta

35091   Direct repair of aneurysm, pseudoaneurysm, or excision (partial or total) and graft insertion, with or without patch graft; for aneurysm, pseudoaneurysm, and associated occlusive disease, abdominal aorta involving visceral vessels (mesenteric, celiac, renal)

35102   Direct repair of aneurysm, pseudoaneurysm, or excision (partial or total) and graft insertion, with or without patch graft; for aneurysm, pseudoaneurysm, and associated occlusive disease, abdominal aorta involving iliac vessels (common, hypogastric, external)

35111   Direct repair of aneurysm, pseudoaneurysm, or excision (partial or total) and graft insertion, with or without patch graft; for aneurysm, pseudoaneurysm, and associated occlusive disease, splenic artery

35121   Direct repair of aneurysm, pseudoaneurysm, or excision (partial or total) and graft insertion, with or without patch graft; for aneurysm, pseudoaneurysm, and associated occlusive disease, hepatic, celiac, renal, or mesenteric artery

35131   Direct repair of aneurysm, pseudoaneurysm, or excision (partial or total) and graft insertion, with or without patch graft; for aneurysm, pseudoaneurysm, and associated occlusive disease, iliac artery (common, hypogastric, external)

35141   Direct repair of aneurysm, pseudoaneurysm, or excision (partial or total) and graft insertion, with or without patch graft; for aneurysm, pseudoaneurysm, and associated occlusive disease, common femoral artery (profunda femoris, superficial femoral)

35151   Direct repair of aneurysm, pseudoaneurysm, or excision (partial or total) and graft insertion, with or without patch graft; for aneurysm, pseudoaneurysm, and associated occlusive disease, popliteal artery

35161   Direct repair of aneurysm, pseudoaneurysm, or excision (partial or total) and graft insertion, with or without patch graft; for aneurysm, pseudoaneurysm, and associated occlusive disease, other arteries

35646   Bypass graft, with other than vein; aortobifemoral

36005   Injection procedure for extremity venography (including introduction of needle or intracatheter)

36400   Venipuncture, under age 3 years; femoral or jugular

36819   Arteriovenous anastomosis, open; by upper arm basilic vein transposition

36823   Insertion of arterial and venous cannula(s) for isolated extracorporeal circulation including regional chemotherapy perfusion to an extremity, with or without hyperthermia, with removal of cannula(s) and repair of arteriotomy and venotomy sites

42970   Control of nasopharyngeal hemorrhage, primary or secondary (eg, postadenoidectomy); simple, with posterior nasal packs, with or without anterior packs and/or cautery

43108   Total or near total esophagectomy, without thoracotomy; with colon interposition or small intestine reconstruction, including intestine mobilization, preparation and anastomosis(es)

43113   Total or near total esophagectomy, with thoracotomy; with colon interposition or small intestine reconstruction, including intestine mobilization, preparation, and anastomosis(es)

43118   Partial esophagectomy, distal two-thirds, with thoracotomy and separate abdominal incision, with or without proximal gastrectomy;

	with colon interposition or small intestine reconstruction, including intestine mobilization, preparation, and anastomosis(es)
43123	Partial esophagectomy, thoracoabdominal or abdominal approach, with or without proximal gastrectomy; with colon interposition or small intestine reconstruction, including intestine mobilization, preparation, and anastomosis(es)
43227	Esophagoscopy, rigid or flexible; with control of bleeding (eg, injection, bipolar cautery, unipolar cautery, laser, heater probe, stapler, plasma coagulator)
43245	Upper gastrointestinal endoscopy including esophagus, stomach, and either the duodenum and/or jejunum as appropriate; with dilation of gastric outlet for obstruction (eg, balloon, guide wire, bougie)
43264	Endoscopic retrograde cholangiopancreatography (ERCP); with endoscopic retrograde removal of calculus/calculi from biliary and/or pancreatic ducts
43265	Endoscopic retrograde cholangiopancreatography (ERCP); with endoscopic retrograde destruction, lithotripsy of calculus/calculi, any method
43361	Gastrointestinal reconstruction for previous esophagectomy, for obstructing esophageal lesion or fistula, or for previous esophageal exclusion; with colon interposition or small intestine reconstruction, including intestine mobilization, preparation, and anastomosis(es)
43847	Gastric restrictive procedure, with gastric bypass for morbid obesity; with small intestine reconstruction to limit absorption
43860	Revision of gastrojejunal anastomosis (gastrojejunostomy) with reconstruction, with or without partial gastrectomy or intestine resection; without vagotomy
44020	Enterotomy, small intestine, other than duodenum; for exploration, biopsy(s), or foreign body removal
44110	Excision of one or more lesions of small or large intestine not requiring anastomosis, exteriorization, or fistulization; single enterotomy
44160	Colectomy, partial, with removal of terminal ileum with ileocolostomy
44202	Laparoscopy, surgical; enterectomy, resection of small intestine, single resection and anastomosis
44322	Colostomy or skin level cecostomy; with multiple biopsies (eg, for congenital megacolon) (separate procedure)
44366	Small intestinal endoscopy, enteroscopy beyond second portion of duodenum, not including ileum; with control of bleeding (eg, injection, bipolar cautery, unipolar cautery, laser, heater probe, stapler, plasma coagulator)
44378	Small intestinal endoscopy, enteroscopy beyond second portion of duodenum, including ileum; with control of bleeding (eg, injection, bipolar cautery, unipolar cautery, laser, heater probe, stapler, plasma coagulator)
44391	Colonoscopy through stoma; with control of bleeding (eg, injection, bipolar cautery, unipolar cautery, laser, heater probe, stapler, plasma coagulator)
44661	Closure of enterovesical fistula; with intestine and/or bladder resection
44700	Exclusion of small intestine from pelvis by mesh or other prosthesis, or native tissue (eg, bladder or omentum)
45190	Destruction of rectal tumor (eg, electrodessication, electrosurgery, laser ablation, laser resection, cryosurgery) transanal approach
45303	Proctosigmoidoscopy, rigid; with dilation (eg, balloon, guide wire, bougie)
45317	Proctosigmoidoscopy, rigid; with control of bleeding (eg, injection, bipolar cautery, unipolar cautery, laser, heater probe, stapler, plasma coagulator)
45334	Sigmoidoscopy, flexible; with control of bleeding (eg, injection, bipolar cautery, unipolar cautery, laser, heater probe, stapler, plasma coagulator)
45382	Colonoscopy, flexible, proximal to splenic flexure; with control of bleeding (eg, injection, bipolar cautery, unipolar cautery, laser, heater probe, stapler, plasma coagulator)
46604	Anoscopy; with dilation (eg, balloon, guide wire, bougie)
46614	Anoscopy; with control of bleeding (eg, injection, bipolar cautery, unipolar cautery, laser, heater probe, stapler, plasma coagulator)

46924	Destruction of lesion(s), anus (eg, condyloma, papilloma, molluscum contagiosum, herpetic vesicle), extensive (eg, laser surgery, electrosurgery, cryosurgery, chemosurgery)
46940	Curettage or cautery of anal fissure, including dilation of anal sphincter (separate procedure); initial
47554	Biliary endoscopy, percutaneous via T-tube or other tract; with removal of calculus/calculi
48100	Biopsy of pancreas, open (eg, fine needle aspiration, needle core biopsy, wedge biopsy)
48160	Pancreatectomy, total or subtotal, with autologous transplantation of pancreas or pancreatic islet cells
48500	Marsupialization of pancreatic cyst
48545	Pancreatorrhaphy for injury
48547	Duodenal exclusion with gastrojejunostomy for pancreatic injury
49220	Staging laparotomy for Hodgkins disease or lymphoma (includes splenectomy, needle or open biopsies of both liver lobes, possibly also removal of abdominal nodes, abdominal node and/or bone marrow biopsies, ovarian repositioning)
49424	Contrast injection for assessment of abscess or cyst via previously placed drainage catheter or tube (separate procedure)
49495	Repair, initial inguinal hernia, full term infant under age 6 months, or preterm infant over 50 weeks postconceptual age and under age 6 months at the time of surgery, with or without hydrocelectomy; reducible
50220	Nephrectomy, including partial ureterectomy, any open approach including rib resection;
50810	Ureterosigmoidostomy, with creation of sigmoid bladder and establishment of abdominal or perineal colostomy, including intestine anastomosis
50815	Ureterocolon conduit, including intestine anastomosis
50820	Ureteroileal conduit (ileal bladder), including intestine anastomosis (Bricker operation)
50825	Continent diversion, including intestine anastomosis using any segment of small and/or large intestine (Kock pouch or Camey enterocystoplasty)
50840	Replacement of all or part of ureter by intestine segment, including intestine anastomosis
51065	Cystotomy, with calculus basket extraction and/or ultrasonic or electrohydraulic fragmentation of ureteral calculus
51590	Cystectomy, complete, with ureteroileal conduit or sigmoid bladder, including intestine anastomosis;
51596	Cystectomy, complete, with continent diversion, any open technique, using any segment of small and/or large intestine to construct neobladder
51940	Closure, exstrophy of bladder
51960	Enterocystoplasty, including intestinal anastomosis
52510	Transurethral balloon dilation of the prostatic urethra
53445	Insertion of inflatable urethral/bladder neck sphincter, including placement of pump, reservoir, and cuff
53447	Removal and replacement of inflatable urethral/bladder neck sphincter including pump, reservoir, and cuff at the same operative session
53449	Repair of inflatable urethral/bladder neck sphincter, including pump, reservoir, and cuff
54065	Destruction of lesion(s), penis (eg, condyloma, papilloma, molluscum contagiosum, herpetic vesicle), extensive (eg, laser surgery, electrosurgery, cryosurgery, chemosurgery)
54405	Insertion of multi-component, inflatable penile prosthesis, including placement of pump, cylinders, and reservoir
56501	Destruction of lesion(s), vulva; simple (eg, laser surgery, electrosurgery, cryosurgery, chemosurgery)
56515	Destruction of lesion(s), vulva; extensive (eg, laser surgery, electrosurgery, cryosurgery, chemosurgery)
57022	Incision and drainage of vaginal hematoma; obstetrical/postpartum
57061	Destruction of vaginal lesion(s); simple (eg, laser surgery, electrosurgery, cryosurgery, chemosurgery)

57065	Destruction of vaginal lesion(s); extensive (eg, laser surgery, electrosurgery, cryosurgery, chemosurgery)
57510	Cautery of cervix; electro or thermal
58140	Myomectomy, excision of leiomyomata of uterus, single or multiple (separate procedure); abdominal approach
58275	Vaginal hysterectomy, with total or partial vaginectomy;
58563	Hysteroscopy, surgical; with endometrial ablation (eg, endometrial resection, electrosurgical ablation, thermoablation)
58611	Ligation or transection of fallopian tube(s) when done at the time of cesarean delivery or intra-abdominal surgery (not a separate procedure) (List separately in addition to code for primary procedure)
59000	Amniocentesis; diagnostic
60000	Incision and drainage of thyroglossal duct cyst, infected
60270	Thyroidectomy, including substernal thyroid; sternal split or transthoracic approach
61026	Ventricular puncture through previous burr hole, fontanelle, suture, or implanted ventricular catheter/reservoir; with injection of medication or other substance for diagnosis or treatment
61055	Cisternal or lateral cervical (C1-C2) puncture; with injection of medication or other substance for diagnosis or treatment (eg, C1-C2)
61618	Secondary repair of dura for cerebrospinal fluid leak, anterior, middle or posterior cranial fossa following surgery of the skull base; by free tissue graft (eg, pericranium, fascia, tensor fascia lata, adipose tissue, homologous or synthetic grafts)
62100	Craniotomy for repair of dural/cerebrospinal fluid leak, including surgery for rhinorrhea/otorrhea
62230	Replacement or revision of cerebrospinal fluid shunt, obstructed valve, or distal catheter in shunt system
62252	Reprogramming of programmable cerebrospinal shunt
62256	Removal of complete cerebrospinal fluid shunt system; without replacement
62272	Spinal puncture, therapeutic, for drainage of cerebrospinal fluid (by needle or catheter)
63707	Repair of dural/cerebrospinal fluid leak, not requiring laminectomy
63709	Repair of dural/cerebrospinal fluid leak or pseudomeningocele, with laminectomy
64555	Percutaneous implantation of neurostimulator electrodes; peripheral nerve (excludes sacral nerve)
64575	Incision for implantation of neurostimulator electrodes; peripheral nerve (excludes sacral nerve)
64755	Transection or avulsion of; vagus nerves limited to proximal stomach (selective proximal vagotomy, proximal gastric vagotomy, parietal cell vagotomy, supra- or highly selective vagotomy)
64820	Sympathectomy; digital arteries, each digit
65235	Removal of foreign body, intraocular; from anterior chamber of eye or lens
65900	Removal of epithelial downgrowth, anterior chamber of eye
65920	Removal of implanted material, anterior segment of eye
65930	Removal of blood clot, anterior segment of eye
66020	Injection, anterior chamber of eye (separate procedure); air or liquid
66982	Extracapsular cataract removal with insertion of intraocular lens prosthesis (one stage procedure), manual or mechanical technique (eg, irrigation and aspiration or phacoemulsification), complex, requiring devices or techniques not generally used in routine cataract surgery (eg, iris expansion device, suture support for intraocular lens, or primary posterior capsulorrhexis) or performed on patients in the amblyogenic developmental stage
67515	Injection of medication or other substance into Tenon's capsule
69310	Reconstruction of external auditory canal (meatoplasty) (eg, for stenosis due to injury, infection) (separate procedure)
69990	Microsurgical techniques, requiring use of operating microscope (List separately in addition to code for primary procedure)
74230	Swallowing function, with cineradiography/videoradiography
74245	Radiologic examination, gastrointestinal tract, upper; with small intestine, includes multiple serial films
74249	Radiological examination, gastrointestinal tract, upper, air contrast, with specific high density barium, effervescent agent, with or without glucagon; with small intestine follow-through
74250	Radiologic examination, small intestine, includes multiple serial films;
74305	Cholangiography and/or pancreatography; through existing catheter, radiological supervision and interpretation
74327	Postoperative biliary duct calculus removal, percutaneous via T-tube tract, basket, or snare (eg, Burhenne technique), radiological supervision and interpretation
74363	Percutaneous transhepatic dilation of biliary duct stricture with or without placement of stent, radiological supervision and interpretation
75898	Angiography through existing catheter for follow-up study for transcatheter therapy, embolization or infusion
75989	Radiological guidance for percutaneous drainage of abscess, or specimen collection (ie, fluoroscopy, ultrasound, or computed axial tomography), with placement of indwelling catheter, radiological supervision and interpretation
76066	Joint survey, single view, two or more joints (specify)
76070	Computerized axial tomography bone density study, one or more sites
76078	Radiographic absorptiometry (eg, photodensitometry, radiogrammetry), one or more sites
76120	Cineradiography/videoradiography, except where specifically included
76125	Cineradiography/videoradiography to complement routine examination (List separately in addition to code for primary procedure)
76355	Computerized axial tomographic guidance for stereotactic localization
76360	Computerized axial tomographic guidance for needle biopsy, radiological supervision and interpretation
76370	Computerized axial tomographic guidance for placement of radiation therapy fields
76375	Coronal, sagittal, multiplanar, oblique, 3-dimensional and/or holographic reconstruction of computerized axial tomography, magnetic resonance imaging, or other tomographic modality
76380	Computerized axial tomography, limited or localized follow-up study
76536	Ultrasound, soft tissues of head and neck (eg, thyroid, parathyroid, parotid), B-scan and/or real time with image documentation
76604	Ultrasound, chest, B-scan (includes mediastinum) and/or real time with image documentation
76645	Ultrasound, breast(s) (unilateral or bilateral), B-scan and/or real time with image documentation
76700	Ultrasound, abdominal, B-scan and/or real time with image documentation; complete
76770	Ultrasound, retroperitoneal (eg, renal, aorta, nodes), B-scan and/or real time with image documentation; complete
76778	Ultrasound, transplanted kidney, B-scan and/or real time with image documentation, with or without duplex Doppler study
76800	Ultrasound, spinal canal and contents
76805	Ultrasound, pregnant uterus, B-scan and/or real time with image documentation; complete (complete fetal and maternal evaluation)
76819	Fetal biophysical profile; without non-stress testing
76830	Ultrasound, transvaginal
76856	Ultrasound, pelvic (nonobstetric), B-scan and/or real time with image documentation; complete
76870	Ultrasound, scrotum and contents
76880	Ultrasound, extremity, non-vascular, B-scan and/or real time with image documentation
76885	Ultrasound, infant hips, real time with imaging documentation; dynamic (requiring physician manipulation)
76886	Ultrasound, infant hips, real time with imaging documentation; limited, static (not requiring physician manipulation)
77300	Basic radiation dosimetry calculation, central axis depth dose calculation, TDF, NSD, gap calculation, off axis factor, tissue inhomogeneity factors, calculation of non-ionizing radiation surface and depth dose, as required during course of treatment, only when prescribed by the treating physician

78195 Lymphatics and lymph nodes imaging

78290 Intestine imaging (eg, ectopic gastric mucosa, Meckels localization, volvulus)

78615 Cerebral vascular flow

78650 Cerebrospinal fluid leakage detection and localization

82270 Blood, occult, by peroxidase activity (eg, guaiac), qualitative; feces, 1-3 simultaneous determinations

82273 Blood, occult, by peroxidase activity (eg, guaiac), qualitative; other sources

82355 Calculus; qualitative analysis

83013 Helicobacter pylori; analysis for urease activity, non-radioactive isotope

83873 Myelin basic protein, cerebrospinal fluid

83916 Oligoclonal immune (oligoclonal bands)

84445 Thyroid stimulating immune globulins (TSI)

85097 Bone marrow, smear interpretation

86325 Immunoelectrophoresis; other fluids (eg, urine, cerebrospinal fluid) with concentration

87045 Culture, bacterial; feces, with isolation and preliminary examination (eg, KIA, LIA), Salmonella and Shigella species

87903 Infectious agent phenotype analysis by nucleic acid (DNA or RNA) with drug resistance tissue culture analysis, HIV 1; first through 10 drugs tested

87904 Infectious agent phenotype analysis by nucleic acid (DNA or RNA) with drug resistance tissue culture analysis, HIV 1; each additional 1 through 5 drugs tested (List separately in addition to code for primary procedure)

88304 Level III - Surgical pathology, gross and microscopic

88305 Level IV - Surgical pathology, gross and microscopic examination

89050 Cell count, miscellaneous body fluids (eg, cerebrospinal fluid, joint fluid), except blood;

90471 Immunization administration (includes percutaneous, intradermal, subcutaneous, intramuscular and jet injections); one vaccine (single or combination vaccine/toxoid)

90732 Pneumococcal polysaccharide vaccine, 23-valent, adult or immunosuppressed patient dosage, for use in individuals 2 years or older, for subcutaneous or intramuscular use

90780 Intravenous infusion for therapy/diagnosis, administered by physician or under direct supervision of physician; up to one hour

92532 Positional nystagmus test

92534 Optokinetic nystagmus test

93609 Intraventricular and/or intra-atrial mapping of tachycardia site(s) with catheter manipulation to record from multiple sites to identify origin of tachycardia (List separately in addition to code for primary procedure)

93619 Comprehensive electrophysiologic evaluation with right atrial pacing and recording, right ventricular pacing and recording, His bundle recording, including insertion and repositioning of multiple electrode catheters, without induction or attempted induction of arrhythmia

93620 Comprehensive electrophysiologic evaluation with right atrial pacing and recording, right ventricular pacing and recording, His bundle recording, including insertion and repositioning of multiple electrode catheters with induction or attempted induction of arrhythmia;

93621 Comprehensive electrophysiologic evaluation with right atrial pacing and recording, right ventricular pacing and recording, His bundle recording, including insertion and repositioning of multiple electrode catheters with induction or attempted induction of arrhythmia; with left atrial pacing and recording from coronary sinus or left atrium (List separately in addition to code for primary procedure)

93622 Comprehensive electrophysiologic evaluation with right atrial pacing and recording, right ventricular pacing and recording, His bundle recording, including insertion and repositioning of multiple electrode catheters with induction or attempted induction of arrhythmia; with left ventricular pacing and recording (List separately in addition to code for primary procedure)

94720 Carbon monoxide diffusing capacity (eg, single breath, steady state)

94750 Pulmonary compliance study (eg, plethysmography, volume and pressure measurements)

95144 Professional services for the supervision of preparation and provision of antigens for allergen immunotherapy; single dose vial(s) (specify number of vials)

95145 Professional services for the supervision of preparation and provision of antigens for allergen immunotherapy (specify number of doses); single stinging insect venom

95165 Professional services for the supervision of preparation and provision of antigens for allergen immunotherapy; single or multiple antigens (specify number of doses)

95180 Rapid desensitization procedure, each hour (eg, insulin, penicillin, equine serum)

95875 Ischemic limb exercise test with serial specimen(s) acquisition for muscle metabolite(s)

95904 Nerve conduction, amplitude and latency/velocity study, each nerve; sensory

96450 Chemotherapy administration, into CNS (eg, intrathecal), requiring and including spinal puncture

97112 Therapeutic procedure, one or more areas, each 15 minutes; neuromuscular reeducation of movement, balance, coordination, kinesthetic sense, posture, and/or proprioception for sitting and/or standing activities

97504 Orthotic(s) fitting and training, upper extremity(ies), lower extremity(ies), and/or trunk, each 15 minutes

97535 Self-care/home management training (eg, activities of daily living (ADL) and compensatory training, meal preparation, safety procedures, and instructions in use of assistive technology devices/adaptive equipment) direct one-on-one contact by provider, each 15 minutes

97601 Removal of devitalized tissue from wound(s); selective debridement, without anesthesia (eg, high pressure waterjet, sharp selective debridement with scissors, scalpel and tweezers), including topical application(s), wound assessment, and instruction(s) for ongoing care, per session

99090 Analysis of clinical data stored in computers (eg, ECGs, blood pressures, hematologic data)

99374 Physician supervision of a patient under care of home health agency (patient not present) in home, domiciliary or equivalent environment (eg, Alzheimer's facility) requiring complex and multidisciplinary care modalities involving regular physician development and/or revision of care plans, review of subsequent reports of patient status, review of related laboratory and other studies, communication (including telephone calls) for purposes of assessment or care decisions with health care professional(s), family member(s), surrogate decision maker(s) (eg, legal guardian) and/or key caregiver(s) involved in patient's care, integration of new information into the medical treatment plan and/or adjustment of medical therapy, within a calendar month; 15-29 minutes

99377 Physician supervision of a hospice patient (patient not present) requiring complex and multidisciplinary care modalities involving regular physician development and/or revision of care plans, review of subsequent reports of patient status, review of related laboratory and other studies, communication (including telephone calls) for purposes of assessment or care decisions with health care professional(s), family member(s), surrogate decision maker(s) (eg, legal guardian) and/or key caregiver(s) involved in patient's care, integration of new information into the medical treatment plan and/or adjustment of medical therapy, within a calendar month; 15-29 minutes

99379 Physician supervision of a nursing facility patient (patient not present) requiring complex and multidisciplinary care modalities involving regular physician development and/or revision of care plans, review of subsequent reports of patient status, review of related laboratory and other studies, communication (including telephone calls) for purposes of assessment or care decisions with health care professional(s), family member(s), surrogate decision maker(s) (eg, legal guardian) and/or key caregiver(s) involved in patient's care, integration of new information into the medical treatment plan and/or adjustment of medical therapy, within a calendar month; 15-29 minutes

99381 Initial comprehensive preventive medicine evaluation and management of an individual including an age and gender appropriate history, examination, counseling/anticipatory guidance/risk factor reduction interventions, and the ordering of appropriate immunization(s), laboratory/diagnostic procedures, new patient; infant (age under 1 year)

99391 Periodic comprehensive preventive medicine reevaluation and management of an individual including an age and gender appropriate history, examination, counseling/anticipatory guidance/risk factor reduction interventions, and the ordering of appropriate immunization(s), laboratory/diagnostic procedures, established patient; infant (age under 1 year)

93607 Left ventricular recording

93737 Electronic analysis of single or dual chamber pacing cardioverter-defibrillator only (interrogation, evaluation of pulse generator status); without reprogramming

93738 Electronic analysis of single or dual chamber pacing cardioverter-defibrillator only (interrogation, evaluation of pulse generator status); with reprogramming

DELETED CODES

00850 Anesthesia for intraperitoneal procedures in lower abdomen including laparoscopy; cesarean section

00855 Anesthesia for intraperitoneal procedures in lower abdomen including laparoscopy; cesarean hysterectomy

00857 Neuraxial analgesia/anesthesia for labor ending in a cesarean delivery (includes any repeat subarachnoid needle placement and drug injection and/or any necessary replacement of an epidural catheter during labor)

00884 Anesthesia for procedures on major lower abdominal vessels; transvenous umbrella insertion

00946 Anesthesia for vaginal procedures (including biopsy of labia, vagina, cervix or endometrium); vaginal delivery

00955 Neuraxial analgesia/anesthesia for labor ending in a vaginal delivery (includes any repeat subarachnoid needle placement and drug injection and/or any necessary replacement of an epidural catheter during labor)

01904 Anesthesia for injection procedure for pneumoencephalography

01906 Anesthesia for injection procedure for myelography; lumbar

01908 Anesthesia for injection procedure for myelography; cervical

01910 Anesthesia for injection procedure for myelography; posterior fossa

01912 Anesthesia for injection procedure for diskography; lumbar

01914 Anesthesia for injection procedure for diskography; cervical

01918 Anesthesia for arteriograms, needle; retrograde, brachial or femoral

01921 Anesthesia for angioplasty

26585 Repair bifid digit

26597 Release of scar contracture, flexor or extensor, with skin grafts, rearrangement flaps, or Z-plasties, hand and/or finger

29815 Arthroscopy, shoulder, diagnostic, with or without synovial biopsy (separate procedure)

29909 Unlisted procedure, arthroscopy

53443 Urethroplasty with tubularization of posterior urethra and/or lower bladder for incontinence (eg, Tenago, Leadbetter procedure)

54402 Removal or replacement of non-inflatable (semi-rigid) or inflatable (self-contained) penile prosthesis

54407 Removal, repair, or replacement of inflatable (multi-component) penile prosthesis, including pump and/or reservoir and/or cylinders

54409 Surgical correction of hydraulic abnormality of inflatable (multi-component) prosthesis including pump and/or reservoir and/or cylinders

54510 Excision of local lesion of testis

80072 Arthritis panel This panel must include the following: Uric acid, blood, chemical (84550) Sedimentation rate, erythrocyte, non-automated (85651) Fluorescent noninfectious agent, screen, each antibody (86255) Rheumatoid factor, qualitative (86430)

85095 Bone marrow; aspiration only

85102 Bone marrow biopsy, needle or trocar

85535 Iron stain (RBC or bone marrow smears)

86683 Antibody; hemoglobin, fecal

88170 Fine needle aspiration; superficial tissue (eg, thyroid, breast, prostate)

88171 Fine needle aspiration; deep tissue under radiologic guidance

93536 Percutaneous insertion of intra-aortic balloon catheter

APPENDIX C—GLOSSARY

Abdominal lymphadenectomy — Cutting out (removing) the lymph node grouping, with or without para-aortic and vena caval nodes, and dissecting away from the surrounding tissue, nerves, and blood vessels.

Absorbable sutures — Strands prepared from collagen or a synthetic polymer and capable of being absorbed by tissue over time. Examples include surgical gut, collagen sutures, or synthetics like polydioxanone (PDS), polyglactin 910 (Vicryl), polylecapron 25 (Monocryl), polyglyconate (Maxon), and polyglycolic acid (Dexon).

Acetabuloplasty — Plastic repair/reconstruction of the acetabulum. The acetabulum is the rounded cavity on the external surface of the innominate bone that receives the head of the femur.

Air conduction — The transportation of sound from the air, through the external auditory canal, to the tympanic membrane, and ossicular chain, ending at, but not including the cochlea. Testing air conduction establishes the patency or nonpatency of these mechanisms.

Air puff device — Measures intraocular pressure by evaluating the force of a reflected amount of air blown against the cornea. A valuable screening tool, but less precise than other methods.

Allograft — Tissue obtained from a nonidentical individual of the same species. Other terms used to identify allografts include: allogenic graft, homologous graft, homoplastic graft.

Amniocentesis — Amniocentesis provides an accurate source of chromosomal information about the fetus. It is usually performed between 16 and 20 weeks gestation.

Anastomosis — Surgically created connection between ducts, blood vessels, or bowel segments to allow flow from one to the other.

Angioplasty — Reconstruction or repair of a diseased or damaged blood vessel.

Annuloplasty — The annuli are thick, fibrous rings and one is found surrounding each of the cardiac chambers. The atrial and ventricular muscle fibers attach to the annuli. In annuloplasty, weakened annuli may be surgically plicated, or tucked, to improve muscular functions.

Anorectal Manometry — Measurement of pressure generated by anal sphincter to help treat incontinence.

Anterior chamber lenses — These are inserted in conjunction with intracapsular cataract extraction and posterior chamber lenses are inserted in conjunction with extracapsular cataract extraction. Anterior chamber lenses are commonly used for secondary insertion.

Applanation tomometer — Measures intraocular pressure by recording the force required to flatten an area of the cornea. It is attached to a slit lamp and is considered the most accurate methodology.

Aspirate — Physician uses a syringe or a suction device to withdraw fluid or air from a cavity.

Atrial septal defect — An atrial septal defect allows oxygenated blood to return to the lungs instead of circulating throughout the rest of the body. This can increase pulmonary blood flow, causing pulmonary hypertension if the defect is not closed.

Auricle — The external ear, or auricle, is a single elastic cartilage covered in skin and normal adnexal features (hair follicles, sweat glands, and sebaceous glands). The ridged nature of the auricle is to channel sounds into the acoustic meatus. The semicircular depression leading into the ear is named the concha, Latin for shell. The lining of the acoustic meatus is skin with ceruminous glands that secrete ear wax.

Autogenous transplant — Transplanted from one part of the patient's body to another. Autogenous bone may be freshly harvested, or preserved and stored in a bone bank for later grafting. Most commonly, the bone is cryogenically preserved. Other terms for autograft include: autogenic graft, autologous graft, autotransplant.

Bankart procedure — This procedure is also referred to as a capsulolabral reconstruction. The procedure is used to treat recurrent dislocation of the shoulder requiring reconstruction of the avulsed capsule and labrum at the glenoid lip.

Bartholin's Gland — Gland on either side of vaginal opening. Also called vestibular glands.

Bartholin's gland abscess — An abscess of the Bartholin's gland is a pocket of pus and surrounding cellulitis caused by infection of the Bartholin's gland. Symptoms include localized swelling and pain in the posterior labia majora. The pain may extend into the lower vagina.

Basic Value or Base Unit (anesthesia services) — The basic value, also referred to as the base unit or relative value, has two components. One component reflects all usual services included in the anesthesia service, including pre-operative and post-operative visits, administration of fluids and/or blood products incident to the procedure, and interpretation of non-invasive monitoring (ECG, temperature, blood pressure, oximetry, capnography, and mass spectrometry). The second component reflects the relative work or cost of the specific anesthesia service. Cost in this context refers to the physician's cost of doing business. For anesthesiologists, the majority of the cost goes to malpractice insurance.

Berman locator — Small, sensitive tool for detecting location of a metallic foreign body.

Bifurcated — Having two branches or divisions, such as the left pulmonary veins that split off from the left atrium to carry oxygenated blood away from the heart.

Biopsy — Tissue or fluid removed for diagnosis. A pathologist confirms a diagnosis through analysis of the cells in the biopsy material.

Blalock-Hanlon procedure — A segment of the right atrium is excised, creating an atrial septal defect. This is a palliative procedure for transposition of great vessels.

Blalock-Taussig procedure — An end-to-side anastomosis of right subclavian artery to right pulmonary artery allows arterial and venous blood to mix and flow through the shunt to the pulmonary artery and into the lungs for oxygenation.

Blepharorrhaphy — Synonym of tarsorrhaphy. See tarsorrhaphy.

Blue baby — A term commonly used for infants that are cyanotic due to oxygen deprivation.

Body positions — There are several body positions for patients during surgical procedures. These include:

- Fowler's position. Position assumed by patient when the head of the bed is raised 18 or 20 inches and the individual's knees are elevated.

- Prone. Lying horizontally when lying face downward.

- Supine. Lying horizontally on the back (also called dorsal decubitus position).

- Trendelenburg position. Position by the patient when the patient's head is lower in relation to the inclined plane of the body and legs.

Bona Fide Emergency Services — The term means services provided in a hospital emergency room after the sudden onset of a medical condition with acute symptoms of sufficient severity (including severe pain) such that the absence of immediate medical attention could result in:

- Placing the patient's health in serious jeopardy

- Serious impairment to bodily functions

- Serious dysfunction of any bodily organ or part

Bone conduction —The transportation of sound through bone. The source of sound is placed on the skull or teeth, and the vibration stimulates the cochlea, bypassing normal air conduction routes. Bone conduction requires operational sensorineural hearing mechanisms.

Bone Mass Measurement — The term means a radiologic or radioisotopic procedure or other procedure approved by the FDA for identifying bone mass, detecting bone loss. or determining bone quality. The procedure includes a physician's interpretation of the results. Qualifying individuals must be an estrogen-deficient woman at clinical risk for osteoporosis with vertebral abnormalities.

Bristow procedure — This procedure transfers the tip of the coracoid process with its muscle attachments across the anteroinferior glenohumeral joint creating a musculotendinous sling.

Buccal mucosa — The mucous membrane on the inside of the cheek.

Caldwell-Luc — A large nasoantral window is created above the canine tooth in this intraoral approach to surgery. This antrostomy is usually limited to adults because of the unerupted teeth in children.

Cardiopulmonary bypass — Venous blood is diverted to a heart-lung machine, which mechanically pumps and oxygenates the blood temporarily so that the heart can be bypassed while an open procedure on the heart or coronary arteries is performed. During bypass, the lungs are deflated and immobile.

Cardioverter-defibrillator — A cardioverter-defibrillator device uses both low energy cardioversion or defibrillating shocks and antitachycardia pacing to treat ventricular tachycardia or ventricular fibrillation. It may be either a single or dual chamber device. Cardioverter-defibrillators may require the placement of multiple leads even for single chamber devices.

Care Plan Oversight Services — The term describes the services of a physician providing ongoing review and revision of a patient's care plan involving complex or multidisciplinary care modalities. Care plan oversight services are reported separately from any necessary office/outpatient, hospital, home, nursing facility, or domiciliary services.

Case Management Services — Physician case management is a process of involving direct patient care as well as coordinating and controlling access to the patient or initiating and/or supervising other necessary health care services.

Cataract extraction — The most common surgical procedure performed on adults. Most ophthalmologists perform cataract surgery in an ambulatory surgical setting. Anterior chamber lenses are inserted in conjunction with intracapsular cataract extraction and posterior chamber lenses are inserted in conjunction with extracapsular cataract extraction.

Certified Nurse Midwife — The term means a registered nurse who has successfully completed a program of study and clinical experience or has been certified by a recognized organization.

Cervical cap — Cervical cap is similar in form and function to the diaphragm, however, it can be left in place for up to 48 hours.

Cervical intraepithelial neoplasia — This classification system is used to report abnormalities in the epithelial cell:

- CIN I. Cervical intraepithelial neoplasia I; low-grade abnormality; mild dysplasia

- CIN II. Cervical intraepithelial neoplasia II; high-grade abnormality; moderate dysplasia

- CIN III. Cervical intraepithelial neoplasia III; carcinoma in situ; severe dysplasia

Choanal atresis — A potentially dangerous congenital defect. Infants unable to breathe through their noses cannot feed properly and have difficulty keeping their air passages clear.

Cholecystectomy — The removal of the gallbladder and its contents is the most common major operation in the United States, and performed as the definitive treatment for gallstones.

Chorionic villi sampling — Chorionic villi sampling provides a rich source of fetal genetic information. Obtained between the eighth week and the twelfth week of gestation, it can provide information to diagnose some enzymatic defects.

Chronic Pain Management Services — The term describes distinct services frequently performed by anesthesiologists who have additional training in pain management procedures. Pain management services include initial and subsequent evaluation and management (E/M) services, trigger point injections, spine and spinal cord injections, and nerve blocks.

Cineplastic amputation — This type of amputation may also be referred to as a cinematic amputation or a kineplasty procedure. In this type of amputation, the muscles and tendons of the remaining portion of the extremity are arranged so that they may be utilized for motor functions. Following this type of amputation, a specially constructed prosthetic device allows the individual to execute more complex movements because the muscles and tendons are able to communicate independent movements to the device.

Circadian — Refers to the 24 hour period.

Classification of surgical wound — Surgical wounds fall into four categories that determine methods of treatment and outcomes:

- Clean wound. No inflammation and procedure performed under sterile operating room conditions with no break in sterile technique. No alimentary, respiratory, oropharyngeal, or genitourinary tracts are involved in the surgery. Infection rate: up to 5 percent.

- Clean-contaminated wound. No inflammation and procedure performed with minor break in surgical technique. No unusual contamination found in alimentary, respiratory, genitourinary, or oropharyngeal cavity entered. Infection rate: up to 11 percent.

- Contaminated wound. Acute nonpurulent inflammation noted and procedure performed with major break in surgical technique. Open wound less than four hours old. Gross contamination from gastrointestinal tract. Infection rate: up to 20 percent.

- Dirty and infected wound. Existing infection and inflammation prior to surgery in a dirty traumatic wound more than four hours old, or an old abscess and/or existing surgical infection. In either case abscess, and nonsterile conditions were present. Wound older than four hours. Perforated viscus, fecal contamination, necrotic tissue, or foreign body may be present. Infection rate: up to 40 percent.

Clinical Social Worker — The term means an individual who possesses a master's or doctor's degree in social work and, after obtaining the degree, has performed at least two years of supervised clinical social work. A clinical social worker must be licensed by the state or, in the case of states without licensure, must completed at least two years or 3,000 hours of post-master's degree supervised clinical social work practice under the supervision of a master's level social worker.

CO2 Laser — A carbon dioxide laser that emits an invisible beam and vaporizes water-rich tissue. The vapor is suctioned from the site.

Colorectal Cancer Screening Tests — The term means any of the following procedures furnished to an individual for the purpose of early detection of colorectal cancer:

- Screening fecal-occult blood test

- Screening flexible sigmoidoscopy

- In the case of an individual at high risk for colorectal cancer, screening colonoscopy

- Other tests or procedures, and modifications to tests and procedures, with such frequency and payment limits

- Individuals are considered at high risk for colorectal cancer because of family history, prior experience of cancer or precursor neoplastic polyps, history of chronic digestive disease condition (i.e., inflammatory bowel disease, Crohn's Disease, or ulcerative colitis), or the presence of any appropriate recognized gene markers for colorectal cancer.

Colostomy — Artificial surgical opening anywhere along the length of the colon to the skin surface for the diversion of feces.

Colpocleisis — Vaginal canal closure.

Commissurotomy — Surgical division or opening of a band of fibrous tissue.

  2001 Ingenix, Inc.

APPENDIX C—GLOSSARY

Community Mental Health Center, Partial Hospitalization Services — The term means the services prescribed and supervised by a physician pursuant to an individualized, written plan of treatment that sets forth the diagnosis and the type, amount, frequency, and duration of care for a patient in a community mental health center. Services must be reasonable and necessary for the diagnosis or active treatment of the individual's condition and to prevent relapse or hospitalization. The items and services include the following:

- Individual and group therapy with physicians, psychologists, or other mental health professionals

- Occupational therapy requiring the skills of a qualified occupational therapist

- Services of social workers, trained psychiatric nurses, and other staff trained to work with psychiatric patients

- Drugs and biologicals for therapeutic purposes that cannot be self-administered)

- Individualized activity therapies that are not primarily recreational or diversionary

- Family counseling

- Patient training and education

- Diagnostic services, and

- Other items and services, excluding meals and transportation

Comprehensive Outpatient Rehabilitation Facility Services (CORF) — The term describes a facility that provides (by or under the supervision of physicians) diagnostic, therapeutic, and restorative services to outpatients. Patients must be under the supervision of a physician and the facility must maintain the medical record of each patient. The following items and services provided by a physician or other qualified professional to an outpatient of a comprehensive outpatient rehabilitation facility under a plan established and periodically reviewed by a physician:

- Physicians' services

- Physical therapy, occupational therapy, speech-language pathology services, and respiratory therapy

- Prosthetic and orthotic devices, including testing, fitting, or training in the use of prosthetic and orthotic devices

- Social and psychological services

- Nursing care provided by or under the supervision of a registered professional nurse

- Drugs and biologicals that cannot be self-administered

- Supplies and durable medical equipment

- Other supplies and services necessary for the rehabilitation of the patient that are ordinarily available through the CORF

A CORF must provide a surety bond in an amount that is not less than $50,000 to ensure the efficiency and effectiveness of its programs.

Conjunctivodacryocystostomy — Surgical connection of the lacrimal sac directly to the conjunctival sac.

Conjunctivorhinostomy — Correction of an obstruction of the lacrimal canal

Consultations — The term describes consulting services provided at the request of another physician or other appropriate source for the purpose of rendering an opinion or advice regarding the evaluation and management of a specific problem. Consultations in CPT fall under four subcategories: office or other outpatient consultations, initial inpatient consultations, follow-up inpatient consultations, and confirmatory consultations.

Costochondral — Pertains to the ribs and the scapula.

Covered Osteoporosis Drug — The term means an injectable drug approved for the treatment of post-menopausal osteoporosis provided to an individual by a home health agency if the individual's attending physician certifies that the individual has suffered a bone fracture related to post-menopausal osteoporosis. The individual must be unable to learn the skills needed to self-administer such drug or is otherwise physically or mentally incapable of self-administering the drug and be confined to home.

Core needle biopsy — A large-bore biopsy needle is inserted into a mass and a core of tissue is removed for diagnostic study.

Craterization — Excision of a portion of bone to create a crater-like depression to facilitate drainage from infected areas of bone.

Cricoid — The circular cartilage around the trachea.

Cryolathe — Tool for reshaping a button of corneal tissue.

Cryosurgery — Local freezing of diseased tissue without causing harm to adjacent tissue. The cold causes tissue necrosis. Frozen tissue may be removed without significant bleeding during the surgical procedure, even in highly vascular tissue. Liquid nitrogen is the most commonly used source for the cold.

Cutdown — The technique of creating a small, incised opening for venipuncture.

Cytogenetic Studies — The term refers to the procedures in CPT 2001 that are related to the branch of genetics that studies cellular (cyto) structure and function as it relates to heredity (genetics). White blood cells, specifically T-lymphocytes, are the most commonly used specimen for chromosome analysis.

Dacryocystorhinostomy — Performed by suturing the posterior flaps while the lacrimal obstruction is removed, preserving the conjunctiva.

Dacryocystotome — Instrument for incising lacrimal duct strictures, also spelled dacryocystitome.

Dacryorhinocystostomy — Synonym to dacryocystorhinostomy.

Debride — Procedure involves the removal of all foreign objects and damaged tissue from a burn or a wound to prevent infection and promote healing.

Dermis graft — Skin graft that has been separated from the epidermal tissue and the underlying subcutaneous fat. Used primarily as a substitute for fascia grafts in plastic surgery.

Desensitization — Administration of extracts of allergens periodically to build immunity in the patient.

Destruction — The term describes the ablation of benign, premalignant, or malignant tissue by any of the following methods used alone or in combination: electrosurgery, cryosurgery, laser, and chemical treatment.

Diabetes Outpatient Self-Management Training Services — The term means educational and training services furnished by a certified provider in an outpatient setting. The physician managing the individual's diabetic condition must certify that the services are needed under a comprehensive plan of care provide the patient with the skills and knowledge necessary for therapeutic program compliance (including skills related to the self-administration of injectable drugs). The provider must meet applicable standards established by the National Diabetes Advisory or be recognized by an organization that represents individuals with diabetes as meeting standards for furnishing the services.

Diagnostic Procedures — Terms describes the procedures performed to evaluate the patient's complaints or symptoms. These procedures help the physician establish the nature of the patient's disease or condition so that definitive care can be provided. Diagnostic procedures include endoscopy, arthroscopy, injection procedures, and biopsies.

Diaphragm — Flexible, dome-shaped rubber cap that fits over the cervix and acts as a barrier to sperm. It must be used in conjunction with spermicidal cream or jelly. It is generally left in place for eight hours after coitus.

Diaphysectomy — Partial removal of a portion of bone, usually a portion of the shaft of a long bone, to facilitate drainage from infected bone.

Diathermy — Heating of tissue using microwave radiation, ultrasound, or electric currents.

Appendixes

Dilation — Artificial increase in the diameter of an opening made by medication or by instrumentation.

Discharge Planning Process — The term defines a plan applicable to services furnished by the hospital to individuals entitled to medical benefits. Upon the request of a patient's physician, the hospital must arrange for the development and initial implementation of a discharge plan for the patient. The discharge planning evaluation must be included in the patient's medical record for use in establishing an appropriate discharge plan and the results of the evaluation must be discussed with the patient or the patient's representative). Plan guidelines and standards should address the following:

- Patients who are likely to suffer adverse health consequences upon discharge in the absence of adequate discharge planning and patients, their physicians, and their representatives requesting a discharge plan

- Appropriate arrangements for post-hospital care made before discharge and to avoid unnecessary delays in discharge

- An evaluation of a patient's likely need for appropriate post-hospital services, including hospice services and the availability of those services, including the availability of home health services

Dissect — A scalpel, a probe, or scissors is used to cut apart tissues for visual or microscopic study.

Dorsal — Pertaining to the back or posterior aspect.

Drugs and Biologicals — The term covers drugs and biologicals included - or approved for inclusion - in the United States Pharmacopoeia, the National Formulary, the United States Homeopathic Pharmacopoeia, in New Drugs or Accepted Dental Remedies, or approved by the pharmacy and drug therapeutics committee of the medical staff of the hospital. Drugs also include those used in an anticancer chemotherapeutic regimen for a medically accepted approved by the FDA. The carrier determines medical acceptance based on supportive clinical evidence.

Durable Medical Equipment (DME) — The term includes iron lungs, oxygen tents, hospital beds, and wheelchairs used in the patient's home, including an institution considered the patient's home. DME also blood-testing strips and blood glucose monitors for individuals with diabetes without regard to Type I or Type II diabetes or use of insulin.

DuToit staple capsulorrhaphy — Reattachment of the capsule and glenoid labrum to the glenoid lip using staples to anchor the avulsed capsule and glenoid labrum.

Eden-Hybinette — This anterior repair utilizes an anterior bone block to augment the bony anterior glenoid lip.

EDTA — Drug used to inhibit damage to the cornea by collagenase. EDTA is especially effective in alkali burns as it neutralizes soluable alkali, including lye.

Effusion — Escape of fluid from within a body cavity.

Electrocautery — Destruction of tissue using high-frequency electrical current. The current produces heat, which destroys cells.

Endarterectomy — Removal of the endothelial lining of a diseased or damaged artery.

Epiphysiodesis — Surgical fusion of an epiphysis performed to prematurely stop further bone growth.

Escharotomy — Removal of the scab caused by the burn, which is constricting blood flow. The procedure allows the edges to separate and restore blood flow to the unburned tissues.

Established Patient — Evaluation and Management guidelines define an established patient as one who has received professional services from the physician, or another physician of the same specialty who belongs to the same group practice, within the past three years.

Exenteration — Radical excision of the contents of a body cavity (e.g., orbit).

Extended Care Services — The term defines the items and services provided to an inpatient of a skilled nursing facility, including nursing care, physical or occupational therapy, speech pathology, drugs and supplies, and medical social services.

External electrical capacitor device — External electrical stimulation device designed to promote bone healing. This device may also promote neural regeneration, revascularization, epiphyseal growth, and ligament maturation.

External pulsating electromagnetic field — External stimulation device designed to promote bone healing. This device may also promote neural regeneration, revascularization, epiphyseal growth, and ligament maturation.

Evaluation and Management (E/M) Codes — E/M codes encompass services that are part of the 99000 series of CPT codes and represent the services most frequently performed by physicians (e.g., office, emergency department, inpatient visits).

Evaluation and Management Service Components — The components of history, examination, and medical decision making are keys to selecting the correct E/M codes. In most cases, all three components must be addressed in the documentation. However, in established, subsequent, and follow-up categories, only two of the three must be met or exceeded for a given code.

Eyre-Brook capsulorrhaphy — Reattachment of the capsule and glenoid labrum to the glenoid lip.

Fascia — The fibrous tissue that envelopes the muscle.

Fasciectomy — Surgical incision through the fascia.

Fasciotomy — Excision of the fascia or strips of fascial tissue.

Fat graft — A graft composed of fatty tissue completely freed from surrounding tissue. Used primarily to fill in depressions.

Fine needle aspiration (FNA) — A 22- or through 25-gauge needle attached to a syringe is inserted into a lesion/tissue and a few cells are aspirated for diagnostic study. Aspiration is also used to remove fluid from a benign cyst.

Fluoroscopy — Radiology technique that allows visual examination of part of the body or a function of an organ using a device that projects an x-ray image on a fluorescent screen.

Focal length — Distance between the object in focus and the lens.

Free flap — Tissue that is completely detached from the donor site and reattached to the recipient site. It receives its blood supply from capillary ingrowth at the recipient site.

Free microvascular flap — Tissue that is completely detached from the donor site following careful dissection and preservation of the blood vessels. The tissue is attached to the recipient site and the transfered blood vessels are anastomosed to vessels in the recipient site.

Fulguration — Destruction of living tissue by sparks from electric current.

Gas tamponade — Absorbable gas may be injected to force the retina against the choroid. Common gases include room air, short-acting sulfahexafluoride, intermediate-acting perfluoroethane, or long-acting perfluorooctane.

Hemilaminectomy — Excision of the right or left lamina.

Hemoperitoneum — The effusion of blood into the peritoneal cavity.

Heterologous transplant — Nonhuman biotissue transplanted into the patient.

Heterotopic transplant — Tissue transplanted from a different anatomical site for usage as is natural for that tissue, for example, buccal mucosa to a conjunctival site.

Home Health Agency — The term means a public agency or private organization providing skilled nursing services and other therapeutic services. Home health agencies receiving federal funds must have policies governing it services and the medical services of a physician or registered professional nurse. According to law, home health agencies must maintain clinical reports of all patients. Provisions of the Balanced Budget Act of 1997, home health agencies must provide, on a continuing basis, surety bonds of $50,000 to guarantee the efficient and effective operation of the agency. The term home health agency does not include any agency or organization that is primarily for the care and treatment of mental diseases.

Home Health Services — The term encompasses the items and services a home health agency provides to an individual, according to a plan developed and reviewed by the patient's physician. Services may include:

- Part-time or intermittent nursing care provided by or under the supervision of a registered professional nurse

- Physical or occupational therapy or speech-language pathology services

- Medical social services under the direction of a physician

- Part-time or intermittent services of a home health aide who has successfully completed a training program

- Medical supplies (including catheters, catheter supplies, ostomy bags, and supplies related to ostomy care, and a covered osteoporosis drug and durable medical equipment

- Medical services provided by an intern or resident-in-training of a hospital affiliated with the home health agency

Homogenous transplant (homograft) — Tissue from another human transplanted to the patient. For bone transplants, the tissue is usually obtained from a cadaver.

Hospice Care — The term specifies the following items and services provided to a terminally ill individual by a hospice program under a written plan established and periodically reviewed by the individual's attending physician and by the medical director:

- Nursing care provided by or under the supervision of a registered professional nurse

- Physical or occupational therapy or speech-language pathology services

- Medical social services under the direction of a physician

- Services of a home health aide who has successfully completed a training program

- Medical supplies (including drugs and biologicals) and the use of medical appliances

- Physicians' services

- Short-term inpatient care (including both respite care and procedures necessary for pain control and acute and chronic symptom management) in an inpatient facility on an intermittent basis and not consecutively over longer than five days

- Counseling (including dietary counseling) with respect to care of the terminally ill individual and adjustment to his death

- Any item or service which is specified in the plan and for which payment may be made

Hospice Program — An Hospice program establishes the care and service plan and ensures that the services are available (as needed) on a 24-hour basis and also provides bereavement counseling for the immediate family of terminally ill individuals. The services may be delivered in an individual's home, on an outpatient basis, and on a short-term inpatient basis, directly or under arrangements made by the agency or organization. The Hospice agency is responsible for all services in an aggregate number of days of inpatient care provided in any 12-month period, as overseen by an interdisciplinary group of personnel that includes at least one physician, one registered professional nurse, and one social worker. A central clinical record must be maintained for each patient.

According to federal law, an Hospice cannot discontinue its services with respect to a patient because of the inability of the patient to pay for care. Volunteers may provide care and services as long as the program maintains records on the cost savings and expansion of care and services achieved through volunteers.

Hospital — The term means an institution that provides, under the supervision of physicians, diagnostic, therapeutic, and rehabilitation services for medical diagnosis, treatment, and care of patients. Hospitals receiving federal funds must maintain clinical records on all patients, provides 24-hour nursing services, and have a discharge planning process in place. The term "hospital" also includes religious nonmedical health care institutions and facilities of 50 beds or less located in rural areas.

Ileostomy — Proximal end of transected ileum is brought out through the peritoneum and muscle of the abdominal wall to the skin. Liquid or semisolid discharge is collected in a bag over the stoma.

Infundibulectomy — Excision of the anterosuperior portion of the right ventricle of the heart.

Institutional Planning — The terms describes the overall plan and budget of a hospital, skilled nursing facility, comprehensive outpatient rehabilitation facility, or home health agency. Plans must be prepared by a governing and submitted to the state health agency. Plans must include:

- An annual operating budget

- A capital expenditures plan for at least a three-year period

Internal direct current stimulator — Electrostimulation device designed to promote bone regeneration by encouraging cellular response in bone and ligaments. It is placed directly into the surgical site.

Intramedullary implants — An intramedullary nail, rod, or pin is placed into the intramedullary canal at the fracture site. Intramedullary implants not only provide a method of aligning the fracture, they also act as a splint and may reduce fracture pain. Implants may be rigid or flexible. Rigid implants are preferred for prophylactic treatment of diseased bone, while flexible implants are preferred for traumatic injuries.

Irrigation — To wash out or cleanse a body cavity wound with water or other fluid.

Jatene procedure — This corrective measure for transposition of the great vessels is used when subaortic stenosis and narrowing of the left aortic ventricular junction are present requiring reconstruction of these sites as well as surgical correction of the transposed aortic and pulmonary arteries. This technique may be used in cases where the transposition is accompanied by a ventricular septal defect or a large patent ductus arteriosus.

Krypton laser — Because the krypton spectrum (red-yellow) is poorly absorbed by hemoglobin, it can be used effectively to treat retinal bleeding, macular lesions, and vessel aberrations of the choroid.

Lacrimal punctum — The opening of the lacrimal papilla of the eyelid through which tears flow to the canaliculi to the lacrimal sac.

Lacrimotome — Knife for cutting the lacrimal sac or duct.

Lacrimotomy — Incision of the lacrimal sac or duct.

Larynx — The larynx is the air passage of the neck area, serving as the voice mechanism as well as the valve to prevent food and other particles from entering the respiratory tract. The larynx is composed of three single cartilages: cricoid, epiglottis, and thyroid; and three paired cartilages: arytenoid, corniculate, and cuneiform.

Laser surgery — Laser beams deliver a sharply defined burn, and the color and wavelength of the laser determines which tissues it can best treat. The argon laser is effective in coagulating blood-rich tissue with heat. CO2 lasers are used to vaporize tissue. Potassium titanyl phosphate (KTP) lasers coagulate tissues. Nd:YAG lasers cut and cauterize.

LEEP — Loop electrosurgical excision prcocedure. This uses a stainless steel or tungsten loop electrode to excise a central core of cervical tissue. This is a therapeutic technique for treatment of premalignant lesions in women of child-bearing age, since future childbearing is unaffected.

Levonorgestrel — Drug inhibiting ovulation and preventing sperm from penetrating cervical mucus. It is delivered subcutaneously in polysiloxone capsules. The capsules can be effective for up to five years, and provide a cumulative pregnancy rate of less than 2 percent. The capsules are not biodegradable, and therefore must be removed. Removal is more difficult than insertion of levonorgestrel capsules because fibrosis develops around the capsules. Normal hormonal activity and a return to fertility begins immediately upon removal.

Ligation — This procedure involves tying off a blood vessel or duct with a suture or a soft, thin wire (ligature wire).

Magnuson-Stack procedure — Recurrent anterior dislocation is treated by tightening and realigning the subscapularis tendon.

Marsupialization — Suturing of cyst walls to the edge of a wound, following evacuation of the wound, so cavity may close by granulation.

Mastectomy — The surgical removal of one or both breasts and is most often performed to remove a malignant tumor. The types of mastectomy include:

- Radical. The breast, all lymph nodes in the axilla, and some muscles of the chest wall are removed.

- Modified radical. The large muscles of the chest that move the arm are preserved.

- Simple. Only breast tissue, nipple, and a small portion of overlying skin are removed.

McDonald Procedure — Polyester tape is placed around the cervix with a running stitch to assist in the prevention of pre-term delivery. Tape is removed at term for vaginal delivery.

Mitral valve — The mitral valve is located between the left atrium and left ventricle of the heart. It has two cusps and is, therefore, frequently referred to as the bicuspid valve.

Moh's Micrographic Surgery — This is a special technique used to treat complex or ill-defined skin cancer and requires a single physician to provide two distinct services. The first service is surgical and involves the destruction of the lesion by a combination of chemosurgery and excision. The second service is that of a pathologist and includes mapping, color coding of specimens, microscopic examination of specimens, and complete histopathologic preparation.

Mustard procedure — This corrective measure for transposition of great vessels involves an intra-atrial baffle made of pericardial tissue or synthetic material. The baffle is secured between pulmonary veins and mitral valve and between mitral and tricuspid valves. The baffle directs systemic venous flow into the left ventricle and lungs and pulmonary venous flow into the right ventricle and aorta.

Myasthenia Gravis — Neuromuscular disorder with symptoms of fatigue and exhaustion with fluctuating severity.

Myotomy — Cutting of a muscle to gain access to underlying tissues or to relieve constriction in a sphincter.

Nasal polyps — Polyps usually are bilateral, but they can be unilateral. Polyps, soft, edematous growths, project from nasal or sinus mucosa and may obstruct the posterior choanae. In addition to obstructing ventilation, they may affect the sense of smell if the olfactory epithelium is blocked. The KTP laser or the CO2 laser is sometimes used in reducing or eliminating polyps.

Nasal sinus — The nasal sinuses are air-filled cavities in the crainal bones that earn their names; all are lined with mucous membrane continuous with the nasal cavity and all drain fluids into the nasal cavity. The ethmoid cells vary in size and number and feature very thin septa, or walls. The maxillary sinuses are the largest and are the most frequently infected.

Nasopharynx — The nasopharynx is the membranous passage above the level of the soft palate; the oropharynx is the region between the soft palate and the edge of the epiglottis; the hypopharynx is the region of the epiglottis to the juncture of the larynx and esophagus; the three regions collectively are called the pharynx.

Nd:YAG laser — Invisible pulsed neodyminum is used for cataract extraction and lysis of vitreous strands. The light used by the Nd:YAG laser does not require the tissues that are being treated to be pigmented.

Neurectomy — The removal of part of a nerve.

New Patient — Evaluation and Management guidelines define a new patient as one who has not received any professional services from the physician, or another physician of the same specialty who belongs to the same group practice, within the past three years.

Nissen fundoplasty — Fundus of the stomach is wrapped around the lower end of the esophagus to treat reflux esophagitis.

Nonabsorable sutures — Strands of natural or synthetic material that resist absorption into living tissue. Skin is usually closed with nonabsorbable sutures. Examples include surgical silk, surgical cotton, linen, stainless steel, surgical nylon, polyester fiber, polybutester (Novafil), polyethylene (Dermalene), and polypropylene (Prolene, Surilene).

Nystagmus — Uncontrolled rapid movement of the eye.

Oophorectomy — Removal of ovary.

Outpatient Physical Therapy Services — The term means the physical therapy services provided to an outpatient of a clinic, rehabilitation agency, or public health agency. The attending physician must establish a plan of physical therapy or periodically review a plan developed by a qualified physical therapist. A group of professional personnel, including one or more physicians (associated with the clinic or rehabilitation agency) and one or more qualified physical therapists must govern services and maintain clinical records of all patients. Outpatient clinics must provide a surety bond of $50,000 to guarantee the efficiency and effectiveness of programs. The term outpatient physical therapy services also includes physical therapy services provided by a physical therapist in office or at the patient's home and speech-language pathology services.

Pacemaker — A pacemaker device is used to artificially stimulate the heart muscle by the use of electric impulses that aid in maintaining normal sinus rhythm.

Paratenon graft — A graft composed of the fatty tissue found between a tendon and its sheath.

Pedicle flap — Tissue that remains partially attached to the donor site by a pedicle or stem. The blood supply is provided by vessels that remain intact in the pedicle or stem of the flap.

Percutaneous skeletal fixation — Treatment that is neither open nor closed. In this procedure, the injury site is not directly visualized. Instead fixation devices (pins, screws) are placed to stabilize the dislocation using x-ray guidance.

Percutaneous Transluminal Coronary Angioplasty (PTCA) — The term describes the procedure used to treat coronary artery obstruction. A balloon catheter is placed in the affected artery and the balloon is inflated to flatten the plaque against the wall of the artery and open the obstruction.

Pericardium — The pericardium is the thin and slippery case in which the heart lies. It is lined with fluid so that the heart is free to pulse and move as it beats.

Physical Status Modifiers (anesthesia services) — Physical status modifiers reflect the patient's state of health. Individuals undergoing surgery may be healthy or may have varying degrees of systemic disease. A patient's health status affects the work related to providing the anesthesia service.

Pleurodesis — The production of adhesions between the parietal and visceral pleura.

Plication — Operation involving folding, shortening, or decreasing the size of a muscle or hollow organ by taking in tucks.

Potts-Smith-Gibson procedure — A side-to-side anastomosis of the aorta and left pulmonary artery creating a shunt that enlarges as the child grows.

Profunda — Denotes a part of a structure that is deeper from the surface of the body than the rest of the structure.

Prolonged Physician Services — Extended pre- or post-operative care provided to a patient whose condition requires services beyond the usual.

Prostate Cancer Screening Tests — The term means a test that consists of any (or all) of the procedures provided for the early detection of prostate cancer to a man over 50 years of age who has not had a test during the preceding year. The procedures are as follows:

- A digital rectal examination

- A prostate-specific antigen blood test

    2001 Ingenix, Inc.

After 2002, the list of procedures may be expanded as appropriate for the early detection of prostate cancer, taking into account changes in technology and standards of medical practice, availability, effectiveness, costs, and other factors.

Provider of Services — The term means a hospital, critical access hospital, skilled nursing facility, comprehensive outpatient rehabilitation facility, home health agency, hospice program.

Psychiatric Hospital — The term means an institution that provides, under the supervision of physicians, services for the diagnosis and treatment of mentally ill persons. Psychiatric hospitals receiving federal funds must maintain clinical records sufficient to determine the type of treatment provided to patients.

Pulmonary artery banding — In this palliative procedure for transposition of great vessels, the pulmonary artery is surgically constricted to prevent irreversible pulmonary vascular obstructive changes. Banding is often performed when a large ventricular septal defect is present.

Putti-Platt procedure — This procedure treats recurrent anterior dislocation by tightening and realigning the subscapularis tendon, thereby partially eliminating external rotation. The anterior capsule is also tightened and reinforced.

Pyloroplasty — Enlargement of the opening between the stomach and duodenum that may be performed in patients with an obstructing pyloric ulcer in combination with a vagotomy to treat bleeding duodenal ulcers.

Radiological Examination — The term in CPT refers to plain films of specific sites. Other terms used to describe plain films include standard or conventional films. Services employing other modalities and additional techniques include the following:

- Computerized Axial Tomography (CT or CAT scan) is a type of imaging that employs basic tomographic technique enhanced by computer imaging. Computer enhancement synthesizes the images obtained from different directions in a given plane, effectively reconstructing a cross-sectional plane of the body.

- Computerized Tomography Angiography (CTA) provides multiple rapid thin section CT scans, a series of x-ray beams taken from different angles to create cross-sectional images of organs, bones, and tissues.

- Magnetic Resonance Imaging (MRI) involves the application of an external magnetic field that forces a uniform alignment of hydrogen atom nuclei in the soft tissue. The nuclei emit radiofrequency signals that are converted into sets of tomographic images and displayed on a computer screen for three-dimensional visualization of the soft tissue structure.

Rashkind procedure — A balloon catheter is inserted into the left atrium, inflated, and pulled across the septum to enlarge the foramen ovale, thus creating an atrial septal defect. This is a palliative procedure for transposition of great vessels.

Repair — Repair is the surgical closure of a wound. The wound may be a result of injury/trauma or it may be a surgically created defect. Repairs are divided into three categories: simple, intermediate, and complex. Simple repair is performed when the wound is superficial and only requires simple, one layer, primary suturing. Intermediate repair is performed for wounds and lacerations in which one or more of the deeper layers of subcutaneous tissue and non-muscle fascia are repaired in addition to the skin and subcutaneous tissue. Complex repair includes repair of wounds requiring more than layered closure. See also Wound repair.

Rural Health Clinic — The term defines a clinic in an area where there is a shortage of health services. The clinic must provide routine diagnostic services, including clinical laboratory services and have prompt access to additional diagnostic services from facilities meeting requirements (i.e., agreements with one or more hospitals for the referral and admission of patients requiring inpatient, diagnostic, or other specialized services not available at the clinic). In addition, the clinic must be able to administer drugs and biologicals as necessary for the treatment of emergency cases and have appropriate procedures or arrangements for storing, administering, and dispensing any drugs and biologicals. Staff must include a nurse practitioner, a physician assistant, or a certified nurse-midwife available for patient care

not less than 50 percent of the time the clinic operates. In the case of a facility that is not a physician-directed clinic, there must be an arrangement with one or more physicians for the periodic review of covered services furnished by physician assistants and nurse practitioners.

Saucerization — Creation of a shallow, saucer-like depression in the bone to facilitate drainage from infected areas of bone.

Schiotz tonometer — Measures intraocular pressure by recording the depth of an indentation on the cornea by a plunger of known weight. The degree of indentation is calibrated on the tonometer to correspond to the intraocular pressure.

Screening Mammography — The term means a radiologic procedure provided to a woman for the purpose of early detection of breast cancer and includes a physician's interpretation of the results of the procedure.

Screening Pap Smear; Screening Pelvic Exam — The term means a diagnostic laboratory test consisting of a routine exfoliative cytology test (Papanicolaou test) provided to a woman for the purpose of early detection of cervical or vaginal cancer. The exam includes a clinical breast examination and a physician's interpretation of the results. Coverage depends on several factors, including the results of an exam during the preceding three years that indicated the presence of cervical or vaginal cancer or other abnormality or is at high risk of developing cervical or vaginal cancer.

Senning procedure — Flaps of intra-atrial septum and right atrial wall are used to create two interatrial channels to divert the systemic and pulmonary venous circulation.

Sensitivity Tests — Describes a number of methods of applying selective suspected allergens to the skin or mucous.

Sensorineural conduction — The transportation of sound from the cochlea to the acoustic nerve and central auditory pathway to the brain.

Separate Procedures — Term in CPT describes services that are commonly carried out as an integral part of a larger service, and as such do not warrant separate identification. These services are noted in CPT with the parenthetical phrase (separate procedure). When this phrase appears before the semicolon, all indented descriptions that follow are covered by it.

Shirodkar Procedure — Mersilene tape is drawn around the internal os and tied. This requires a small incision in the vaginal mucosa and usually predicates cesarean section.

Sinus of Valsalva — Small cavity in the aorta just superior to the aortic valve. It is the origin of the coronary arteries. This area may also be referred to as the aortic sinus.

Speech-Language Pathology Services; Audiology Services — The term means such speech, language, and related function assessment and rehabilitation services furnished by a qualified speech-language pathologist. Audiology services include hearing and balance assessment services furnished by a qualified audiologist. A qualified speech pathologist and audiologist must have a master's or doctoral degree in their respective fields and be licensed to serve in the state. Speech pathologists and audiologists practicing in states without licensure must complete 350 hours of supervised clinical work and perform at least nine months of supervised full-time service after earning their degrees.

Speech prosthetics — Electronic speech aids are covered by Medicare under Part B as prosthetic devices when the patient has had a laryngectomy. One operates by placing a vibrating head against the throat; the other amplifies sound waves through a tube which is inserted into the user's mouth.

Sphinteroplasty — Plastic surgery done to correct, augment, or improve the function of the muscular sphincter fibers founds in organs such as the anus or intestines.

Spirometry — Measurement of the lungs' breathing capacity.

Staghorn Calculus — A concretion of the renal pelvis that often fills several calices.

Surgical Package — The majority of the CPT surgical codes are "package" services; they include the actual surgical procedure, local infiltration, metacarpal and digital block or topical anesthesia (when used), and the normal, uncomplicated postoperative care.

Suture — There are numerous suturing techniques employed in wound closure. Among these are:

- Buried suture. A suture placed under the skin for a layered closure. It may be continuous or interrupted.

- Continuous suture. A running stitch with tension evenly distributed across the single strand so that it provides a leak proof suture line.

- Interrupted suture. A series of single stitches with tension isolated at each stitch. If one stitch loosens, the others may not be affected, and in the presence of infection, the isolated sutures cannot act as a wick to transport the infection.

- Purse-string suture. A continuous suture placed around a lumen and tightened to reduce or close the lumen.

- Retention suture. A secondary suture bridging the primary suture. Functionally, it provides support to the primary repair. A plastic or rubber bolster may be placed over the primary repair and under the retention sutures.

Tarsocheiloplasty — Plastic operation upon the edge of the eyelid for the treatment of trichiasis.

Tarsorrhaphy — Suture of a portion or all of the opposing eyelids for the purpose of shortening the palpebral fissure, or closing it entirely. External tarsorrhaphy involves the suture of the outer edges of the eyelid margins; median tarsorraphy involves the middle eyelid margins; and internal tarsorrhaphy involves the inner eyelid margins.

Tendon allograft — Allografts are tissues obtained from another individual of the same species. Tendon allografts are usually obtained from cadavers and frozen or freeze dried for later use in soft tissue repairs where the physician elects not to obtain an autogenous graft (a graft obtained from the individual on whom the surgery is being performed).

Tendon suture material — Tendons are composed of fibrous tissue consisting primarily of collagen and containing few cells or blood vessels. This tissue heals more slowly than tissues with more vascularization. Because of this, tendons are usually repaired with nonabsorbable suture material. Examples include surgical silk, surgical cotton, linen, stainless steel, surgical nylon, polyester fiber, polybutester (Novafil), polyethylene (Dermalene), and polypropylene (Prolene, Surilene).

Tenon's capsule — Connective tissue that forms the capsule enclosing the posterior eyeball, extending from the conjunctival fornix and continuous with the muscular fascia of the eye, also called the bulbar fascia, capusula bulbi, bulbar sheath, Bonnet's ocular, or sheath of eyeball.

Tensilon — Edrophonium chloride. An agent used for evaluation and treatment of myasthenia gravis.

Terminally Ill — An individual is considered to be "terminally ill" if the medical prognosis for life expectancy is six months or less.

Tetralogy of Fallot — A combination of congenital cardiac defects that include interventricular defect, pulmonary stenosis, right ventricular hypertrophy, and malpositioning of the aorta so that it receives venous as well as arterial blood.

Therapeutic Services — Term describes the procedures performed for treatment of a specific diagnosis. These services include performance of the procedure, various incidental elements, and normal, related follow-up care.

Thoracentesis — Using a needle to perforate the chest wall and pleural space for the aspiration of fluid for diagnostic or therapeutic purposes, or for biopsy.

Thoracic lymphadenectomy — Procedure to cut out the lymph nodes near the lungs, around the heart, and behind the trachea.

Thoracostomy — Making an incision into the chest wall to provide an opening for drainage.

Thyroglossal duct — An embryonic duct through which the thyroid gland descends during fetal development. The duct may form a cyst or sinus in adulthood. It is found at the front of the neck, within the hyoid bone.

Total shoulder replacement — Prosthetic replacement of the entire shoulder joint, including the humeral head and the glenoid fossa.

Trabeculae carneae cordis — Bands of muscular tissue that line the walls of the ventricles in the heart.

Tracheostomy — Formation of a tracheal opening to create a path for respiration. This is performed to relieve obstruction or improve patency of an airway. This is generally a more long-term measure.

Tracheotomy — Incision into the trachea below the larynx. This may be a controlled procedure or an emergency procedure, but is generally considered a temporary measure.

Trephine — A saw for removing a circular disk of bone used on the skull.

Tricuspid atresia — Tricuspid atresia is the congenital absence of the valve and it may occur with other defects, such as atrial septal defect, pulmonary atresia, and transposition of great vessels.

Tympanic membrane — The tympanic membrane is a thin, sensitive tissue and is the gateway to the middle ear. The membrane vibrates in response to sound waves and the movement is transmitted via the ossicular chain to the internal ear. The tympanic membrane may be punctured and tympanum penetrated by objects placed in the ear canal or entering the canal accidentally.

Urodynamics — The term describes a diagnostic service performed to evaluate the storage of urine and urine flow through the urinary tract.

Vagotomy — Division of the vagus nerves in the treatment of chronic gastric, pyloric, and duodenal ulcers that can cause severe pain and difficulties in eating and sleeping. Procedure interrupts nerve impulses to lower gastric acid production and hastens gastric emptying.

Vasectomy — Male sterilization achieved through removal of a portion of the vas deferens (route spermatozoa must take).

VBAC — (Vaginal Birth After Cesarean) Denotes a successful vaginal delivery after a previous cesarean delivery.

Ventricular septal defect — In a large ventricular septal defect, oxygenated blood flows back into the lungs, causing pulmonary hypertension. Small defects may be asymptomatic, and treatment may be unnecessary.

Vertebral interspace — The non-bony space between two vertebral bodies containing the intervertebral disk. It includes the nucleus pulposus, annulus, fibrosus, and the two cartilagenous endplates.

Volar — Pertaining to the palm of the hand or sole of the foot. Also may refer to the flexor surface of the forearm, wrist, or hand.

Waterston procedure — Anastomosis of aorta and right pulmonary artery placed on the posterior aspect of the aorta.

Wharton's Ducts — The salivary ducts below the mandible.

Wick catheter — A device used to monitor interstitial fluid pressure. It provides continuous measurement of interstitial fluid pressure. It may also be used intraoperatively during fasciotomy procedures to evaluate the effectiveness of the decompression.

Wound Repair — Repairs in CPT are divided into three categories: simple, intermediate, and complex. They are further described by anatomic site and wound size.

- Simple repair is performed when the wound is superficial, e.g., involving partial or full-thickness damage to the skin and/or subcutaneous tissues. No deeper structures are involved and only simple, one layer, primary suturing is required. This procedure includes local anesthetic and chemical or electrocauterization of wounds not closed.

- Intermediate repair is performed for wounds and lacerations in which one or more of the deeper layers of subcutaneous tissue and non-muscle fascia are repaired in addition to the skin and subcutaneous tissue. Single-layer closure can also be coded as an intermediate repair if the wound is heavily contaminated and requires extensive cleaning or removal of particulate matter.

- Complex repair includes repair of wounds requiring more than layered closure. Wounds coded from this category include those requiring revision, debridement, extensive undermining, and placement of stents or retention sutures. Complex repairs also include those requiring creation of a defect (e.g., extending excision) and special preparation of the site.

Xenograft — Tissue obtained from an animal of another species. Other terms for xenograft include heterograft, heterologous graft, xenogeneic graft.

Z-plasty — A plastic surgery technique used primarily to release tension or elongate contracted scar tissue. A Z-shaped incision is made with the middle line of the Z crossing the area of greatest tension. The triangular flaps are then rotated so that they cross the incision line in the opposite direction creating a reversed Z.

APPENDIX D— CPT CODES MOST OFTEN MISCODED AND WHY

E AND M SERVICES

99201–99215 The most common mistake when reporting Evaluation and Management services is not adequately documenting the service billed. This generally happens more with the higher level codes, where the documentation indicates a lower level of service than what is being billed. This is more an education issue on how to document.

99241–99255 Consultation codes are not to be used when the intent of the visit is a transfer of the patient for one or all of the patients' health issues from one provider to another. The patient medical record should contain documentation of the request for consultation by a health care provider or other appropriate source. The medical record should also contain documentation that the assessment and plan of the consulting provider was communicated to the provider or appropriate source that requested the consultation.

99300–99303 These codes are used for the admission or readmission of a patient to a nursing facility as well as for annual assessments. Any Evaluation and Management services rendered by the physician on the same date as the admission or readmission at another site of service should be taken into account when coding the level of nursing facility admission and not reported separately. Only hospital or observation discharge services performed on the same day as the nursing facility admission or readmission may be reported separately.

99354–99357 There must be direct (face-to-face) patient contact to report these services. Prolonged service of less than thirty minutes is included in the evaluation and management codes and not separately reportable. Prolonged service of less than fifteen minutes beyond the first hour or final half hour is not separately reported.

99374–99380 Only the physician who has the predominant supervisory role for the patient's care should bill these services for a given period of time. These codes are reported based on the physician time spent in a calendar month and should be billed only once per month based on the accumulated time spent that month.

DERMATOLOGY

11400–11446 These codes are used to report the surgical excision of benign lesions, if another method is used to destroy the lesion see code range 17000-17250 based on the type and number of lesions. Excision of benign lesions includes the simple closure of the excision site and local anesthesia. Simple closure is non-layered closure of the epidermis or dermis without involvement of deeper structures. If intermediate or complex closure is required to repair the excision site they may be reported separately with the appropriate code from range 12031-12057 for intermediate repair and 13100-13153 for complex repair.

11600–11646 These codes are used to report the surgical excision of malignant lesions, if another method is used to destroy the lesion see code range 17260-17286 based on the size and location of the lesion. Excision of benign lesions includes the simple closure of the excision site and local anesthesia. Simple closure is non-layered closure of the epidermis or dermis without involvement of deeper structures. If intermediate or complex closure is required to repair the excision site they may be reported separately with the appropriate code from range 12031-12057 for intermediate repair and 13100-13153 for complex repair.

11750 This service is often miscoded when billing 2 units for one toenail excision. Providers often bill for each nail border on one toe, when the code reads "partial or complete". Only one unit should be reported per toe no matter whether 1 or two nail borders are excised.

12001–12021 These codes are used to report the simple repair of wounds, to include those surgically created due to the excision of a lesion. Simple repair is non-layered closure. If multiple wounds are repaired with simple closure and are located on the body in the same anatomical site grouping defined by CPT, the lengths are added together to make one wound closure length when choosing a CPT code.

Example A: 2.5 cm wound right arm, closed by simple repair

1.5 cm wound left arm, closed by simple repair

4.0 cm wound total, closed by simple repair = CPT code 12002 for coding and billing purposes

Example B: 2.0 cm wound right side of neck, closed by simple repair cm wound right cheek, closed by simple repair

Do not total wounds together for code selection. Even though these wounds were both repaired by simple closure, they are not located in the same CPT anatomical grouping, so each wound is coded individually for coding and billing purposes.

Example C: 2.5 cm wound, right arm, closed by simple repair

3.0 cm wound right leg, closed by intermediate repair

Do not total wounds together for code selection. Even though these wounds are in the same CPT anatomical grouping, the method of closure is different, so each wound is coded individually for coding and billing purposes.

12031–12057 These codes are used to report the intermediate repair of wounds, to include those surgically created due to the excision of a lesion. If multiple wounds are repaired with intermediate closure and are located on the body in the same anatomical site grouping defined by CPT, the lengths are added together to make one wound closure length when choosing a CPT code.

Example A: 7.0 cm wound right arm, closed by intermediate repair

1.5 cm wound left arm, closed by intermediate repair

8.5 cm wound total, closed by intermediate repair = CPT code 12034 for coding and billing purposes

Example B: 2.8 cm wound of scalp, closed by intermediate repair cm wound right cheek, closed by intermediate repair

Do not total wounds together for code selection. Even though these wounds were both repaired by intermediate closure, they are not located in the same CPT anatomical grouping, so each wound is coded individually for coding and billing purposes.

Example C: 2.5 cm wound, cheek, closed by simple repair

4.2 cm wound left foot, closed by intermediate repair

Do not total wounds together for code selection. Even though these wounds are in the same CPT anatomical grouping, the method of closure is different, so each wound is coded individually for coding and billing purposes.

APPENDIX D— CPT CODES MOST OFTEN MISCODED AND WHY

17000–17004	These lesion destruction procedures are often miscoded when it comes to identifying the number of lesions destroyed. Code 17000 is used to report the destruction of only one lesion. For the destruction of two through 14 lesions code 17003 is reported only once regardless of whether 3 or 10 lesions are destroyed. And the remaining code in the series 17004 is reported for 15 or more lesions. So the first issue to resolve when coding these services is the number of lesions destroyed. If it is 15 or more only code 17004 is reported. If it is less than 15 lesions than both codes 17000 for the first lesion and 17003 for lesion two through fourteen are to be reported.
17106–17108	The codes in range 17106-17108 are used explicitly for laser removal of cutaneous vascular proliferative lesions. These codes are often misreported for laser removal of warts and various other types of lesions. These codes are reported based on the specific type of lesion destroyed and not the method.

ORTHOPEDICS

20600–20610	A common miscoding scenario involving arthrocenteses is when providers report both the aspiration of fluid from and the injection of medication into the same joint or bursa. These codes include both as indicated by the terms "and/or" in the narrative. For example, if a provider were to aspirate fluid from a patient's knee and then inject cortisone they should be reporting only code 20610.
22554–22585	A major mistake is not coding for the diskectomy. While these codes include "minimal diskectomy," code complete diskectomies separately. These procedures more often than not require the work of two surgeons who perform different parts of the same procedure. In these cases both surgeons should be reporting the same procedure code with the –62 Two Surgeons modifier. In addition any appropriate add-on codes should be reported by both surgeons with the –62 modifier as long as both participated in that aspect of the surgery together.
22590–22632	The most common miscoding is not coding for all appropriate procedures. For example bone graft procedures should be reported separately as well as spinal instrumentation procedures when appropriate. Often, providers fail to report all the services rendered when billing for arthrodesis procedures.
22851	As stated in code range 22590-22632 this is one of those procedures often not coded when it should be. The caution here is to report only the number of vertebral defects or interspaces treated not the number of devices used. For example if one interspace is treated with two biomechanical devices code 22851 should be reported only once.
28285	This code is reported exclusively for the correction of hammertoe deformity. It includes any method used to correct the deformity. Providers often inappropriately bill for the removal of bone (phalangectomy) in addition to code 28285 that is all inclusive of any method used to repair the hammertoe.

28290–28299	This range of codes describes bunionectomies. They are rather specific in their narratives regarding what is included in them. All codes in the range include a sesamoidectomy that should not be reported separately. Carefully read all the code narratives when billing this procedure and be sure you code the appropriate service based on the medical record documentation. When billing these procedures, especially on multiple toes, performed at the same operative session, be sure to report the appropriate anatomical modifiers (T1-TA) to identify the specific digits on which the procedure(s) were performed.

ENT

31256–31267	Miscoding of endoscopies often occurs due to upcoding with regards to the documentation. You can only code what is documented in the medical record. If the operative report does not clearly indicate a maxillary antrostomy was performed then you cannot report it. Or in the case of code 31267 if you do not have documentation that states tissue was actually removed from the maxillary sinus you may not report this code.

CARDIOVASCULAR /THORACIC SURGERY

36011–36015	These catheterizations procedures are often misused in conjunction with cardiac catheterization procedures. The cardiac catheterization procedures include catheter placement and these services should not be reported separately.
36215–36248	These selective vascular catheterizations include local anesthesia, introduction of the catheter(s), injection of the contrast media and any necessary pre- or postinjection care related to the procedure. To accurately code these services one must have at least a basic understanding of the vascular system hierarchy. The two biggest areas of miscoding are either listing too many codes (eg, billing for a 2nd order and a 3rd order when only the 3rd order should be billed) or not listing enough codes. These catheterizations procedures are often misused in conjunction with cardiac catheterization procedures. The cardiac catheterization procedures include catheter placement and these services should not be reported separately.
36430	The most common miscoding scenario regarding transfusion is reporting it at all. The risk of excessive bleeding is inherent is numerous procedures and having to provide a blood transfusion to a surgical patient does not warrant additional reimbursement and as such should not be reported.
36489	This service is distinguished from code 36491 and 36533 based on the method of catheter placement. In the case of code 36489 it is percutaneous (through the skin) placement of the catheter. The medical documentation must be clear regarding the method of catheter placement before you can accurately code this service. In addition if radiological guidance is used to perform the procedure, report the appropriate code from 76000, 76003, 76942.
36491	This procedure is performed by an incision of the blood vessel, to facilitate catheter placement. In the case of 36489 the catheter is placed through the skin. This procedure differs from 36533 in that there is no tunneling performed to create a passageway from the skin to the point of venous access and there is generally a longer distance between the two.

36533	This code is used to report both partially and completely implantable venous access devices. Partially implanted devices do not have reservoirs. During the insertion of a catheter, a tunnel will be created so that the catheter can be advanced to the point of venous access. In addition if radiological guidance is used to perform the procedure, report the appropriate code from 76000, 76003, 76942.
36535	This code is often inappropriately reported for the removal of a central venous catheter. It should be used only to report the removal of implantable venous access device with or without the reservoir. If radiological imaging is used to assist in the removal, report code 76000 additionally.
37700–37730	These services are often miscoded in conjunction with code for coronary artery bypass grafting. The procurement of the saphenous veins used during coronary artery bypass is included in the bypass procedure codes and should not be separately reported with these codes.

GENERAL SURGERY OR GASTROENTEROLOGY

44005	The biggest issue regarding miscoding of this procedure involves when to use it with other open abdominal procedure codes or whether to use it at all. When appropriate, there are a number of ways to report this service, add the –22 Unusual Procedural Service modifier to the primary open abdominal procedure. Or use 44005 with the –59 Distinct Procedural Service modifier. In the case of code 44005 it is best to check with your carrier for specific guidelines for use.
44200	The biggest issue regarding miscoding of this procedure involves when to use it with other laparoscopic abdominal procedure codes or whether to use it at all. When appropriate, there are a number of ways to report this service, add the –22 Unusual Procedural Service modifier to the primary laparoscopic abdominal procedure. Or use 44200 with the –59 Distinct Procedural Service modifier. In the case of code 44200 it is best to check with your carrier for specific guidelines for use.
49010	The miscoding of this service is due to the uncertainty of when it can or can't be billed. Most of the time this is included in all other abdominal procedures. However, there may be exceptions for some surgical scenarios. Traumas are a good example. A splenectomy may be performed and then an hour spent running the bowel, checking the liver, etc. A –22 modifier applied to the splenectomy code doesn't accurately reflect the work involved. In that type of case, check your carrier's policy on using 49010 with a –59 modifier.
49568	This code is very explicit in its narrative regarding which hernia repair codes it can be used in conjunction with. It is only to be reported with codes 49560–49566. The implantation of mesh or other prosthesis is included in all other hernia repair procedures and should not be reported separately.

UROLOGY

52005	This procedure is over-reported when it comes to reporting cystourethoscopies. Often it is mistakenly used in lieu of 52000. The difference is the urethral catheterization. It is imperative that medical record documentation clearly identifies the catheterization in order to report this procedure.

52310–52315	When this service is reported for the removal of a previously placed stent, it is crucial to know the date of the placement and your carriers postoperative period for the procedure. Often this service is denied as being performed during the postoperative period because the provider has neglected to use the –58 modifier when needed.
52320	This service includes the insertion and removal of a temporary stent during the procedure and, therefore, the stent should not be reported separately. The insertion of a self-retaining, indwelling stent during cystourethroscopy (52320) should be reported with code 52332 and the –51 modifier in addition to code 52320.
52332	This service is for the insertion of a self-retaining, indwelling urethral stent. When performed during any diagnostic or therapeutic cystourethroscopy (52320-52355) code 52332 should be reported additionally with the –51 modifier.
52606	This procedure is often overused only because most providers don't keep track of the carrier's postoperative periods. This procedure should not be reported when performed within the postoperative period. Know your carrier's policies, repeatedly billing the same inappropriate procedures will make it appear as though you are trying to get away with something, and raise concerns with your carrier.
53670	This is another overly used procedure code. The basic catheterization described in this code is inherent in most other urinary system procedures, and as such should not be reported separately.

GYNECOLOGY AND OB

57240–57260	These services 57240 and 57250 are never to be billed together. In the case of combined anterior and posterior colporrhaphy the correct code to report is 57260.

NEUROLOGY/PAIN MANAGEMENT

64450	we see a lot of podiatrists and hand surgeons using this code for the anesthetic. We also see a lot of surgeries where a pain management block is performed and NOT coded.
64470–64484	the radiological portion of the services often goes unreported. If fluoroscopic guidance is used for needle placement, report code 76005 in addition to the appropriate code from range 64470-64478.

OPTHALMOLOGY

67005	This service is often miscoded as a vitrectomy when in essence it is the removal of a small amount of vitreous fluid. They are never going deep into the vitreous cavity. Vitrectomies remove blood, vitreous and/or membranes and are not held to just vitreous fluid. In this case, report the appropriate vitrectomy code from range 67036-67040.
67036–67040	Vitrectomy is often performed in the course of another ocular procedure and as such is part of that procedure and should not be reported with a code from range 67036-67040. Vitrectomy preformed in the course of retinal detachment surgery report code 67108,
67101	This service is often miscoded multiple times based on the number of sessions. This code is to be reported only once regardless of how many sessions are required to complete the treatment. This service is reported for treatment of a retinal detachment for prophylactic treatment to prevent detachment report code 67141.

67105 This service is often miscoded multiple times based on the number of sessions. This code is to be reported only once regardless of how many sessions are required to complete the treatment. If multiple modalities are used only the primary treatment should be reported. This service is reported for treatment of a retinal detachment for prophylactic treatment to prevent detachment report code 67141.

67141 This service is reported for prophylactic treatment to prevent impending retinal detachment for treatment of a confirmed retinal detachment report code 67101.

67145 This service is reported for prophylactic treatment to prevent impending retinal detachment for treatment of a confirmed retinal detachment report code 67105.

67208–67218 This service is often miscoded multiple times based on the number of sessions. This code is to be reported only once regardless of how many sessions are required to complete the treatment.

67227–67228 This service is often miscoded multiple times based on the number of sessions. This code is to be reported only once regardless of how many sessions are required to complete the treatment.

RADIOLOGY

76000–76001 These procedures are often miscoded due to the simple fact that they are coded at all. Fluoroscopy is an inherent part of nearly all diagnostic radiology procedures and should not be reported separately.

78460–78465 Myocardial perfusion imaging can be performed at rest or with stress. When performed with stress the stress can be either exercise or pharmacologically induced. The stress testing is not included in the perfusion testing and should be reported separately with the appropriate code from range 93015-93018.

LAB /PATH

88141 This service is often not reported when it should be. If physician interpretation is required this code 88141 should be reported, without the –51 modifier, in addition to the appropriate code from ranges 88142-88154 or 88164-88167.

88142–88145 It is essential to know the screening system used when coding Pap smears. This code range is often used to report cytopathology smears screened by automated system, when in fact these codes are for manual screening of specimens collected in preservative fluid, with automated thin-layer prep.

88147–88148 This code range is used to report cytopathology smears screened by automated system. Manual screening is reported with a code from range 88142-88145, 88150-88154 or 88164-88167.

88150–88154 it is essential to know the screening system used when coding Pap smears. This code range is often used to report cytopathology smears screened by automated system, when in fact these codes are for manual screening of specimens. Pap smears examined using the Bethesda reporting system should be billed using a code from range 88164-88167.

88155 This service is often not reported when it should be. If physician interpretation is required this code 88155 should be reported, without the –51 modifier, in addition to the appropriate code from ranges 88142-88154 or 88164-88167.

88160–88162 This range of codes is used to report cytopathology screening of other than cervical or vaginal specimens.

88164– 88167 it is essential to know the screening system used when coding Pap smears. This code range is often used to report cytopathology smears screened by automated system, when in fact these codes are for manual screening of specimens. Pap smears examined using the non-Bethesda reporting system should be billed using a code from range 88150-88154.

GENERAL MEDICINE

92960 This service is often miscoded as emergency defibrillation. This is an elective procedure and should not be used to report an emergency defibrillation. There is not a current CPT code for reporting emergency defibrillation; this service is included in critical care services.

CARDIOLOGISTS

93040–93042 These procedures are often miscoded due to the simple fact that they are coded at all. Rhythm strips are an inherent part of nearly all diagnostic cardiology procedures and should not be reported separately.

93501–93533 Cardiac catheterization procedures do not include either the injection procedures (93539-93544) or the imaging supervision, interpretation and report (93555-93556) when performed an appropriate code from all three series 93501-93533, 93539-93544 and 93555-93556 should be reported. All listed services are exempt from modifier –51 reporting. Indicator dilution studies 93561 and 93562 are included in all cardiac catheterizations services and should not be reported separately.

93539–93545 The most common miscoding scenario regarding these injection procedures is that they are often not coded when they should be. The associated cardiac catheterization procedures do not include these injection procedures and when performed they can both be reported. All listed services are exempt from modifier –51 reporting.

93555–93556 Cardiac catheterization procedures do not include either the injection procedures (93539-93544) or the imaging supervision, interpretation and report (93555-93556) when performed an appropriate code from all three series 93501-93533, 93539-93544 and 93555-93556 should be reported. All listed services are exempt from modifier –51 reporting.

93561–93562 Indicator dilution studies 93561 and 93562 are included in all cardiac catheterizations services and should not be reported separately.

PULMONARY/RESPIRATORY

94656 This service is often miscoded by anesthesiologists that bill this for the time spent transporting a patient to the ICU. This is part of the anesthesia time they are billing and should not be reported separately.

94760–94762 These services are included in critical care services 99291-99292 and conscious sedation services 99141-99142 as such should not be reported in addition to the critical care service.